Cerebral Revascularization

Techniques in Extracranial-to-Intracranial Bypass Surgery

Cerebral Revascularization

Techniques in Extracranial-to-Intracranial Bypass Surgery

Saleem I. Abdulrauf, MD, FACS

Neurosurgeon-in-Chief
Saint Louis University Hospital
Professor, Neurological Surgery
Director, Saint Louis University Center for Cerebrovascular
and Skull Base Surgery
Saint Louis University School of Medicine
Vice President, Congress of Neurological Surgeons
Chairman, International Division of the Congress of Neurological
Surgeons
Secretary, North American Skull Base Society
Secretary General, World Federation of Skull Base Societies
St. Louis, MO

ELSEVIER
SAUNDERS

ELSEVIER
SAUNDERS

1600 John F. Kennedy Blvd.
Ste 1800
Philadelphia, PA 19103-2899

CEREBRAL REVASCULARIZATION: TECHNIQUES IN   ISBN: 978-1-4377-1785-3
EXTRACRANIAL-TO-INTRACRANIAL BYPASS SURGERY

Notices

Knowledge and best practice in this field are constantly changing. As new research and experience broaden our understanding, changes in research methods, professional practices, or medical treatment may become necessary.

Practitioners and researchers must always rely on their own experience and knowledge in evaluating and using any information, methods, compounds, or experiments described herein. In using such information or methods they should be mindful of their own safety and the safety of others, including parties for whom they have a professional responsibility.

With respect to any drug or pharmaceutical products identified, readers are advised to check the most current information provided (i) on procedures featured or (ii) by the manufacturer of each product to be administered, to verify the recommended dose or formula, the method and duration of administration, and contraindications. It is the responsibility of practitioners, relying on their own experience and knowledge of their patients, to make diagnoses, to determine dosages and the best treatment for each individual patient, and to take all appropriate safety precautions.

To the fullest extent of the law, neither the Publisher nor the authors, contributors, or editors, assume any liability for any injury and/or damage to persons or property as a matter of products liability, negligence or otherwise, or from any use or operation of any methods, products, instructions, or ideas contained in the material herein.

Library of Congress Cataloging-in-Publication Data
Cerebral revascularization : techniques in extracranial-to-intracranial
bypass surgery / [edited by] Saleem I. Abdulrauf.
       p. ; cm.
Includes bibliographical references and index.
ISBN 978-1-4377-1785-3 (hardcover : alk. paper)
1. Cerebral revascularization. 2. Cerebrovascular disease—Surgery. I. Abdulrauf, Saleem I.
[DNLM: 1. Cerebral Revascularization—methods. 2. Cerebrovascular Disorders—surgery.
WL 355]
  RD594.2.C485 2011
  617.4'81—dc22   2010043228

Acquisitions Editor: Julie Goolsby
Developmental Editor: Taylor Ball
Publishing Services Manager: Anne Altepeter
Project Manager: Cindy Thoms
Senior Book Designer: Louis Forgione

Printed in the United States of America

Last digit is the print number: 9 8 7 6 5 4 3 2 1

To my mother and father for their lifelong sacrifices for their children.

To my sister, Mona, and my brothers, Badr and Salman, for always being there for me.

To my wife, Anne Marie Abdulrauf, my heart and my rock.

To my mentors, Professors Ossama Al-Mefty, Issam Awad, Dennis Spencer, Jack Rock, Ghaus Malik, Kenneth Smith, Albert Rhoton, Jon Robertson, Mark Rosenblum, and Laligam Sekhar; I stand on the shoulders of giants.

To my teacher, Professor M. Gazi Yasargil; I will always be your apprentice.

—*Saleem I. Abdulrauf*

CONTRIBUTORS

Saleem I. Abdulrauf, MD, FACS
Neurosurgeon-in-Chief
Saint Louis University Hospital
Professor, Neurological Surgery
Director, Saint Louis University Center for Cerebrovascular
    and Skull Base Surgery
Saint Louis University School of Medicine
Vice President, Congress of Neurological Surgeons
Chairman, International Division of the Congress of
    Neurological Surgeons
Secretary, North American Skull Base Society
Secretary General, World Federation of Skull Base Societies
St. Louis Missouri
*Chapter 11: Radial Artery Harvest for Cerebral
Revascularization: Technical Pearls*
*Chapter 15: Minimally Invasive EC-IC Bypass Procedures
and Introduction of the IMA-MCA Bypass Procedure*
Chapter 23: EC-IC Bypass for Giant ICA Aneurysms

Ali Alaraj, MD
Assistant Professor, Department of Neurosurgery
University of Illinois at Chicago
Chicago, Illinois
Chapter 17: EC-IC Bypass for Posterior Circulation Ischemia

Felipe C. Albuquerque, MD
Assistant Director, Endovascular Neurosurgery
Division of Neurological Surgery
Barrow Neurological Institute
Phoenix, Arizona
Chapter 20: Endovascular Therapies for Cerebral Revascularization

Jorge Alvernia, MD
Neurosurgery Department
Saint Edward Mercy Medical Center
Fort Smith, Arkansas
Chapter 32: Intracranial Venous Revascularization

Sepideh Amin-Hanjani, MD, FACS, FAHA
Associate Professor and Program Director
Co-Director, Neurovascular Surgery
Department of Neurosurgery
University of Illinois at Chicago
Chicago, Illinois
*Chapter 5: Decision Making in Cerebral Revascularization
Surgery Using Intraoperative CBF Measurements*
Chapter 17: EC-IC Bypass for Posterior Circulation Ischemia

Daniel L. Barrow, MD
MBNA Bowman Professor and Chairman
Department of Neurosurgery
Director, Emory Stroke Center
Emory University School of Medicine
Atlanta, Georgia
Chapter 22: Natural History of Giant Intracranial Aneurysms

H. Hunt Batjer, MD
Professor and Chair
Northwestern University, Feinberg School of Medicine
Chairman, Department of Neurological Surgery
Northwestern Memorial Hospital
Chicago, Illinois
*Chapter 12: Saphenous Vein Grafts for High-Flow Cerebral
Revascularization*

Bernard R. Bendok, MD, FACS
Associate Professor of Neurosurgery
Department of Neurosurgery
Northwestern University, Feinberg School of Medicine
Northwestern Memorial Hospital
Chicago, Illinois
*Chapter 12: Saphenous Vein Grafts for High-Flow Cerebral
Revascularization*

John D. Cantando, DO
Division of Neurosurgery
Arrowhead Regional Medical Center
Colton, California
*Chapter 15: Minimally Invasive EC-IC Bypass Procedures and
Introduction of the IMA-MCA Bypass Procedure*
Chapter 23: EC-IC Bypass for Giant ICA Aneurysms

Andrew Carlson, MD
Chief Resident
Department of Neurosurgery
University of New Mexico
Albuquerque, New Mexico
*Chapter 2: Using Cerebral Vaso-Reactivity in the Selection of
Candidates for EC-IC Bypass Surgery*

C. Michael Cawley, MD
Associate Professor
Emory University
Atlanta, Georgia
Chapter 22: Natural History of Giant Intracranial Aneurysms

Shamik Chakraborty, BS
State University of New York
Downstate College of Medicine
Brooklyn, New York
Chapter 14: EC-IC Bypass Using ELANA Technique

Fady T. Charbel, MD
Professor and Head
Department of Neurosurgery
University of Illinois at Chicago
Chicago, Illinois
*Chapter 5: Decision Making in Cerebral Revascularization
Surgery Using Intraoperative CBF Measurements*
*Chapter 17: EC-IC Bypass for Posterior Circulation
Ischemia*

Harry J. Cloft, MD
Departments of Radiology and Neurosurgery
Mayo Clinic College of Medicine
Rochester, Minnesota
*Chapter 21: Exploring New Frontiers: Endovascular
Treatment of the Occluded ICA*

E. Sander Connolly, Jr., MD
Bennett M. Stein Professor and Vice-Chair
Department of Neurological Surgery
Columbia University
New York, New York
Chapter 16: EC-IC Bypass Evidence

Jeroen R. Coppens, MD
Department of Neurosurgery
University of Utah
Salt Lake City, Utah
*Chapter 15: Minimally Invasive EC-IC Bypass Procedures and
Introduction of the IMA-MCA Bypass Procedure*

William Couldwell, MD, PhD
Professor
Attending Physician
Department of Neurosurgery
University of Utah
Salt Lake City, Utah
*Chapter 31: Decision-Making Strategies for EC-IC Bypass in the
Treatment of Skull Base Tumors*

Mark J. Dannenbaum, MD
Cerebrovascular Fellow
Department of Neurosurgery
Emory University
Atlanta, Georgia
*Chapter 22: Natural History of Giant Intracranial
Aneurysms*

Colin Derdeyn, MD
Professor of Radiology, Neurology and Neurological Surgery
Director, Center for Stroke and Cerebrovascular Disease
Washington University School of Medicine
St. Louis, Missouri
*Chapter 3: PET Measurements of OEF for Cerebral
Revascularization*

Gavin P. Dunn, MD, PhD
Harvard Medical School
Neurosurgery Service
Massachusetts General Hospital
Boston, Massachusetts
Chapter 25: Bypass Surgery for Complex MCA Aneurysms

Christopher S. Eddleman, MD, PhD
Cerebrovascular Fellow
UT Southwestern Medical Center
Dallas, Texas
*Chapter 12: Saphenous Vein Grafts for High-Flow Cerebral
Revascularization*

Mohamed Samy Elhammady, MD
Department of Neurological Surgery
University of Miami, Miller School of Medicine
Miami, Florida
Chapter 9: OA-PICA Bypass

Christopher C. Getch, MD
Professor
Department of Neurological Surgery
Northwestern University, Feinberg School of Medicine
Chicago, Illinois
*Chapter 12: Saphenous Vein Grafts for High-Flow Cerebral
Revascularization*

Basavaraj Ghodke, MD
Assistant Professor
Department of Neuroradiology and Neurological Surgery
Director, Neuro-Interventional Radiology
Co-Director, UW Brain Aneurysm Center
Attending Neuro-Interventional Radiologist
Vascular Anomalies Clinic—Childrens Hospital and
    Research Center
Seattle, Washington
Chapter 27: Surgical Revascularization of the Posterior Circulation

Paul R. Gigante, MD, BS
Resident
Department of Neurological Surgery
Columbia University
New York, New York
Chapter 16: EC-IC Bypass Evidence

Danial Hallam, MD
Associate Professor, Radiology and of Neurological Surgery
University of Washington
Seattle, Washington
Chapter 27: Surgical Revascularization of the Posterior Circulation

Joshua E. Heller, MD
Chief Neurosurgery Resident
Department of Neurosurgery
Temple University Hospital
Philadelphia, Pennsylvania
Chapter 19: Carotid Endarterectomy

Juha Hernesniemi, MD, PhD
Professor and Chairman
Department of Neurosurgery
Helsinki University Central Hospital
Helsinki, Finland
Chapter 6: New Days for Old Ways in Treating Giant Aneurysms—From Hunterian Ligation to Hunterian Closure?
Chapter 10: The State of the Art in Cerebrovascular Bypasses: Side-to-Side in situ PICA-PICA Bypass

L. Nelson Hopkins, MD, FACS
Professor and Chairman of Neurosurgery
Professor of Radiology
School of Medicine and Biomedical Sciences
University at Buffalo, State University of New York
Buffalo, New York
Chapter 29: Endovascular Techniques for Giant Intracranial Aneurysms

Yin Hu, MD
Department of Neurological Surgery
Barrow Neurological Institute
Phoenix, Arizona
Chapter 20: Endovascular Therapies for Cerebral Revascularization

Shady Jahshan, MD
Clinical Assistant Professor of Health Sciences
Department of Neurosurgery
School of Medicine and Biomedical Sciences
University at Buffalo, State University of New York
Buffalo, New York
Chapter 29: Endovascular Techniques for Giant Intracranial Aneurysms

David H. Jho, MD, PhD
Harvard Medical School
Neurosurgical Service
Massachusetts General Hospital
Boston, Massachusetts
Chapter 25: Bypass Surgery for Complex MCA Aneurysms

Masatou Kawashima, MD, PhD
Associate Professor
Department of Neurosurgery
Saga University Faculty of Medicine
Saga, Japan
Chapter 7: Surgical Anatomy of EC-IC Bypass Procedures

Christopher P. Kellner, BA, MD
Resident
Department of Neurological Surgery
Columbia University Medical Center
New York, New York
Chapter 16: EC-IC Bypass Evidence

Alexander A. Khalessi, MD, MS
Clinical Instructor and Resident Supervisor
Department of Neurological Surgery
University of Southern California
Los Angeles, California
Chapter 29: Endovascular Techniques for Giant Intracranial Aneurysms

Nadia Khan, MD
Clinical Instructor
Stanford University
Department of Neurosurgery
Stanford University School of Medicine
Stanford, California
Chapter 8: STA-MCA Microanastomosis: Surgical Technique
Chapter 18: Cerebral Revascularization for Moyamoya Disease

Louis Kim, MD
Assistant Professor of Neurological Surgery and Radiology
University of Washington School of Medicine
Seattle, Washington
Chapter 27: Surgical Revascularization of the Posterior Circulation

Leena Kivipelto, MD, PhD
Assistant Professor
Department of Neurosurgery
Hospital District of Helsinki and Uusimaa
Helsinki, Finland
Chapter 6: New Days for Old Ways in Treating Giant Aneurysms—From Hunterian Ligation to Hunterian Closure?
Chapter 10: The State of the Art in Cerebrovascular Bypasses: Side-to-Side in situ PICA-PICA Bypass
Chapter 14: EC-IC Bypass Using ELANA Technique

Miikka Korja, MD, PhD
Neurosurgeon
Department of Neurosurgery
Helsinki University Central Hospital
Helsinki, Finland
Chapter 6: New Days for Old Ways in Treating Giant Aneurysms—From Hunterian Ligation to Hunterian Closure?
Chapter 10: The State of the Art in Cerebrovascular Bypasses: Side-to-Side in situ PICA-PICA Bypass

David J. Langer, MD
Associate Professor
Department of Neurosurgery
Harvey Cushing Institutes of Neuroscience
Hofstra University School of Medicine
Manhasset, New York
Chapter 10: The State of the Art in Cerebrovascular Bypasses: Side-to-Side in situ PICA-PICA Bypass
Chapter 14: EC-IC Bypass Using ELANA Technique

Giuseppe Lanzino, MD
Professor of Neurologic Surgery
Mayo Clinic
Rochester, Minnesota
Chapter 21: Exploring New Frontiers: Endovascular Treatment of the Occluded ICA

Michael Lawton, MD
Professor and Vice-Chairman
Chief, Vascular and Skull Base Neurosurgery
Tong-Po Kan Endowed Chair
University of California, San Francisco
San Francisco, California
Chapter 13: IC-IC Bypasses for Complex Brain Aneurysms

Jonathon J. Lebovitz, MS
Medical Student
Saint Louis University Medical School
Center for Cerebrovascular and Skull Base Surgery
St. Louis, Missouri
Chapter 23: EC-IC Bypass for Giant ICA Aneurysms

Martin Lehecka, MD, PhD
Department of Neurosurgery
Helsinki University Central Hospital
Helsinki, Finland
Chapter 6: New Days for Old Ways in Treating Giant Aneurysms—From Hunterian Ligation to Hunterian Closure?

Hanna Lehto, MD
Department of Neurosurgery
Helsinki University Central Hospital
Helsinki, Finland
Chapter 6: New Days for Old Ways in Treating Giant Aneurysms—From Hunterian Ligation to Hunterian Closure?

Elad I. Levy, MD, FACS, FAHA
Professor of Nerosurgery and Radiology
School of Medicine and Biomedical Sciences
University at Buffalo, State University of New York
Buffalo, New York
Chapter 29: Endovascular Techniques for Giant Intracranial Aneurysms

Gordon Li, MD
Neurosurgery Resident
Stanford University
Department of Neurosurgery
Stanford University School of Medicine
Stanford, California
Chapter 18: Cerebral Revascularization for Moyamoya Disease

Michael Lim, MD
Assistant Professor of Neurosurgery, Oncology and Institute for NanoBiotechnology
Johns Hopkins University School of Medicine
Baltimore, Maryland
Chapter 18: Cerebral Revascularization for Moyamoya Disease

Christopher M. Loftus, MD, DrHC, FACS
Professor and Chairman
Department of Neurosurgery
Assistant Dean for International Affiliations
Temple University School of Medicine
Philadelphia, Pennsylvania
Chapter 19: Carotid Endarterectomy

Daniel M. Mandell, MD
Chief Fellow
Diagnostic Neuroradiology
University of Toronto
Toronto, Ontario, Canada
Chapter 4: Assessment of Cerebrovascular Reactivity Using Emerging MR Technologies

Cameron G. McDougall, MD
Department Neurological Surgery
Barrow Neurological Institute
Phoenix, Arizona
Chapter 20: Endovascular Therapies for Cerebral Revascularization

David J. Mikulis, MD
Professor and Co-Director of Medical Imaging Research
Department of Medical Imaging
University of Toronto
Neuroradiologist
Department of Medical Imaging
Toronto Western Hospital, University Health Network
Toronto, Ontario, Canada
Chapter 4: Assessment of Cerebrovascular Reactivity Using Emerging MR Technologies

Yedathore S. Mohan, MD, MS
Department of Neurosurgery
Henry Ford Hospital
Detroit, Michigan
Chapter 15: Minimally Invasive EC-IC Bypass Procedures and Introduction of the IMA-MCA Bypass Procedure
Chapter 23: EC-IC Bypass for Giant ICA Aneurysms

Jacques J. Morcos, MD, FRCS (Eng), FRCS (Ed)
Department of Neurosurgery
University of Miami School of Medicine
Miami, Florida
Chapter 9: OA-PICA Bypass

Sabareeh K. Natarajan, MD, MS
Clinical Assistant Professor of Health Sciences
Department of Neurosurgery
School of Medicine and Biomedical Sciences
University at Buffalo, State University of New York
Buffalo, New York
Chapter 29: Endovascular Techniques for Giant Intracranial Aneurysms

C. Benjamin Newman, MD
Department Neurological Surgery
Barrow Neurological Institute
Phoenix, Arizona
Chapter 20: Endovascular Therapies for Cerebral Revascularization

Mika Niemelä, MD, PhD
Department of Neurosurgery
Helsinki University Central Hospital
Helsinki, Finland
Chapter 6: New Days for Old Ways in Treating Giant Aneurysms—From Hunterian Ligation to Hunterian Closure?

Christopher S. Ogilvy, MD
Director, Endovascular and Operative Neurovascular Surgery
Massachusetts General Hospital
Robert G. and A. Jean Ojemann Professor of Neurosurgery
Harvard Medical School
Boston, Massachusetts
Chapter 25: Bypass Surgery for Complex MCA Aneurysms

Hideki Oka
Department of Neurosurgery
Helsinki University Central Hospital
Helsinki, Finland
Chapter 6: New Days for Old Ways in Treating Giant Aneurysms—From Hunterian Ligation to Hunterian Closure?

Raul Olivera, MD
Saint Louis University
Center for Cerebrovascular and Skull Base Surgery
St. Louis, Missouri
Chapter 23: EC-IC Bypass for Giant ICA Aneurysms

Sheri K. Palejwala
Medical Student
Saint Louis University Medical School
Center for Cerebrovascular and Skull Base Surgery
St. Louis, Missouri
Chapter 15: Minimally Invasive EC-IC Bypass Procedures and Introduction of the IMA-MCA Bypass Procedure

Aditya S. Pandey, MD
Assistant Professor of Neurosurgery
Department of Neurosurgery
University of Michigan School of Medicine
Ann Arbor, Michigan
Chapter 24: Cerebral Bypass in the Treatment of ACA Aneurysms

William Powers, MD
H. Houston Merritt Distinguished Professor and Chair
Department of Neurology
University of North Carolina School of Medicine
Chapel Hill, North Carolina
Chapter 1: Autoregulation and Hemodynamics in Human Cerebrovascular Disease

Alejandro A. Rabinstein, MD
Associate Professor of Neurology
Department of Neurology
Mayo Clinic
Rochester, Minnesota
Chapter 21: Exploring New Frontiers: Endovascular Treatment of the Occluded ICA

Scott Y. Rahimi, MD
Cerebrovascular Fellow
Emory University
Atlanta, Georgia
Chapter 22: Natural History of Giant Intracranial Aneurysms

Dinesh Ramanathan, MD, MS
Fellow
Department of Neurological Surgery
University of Washington
Seattle, Washington
Chapter 27: Surgical Revascularization of the Posterior Circulation

Luca Regli, MD
Professor and Chairman
Department of Neurosurgery
Rudolf Magnus Institute of Neurosciences
University Medical Center
Utrecht, Netherlands
Chapter 8: STA-MCA Microanastomosis: Surgical Technique
Chapter 28: EC-IC and IC-IC Bypass for Giant Aneurysms Using the ELANA Technique

Albert L. Rhoton, Jr., MD
Professor
Department of Neurological Surgery
University of Florida
Gainesville, Florida
Chapter 7: Surgical Anatomy of EC-IC Bypass Procedures

Rossana Romani, MD
Department of Neurosurgery
Helsinki University Central Hospital
Helsinki, Finland
*Chapter 6: New Days for Old Ways in Treating Giant
Aneurysms—From Hunterian Ligation to Hunterian
Closure?*

Duke Samson, MD
Professor and Chair
Department of Neurological Surgery
University of Texas Southwestern Medical Center
Dallas, Texas
*Chapter 30: Fusiform Intracranial Aneurysms: Management
Strategies*

Nader Sanai, MD
Director, Neurosurgical Oncology
Division of Neurological Surgery
Barrow Neurological Institute
Phoenix, Arizona
Chapter 13: IC-IC Bypasses for Complex Brain Aneurysms
*Chapter 26: Bypass Surgery for Complex Basilar Trunk
Aneurysms*

Deanna M. Sasaki-Adams, MD
Saint Louis University
Center for Cerebrovascular and Skull Base Surgery
St. Louis, Missouri
*Chapter 11: Radial Artery Harvest for Cerebral
Revascularization: Technical Pearls*

Albert J. Schuette, MD
Chief Resident
Department of Neurosurgery
Emory University
Atlanta, Georgia
Chapter 22: Natural History of Giant Intracranial Aneurysms

Laligam N. Sekhar, MD, FACS
William Joseph Leedom and Bennett Bigelow Professor
Vice Chairman, Neurological Surgery
Director, Cerebrovascular Surgery
Director, Skull Base Surgery
University of Washington
Seattle, Washington
*Chapter 27: Surgical Revascularization of the Posterior
Circulation*

Chandranath Sen, MD
Department of Neurosurgery
Roosevelt Hospital
New York, New York
*Chapter 10: The State of the Art in Cerebrovascular
Bypasses: Side-to-Side in situ PICA-PICA Bypass*

Adnan H. Siddiqui, MD, PhD
Assistant Professor of Neurosurgery and Radiology
School of Medicine and Biomedical Sciences
University at Buffalo, State University of New York
Buffalo, New York
*Chapter 29: Endovascular Techniques for Giant Intracranial
Aneurysms*

Marc Sindou, MD, DSc
Professor of Neurosurgery
Department of Neurosurgery
Hopital Neurologique P. Wertheimer
University Claude-Bernard of Lyon
Lyon, France
Chapter 32: Intracranial Venous Revascularization

Robert F. Spetzler, MD
Director and J.N. Harber Chair of Neurological Surgery
Barrow Neurological Institute
Phoenix, Arizona
Professor
Department of Surgery
Section of Neurosurgery
University of Arizona College of Medicine
Tucson, Arizona
Chapter 26: Bypass Surgery for Complex Basilar Trunk Aneurysms

Gary K. Steinberg, MD
Department of Neurosurgery and the Stanford Stroke Center
Stanford University School of Medicine
Stanford, California
Chapter 18: Cerebral Revascularization for Moyamoya Disease

Justin M. Sweeney, MD
Saint Louis University
Center for Cerebrovascular and Skull Base Surgery
St. Louis, Missouri
*Chapter 11: Radial Artery Harvest for Cerebral
Revascularization: Technical Pearls*
*Chapter 15: Minimally Invasive EC-IC Bypass Procedures and
Introduction of the IMA-MCA Bypass Procedure*

Tiziano Tallarita, MD
Carotid Disease Fellow
Department of Neurosurgery
Mayo Clinic
Rochester, Minnesota
*Chapter 21: Exploring New Frontiers: Endovascular Treatment
of the Occluded ICA*

Philipp Taussky, MD
Fellow
Department of Neurosurgery
University of Utah
Salt Lake City, Utah
Chapter 31: Decision-Making Strategies for EC-IC Bypass in the Treatment of Skull Base Tumors

B. Gregory Thompson, MD
Professor and JE McGillicuddy Chair
Departments of Neurosurgery, Radiology, and Otolaryngology
University of Michigan
Ann Arbor, Michigan
Chapter 24: Cerebral Bypass in the Treatment of ACA Aneurysms

Cees A.F. Tulleken, MD, PhD
Department of Neurosurgery
Rudolf Magnus Institute of Neurosciences
University Medical Center
Utrecht, Netherlands
Chapter 28: EC-IC and IC-IC Bypass for Giant Aneurysms Using the ELANA Technique

Albert van der Zwan, MD, PhD
Department of Neurosurgery
Rudolf Magnus Institute of Neurosciences
University Medical Center
Utrecht, Netherlands
Chapter 28: EC-IC and IC-IC Bypass for Giant Aneurysms Using the ELANA Technique

Tristan P.C. van Doormaal, MD, PhD
Neurosurgery Resident
Department of Neurosurgery
University Medical Center
Utrecht, Netherlands
Chapter 14: EC-IC Bypass Using ELANA Technique
Chapter 28: EC-IC and IC-IC Bypass for Giant Aneurysms Using the ELANA Technique

Jouke van Popta, MD
Department of Neurosurgery
Helsinki University Central Hospital
Helsinki, Finland
Chapter 6: New Days for Old Ways in Treating Giant Aneurysms—From Hunterian Ligation to Hunterian Closure?

Babu G. Welch, MD
Assistant Professor
Departments of Neurosurgery and Radiology
University of Texas Southwestern Medical Center
Dallas, Texas
Chapter 30: Fusiform Intracranial Aneurysms: Management Strategies

Howard Yonas, MD
Chairman
Department of Neurological Surgery
University of New Mexico
Albuquerque, New Mexico
Chapter 2: Using Cerebral Vaso-Reactivity in the Selection of Candidates for EC-IC Bypass Surgery

FOREWORD: REMARKS ON THE HISTORY OF BRAIN REVASCULARIZATION

The stroke and arterial bleeding, and their unfavorable sequelae, have been a source of deep fear among the population of all cultures for millennia. Even today, these drastic events pose challenging problems for medicine and surgery. The maturation of dietetic and pharmacologic treatments, coupled with the advancing surgical techniques that we are striving toward in order to achieve satisfactory treatment of vascular diseases, are all closely related to the cultural evolution of societies in all continents. The developments are a non-linear but incessant process. The history of medicine teaches us how to focus our attention on scientific endeavors in order to differentiate between the manifold symptoms and syndromes of the closely intertwined cardiovascular and blood organs, and their interaction with other bodily organs, particularly with the central nervous system.[1-8]

Generations of surgeons have been involved in developing procedures to eliminate and control arterial bleedings, especially for amputations. In 97 A.D., **Archigenes** pioneered the ligature technique for limb amputation. During the 2nd century A.D., **Antyllus** performed proximal and distal ligature of the popliteal artery for the treatment of saccular and fusiform aneurysms (see History of Medicine, pp. 247–249, A. Castiglioni, translated into English by E.B. Krumbhaar, published by A. Knopf, 1947). Throughout the next 1500 years, the ligature technique for the treatment of aneurysms was called the **Antyllus procedure**.

John Hunter was among the first to study collateral flow. In 1785, after ligating the main artery to the rapidly growing antler of a stag, he noted no cessation of growth and observed the early appearance of enlarged superficial vessels that carried blood around the obstruction. He explained this phenomenon on the principle that "the blood goes where it is needed." In treating a patient who had a popliteal aneurysm, Hunter applied his experiment by ligating the femoral artery (1786). The limb remained viable.[2] Since the 19th century arterial ligature for the treatment of aneurysm has been called **Hunterian ligature**.

Between 1885 and 1965 the ligature technique of arteries remained the main armamentarium of surgery, including neurosurgery. It is left to our imaginations to estimate the innumerable cases of injured neck and limb vessels that accumulated in ancient wars and in civil life, and to envision their surgical treatments. No documentation exists, although some reports begin to appear at the beginning of the 18th century.

in St. Louis and particularly of Carrel (1901–1940) at the Rockefeller Institute in New York. Carrel was able to resolve virtually all the problems of reconstructive vascular surgery. His refined suturing methods contributed greatly to successful resection, transplantation, and replacement of autogenic, homogenic, and allogenic arteries, veins, and even organs. The accomplishment of Carrel is to be greatly admired, realizing he was lacking in facilities such as angiography, flowmetry, magnification, microsutures, and anticoagulentia. He was a keen advocate of strict asepsis and antiseptic surgical conditions in his animal laboratory. With his co-worker Dawkins, he developed the effective antiseptic solution of sodium chlorate, so-called Dakins solution, which was adopted for clinical use.

The surgical accomplishments in the treatment of human vascular disease and injuries in the 18th and 19th centuries and in the first quarter of the 20th century (Thompson,[7] Burkhard; see additional suggested reading) failed, however, to broaden the scope of vascular surgical management until 1945.

During World War II (1938–1945), the majority of injured vessels of limbs were ligated and the limbs were amputated; this was also the case later in the Korean War (1950–1953). However, during the Vietnam War (1965–1973), the situation changed positively. According to a report by de Bakey et al.,[8a] 70% of patients with injured limbs underwent reconstructive vessel surgery instead of amputation. Systematic reconstructive cardiovascular surgery began in the 1940s, and on the extracranial segment of the carotid artery in 1951.

To further pursue the broad-scale application of vascular surgery, further maturation was needed in the sciences, technologies, and socioeconomic condition of societies. Advances in mathematics, basic sciences, and scientific technology began in the 17th century, developed with consequence in the following centuries, and accelerated, bringing dynamic progress, in the second half of the 20th century. The breakthroughs in physics, chemistry, pharmacology, microbiology, molecular biology, hematology, genetics, immunology, recording and visualization technologies, and sophisticated medical equipment provided a strong foundation for modern medicine and sub-specialties in surgery.

The dynamics evolving in neurovisualization, in neurorecording technologies, and in cardiovascular surgery opened an avenue of opportunity for the successful development of microsurgery and endovascular procedures. In Tables 1 through 8, the developments in surgery are summarized chronologically.

EXPERIMENTAL VASCULAR SURGERY

Systematic experimental vascular surgery in the laboratory began around 1875 (Eck, Gluck, and Jassinowsky). This culminated in the laboratory work of A. Carrel and C.C. Guthrie

MICROVASCULAR SURGERY

In 1953, a universal operating microscope (OPMI 1) was constructed and marketed by Carl Zeiss Company, Oberkochen, Germany. It found immediate and positive appreciation by

Table 1. SCIENTIFIC AND TECHNICAL DEVELOPMENTS INFLUENCING THE EVOLUTION IN MEDICINE AND SURGERY

- Mathematics
- Physics
- Chemistry
- Pharmacology
- Radiology
- Nuclear medicine
- Medical
- Computer
- Robotic techniques
- Communication (cellular telephone)
- Micro-mechanics
- Electric
- Optic
- Laser
- Ultrasound
- Photography, movies, TV (2-D, 3-D)
- Bio-engineering

Table 2. DIAGNOSTIC TECHNOLOGY SINCE 1845 VISUALIZATION OF MORPHOLOGY AND FUNCTION OF LIVING ORGANISMS = VLO

- Ophthalmoscope
- ECG
- Sphygmomanometer
- Riva-Rocci
- Thermometer
- Laboratory examination
- Plain x-ray
- EEG, EMG, ENG, MEG
- Pneumoencephalography
- Myelography
- Angiography
- Kety-Schmidt clearance
- Regional brain blood flow
- Plethysmography
- RISA
- CT, MRI, MRA, MRV
- 3-D CT, 3-D MRI
- MRI spectography, functional MRI
- SPECT, PET
- Xenon CT
- Ultrasound—flowmetry-extracranial-intracranial
- Ultrasound—imaging
- Neuromonitoring
- NIR-ICG videography

Table 3. ACTION FIELDS OF VASCULAR SURGERY

- Hemostasis in cases of spontaneous or traumatic rupture
- Removal of hematoma (cavities, parenchymal)
- Repair, reconstruction of diseased or injured vessels
- Elimination of aneurysm, malformation, fistulas
- Revascularization of organs: heart, brain, limbs, skin, penis
- Organ transplantation
- Cosmetic surgery

Table 4. GOALS OF VASCULAR SURGERY

- Restoration of vessel anatomy and function
- Reestablishment of hemodynamics
- Secure vessel patency
  - care of adequate diameter of vessel lumen
  - avoidance of clotting, pseudoaneurysms, infection
  - care for the nutrition of vessel wall (vasa vasorum)
- Avoidance of hypoxia, ischemia, infarct of related organ or remote organs
- Maintenance of homeostasis

Table 5. VASCULAR SURGERY

- Atraumatic, non-invasive exploration, dissection (care for OR temperature, applied fluids temperature)
- Recognition of anatomy and geometry of the lesion and lesional area
- Possibility to control the hemodynamics
- Hemostasis
  - vascular clamp, clips, balloon
  - bipolar coagulation
  - repair
  - adjuvant: muscle, fibrin, collagen, gelatin, cellulose, vitamin K, FFP, induced hypotension, hypothermia

Table 6. VASCULAR SURGERY

- Repair
- Reconstruction
- Replacement
- Transplantation
- Implantation
- Bypass
- Disobliteration
- Obliteration
- Suture: interrupted, continuous sleeve, partial sleeve
- Anastomosis: suture, staple
- Patch
- Graft (auto, homo, hetero, allo)
- Stents
- Clamp, clip, balloon, coil
- Embolization
- Ligature

Table 7. VASCULAR SURGERY

- Homeostasis
  - infusion
  - transfusion
  - induced blood pressure (hypotension, hypertension)
  - induced temperature (hypothermia, hyperthermia)
  - hyperemia (sympathectomy)
  - vasodilatation: local, focal, systemic
  - coagulopathy: increased, decreased
  - anti-edematous, anti-inflammatory
  - antipyretic, antibiotic
  - analgetic, sedative

Table 8. VASCULAR SURGERY

- Vitamin K, FFP, thrombocyte transfusion antifibrinolytic (AMCA) protamine (reverse heparin)
- Hirudin, heparin (discovered 1916, clinical use 1936), warfarin TPA, protein-C anti-aggregation: aspirin, Plavix, Aggrenox, non-steroid (ibuprofen, Ticlid) improvement of rheology: Rheomacrodex, Dextran
- Thrombogenic: Amino-capron-acid
- Fibrin glue, thrombin spray
- Gelfoam, Avitene
- Flow seal, Angio-Seal

ENT and eye surgeons. In 1957, observing the ENT surgical procedures performed by Dr. W. House at the Southern California Medical Center, Dr. T. Kurze envisioned the use of the operating microscope in neurosurgery. He began to train himself in the laboratory in order to perfect exploration of the cerebellopontine angle. He was not interested in pursuing microvascular surgery.

In 1960, Dr. J. Jacobson was appointed associate professor and director of surgical research at the Mary Fletcher Hospital, Burlington, Vermont. The pharmacologists were interested in evaluating the effect of certain drugs on the denervated extracranial carotid artery of dogs. Dr. Jacobson agreed to study this project and began the task of severing and rejoining the artery of 3.0-mm diameter, applying the end-to-end anastomosis (EEA) technique of Carrel. The results of these anastomoses were unsatisfactory. Dr. Jacobson and Dr. E. Suarez, his fellow, discovered in a corner of the laboratory area, in the corridor, an OPMI 1 microscope, and decided that an attempt to achieve an improved patency of the carotid artery under the operating microscope was a viable solution. The experience was inspiring, likened to observing for the first time the surface of the moon through a telescope. An anastomosis on the carotid artery could be completed with precision at each step of the procedure. This success removed a barrier to progress in the field of microvascular surgery. The microvascular techniques were soon adapted and advanced by vascular, plastic, cosmetic, and transplant surgeons, who began to perform free transplantations of ears, and thumb-to-finger on animals. Subsequently, microsurgery on humans with free transplantation of skin and reimplantation of fingers, hands, and whole extremities became successful (Tables 9 and 10, Figure 1).

Dr. Donaghy, chairman of neurosurgery in Burlington, Vermont, observing closely in Burlington the work of Jacobson and Suarez, began in 1961 to train himself, performing microvascular surgery on the femoral arteries of rabbits, and on the radial and saphenous arteries of dogs.[1] He was followed soon by Khodadad and Lougheed in Toronto, Canada,[9–11] and Sundt in Memphis, Tennessee.[12]

At the beginning of 1960, the majority of neurosurgeons were not attracted to spending long hours exercising reconstructive microvascular surgery in the laboratory. However, some attempts were made to reconstruct the occluded M1 segment of MCA in children and adults with some success—and this without the use of an operating microscope (Welch,

Table 9. MICROVASCULAR SURGERY

1961 – J.H. Jacobson, E.I. Suarez	
1961 – R.M.P. Donaghy	
1963 – M. Mozes, et al.	
1963 – A. Zwaveling	
1964 – G.K. Khodadad	
1965 – J.H. Buncke	Extracranial arteries
1965 – J. Cobbett	
1966 – G.E. Green, et al.	
1966 – J.W. Smith	

Table 10. MICROVASCULAR SURGERY FOR TRANSPLANTATION

1960 – H.J. Buncke	Digital and ear implantation
1965 – S. Kamatsu, S. Tamai	Toe-thumb
1965 – C. Zhong Wei, et al.	Finger-hand (315 cases)
1966 – B.R. Vogt	Arm transplantation
1967 – H.J. Buncke, A.I. Daniller	Whole joint transplantation
1969 – J.R. Cobbet	Toe-thumb
1973 – R.K. Daniel, G.I. Taylor	Island flap
1974 – V.E. Meyer	Hand, finger

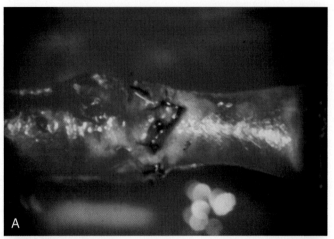

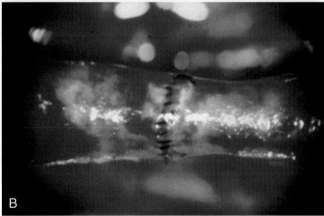

Figure 1. These photos were given to me by Dr. Julius Jacobson in 1966. **A,** End-to-end anastomosis on a dog's extracranial internal carotid artery performed without using an operating microscope. **B,** Same procedure performed by Dr. Julius Jacobson under an operating microscope, which proves the proper suturing technique.

Shillito, Scheibert, Driesen, Chou). In 1962, Woringer (neurosurgeon in Colmar, France) and Kunlin (vascular surgeon in Paris, France) achieved a high-flow bypass between the left common carotid artery and the intracranial segment of internal carotid artery.[13] They also lacked the facility of an operating microscope. In 1963, Dr. Jacobson and Dr. Donaghy accomplished, under the operating microscope, reconstructive surgery on the M1 segment of MCA on several patients.[14] In Toronto, Canada, 1965, Lougheed and his team also accomplished microvascular surgery on the occluded ICA, MCA, and ACA.[15]

In retrospect, these initial attempts of reconstructive microvascular surgery on brain arteries of patients can be evaluated as courageous, but they can also be considered as premature. The fact is that microvascular surgery practiced in the laboratory on extracranial arteries cannot be transferred unconditionally to intracranial arteries in animals and humans. Intracranial vessels are embedded in cisterns and are therefore "aquatic," suspended within the surrounding cisternal wall by a myriad of arachnoidal-pial fibers. Their dissection and manipulation require meticulous bipolar coagulation technology, atraumatic temporary vessel clips, and refined microsutures (Figure 2, Table 11).

RECONSTRUCTIVE MICROVASCULAR SURGERY ON BRAIN ARTERIES IN THE LABORATORY

The drive to establish techniques for reconstructive microvascular surgery on brain arteries at the department of neurosurgery at the University Hospital in Zurich, Switzerland, came in 1963 by cardiac surgeon Ake Senning, who, in 1961, had pioneered endarterectomy on coronary arteries (Figure 3). One of his patients, a 17-year-old female, on awakening after open-heart surgery, right-sided hemisyndrome. The left carotid angiography revealed occlusion only of the left central sulcal artery by an embolus. An immediate embolectomy on this small-caliber artery (0.8–1.0 mm) was impossible due to

Table 11. STRUCTURAL DIFFERENCES BETWEEN THE EXTRACRANIAL AND INTRACRANIAL ARTERIES		
	EXTRACRANIAL	INTRACRANIAL
Muscle layers	55	20
Collagen fibers	33%	22%
Elastic fibers	4%	1%–2%
External elastic membrane	+	–
Tunica externa	+	Spinal fluid
Vena comitans	+	–
Lymphatic vessel	+	– (Spinal fluid)
Vasa vasorum	+	–
Nerves	+	(+)
Vasomotor behavior	+++	(+)

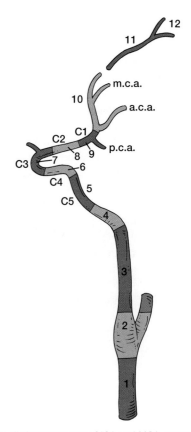

Figure 3. Twelve distinct segments of ICA and MCA according to structural differences of the wall.

our lack of previous laboratory training in microvascular surgery and the non-existence of microinstruments and particularly of microsuture. Fortunately the young patient of Dr. Senning recovered in the following weeks, thanks to the good functioning of the arterial collaterals of her brain. Nevertheless, the discourse continued in our department, revolving around the issue of microvascular surgery of brain arteries (Figures 4 and 5).

Finally, in 1965, I was delegated to Burlington, Vermont, to learn microsurgical techniques. Beginning in October 1965, Dr. Donaghy; his resident, Dr. John Slater; and his first scrub

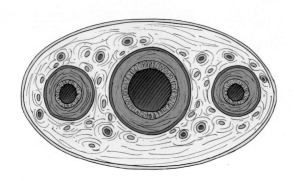

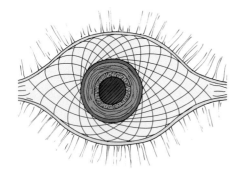

Figure 2. The extracranial vascular organ: an artery accompanied by two veins, having arterial and venous vasa vasorum, lymph vessels, and rich network of sympaticus and parasympaticus nerves. The intracranial "aquatic" artery, suspended by a myriad of arachnoidal-pial fibers within a cistern, having no vaso vasorum and lymph vessels.

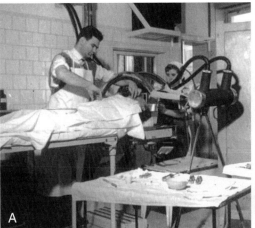
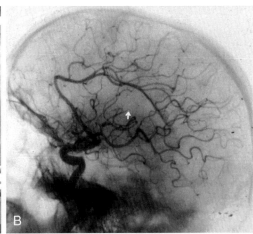

Figure 4. A, Percutaneous carotid angiography in the 1950s. **B,** Left carotid arteriography showing the occlusion of the central sulcus artery *(arrow)* by embolus on a 17-year-old female.

nurse, Mrs. Esther Roberts, were great assistance and support introducing me to the finesse of microvascular surgical techniques (Figure 6). I learned to accomplish EEA, ESA, and the challenging duplication of the femoral arteries of rabbits, but mostly I worked on the radial and saphenous arteries of mongrel dogs, using OPM 1 microscope, fine jewelers' forceps, and 8.0 nylon sutures. After completing 120 such procedures on extracranial arteries, I insisted on transferring my learned techniques to the brain arteries of dogs. My assumption that this would present no problems was an illusion, for the frontal

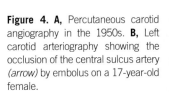

Figure 5. Professor Ake Senning, Chairman of the Cardio-Vascular Department of the University Hospital, Zurich, Switzerland.

and temporal cortical arteries were too small (0.4–0.6 mm in diameter) for repair with 8.0 nylon suture. However, the basilar artery measured 1.0 to 1.2 mm in diameter, and, in December 1965, I began to explore the basilar artery of mongrel dogs under general anesthesia, via a transcervical-submandibular-transclival approach. After longitudinal opening of the arachnoid membrane along the basilar trunk, two Scoville clips were applied and an incision 5.0 to 6.0 mm in length was made in the basilar artery. A T-tube was inserted and secured, and the clips removed. The incision was closed with a small arterial patch using 8.0 nylon suture. Local papaverine application on the basilar artery was very effective to dilate the artery for at least 1 hour. The first dog survived the procedure without complications and the artery remained patent for many months. In 32 other dogs, patch and graft procedure was accomplished with 70% patency[16] (Figures 7 and 8).

In February 1966, bipolar coagulation equipment of L. Malis was purchased with the technology of meticulous hemostasis, thus the operating field was maintained clean and clear, greatly facilitating the progress of procedures. In February 1966, I attempted to perform a high-flow bypass using a femoral artery autologous graft between the left common carotid artery and left MCA. The initial strong pulsations of the graft lessened in the following hour, and a thrombus the entire length of the graft occurred. In four other dogs, the grafts thrombosed within a short time (two times from the femoral artery, two times from saphenous veins). I assumed that in long grafts the vasovasorium of the grafts is affected, causing nutritional damage to the vessel wall and resulting in thrombosis. Fairly disappointed, I gave up the high-flow EC-IC anastomosis experiments.

In March 1966, 9.0 nylon suture became available, which allowed me to exercise on the frontal and temporal cortical arteries of dogs to perform patches, EEA, and short intracranial arterial grafts (1.0–2.0 cm long). Bipolar coagulation technology was indispensable in maintaining precise hemostasis and a clean operating field. In March 1966, the first extra-intracranial bypass was accomplished on a dog, joining the left superficial temporal artery to MCA (STA-MCA). In the

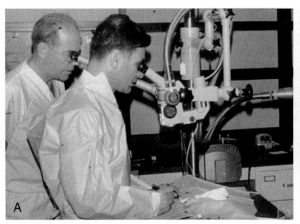 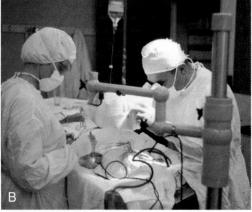

Figure 6. Professor R.M.P Donaghy (**A**) and chief scrub nurse Mrs. E. Roberts (**B**) instructing me in October 1965 on the first steps of microvascular surgery.

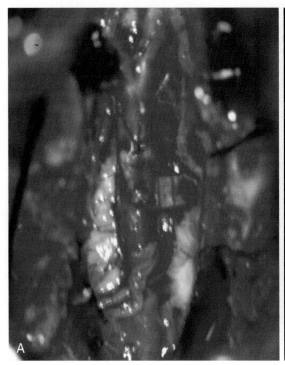 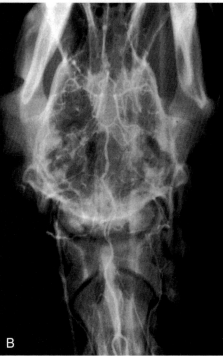

Figure 7. A, Transcervical-trans-clival explored, incised, and patched basilar artery of mongrel dog. **B,** Postoperative angiography verifies the patency of the basilar artery. The dog survived the surgical procedure well and could stand on his legs, eat, and drink the next morning.

following months, STA-MCA bypass was performed on 29 dogs; in 12 cases the adventitia of the superficial temporal artery was stripped for 4.0 to 6.0 cm. The bypass remained patent in only 33% of dogs. In 17 dogs the donor artery was stripped only 3.0 to 4.0 mm, which improved the patency rate of the bypass to 76%[17] (Figure 9).

My 14 months of laboratory experience verified the feasibility of systematically applying microtechniques for the reconstruction of brain arteries in an experimental setting, in preparation and anticipation of success in the clinical arena. This reality caused me to reevaluate my concept of neurosurgery, which had been based on my 12 previous years of involvement (1953–1965) in a clinical setting. I was strongly

convinced of the significance and opportunity microtechniques would offer to advance and broaden the possibilities of neurosurgical procedures. An entirely new vista was unfolding, with the realization that neurosurgery was verging on a venture that would change our perspective of the achievable and the potential of our surgical skills. My laboratory work also resulted in the rediscovery of the cisternal compartments of the brain, which had been precisely studied and documented by Key and Retzius in 1875. The relevance and significance of understanding the detailed anatomy of the cisterns became apparent as the microneurosurgical era began (see Yaşargil, Microneurosurgery, vol 1, G. Thieme, pp. 5–53, 1984). Learning to surgically approach these delicate structures,

Figure 8. A, Bipolar coagulation apparatus in 1966. **B,** Professor Len Malis, chairman of the Neurosurgical Department of Mount Sinai Hospital, New York, who perfected the bipolar coagulation apparatus of Dr. Greenwood, Houston, Texas.

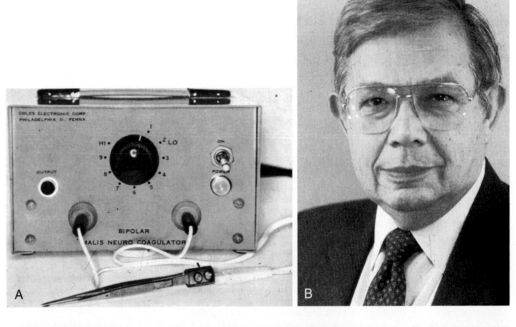

Figure 9. First reconstructive microvascular surgery of leptomeningeal (pial) artery of mongrel dog. **A,** Explored temporal artery (0.8mm in diameter). **B,** Micro-T-tube (Silastic) introduced into the artery to maintain the hemodynamics. **C,** First time successful arterial-patch surgery on a brain artery of a dog in February 1966. **D,** EEA of a graft with 9.0 suture in March 1966. **E,** Completed arterial graft. **F,** Extra-intracranial (STA-TA bypass) on a mongrel dog in March 1966.

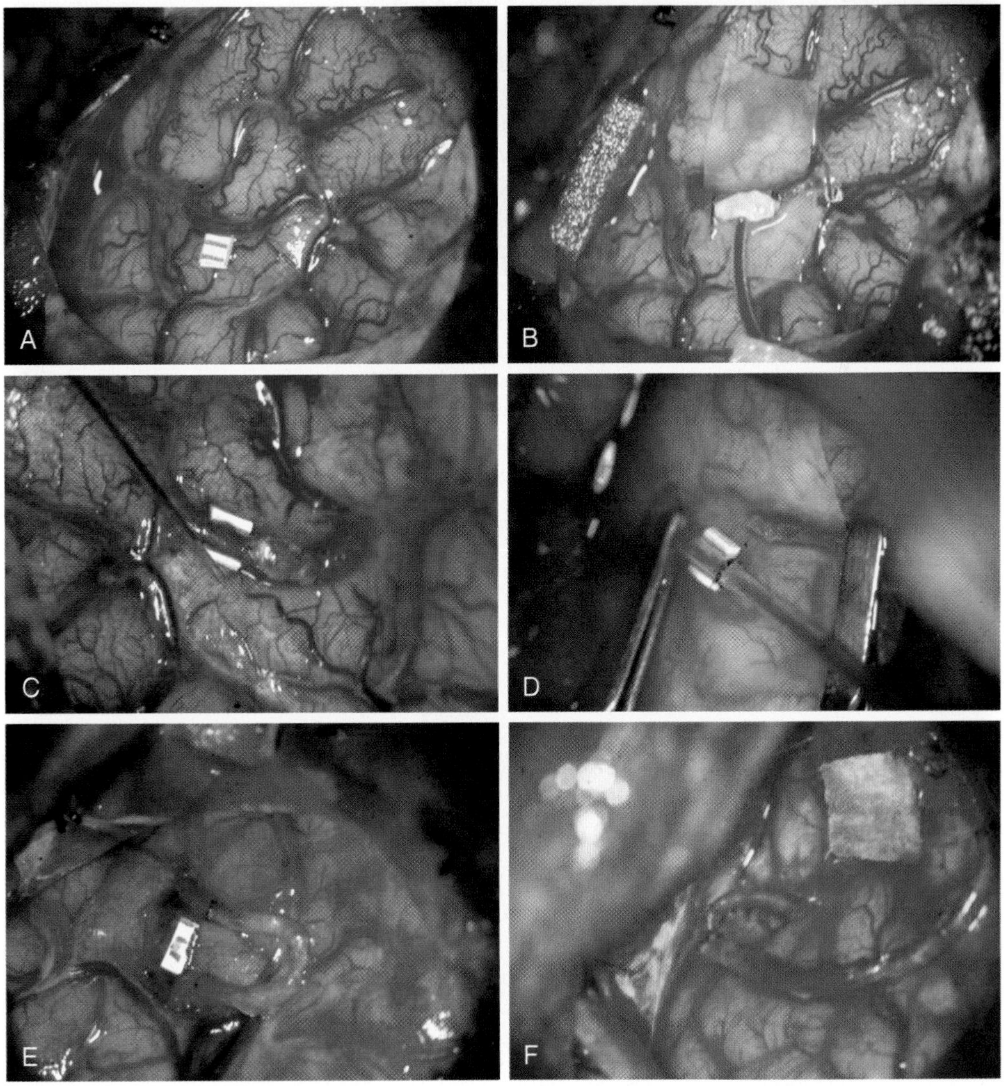

applying microtechniques, and to respect the significance of these fine anatomical structures is an integral part of accomplishing a microneurosurgery, avoiding damage to normal tissue. In laboratory work two goals have been realized:

1. Reconstruction of intracranial brain arteries
2. Recognition of the significance of the cisternal compartments

During my laboratory work, I conceived the concept that lesions in each location of the CNS could be explored along the cisternal pathways, dissecting the veins and arteries within the cisterns, without using any retraction to the brain. The availability of bipolar coagulation, equipment for precise and punctual hemostasis without heating the surrounding normal tissue, pressure-regulated suction system, atraumatic temporary vessel clips, microsutures, and the opportunity to acquire appropriate laboratory training provided the effective instrumentation and sound foundation to develop microneurosurgery.

A perfected microtechnique, skillfully performed, would certainly contribute to creating an effective treatment to eliminate intracranial saccular aneurysms, AVMs, cavernomas, hematomas, extrinsic and intrinsic tumors, craniospinal traumas, and spinal discs injuries. Microtechniques present to neurosurgeons the necessary tactics to become proficient in the repair of iatrogenic injured arteries, veins, and venous sinuses, and to perform intracranial and extra-intracranial bypass surgery in cases of giant saccular or fusiform aneurysms, cavernous fistulas, extrinsic and intrinsic tumors, and malignant neck and skull base tumors, which may encage the principle cranial nerves and brain vessels.

On January 18, 1967, with the support of my esteemed teacher, Professor Hugo Krayenbühl, I began to apply all microtechniques that I had developed, reviewed, and practiced in the laboratory. My 25 years of experience in this field (1967–1992) at the Neurosurgery Department, University Hospital, Zurich, have been published in six volumes titled *Microneurosurgery*. A total of 6000 patients have been operated on for aneurysms, AVMs, cavernoma, and extrinsic and intrinsic tumors. In only 45 patients with cerebrovascular occlusive disease were there true and valid indications for microvascular surgery. In a further 14 patients, brain arteries were repaired, and in 24 patients, the venous sinuses were repaired in situ.

MICROSURGICAL TECHNIQUES APPLIED TO NEUROSURGERY

On my return to Zurich in December 1966, I was informed by our cardiac surgeon that the problem with cerebral emboli had been solved, thanks to the introduction of an improved blood exchanger. In the following years, I had the opportunity to operate on only one patient after open-heart surgery (1968). This 42-year-old male developed complete right-sided hemisyndrome 5 days after his heart surgery, despite anticoagulent

therapy. The embolus was successfully removed from the M1 segment of the left MCA (see case 6 in Table XI, Microneurosurgery applied to Neurosurgery, 1969). From 1967 to 1973, I operated on 11 patients with vascular occlusion; six patients had suffered thrombus, and five had embolus of the M1 segment of the MCA. The incision in MCA (10–20 mm in length) was sutured with 9.0 nylon. The artery was found to be patent in nine cases, but again occluded in two cases. The clinical outcome was excellent in two, good in four, fair in three, and poor in two (see Table XIII in Microsurgery applied to Neurosurgery 1969)[18] (Figure 10). We had to recognize that the recanalization of occluded brain arteries will not help the restitution of microcirculation and the already manifested metabolic disorders.

However, the microvascular techniques acquired during laboratory training were effectively applied in the following procedures; five patients with ruptured intracranial saccular aneurysms (A.Co.A., P.Co.A., ICA, MCA, and pericallosal artery), which evulsed on dissection from the parent artery, and could be repaired immediately with application of temporary clip to the parent artery and suturing with 9.0 nylon thread. In two other patients, the internal carotid artery was inadvertently injured by high-speed drilling of the posterior clinoid process. The artery could not be repaired, and EC-IC bypass was made, which unfortunately did not help to rescue this patient with basilar bifurcation aneurysm. In a further case the carotid artery was injured during dissection of a basal dermoid, and the artery had to be ligated. An EC-IC bypass was instrumental in securing recovery in this young patient.

In two patients the short temporal polar artery, at its origin with a very proximal M1 segment, was injured as a clip was applied to an aneurysm on the posterior communicating artery. The opening on the wall of the M1 could be repaired with a few sutures. In one of these two cases the repaired M1 segment was slightly narrowed; therefore an EC-IC bypass was done.

In five patients with large sclerotic, partially calcified aneurysm on MCA bifurcation and in one patient with pericallosal artery aneurysm, the aneurysm was resected after application of temporary clips on the parent artery. The adjacent intraluminal segment of the parent artery was then cleaned of calcification and the artery repaired with microsuture (see Microneurosurgery, vol II).

REPAIR OF VENOUS SINUSES

In four patients with parasagittal meningiomas and in two patients with interhemispheric approach to intraventricular tumors, the superior sagittal sinus was marginally opened and could be repaired speedily with running sutures. In one case of a large meningioma that had invaded the torcular Herophili, the tumor could be removed completely and the lateral opening of the sinus repaired with a periostal patch. From 1200 infratentorial approaches, a marginal injury of

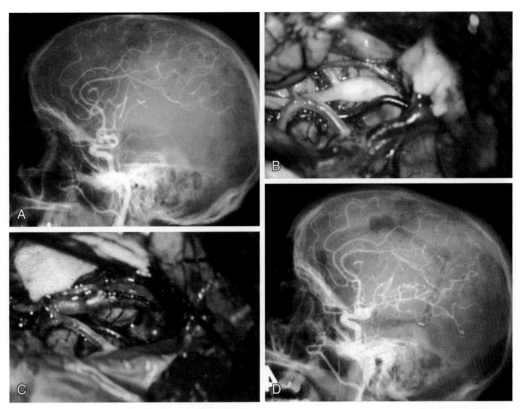

Figure 10. A, Left carotid arteriography shows the occlusion of the inferior trunk of MCA by 42-year-old male who suffered right-sided hemisyndrome and aphasia. Nonsmoker. **B,** The left inferior M2 segment has been explored by pterional trans-Sylvian approach and a thrombus removed. **C,** The incised artery was closed with single sutures (8.0). **D,** Post-operative left carotid angiography verifies patency of the repaired artery, full recovery of the patient, and no recurrence in the following decades.

the transverse or sigmoid sinus occurred on opening of the dura in 18 patients and could be repaired with a 4.0 nylon running suture. (See page 117 in Microsurgery applied to Neurosurgery, 1969.[18–30])

INTRACRANIAL BYPASS (IC-IC)

A 68-year-old male suffered left-sided exophthalmus with palsy of the III, IV, and VI nerves. The left carotid angiography revealed a giant cavernous aneurysm of ICA. The right carotid and vertebral angiography failed to visualize the vessels of the left hemisphere. The patient could not tolerate compression of the extracranial left carotid artery, immediately developing transient right hemiparesis and aphasia. Dr. Krayenbühl asked me to create an anterior communicating artery before attempting ligature of the ICA. In August 1967, I explored via a pterional craniotomy the region of the anterior communicating artery and found that this artery did not exist. To avoid harming both A2 segments, I performed an anastomosis between two branches (0.8 mm in diameter) of the frontopolar arteries (10.0 nylon). It so happened that Dr. J. Jacobson visited us on this day and observed the entire surgical procedure, offering supportive advice. The postoperative course was uneventful, and the intracranial bypass seemed to function as the patient recovered very well. Three days following surgery he tolerated well the compression of the extracranial carotid artery (see Figure 63a-c, p. 118, Microsurgery applied to Neurosurgery).[18] Unfortunately, on the fourth day, the patient developed phlebitis from the vena cava catheter that rapidly

progressed to infection of the frontal flap and bone. The bone flap had to be removed. He recovered from this complication within 2 weeks, but he could no longer tolerate digital compression of the left carotid artery on his neck.

Finally, I wish to mention another unique experience with a large, temporal neopallial AVM, which presented on serial angiographic studies with only one large draining vein. On exploration, the vein was found circulating almost the entire surface of the malformation, affording no opportunity for my usual helical exploration of a malformation. Studying the perplexing situation, I finally performed a venovenous bypass between a vein of the malformation on the surface and a superficial temporal vein, which immediately began to drain the AVM. I explored and removed the lesion, having now some confidence on the substitute hemodynamics of the malformation. Such a venovenous bypass procedure was not necessary in 529 other brain AVM surgeries.

EXTRACRANIAL-TO-INTRACRANIAL ARTERIAL BYPASS (EC-IC)

Since 1953, research activities in laboratories and publications in the literature studying methods to measure precisely the hemodynamics and metabolism of the brain have determined that the indications for reconstructive cerebrovascular surgery are based on uncertainties. In 1960, I visited Dr. Lassen in Copenhagen. He had pioneered the specific measurements of cerebral hemodynamics applying radioactive Xenon and

Krypton technology. He recommended waiting until the PET technology would be available for clinical use. Unfortunately, the purchase of PET equipment was delayed for decades; therefore we placed our reliance on clinical experience and the available investigations to conclude our evaluation and establish sound indications for surgical intervention.

According to the following indications, I performed EC-IC bypasses between the superficial temporal artery and the anterior temporal branch (M4) of the MCA on 34 patients in Zurich:

- Out of 2100 patients with intracranial saccular aneurysms, 30 patients had giant intracranial aneurysms (see Table 124, Microneurosurgery, vol II, p. 303). In six patients, an EC-IC bypass was successfully accomplished, the first case in December 1968 on a 19-year-old female with right-sided ICA bifurcation giant aneurysm and ligation of ICA distal to the origin of the anterior choroidal artery (see Microsurgery applied to Neurosurgery, 1969, Table XIII, Case 6, Figure 62a-h) (Figure 11). In nine other patients, a trapping procedure was performed (five patients with giant aneurysms at the basilar bifurcation) (see Table 124, p. 303, Microneurosurgery, vol II, 1989).

- In another patient in May 1973 with recurrent sphenopetroclival meningioma, the injured ICA in the petrosal segment could be tangentially clipped and a supportive EC-IC bypass was made. The clinical course was successful, but the patient refused postoperative angiography study (Case 1, Table XIII). In 27 patients (2 children under 10 years of age) who suffered recurrent TIAs, RINDs, and progressive hemisyndrome, four-vessel angiography revealed severe stenosis or occlusion of the ICA and MCA with poor or no visualized collateral.

- On October 30, 1967, I performed my first EC-IC bypass procedure in a 20-year-old man with Marfan's syndrome who had suffered a stroke with right-sided hemisyndrome and showed, on left-sided carotid artery angiography, occlusion of the M1 segment. His postoperative course was uneventful, but he and his parents refused a control angiography study. He survived for decades and had good palpable pulsation of the left STA (see Case 1, Table XIII).

- A 61-year-old male with bilateral occlusion of extracranial ICA and right vertebral artery suffered TIAs when turning his neck to the right. Temporal artery EC-IC bypass was performed in November 1967; the bypass was angiographically and clinically successful (see Microsurgery applied to Neurosurgery, 1969, Table XIII, Case 2, p. 183) (Figures 12 and 13).

- On December 5, 1971, a 5-year-old boy was found comatose in bed one morning by his parents. Four-vessel angiography revealed stenosis of bilateral ICA, ACA, and MCA. Moyamoya disease was diagnosed. On admission to the neurosurgical department of the University Hospital Zurich in June 1972, the 6-year-old boy had pronounced hemisyndrome and motor aphasia. A left-sided STA-TA bypass was performed in June 1972 and the postoperative course was rewarding (see paper of Dr. Krayenbühl, 1975, Case 2)[31–34] (Figure 14).

The indications for EC-IC bypass surgery in 34 patients operated on by myself (1967–1972), and in 159 patients operated on from 1973 to 1992 by Drs. Y. Yonekawa, B. Zumstein, and H.G. Imhof were determined during the first 5 years, according to the amnesia results of neurologic examination, EEG, and three-dimensional serial angiography. The computer tomography, transcranial Doppler flowmetry, and scintigraphy became available after 1973; SPECT and MRI technology, after 1985. Regional blood flow studies with Xenon and Krypton and PET were not available at that time. Intraoperative quantitative flow measurements and ICG technologies are recent advances. In 1992, Dr. Imhof submitted his habilitation paper, describing a detailed and thorough analysis on 193 (13 bilateral) patients operated on during a span of 22 years (1967–1989) at the Department of Neurosurgery, University Hospital, Zurich. Unfortunately, this valuable document remained unpublished. Dr. Imhof came to the following conclusion: "Alas, the negative results of this study (Barnett-Peerless) no longer allow us to believe bypass surgery is an instrument of consequence in the prevention of stroke."[35,36] This opinion of Barnett et al., according to studies of Imhof, cannot be supported. The EC-IC bypass procedure is an effective treatment to improve the territorial and hemispheric cerebral hemodynamics and reduce the incidence of recurrent stroke. In Dr. Imhof's opinion, the EC-IC bypass should not be entirely rejected, nor should it be applied indiscriminately. The decision to proceed with the procedure is wholly dependent on thorough evaluation of the patient, and critical, skillful judgment when forming an opinion and defining surgical indication. This concept is valid even today in 2010 (Tables 12 and 13).[9–11,16,37–105]

For the past 43 years, in numerous microsurgical courses, meetings, and conferences, as well as in my publications, I have tried to convince colleagues that although the surgical technique is feasible, the indications for brain revascularization and flow augmentation have not been clearly defined. The indications for reconstructive cerebrovascular surgery cannot be set down as a definite or general rule, even with availability of stable xenon/CO_2 CT, MRI, SPECT, and PET. Until now, our decisions in this field have been little more than vague guesswork (Table 14).

DISCUSSION

Scientific research activities within the past two centuries have revealed the integral functions of cardiovascular, blood, and respiratory organs. These are closely intertwined with other unimorph and unifunctional body organs, all under the auspicious direction of the CNS. Neuroscientific endeavors

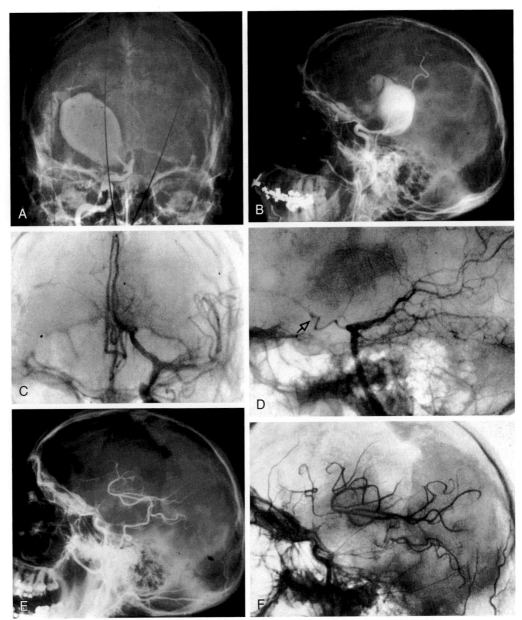

Figure 11. A, Anterior-posterior view of the right carotid arteriography showing a broad-based giant aneurysm at the ICA bifurcation. **B,** Lateral view. **C,** Left carotid angiography with aneurysm of the right common carotid artery shows following of both A2 segments but not the right A1 segment. **D,** Vertebral angiography with compromise of the right common carotid artery shows following of no hypoplastic posterior communicating artery (*arrow*). The aneurysm is not visualized. **E, F,** A 19-year-old female had developed a progressive left-sided hemisyndrome. On December 18, 1968, an STA-TA bypass was performed and the ICA distal to the origin of the anterior choroidal artery ligated; the aneurysm was incised and deflated, not removed. Full recovery from left hemiparesis was achieved in the following days. She survived this episode for decades, married, and gave birth to two healthy children.

have disclosed that the CNS is not an unimorph and unifunctional organ, but is an assembly of multitudes of distinct organs and functional systems:

1. The heterogenous, heteromorph, and heterofunctional parenchyma of the brain is composed of a great number of different types of neurons, glial cells, microglial cells, and ependymal cells, with vertical and horizontal connections organized and arranged in a precise strata within numerous distinct compartments.

2. Myelinized and unmyelinated connective fiber system and synapses.

3. A total of 6 sense organs (olfactory, optic, auditive, vestibular, gustatory, and haptic) and 7 other pairs of cranial and 32 pairs of spinal nerves.

4. Central and peripheral autonomous nervous organ.

5. Chief endocrine organ in the hypothalamic and hypophyseal axis.

6. Vascular organ: segmentally organized aquatic (cisternal) arteries and veins; intraparenchymal arterioles, capillaries, and venules.

7. Still incompletely discovered cerebrospinal fluid production, circulation, and resorption, and circumventricular organs.

8. Phylogenetically and ontogenetically regulated and selectively active fluidal and cellular immune system.

9. Protection organ of meninges (dura, arachnoidea, pia) with unique architecture of cisternal compartments.

10. Biophysical and triochemical compartmental activities.

11. Neurogenetics.

12. Neurostem cells.

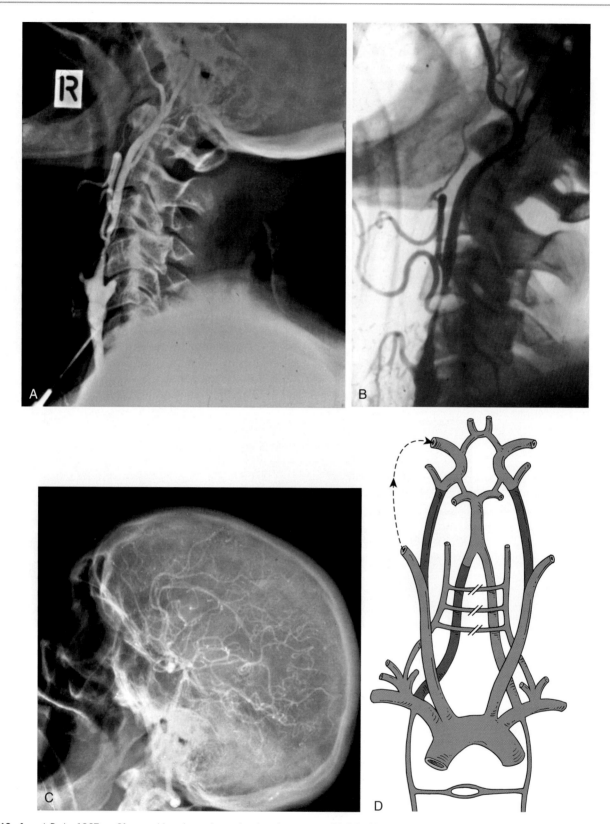

Figure 12. A and **B,** In 1967, a 61-year-old male engineer developed syncope with left-sided hemisyndrome upon turning his head. The four-vessel angiography showed occlusion of bilateral carotid and right vertebral artery. **C,** The blood supply of his entire left brain was secured by left vertebral artery. **D,** Diagram showing the triple occlusion of the brain arteries.

(Continued)

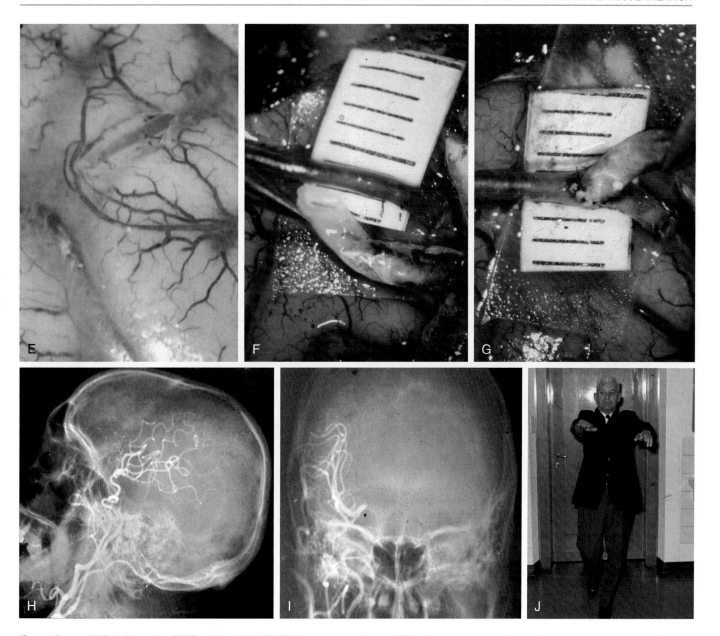

Figure 12—cont'd E, In November 1967, a right-sided STA-TA bypass was performed. This photograph shows the explored right anterior temporal region. **F,** Microsurgically dissected right anterior temporal artery. **G,** End-to-side anastomosis between the right STA and anterior temporal artery. **H, I,** Postoperative right-sided common carotid angiogram verifies well-developed collateral to the right MCA through the bypass. **J,** Excellent postoperative course. The patient no longer had any problems turning his head to the right and left sides.

The brain is generally known as an electrical and electromagnetic organ but is less appreciated in its essential instant and periodic biochemical functions which oscillate with synchronic-isodynamic and heterochronical-heterodynamic functions. The brain is capable of single or multiple, partial or unified, subtotal or even global activities, which require high energy consumption for the integrity of membrane potentials, ionic transport, biosynthesis, and transport of neurotransmitters and cellular elements.

Since storage of substrates for energy metabolism in the brain is minimal, the brain is highly dependent on a continuous supply of oxygen and glucose from the blood for its functional and structural integrity (Jones and Carlson). Although the brain is only 1/20 of the body weight, it receives 1/5 of cardiac output. The blood flows where it is needed, provided by open channel system of the vessels.

In 1561 Fallopius reported for the first time the arterial circle at the base of the brain. In 1632 Cascesirio provided the first illustration of the circle. In 1660 Willis and Lower demonstrated the efficiency and function of the arterial circle at the base of the brain, to maintain the cerebral circulation even when three of the four arteries supplying the brain are blocked or have been ligated. For their physiologic study on cadavers, they injected dye into one internal carotid artery and ligated the contralateral internal carotid artery (Figure 15).

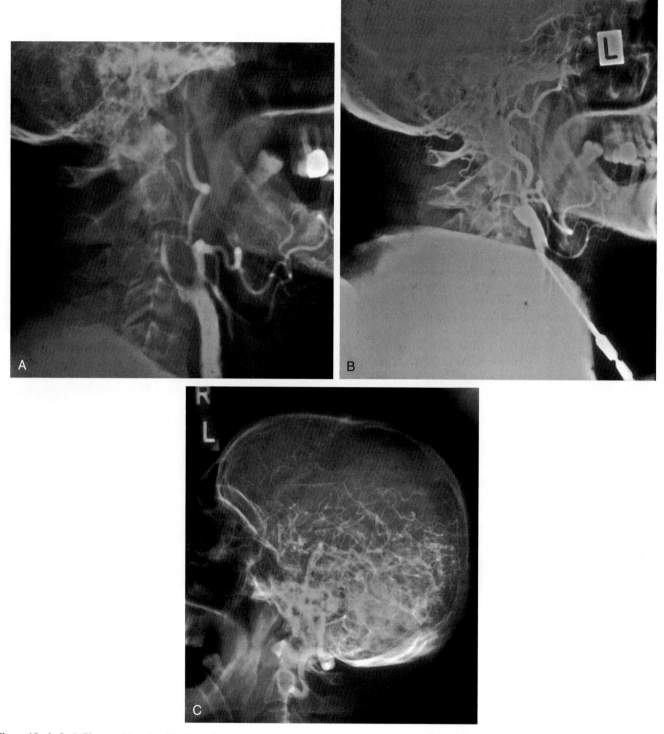

Figure 13. A, B, A 61-year-old male with alternating hemisyndrome showed bilateral occlusion of the carotid and right vertebral artery on a four-vessel angiography study. **C,** The left vertebral angiogram supplies the entire brain. In 1970, Dr. Imhof performed bilateral STA-TA bypass in two sessions within 3 months, resulting in an excellent postoperative course. The postoperative angiogram shows excellent quality of the STA-TA bypass.

(Continued)

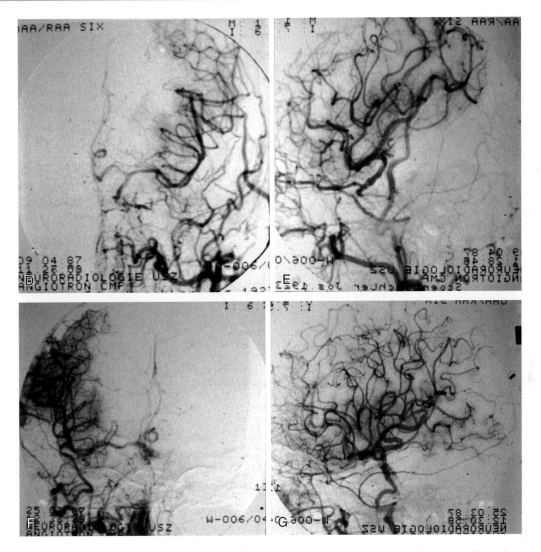

Figure 13—cont'd D, E, Postoperative left-sided common carotid arteriogram. **F, G,** Postoperative right-sided common carotid arteriogram.

Alpers and Berry (1959) studied the circle in 350 cadavers brains and in 53.3% found it to be well developed.[106] In 1794, Frederick Ruysch demonstrated with his injection-maceration technique the subarachnoidal anastomosis between major cerebral arteries. The concept of Cohnheim (1872) that brain arteries are "end arteries" was opposed by anatomists (Heubner 1872, Duret 1876, Fay 1925, R.A. Pfeifer 1935, van der Eecken-Adams 1953). Cerebral angiographic studies, culminating with endovascular superselective angiography technology, confirmed the cascade of craniospinal and spinal cord-brain arterial and venous collaterals.[97] We recognize that the leptomeningeal (pial) arteries have the potential for profuse/abundant collaterals. However, the quantity and quality of these collaterals demonstrate remarkable individual variations, and their functionality is limited with time. The complex hemodynamics of the CNS require the development of more advanced technology to measure and evaluate flow sequences. Kety[113] pioneered the measuring of cerebral blood flow in laboratory animals using inert gas. Lassen et al. (1960) introduced

radioactive Xenon and Krypton to measure the regional cerebral blood flow, which attracted great attention worldwide. The introduction of Xenon/CT, transcranial Doppler flowmetry, SPECT, PET, functional MRI, perfusion and diffusion MRI, quantitative extracranial and intracranial blood flow measurements, and ICG offer great advances in the evaluation of our patients. Immense research in animal laboratories and intense working with patients is making progress, measuring the brain blood flow, brain metabolism, and related parameters, such as the cerebral blood volume (CBV), arterial oxygen content (CaO_2), oxygen extraction factor (OEF), glucose extraction factor (GEF), cerebral metabolic rate ($CMRO_2$), and cerebral vasoreactivity (reserve, resistoma) (CVR) (Figure 16).

There are excellent, informative publications providing abundant data, which are essential for further research endeavors and are beneficial and practical for clinical use.[121–124] Proton emission tomography measurements[111] are summarized in Table 2, p. 534,[93] showing the results of regional measurements in 18 superficial, deep gray and white matter

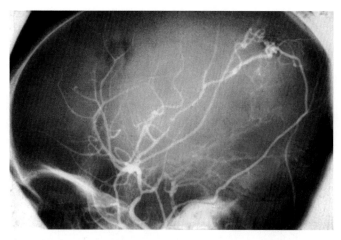

Figure 14. A unique arteriogram was sent to me from Nairobi, Kenya, by a surgeon who was trained by Professor Senning in Zurich. The young male patient with stenosis of the ICA showed the development of a spontaneous EC-IC arterial bypass.

Table 12. RESULT OF EC-IC BYPASS OPERATION IN 190 PATIENTS BETWEEN 1967–1990 (UNIVERSITY HOSPITAL, NEUROSURGICAL DEPARTMENT, ZURICH)

195 anastomoses in 190 patients:	
Mortality	2.1%
Morbidity (serious)	2.1%
Patency of EIAB ($n = 195$)	90%
Follow-up (mean 8.5 years) completed stroke:	
Overall	13.3%
Ipsilateral to EIAB	6.7%

Table 13. CEREBRAL REVASCULARIZATION (EC-IC BYPASS)

1939 – W.S. German, N. Taffel (in animal)	(in human)	Encephalomyo-synangiose
1942 – F.E. Kredel		
1944 – C. Henschen		
1963 – E. Woringer, J. Kunlin		Saphenous vein to ICA
1963 – J.H. Jacobson, R.M.P. Donaghy		Repair of MCA
1965 – J.L. Pool, D.G. Potts		Prosthetic graft (STA-PA)
1965 – W.M. Lougheed, G. Khodadad		Repair of MCA, ICA
1967 – M.G. Yaşargil, R.M.P. Donaghy		EC-IC anastomosis (STA-MCA) in cases of occlusive arterial diseases
1968 – M.G. Yaşargil		EC-IC for giant aneurysm
1972 – M.G. Yaşargil		EC-IC in a male child with Moyamoya disease
1976 – D.H. Reichmann		
1976 – Y. Yonekawa, M.G. Yaşargil		
1977 – H. Kikuchi, J. Karasawa		
1977 – S.J. Peerless		
1978 – T. Sundt		Series of EC-IC bypass
1978 – J.L. Ausman		
1980 – R.F. Spetzler		
1983 – N. Chater		
1985 – H.J. Barnett (cooperative study)		
1989 – K. Kinugasa, et al.		Contralateral ECA-ipsilateral MCA
1989 – C.A. East, et al.		Saphenous vein—MCA
1996 – C.F. Tulleken, et al.		Excimer laser

cerebral regions. In contrast to the observation of static CBF and PET studies, dynamic interactions between brain regions have been revealed using resting-state functional magnetic resonance imaging (fMRI).[108,109,119,130] The data show that static CBF was significantly higher in PCG (posterior cingulated gyrus), thalamus, insula, STG (superior temporal gyrus), and MPFC (medial prefrontal cortex) than the global brain blood flow average, which is consistent with previous PET observations.[74,107–130]

In their 1985 publication, Lassen et al.[115] discuss their experiences as follows:

> The normal brain has a high and rather stable global metabolic rate of oxygen in sleep, in resting, in wakefulness, and while performing motor and/or sensory work. Cerebral blood flow, a main determinant of the oxygen supply, also is relatively high, approximately 50 ml/100 g/min, and is stable with increases in pain and anxiety of the same magnitude as indicated. However, this picture of a fairly constant level of energy production and of energy delivery to the brain is somewhat misleading. Because, at a *regional* level, the physiologic variations in brain activity produce corresponding changes in flood flow and metabolism; more work results in a higher level of oxidative metabolism and a higher blood flow. As an example, during voluntary movements of the hand, both CBF and cerebral oxygen uptake increase within

Table 14. INITIAL MICROSURGICAL SYMPOSIUM AND HANDS-ON COURSES

Oct. 6–7, 1966	Microvascular Symposium, Burlington
April 13–15, 1967	Microneurosurgical Symposium, Los Angeles
Nov. 14–20, 1968	Microneurosurgical Symposium, Zurich
1968–2010	Permanent Microsurgical Training Laboratory
1969–1973	Microsurgical Courses in New York (L. Malis) (Annual)
1971–1977	Microsurgical Courses in Cincinnati (J. Tew) (Annual)
1985–1990	Microsurgical Courses in San Francisco, Chicago, New York (P. Young)
1995	Microsurgical Courses in St. Louis (P. Young) (Annual)
1970	Microsurgical Courses in Tokyo (Shigasaki, Ischii)
1970	Microsurgical Courses in Kyoto (Handa, Kikuchi)
1970	Microsurgical Courses in Brasilia (Mello)

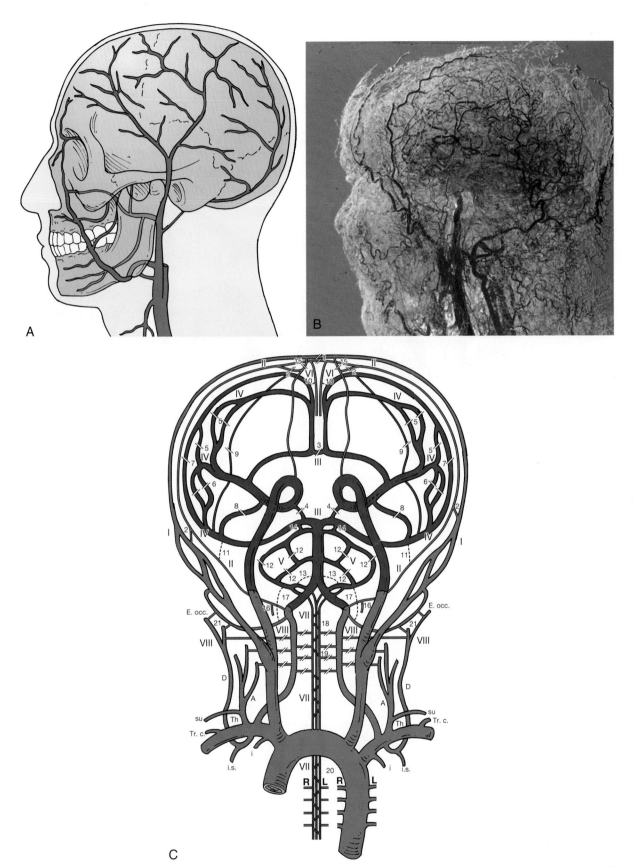

Figure 15. A, Diagram of the left-sided external carotid artery and its branches. **B,** Injected arteries of head and brain, performed by Mr. Lang, Institute of Anatomy, University of Zurich, Switzerland. **C,** Extracranial and intracranial cascades of arterial circles and the known collaterals in 1970. In the meantime, the interventional neuroradiologists discovered even more distinct collaterals. The schematic drawing was based on one made by scientific artist, Mr. P. Roth, Neurosurgical Department, University Hospital, Zurich, Switzerland. Diagram to show the possible collaterals between the intracranial and extracranial arteries and their connection to the spinal medullary arteries – especially to the aorta. A, ascending cervical artery; D, deep cervical artery; E. occ., external occipital artery; I, internal thoracic artery; i.s., supreme intercostals artery; Su, supraclavicular artery; Th, thyrocervical truncus; Tr.c., transverse colli artery.

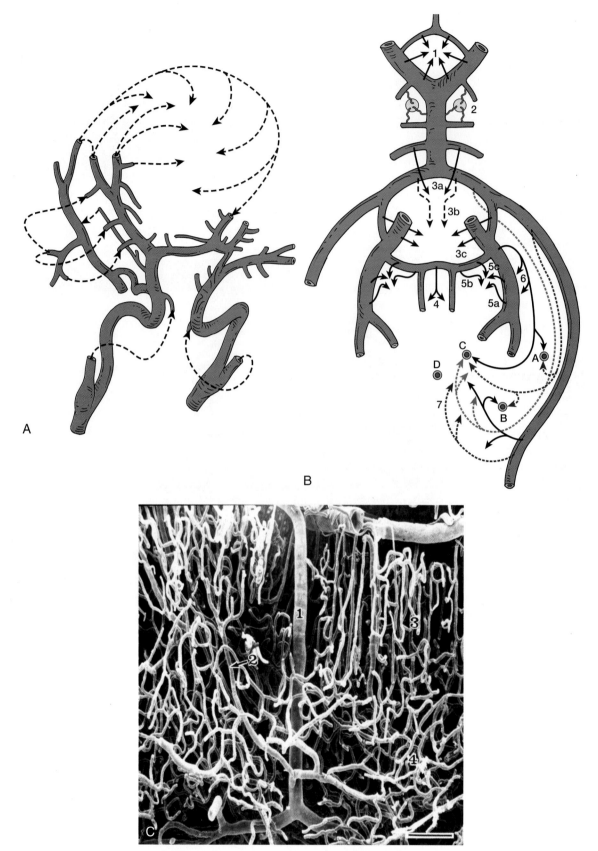

Figure 16. A, This schematic drawing presents right-sided leptomeningeal arteries (MCA, ACA, and PCA) and their possible collaterals. Based on drawing by Mr. P. Roth. **B,** This schematic drawing illustrates the origin and course of the basal perforators, which do not have collaterals. In some cases of AVMs and Moyamoya disease, collaterals may develop. **C,** The network of the cortical capillaries perfectly worked out by Professor H.M. Duvernoy, Besançon, France.

a few seconds by about 30% in the contralateral primary (rolandic) sensory-motor hand area. The technique of measurement causes a damping effect because nonactivated cortical areas are simultaneously recorded. The true amplitude of the effect is therefore two to three times greater. Thus, regional increases of CBF of 50% to 100% may occur locally during normal neuronal activity. Sensory perception increases flow in the corresponding cortical areas. More complex tasks activate many areas simultaneously. Reading tasks activate at least 14 discrete areas—seven in each hemisphere. It is therefore apparent that the observed stability of the overall CBF mainly reflects the small size of the cortical areas intensely activated in the types of brain work studied.

In this context, the question arises with regard to the regulation and safety of hemodynamics and metabolism in the vascular territories of the so-called basal perforating arteries. Phylogenetically and ontogenetically elder and functionally highly vital compartments of the brain such as the medulla oblongata, pons, mesencephalon, diencephalon, lentiform nuclei, and internal third of the white matter receive their blood supply from basal perforating arteries, which have no collaterals. In some cases of AVMs and Moyamoya disease, the ventriculofugal segment of basal perforators developed collaterals to transcortical perforators.

Paying attention to the essential "pacemaker" functions of the astrocytes, which are located between the neurons and the walls of arterioles, there may be distinct functional differences in the various areas of the brain, partially between astrocytes of phylogenetic and ontogenetic elder brain areas and astrocytes of the newer brain areas. The astrocytes are oversimplified in their definition, naming all of them only according to histologic criteria as *astrocytes*. The regulatory function of astrocytes and pericytes in hemodynamics and metabolism of the CNS require our particular investigation (Figure 17).

In this context, the research trend of Yemişci et al.,[126] that ischemia induces sustained contraction of pericytes on microvessels in the intact mouse brain, is of great promise. Pericyte contractions cause capillary constriction and obstruct erythrocyte flow. Suppression of oxidative-nitrative stress relieves pericyte contraction. The authors could show that the microvessel wall is the major source of oxygen and nitrogen radicals that cause ischemia and reperfusion-induced microvascular dysfunction.[128]

The heterogenous, heteromorphic, and heterofunctional brain with its numerous phylogenetic and ontogenetic compartments is not completely understood. The refinement of measuring technology to adequately and appropriately evaluate the global and regional hemodynamics, and the metabolism of the brain, and to trace deficiencies and calculate needs is a priority.

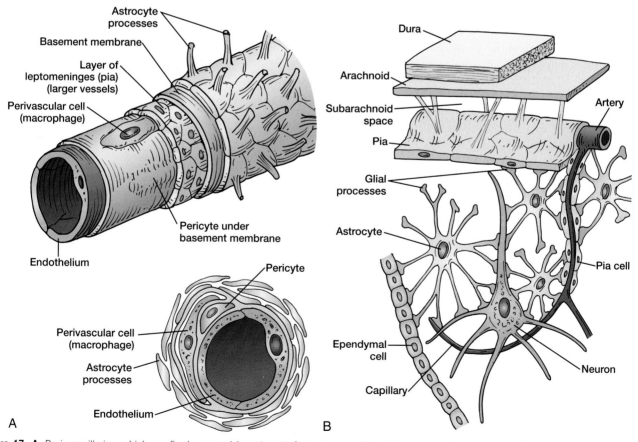

Figure 17. A, Brain capillaries, which are firmly covered by astrocyte foot processes (blue), the basement membrane (red), layer of pia (purple; larger vessels), and pericytes (orange). **B,** Illustration presenting the essential position and function of an astrocyte between the meninges, artery, neuron, and ependyma.

CONCLUSION

Definite or general rules to guide our evaluation process and point with certainty to correct indications for a particular treatment currently elude us, despite the availability of stable Xenon/CO_2, MRI, SPECT, and PET.

In 1966, microvascular surgery on brain arteries of dogs proved to be a breakthrough, confirming the capability to perform reconstructive microneurovascular surgery and other procedures on patients. The EC-IC bypass is an excellent surgical option, but only for those select cases with occlusive brain artery diseases, having verified there are insufficient collaterals. Reconstructive microvascular surgery certainly contributed positively to the treatment of intracranial saccular and fusiform aneurysms, AVMs,[129,131–141] cavernomas, and extrinsic and intrinsic tumors.[18] In the treatment of large, giant, and fusiform aneurysms[90,142,143]; AVMs; cavernous fistulas[43]; vasospasm[42]; invasive neck and skull base tumors; tumors invading and encasing brain arteries, veins,[23,144–151] and venous sinuses[17,38,92,136,142,145–152]; and reconstructive microvascular surgery such as the in situ repair, intracranial bypass, or extracranial bypass (which are already effectively practiced) will be used on a broader scale in the future.

Basic sciences, scientific technology, and the medical and surgical industry undoubtedly provide sophisticated equipment and materials to promote neurosurgical treatments. I am more than satisfied and encouraged to learn of these advances described in the publications of the young colleagues included in this monograph. The coming generations of neurosurgeons will be well equipped to cope with the variations in hemodynamics in the field of neuroscience.

Intense laboratory exercise and practice will stimulate the creation of fresh avenues into research and clinical treatments, and will guide young generations of colleagues toward innovative and effective concepts in vascular neurosurgery.

M. Gazi Yaşargil, MD

REFERENCES

1. Donaghy RMP, Wallman LJ, Flanagan MJ, et al: Sagittal sinus repair. Technical note, *J Neurosurg* 38:244–248, 1973.
2. Fields WS, Lemak NA: *A history of stroke: Its recognition and treatment*, New York, Oxford, 1989, Oxford University.
3. Fein JM, Flamm ES: *Cerebrovascular surgery*. 4 volumes, New York, 1985, Springer.
4. Garrison FH: *History of neurology*. Revised and enlarged by McHenry LC Jr, Springfield, IL, 1969, Charles C Thomas.
5. Rob CG: Principles of vascular surgery. In Fein JM, Flamm ES, eds: *Cerebrovascular surgery*, vol. 2, New York, 1985, Springer, pp 383–397.
6. Thompson JE: Carotid Endarterectomy, *Br J Surg* 70:371–376, 1983.
7. Thompson JE: The evolution of surgery for the treatment and prevention of stroke, *Stroke* 27:1427–1434, 1996.
8. Yaşargil MG: History of the microneurosurgery. In Spetzler RF, Carter LP, Selman WR, Martin NA, eds: *Cerebral revascularization for stroke*, New York, 1985, Thieme-Stratton.
8a. De Bakey ME, Crawford ES, Morris GC Jr, et al: Surgical considerations of occlusive disease of the innominate, carotid, subclavian and vertebral arteries, *Ann Surg* 154:698, 1961.
9. Khodadad G: Short-and long-term results of microvascular anastomosis in the vertebrobasilar system, a critical analysis, *Neurol Res* 3:33–65, 1981.
10. Khodadad G, Lougheed WM: Repair and replacement of small arteries, microsuture technique, *J Neurosurg* 21:61–69, 1964.
11. Khodadad G, Lougheed WM: Repair of small arteries with contact cement and Teflon graft, *J Neurosurg* 21:552–560, 1964.
12. Sundt TM Jr, Nofzinger JD, Murphey F: Arteriotomy patching by means of intraluminal pressure sealing venous autografts, *J Neurosurg* 23:452–454, 1965.
13. Woringer E, Kunlin J: Anastomose entre la carotid primitive et la carotid intracrânienne ou de la sylvienne par greffon selon la technique de la suture suspendue, *Neurochirurgie (Stuttg)* 9:181–188, 1963.
14. Jacobson JH II, Wallman LJ, Schumacher GH, et al: Microsurgery as an aid to middle cerebral artery endarterectomy, *J Neurosurg* 19:108–115, 1962.
15. Lougheed WM, Gunton RW, Barnett HJM: Embolectomy of internal carotid, middle and anterior cerebral arteries, Report of a case, *J Neurosurg* 22:607–609, 1965.
16. Donaghy RMP, Yaşargil MG: *Microvascular surgery*, St Louis, 1967, G. Thieme.
17. Donaghy RMP: Patch and by-pass in microangeoinal surgery. In Donaghy RMP, Yaşargil MG, eds: *Microvascular surgery*, St Louis, 1967, G. Thieme, pp 75–86.
18. Yaşargil MG: *Microsurgery applied to neurosurgery*, Stuttgart, New York, 1969, Thieme.
19. Brotchi J, Patay Z, Baleriaux D: Surgery of the superior sagittal sinus and neighbouring veins. In Hakuba A, ed: *Surgery of the Intracranial Venous System*. Proceedings of the First International Workshop on Surgery of the Intracranial Venous System, Osaka, September 1994, Tokyo, 1996, Springer-Verlag, pp 207–219.
20. Donaghy RMP: The history of microsurgery in neurosurgery, *Clin Neurosurg* 58:829–831, 1983.
21. Hakuba A: Reconstruction of dural sinus involved in meningiomas. In Al-Mefty O, ed: *Meningiomas*, New York, 1991, Raven Press, pp 371–382.
22. Hakuba A, ed: *Surgery of the Intracranial Venous System*. Proceedings of the First International Workshop on Surgery of the Intracranial Venous System, Osaka, September 1994, Tokyo, 1996, Springer-Verlag, p 619.
23. Nagashima H, Kobayashi S, Takemae T, et al: Total resection of torcular herophili hemangiopericytoma with radial artery graft case report, *Neurosurgery* 36:1024–1027, 1995.
24. Sindou M, Alaywan F, Hallacq P: Main dural sinuses surgery, *Neurochirurgie (Suppl)*:45–87, 1996 [French].
25. Sindou M, Alvernia J: Results of attempted radical tumor removal and venous repair in 100 consecutive meningiomas involving the major dural sinuses, *J Neurosurg* 105:514–1225, 2006.
26. Sindou M, Auque J, Jouanneau E: Neurosurgery and the intracranial venous system, *Acta Neurochir (Wien)* 94(Suppl):1686–1692, 2005.
27. Sindou M, Grunewald P, Guegan Y, et al: Cerebral revascularization with extra-intracranial anastomoses for vascular lesions of traumatic, malformative, and tumorous origin. (Cooperative Study: 20 cases), *Acta Neurochir (Suppl 28)*:282–286, 1979.
28. Sindou M, Hallacq P: Venous reconstruction in surgery of meningiomas invading the sagittal and transverse sinuses, *Skull Base Surgery* 8:57–64, 1998.
29. Sindou M, Mercier P, Bokor J, et al: Bilateral thrombosis of the transverse sinuses: Microsurgical revascularization with venous bypass, *Surg Neurol* 13:215–220, 1980.
30. Steiger HJ, Reuben HJ, Huber P, et al: Radical resection of superior sagittal sinus meningioma with venous interposition graft and reimplantation of the rolandic veins. Case report, *Acta Neurochir (Wein)* 100:108–111, 1989.
31. Krayenbühl H: The Moyamoya syndrome and the neurosurgeon, *Surg Neurol* 4:353–360, 1975.
32. Matsushima Y, Inaba Y: Moyamoya disease in children and its surgical treatment, *Child's Brain* 2:155–170, 1984.

33. Yonekawa Y, Handa H, Moritake K, et al: Revascularization in children with Moyamoya disease: Low-density areas and regional cerebral blood flow after operation. In Handa H, Kikuchi H, Yonekawa Y, eds: *Microsurgical anastomoses for cerebral ischemia*, New York, 1985, Igaku-Shoin Ltd, pp 272–274.

34. Yonekawa Y, Okuno T, Handa H: 'Moyamoya' disease: Clinical review and surgical treatment. In Fein JM, Flamm ES, eds: *Cerebrovascular surgery,* New York, 1985, Springer-Verlag, pp 557–580.

35. Barnett HJM, Peerless SJ, McCormick CW: In answer to the question: 'As compared to what?' A progress report on the EC/IC bypass study, *Stroke* 11:137–140, 1980.

36. Barnett HJM, the EC/IC bypass study group: Failure of extracranial intracranial arterial bypass to reduce the risk of ischemic stroke. Results of an international randomized trial, *N Engl J Med* 313:1191–1200, 1985.

37. Ausman JI, Diaz FG: Critique of the extracranial-intracranial bypass study, *Surg Neurol* 26:218–221, 1986.

38. Ausman JI, Diaz FG, DeLosReyes RA, et al: Anastomosis of occipital artery to anterior inferior cerebellar artery for vertebrobasilar junction stenosis, *Surg Neurol* 16:999–1102, 1981.

39. Ausman JI, Diaz FG, DeLosReyes RA, et al: Superficial temporal to superior cerebellar artery anastomosis for basilar artery stenosis, *Neurosurgery* 9:56–60, 1981.

40. Ausman JI, Nicoloff D, Chou S: Posterior fossa revascularization: Anastomosis of vertebral artery to posterior inferior cerebellar artery with interposed radial artery graft, *Surg Neurol* 9:281–285, 1978.

41. Bannister CM, Hillier VF: Results of extracranial-intracranial bypass performed in a single British neurosurgical unit. In Gagliardi R, Benvenuti L, eds: *Controversies in EIAB for cerebral ischemia.* 8th International Symposium on Microsurgical Anastomoses for Cerebral Ischemia, Florence, Italy. Bologna, 1987, Monduzzi Editore, pp 29–38.

42. Batjer H, Samson D: Use of extracranial-intracranial bypass in the management of symptomatic vasospasm, *Neurosurgery* 19:235–243, 1986.

43. Barrow DL, Spector RH, Braun IF, et al: Classification and treatment of spontaneous carotid cavernous fistulas, *J Neurosurg* 56:248–256, 1985.

44. Benvenuti L, Gagliardi R: Acute cerebral revascularization: long-term results. In Gagliardi R, Benvenuti L, eds: *Controversies in EIAB for cerebral ischemia.* 8th International Symposium on Microsurgical Anastomoses for Cerebral Ischemia, Florence, Italy. Bologna, 1987, Monduzzi Editore, pp 475–480.

45. Candon E, Marty-Ane C, Pieuchot P, et al: Cervical-to-petrous internal carotid artery saphenous vein in situ bypass for the treatment of a high cervical dissecting aneurysm: technical case report, *Neurosurgery* 39:863–866, 1996.

46. Chater N: Patient selection and results of extra to intracranial anastomosis in selected cases of cerebrovascular disease, *Clin Neurosurg* 23:287–309, 1976.

47. Chater N, Popp J: Microsurgical vascular bypass for occlusive cerebrovascular disease. Review of 100 cases, *Surg Neurol* 6:115–118, 1976.

48. Crowell RM, Olsson Y: Effect of extra-intracranial vascular bypass graft on experimental acute stroke in dogs, *J Neurosurg* 38:26–31, 1973.

49. Diaz FG, Umansky F, Metha B, et al: Cerebral revascularization to a main limb of the middle cerebral artery in the Sylvian fissure. An alternative approach to conventional anastomosis, *J Neurosurg* 59:384–388, 1985.

50. Ferguson GG, Peerless SJ: Extracranial-intracranial arterial bypass in the treatment of dementia and multiple extracranial arterial occlusion, *Stroke* 7:13, 1976.

51. Fox AJ, Taylor DW, Peerless SJ: Preexisting collateral pathways: a factor in determining success in EC-IC bypass surgery? In Handa H, Kikuchi H, Yonekawa H, eds: *Microsurgical anastomoses for cerebral ischemia*, New York, 1985, Igaku-Shon Ltd, pp 153–157.

52. Friedman JA, Piepras DG: Current neurosurgical indications for saphenous vein graft bypass, *Neurosurg Focus* 14:e1, 2003.

53. Gagliardi R, Benvenutti L, Onesti S: Seven years experience with extracranial-intracranial arterial bypass for cerebral ischemia. In Spetzler RF, Carter LP, Selman WR, Martin NA, eds: *Cerebral revascularization for stroke,* New York, 1985, Thieme-Stratton, pp 41–44.

54. Goldring S, Zervas N, Langfitt T: The Extracranial-Intracranial Bypass Study. A report of the committee appointed by the American Association of Neurological Surgeons to examine the study, *N Engl J Med* 316:817–820, 1987.

55. Gratzl O, Schmiedek P: STA-MCA bypass: Results 10 years postoperatively, *Neurol Res* 5:11–18, 1983.

56. Gratzl O, Schmiedek P, et al: Clinical experience with extra-intracranial arterial anastomosis in 65 cases, *J Neurosurg* 44:313–324, 1976.

57. Gratzl O, Schmiedek P, Spetzler R: Extracranial-intracranial arterial bypass for cerebral ischemia. In Krayenbühl H, Maspes PE, Sweet WH, eds: *Progress in neurological surgical,* Basel, 1978, Karger S, pp 1–29.

58. Gross RE: Complete division for patent ductus arteriosus, *J Thoracic Surg* 16:314, 1947.

59. Haase J: Extracranial-intracranial bypass surgery in cerebrovascular diseases, *Neurosciences* 6(1):7–15, 2001.

60. Hadeishi H, Yasui N, Okamoto Y: Extracranial-intracranial high-flow bypass using the radial artery between the vertebral and middle cerebral arteries. Technical note, *J Neurosurg* 85:976–979, 1996.

61. Hayden MG, Lee M, Guzman R, et al: The evolution of cerebral revascularization surgery, *Neurosurg Focus* 26(5):E17, 2009.

62. Heros RC, Sekhar LN: Diagnostic and therapeutic alternatives in patients with symptomatic 'carotid occlusion' referred for extracranial-intracranial bypass surgery, *J Neurosurg* 54:790–796, 1981.

63. Imhof HG, Keller HM, Yaşargil MG: Clinical experience with the anastomoses between the superficial temporal artery and the middle cerebral artery. A survey of 15 years, *Acta Neurochir (Wien)* 72:112–113, 1984.

64. Kletter G: Indications for extra-intracranial bypass procedure: Clinical aspects. In Kletter G, ed: *The extra-intracranial bypass operation for prevention and treatment of stroke*, New York, 1979, Springer-Verlag, Wien, pp 112–129.

65. Koos WT, Kletter G, Schuster H: Microsurgical extra-intracranial arterial bypass (EIAB) in patients with completed stroke. In Meyer JS, Lechner H, Reivich M, eds: *Cerebral vascular disease,* International congress series 449, Amsterdam, 1979, Excerpta Medica, pp 241–244.

66. Laurent JP, Lawner PM, O'Connor M: Reversal of intracerebral steal by STA-MCA anastomosis, *J Neurosurg* 57:629–632, 1982.

67. Lemole GM, Henn J, Javedan S, et al: Cerebral revascularization performed using posterior inferior cerebellar artery-posterior inferior cerebellar artery bypass. Report of four cases and literature review, *J Neurosurg* 97:219–223, 2002.

68. Mendelowitsch A, Taussky P, Rem JA, et al: Clinical outcome of standard extracranial-intracranial bypass surgery in patients with symptomatic atherosclerotic occlusion of the internal carotid artery, *Acta Neurochir (Wien)* 146(2):95–101, 2004.

69. Morgan MK, Sekhon LH: Extracranial-intracranial saphenous vein bypass for carotid or vertebral artery dissections: a report of six cases, *J Neurosurg* 80:237–246, 1994.

70. Peerless SJ: Indications for the extracranial-intracranial arterial bypass in light of the EC-IC bypass study, *Clin Neurosurg* 33:307–326, 1986.

71. Peerless SJ: Techniques of cerebral revascularization, *Clin Neurosurg* 23:258–269, 1976.

72. Peerless SJ, Chater NL, Ferguson GF: Multiple-vessel occlusions in cerebrovascular disease. A further follow-up of the effects of microvascular by-pass on the quality of life and the incidence of stroke. In Schmiedek P, ed: *Microsurgery for stroke*, New York, 1977, Springer-Verlag, pp 251–259.

73. Peerless SJ, Ferguson GG, Drake CG: Extracranial-intracranial (EC/IC) bypass in the treatment of giant intracranial aneurysms, *Neurosurg Rev* 5:77–81, 1982.

74. Piepgras A, Schmiedek P, Leinsinger G, et al: A simple test to assess cerebrovascular reserve capacity using transcranial Doppler sonography and acetazolamide, *Stroke* 21(9):1306–1311, 1990.

75. Reichman OH: Complications of cerebral revascularization, *Clin Neurosurg* 23:318–335, 1976.

76. Reichman OH: Estimation of flow through STA by-pass graft. In Fein JM, Reichman OH, eds: *Microvascular anastomosis for cerebral ischemia*, New York, 1978, Springer, pp 220–240.

77. Reichman OH: Extracranial to intracranial arterial anastomosis. In Youmans JR, ed: *Neurological surgery*, vol. 3, Philadelphia, 1982, WB Saunders, pp 1584–1618.

78. Reichman OH: Neurosurgical microsurgical anastomosis for cerebral ischemia: Five years experience. In Sheinberg B, ed: *Cerebrovascular diseases*, New York, 1976, Raven Press, pp 311–337.

79. Reichman OH: Selection of patients and clinical results following STA-cortical MCA anastomosis. In Austin GM, ed: *Microneurosurgical anastomosis for cerebral ischemia*, Springfield, 1976, Thomas, pp 275–280.

80. Rivet DJ, Wanebo JE, Roberts GA, et al: Use of a side branch in a saphenous vein interposition graft for high-flow Extracranial-intracranial bypass procedures. Technical note, *J Neurosurg* 103:186–187, 2005.

81. Samson DS, Boone S: Extracranial-intracranial (EC-IC) arterial bypass: Past performance and current concepts, *Neurosurgery* 3:79–86, 1978.

82. Samson DS, Gewertz BL, Beyer CW, et al: Saphenous vein interposition grafts in the microsurgical treatment of cerebral ischemia, *Arch Surg* 116:1578–1582, 1981.

83. Schmiedek P, Gratzl O, Spetzler R, et al: Selection of patients for extra-intracranial by-pass surgery based on rCBF measurements, *J Neurosurg* 44:303–312, 1976.

84. Schmiedek P, Olteanu-Nerbe V, Gratzl O, et al: Extra-intracranial arterial bypass surgery for cerebral ischemia in patients with normal cerebral angiograms. In Peerless SJ, McCormick CW, eds: *Microsurgery for cerebral ischemia*, New York, 1980, Springer-Verlag, pp 268–274.

85. Spetzler RF: Extracranial-intracranial arterial anastomosis for cerebrovascular disease, *Surg Neurol* 11:157–161, 1979.

86. Spetzler RF, Chater N: Microvascular bypass surgery. Part 2: Physiological studies, *J Neurosurg* 45:508–513, 1976.

87. Spetzler RF, Chater N: Occipital artery-middle cerebral artery anastomosis for cerebral artery occlusive disease, *Surg Neurol* 2:235–238, 1974.

88. Sundt TM Jr, Piepgras DG: Occipital to posterior inferior cerebellar artery bypass surgery, *J Neurosurg* 48:916–928, 1978.

89. Sundt TM Jr, Whisnant JP, Fode NC, et al: Results, complications and follow-up of 415 bypass operations for occlusive disease of the carotid system, *Mayo Clin Proc* 60:230–260, 1985.

90. Suzuki S, Takahashi T, Ohkuma H, et al: Management of giant serpentine aneurysms of the middle cerebral artery. Review of the literature and report of a case successfully treated by STA-MCA anastomosis only, *Acta Neurochir (Wien)* 117:23–39, 1992.

91. Tew JM Jr, Comment on: Story JL, et al: Cerebral revascularization: Proximal external carotid to distal middle cerebral artery bypass with a synthetic tube graft, *Neurosurgery* 3:64–65, 1978.

92. Tew JM Jr: Techniques of supratentorial cerebral revascularization, *Clin Neurosurg* 26:330–345, 1979.

93. The EC/IC Bypass Study Group: The international cooperative study of extracranial/intracranial arterial anastomosis (EC/IC bypass study): Methodology and entry characteristics, *Stroke* 16:397–406, 1985.

94. Umansky F, Diaz FG, Dujovny M, et al: Superficial temporal artery to middle cerebral artery anastomoses in the sylvian fissure. Case report, *Vasc Surg* 18:244–249, 1984.

95. Weinstein PR, Comment on: Samson DS, Neuwelt EA, Beyer CW, Ditmore QM: Failure of extracranial-intracranial arterial bypass in acute middle cerebral artery occlusion: Case report, *Neurosurgery* 6:187–188, 1980.

96. Weinstein PR, Charter NL, Yaşargil MG: Microsurgical treatment of intracranial cerebrovascular occlusive disease. In Weinstein PR, Charter NL, Yaşargil MG, eds: *Practice of neurosurgery*, Hagerstown, Maryland, 1978, Harper & Row, pp 1–33.

97. Weinstein PR, Rodriguez Y, Bacna R, et al: Results of extracranial-intracranial arterial bypass for intracranial internal carotid artery stenosis: Review of 105 cases, *Neurosurgery* 15:787–794, 1984.

98. Whisnant JP, Sundt TM, Fode NC: Long-term mortality and stroke morbidity after superficial temporal artery-middle cerebral artery bypass operation, *Mayo Clin Proc* 60:241–246, 1985.

99. Yaşargil MG, Chater NL: Surgical results of Professor Yaşargil's series. In Austin GM, ed: *Microsurgical anastomoses for cerebral ischemia*, Springfield, IL, 1976, Thomas, pp 359–367.

100. Yaşargil MG, Krayenbühl H, Jacobson JH: Microneurosurgical arterial reconstruction, *Surgery* 67(1):221–233, 1970.

101. Yaşargil MG, Yonekawa Y: Results of microsurgical extra-intracranial arterial bypass in the treatment of cerebral ischemia, *Neurosurgery* 1:22–24, 1977.

102. Yonekawa Y, Handa H, Moritake K, et al: Single-stage bilateral STA-MCA bypass. In Spetzler RF, Carter LP, Selman WR, Martin NA, eds: *Cerebral revascularization for stroke*, New York, 1985, Thieme-Stratton, pp 348–352.

103. Yonekawa Y, Yaşargil MG: Extra-intracranial arterial anastomosis. Clinical and technical aspects. Results. In Krayenbühl H, ed: *Advances and technical standards in neurosurgery*, New York, 1976, Springer-Verlag, Wien, pp 47–48.

104. Zumstein B, Yaşargil MG, Keller HM: *Prevention of cerebral ischemia by extra-intracranial micro-anastomosis*, New York, Springer, pp 334–342. Fourth International Symposium.

105. Zumstein B, Yonekawa Y, Yaşargil MG: Extra-intracranial arterial anastomosis for cerebral ischemia: Technique and results in 90 cases. In Carlson LA, Paoletti R, Sirtori CR, eds: *International Conference on Atherosclerosis*, New York, 1978, Raven Press, pp 257–263.

106. Alpers BJ, Berry RG, Paddison RM: Anatomical studies of the circle of Willis in normal brain, *Arch Neurol Psychiat (Chic)* 81:409–418, 1959.

107. Biswall BB, Van Kylen J, Hyde JS: Simultaneous assessment of flow and BOLD signals in resting-state functional connectivity maps, *NMR Biomed* 10:165–170, 1997.

108. Biswal BB, Yetkin FZ, Haughton VM, et al: Functional connectivity in the motor cortex of resting human brain using echo-planar MRI, *Magn Reson Med* 34:537–541, 1995.

109. Fox MD, Raichle ME: Spontaneous fluctuations in brain activity observed with functional magnetic resonance imaging, *Nat Rev Neurosci* 8:700–711, 2007.

110. Herscovitch P, Raichle ME: Effect of tissue heterogeneity on the measurement of cerebral blood flow with the equilibrium $C^{15}O_2$ inhalation technique, *J Cereb Blood Flow Metab* 3:407–415, 1983.

111. Herscovitch P, Raichle ME, Kilbourn MR, et al: Positron emission tomographic measurement of cerebral blood flow and permeability—Surface area product of water using [^{15}O]water and [^{11}C] butanol, *J Cereb Blood Flow Metab* 7:527–542, 1987.

112. Kety SS: Regional cerebral blood flow: estimation by means of nonmetabolized diffusible tracers—an overview, *Semin Nucl Med* 15:324–328, 1985.

113. Kety SS: The theory and applications of the exchange of inert gas at the lungs and tissues, *Pharmacol Rev* 3:1–41, 1951.

114. Landau WM, Freygang WH, Rowland LP, et al: The local circulation of the living brain; values in the unanesthetized and anesthetized cat, *Trans Am Neurol Assoc* 96:72–82, 1955.

115. Lassen NA, Astrup J: Cerebrovascular physiology. In Fein JM, Flamm ES, eds: *Cerebrovascular surgery*, New York, 1985, Springer, pp 75–87.

116. Lassen NA, Sveinsdottir E, Kanno I, et al: A fast single photon emission tomograph for regional cerebral blood flow studies in man (Abstr.), *J Comput Assist Tomogr* 2:661, 1978.

117. Mortake K, Handa H, Yonekawa Y, et al: Ultrasonic Doppler assessment of hemodynamics in superficial temporal artery-middle cerebral artery anastomosis, *Surg Neurol* 13:249–257, 1980.

118. Plum F: Extracranial-intracranial arterial bypass and cerebral vascular disease, *N Engl J Med* 313:1221–1223, 1985.

119. Raichle ME, MacLeod AM, Snyder AZ, et al: A default mode of brain function, *Proc Natl Acad Sci U S A* 98:676–682, 2001.

120. Sakurada O, Kennedy C, Jehle J, et al: Measurement of local cerebral blood flow with iodo[^{14}C]antipyrine, *Am J Physiol* 234(1):H59–H66, 1978.
121. Sokoloff L: Local cerebral circulation at rest and during altered cerebral activity induced by anesthesia or visual stimulation. In Kety SS, Elkes J, eds: *The Regional Chemistry, Physiology and Pharmacology of the Nervous System*, Oxford, 1961, Pergamon, pp 107–117.
122. Sokoloff L, Reivich M, Kennedy C, et al: The [^{14}C]deoxyglucose method for the measurement of local cerebral glucose utilization: theory, procedure, and normal values in the conscious and anesthetized albino rat, *J Neurochem* 28:897–916, 1977.
122a. Mazziotta JC, Phelps ME, Plummer D, et al: Quantitation in positron emission computed tomography: 5 physical-anatomical effects, *J Comput Assist Tomog* 5:734–743, 1981.
123. Ter-Pogossian MM, Ficke DC, Hood JT Sr, et al: PETT VI: a positron emission tomography utilizing cesium fluoride scintillation detectors, *J Comput Assist Tomogr* 6:125–133, 1982.
124. Umemura A, Suzuka T, Yamada K: Quantitative measurement of cerebral blood flow by (99m)Tc-HMPAO SPECT in acute ischaemic stroke: usefulness in determining therapeutic options, *J Neurol Neurosurg Psychiatry* 200;69(4):427–428.
125. Yamamoto YL, Little J, Thompson C, et al: Positron emission tomography following EC-IC bypass surgery, *Acta Neurol Scand* 60(Suppl 72):522–523, 1979.
126. Yemisci M, Gursoy-Ozdemir Y, Vural A, et al: Pericyte contraction induced by oxidative-nitrative stress impairs capillary reflow despite successful opening of an occluded cerebral artery, *Nat Med* 15(9):1031–1037, 2009.
127. Yonas H, Wolfson SK Jr, Gur D, et al: Clinical experience with the use of xenon-enhances CT blood flow mapping in cerebral vascular disease, *Stroke* 15:443–450, 1984.
128. Yonekawa Y, Yaşargil MG, Klaiber R: Intra-operative intra-arterial measurement of cerebral ischemia. In Meyer JS, Lechner H, Reivich M, eds: *Cerebral vascular disease*, Stuttgart, 1976, Georg Thieme Verlag, pp 177–180.
129. Zhang YJ, Barrow DL, Day AL: Extracranial-intracranial vein graft bypass for giant intracranial aneurysm surgery for pediatric patients: two technical case reports, *Neurosurgery* 50:663–668, 2002.
130. Zou Q, Wu CW, Stein EA, et al: *Static and dynamic characteristics of cerebral blood flow during the resting state* 48:515–524, 2009.
131. Amin-Hanjani S, Chen PR, Chang SW, et al: Long-term follow-up of giant serpentine MCA aneurysm treated with EC-IC bypass and proximal occlusion, *Acta Neurochir (Wien)* 148(2):227–228, 2006.
132. Bederson JB, Spetzler RF: Anastomosis of the anterior temporal artery to a secondary trunk of the middle cerebral artery for treatment of a giant M1 segment aneurysm. Case Report, *J Neurosurg* 76: 863–866, 1992.
133. Evans JJ, Sekhar LN, Rak R, et al: Bypass grafting and revascularization in the management of posterior circulation aneurysms, *Neurosurgery* 55(5):1036–1049, 2004.
134. Kato Y, Sano H, Imizu S, et al: Surgical strategies for treatment of giant of large intracranial aneurysms: our experience with 139 cases, *Minim Invasive Neurosurg* 46:339–343, 2003.
135. Lawton MT, Hamilton MG, Morcos JJ, et al: Revascularization and aneurysm surgery: current techniques, indications, and outcome, *Neurosurgery* 38:83–92, 1996; discussion 92–94.
136. Liu JK, Couldwell WT: Interpositional carotid artery bypass strategies in the surgical management of aneurysms and tumors of the skull base, *Neursurg Focus* 14(3):e2, 2003.
137. Mohit AA, Sekhar LN, Natarajan SK, et al: High-flow bypass grafts in the management of complex intracranial aneurysms, *Neurosurgery* 60:ONS105–ONS122, ONS122–ONS123, 2007.
138. Morimoto T, Sakaki T, Kakizaki T, et al: Radial artery graft for an extracranial-intracranial bypass in cases of internal carotid aneurysms, *Surg Neurol* 30:293–297, 1988.
139. Quinones-Hinojosa A, Lawton MT: In situ bypass in the management of complex intracranial aneurysms: technique application in 13 patients, *Neurosurgery* 57:140–145, 2005; discussion 140–145.
140. Sanai N, Zador Z, Lawton MT: Bypass surgery for complex brain aneurysms: an assessment of intracranial-intracranial bypass, *Neurosurgery* 65:670–683, 2009; discussion 683.
141. Spetzler RF, Carter LP: Revascularization and aneurysm surgery: current status, *Neurosurgery* 16:111–116, 1985.
142. Anson JA, Lawton MT, Spetzler RF: Characteristics and surgical treatment of dolichoectatic and fusiform aneurysms, *J Neurosurg* 84(2):185–193, 1996.
143. O'Shaughnessy BA, Getch CC, Bendok BR, et al: Progressive growth of a giant dolichoectatic vertebrobasilar artery aneurysm after complete Hunterian occlusion of the posterior circulation: Case report, *Neurosurgery* 55(5):1223, 2004.
144. Di Meco F, Li KW, Casali C, et al: Meningiomas invading the superior sagittal sinus: surgical experience in 108 cases, *Neurosurgery* 55:1263–1274, 2004.
145. Eliason JL, Netterville JL, Guzman RJ, et al: Skull base resection with cervical-to-petrous carotid artery bypass to facilitate repair of distal internal carotid artery lesions, *Cardiovasc Surg* 10(1):31–37, 2002.
146. Feiz-Erfan I, Han PP, Spetzler RF, et al: Salvage of advanced squamous cell carcinomas of the head and neck: internal carotid artery sacrifice and extracranial-intracranial revascularization, *Neurosurg Focus* 14(3):e6, 2003.
147. Lawton MT, Spetzler RF: Internal carotid artery sacrifice for radical resection of skull base tumors, *Skull Base Surg* 6(2):119–123, 1996.
148. Saito K, Fukuta K, Takahashi M, et al: Management of the cavernous sinus in en bloc resections of malignant skull base tumors, *Head Neck* 21(8):734–742, 1999.
149. Sekhar LN, Natarajan SK, Ellenbogen RG, et al: Cerebral revascularization for ischemia, aneurysms, and cranial base tumors, *Neurosurgery* 62:SHC1373–SHC1408, 2008; discussion SCH1408–1310.
150. Sekhar LN, Tzortzidis FN, Bejjani GK, et al: Saphenous vein graft bypass of the sigmoid sinus and jugular bulb during the removal of glomus jugular tumors. Report of two cases, *J Neurosurg* 86:1036–1041, 1997.
151. Wolfe SQ, Tummala RP, Morcos JJ: Cerebral revascularization in skull base tumors, *Skull Base* 15(1):71–82, 2005.
152. Sen C, Sekhar LN: Direct vein graft reconstruction of the cavernous, petrous, and upper cervical internal carotid artery: lessons learned from 30 cases, *Neurosurgery* 30(5):732–742, 1992; discussion 742–743.

ADDITIONAL SUGGESTED READINGS

Amin-Hanjani S, Du X, Zhao M, et al: Use of a quantitative magnetic resonance angiography to stratify stroke risk in symptomatic vertebrobasilar disease, *Stroke* 36:1140–1145, 2005.
Bier A: Chirurgie der Gefässe, Aneurysmen, *Deutsche Med. Wochenshcrift* 41(5):157, 121 Nr. 6:157, 1915.
Buncke HJ, Schulz WP: Experimental digital amputation and reimplantation, *Plast Reconstr Surg* 36:62–70, 1965.
Burkhard-Zehnder KM: *Geschicte der Gefässchirurgie*. Medical dissertation, Zürich, Switzerland, 1990, University of Zürich.
Carrel A: Results of the transplantation of blood vessels, organs and limbs, *J Am Med Ass* 51:1662–1667, 1908.
Carrel A: The surgery of blood vessels, *Johns Hopkins Hospital Bull* 18:18, 1909.
Couldwell WT, Liu JK, Amini A, et al: Submandibular-infratemporal interpositional carotid artery bypass for cranial base tumors and giant aneurysms, *Neurosurgery* 59(4 Suppl 2):ONS353–ONS359, 2006; discussion ONS359–360.
Fitzpatrick BC, Spetzler RF, Ballard JL, et al: Cervical-to-petrous internal carotid artery bypass procedure. Technical note, *J Neurosurg* 79(1):138–141, 1993.
Garret HE, Dennis EW, DeBakey ME: Aorto-coronary bypass with saphenous vein graft: Seven year follow up, *JAMA* 223(7):792–794, 1973.
Gluck TG: Zwei Fälle von Aortenaneurysmen nebst Bemerkungen über die Naht der Blutgefässe, *L Arch Klin Chir* 28:548, 1883.

Haberer H: Kriegsaneurysmen, *Arch Klin Chir* 107:611, 1916.

Handley WS: An operation for embolism, *Brit Med J* 2:712, 1907.

Henschen C: Operative revascularization des zirkulatorisch geschädigten Gehirn durch Anlagen gestielter Muskellappen. (Encephalo-Myo-Synangiose), *Langenbeck's Arch Dtsch 2 Chir* 264:392–401, 1950.

Heubner D: *Die Luetische Erkrankung der Hirnarterien*, Leipzig, 1874, Vogel.

Ho Y-CL, Peterson ET, Golay X: Measuring arterial and tissue responses to functional challenges using arterial spin labeling, *NeuroImage* 49:478–487, 2010.

Höpfner E: Über Gefässtransplantationen und Replantation, *L Arch Klin Chir* 70:417, 1903.

Hunter J: *The reluctant surgeon* (cited by J. Kobler), New York, 1960, Doubleday.

Jacobson JH, Suarez EL: Microsurgery in anastomoses of small vessels, *Surg Forum* 11:243–245, 1960.

Jassinowsky A: Ein Beitrag zur Lehre von der Gefässnaht, *L Arch Klin Chir* 42:816, 1891.

Karasawa J, Kikuchi H, Furuse S, et al: Enlarged anterior spinal artery as collateral circulation, *J Neurosurg* 41:356–359, 1974.

Karasawa J, Kikuchi H, Furuse S, et al: Treatment of Moyamoya disease with STA-MCA anastomosis, *J Neurosurg* 49:679–688, 1978.

Kurze T: Microtechniques in neurological surgery, *Clin Neurosurg, Proceeding of congress of Neurological Surgeons* 1963/1964.

Lassen NA, Henriksen L, Paulson O: Regional cerebral blood flow in stroke by 133-xenon inhalation and emission tomography, *Stroke* 12:284–288, 1981.

Lassen NA, Hoedt-Rasmussen K, Sorensun SC, et al: Regional cerebral blood flow in man determined by Krypton-85, *Neurology* 13:719–725, 1963.

Leriche R: *Physiologie Pathologique et Traitement chirurgical des Maladies artérielles de la Vasomotricité*, 1945, Masson.

Lexer E: 20 Jahre Transplantationsforschung in der Chirurgie, *Arch Klin Chir* 138:298, 1925.

Lougheed WM, Marshall BM, Michel ER, et al: Common carotid to intracranial carotid by-pass venous graft: technical note, *J Neurosurg* 34:114–118, 1971.

Oudot J: La greffe vasculaire dans les thromboses de carrefour aortique, *Presse Med* 59:234, 1951.

Payr E: Beiträge zur Technik der Blutgefäss-und Nervennaht, *L Arch Klin Chir* 62I:67, 1900.

Petropoulos P: Gefässrekonstruktion mit autologer Faszie, *Inaug Diss* Zürich 1972.

Pirovano MA: Un cas de greffe artérielle, *Press Med* 19:55, 1911.

Quarles RP, Mintun MA, Larson KB, et al: Measurement of regional cerebral blood flow with positron emission tomography: A comparison of (^{15}O)water to (^{11}C)butanol with distributed-parameter and compartmental models, *J Cereb Blood Flow Metab* 13:733–747, 1993.

Quinones-Hinojosa A, Du R, Lawton MT: Revascularization with saphenous vein bypasses for complex intracranial aneurysms, *Skull Base* 15:119–132, 2005.

Smith JW: Microsurgery: Review of the literature and discussion of microtechniques, *Plast Reconstr Surg* 37:227–245, 1966.

Strully KJ, Hurwitt ES, Blankenberg HW: Thromboendarterectomy for thrombosis of the internal carotid artery in the neck, *J Neurosurg* 10:474, 1953.

Suarez EL, Jacobson JH II: Results of small artery endarterectomy microsurgical technique, *Surg Forum* 12:256–259, 1961.

Sundt TM Jr: Was the international randomized trial of extracranial-intracranial arterial bypass representative of the population at risk? *N Engl J Med* 316:814–816, 1987.

Sundt TM Jr, Piepgras DG: Surgical approach to giant intracranial aneurysms: Operative experience with 80 cases, *J Neurosurg* 51:731–742, 1979.

Tuffier M: De l'intubation dans les plaies des grosses artères, *Bull Acad Méd* 74:455, 1915.

Urschel HC Jr, Roth EJ: Small arterial anastomosis II suture, *Ann Surg* 153 (4):611–616, 1961.

Yaşargil MG: Experimental small vessel surgery in the dog including patching and grafting of cerebral vessels and the formation of functional extra-intracranial shunts. In Donaghy RMP, Yaşargil MG, eds: *Microvascular surgery*, St Louis, 1967, Thieme, pp 87–126.

Yaşargil MG: Extra-intracranial arterial anastomosis for transient cerebral ischemic attacks. Proceedings of the Symposia of the Fifth International Congress of Neurological Surgery Tokyo, Japan, October 1973, *Prog Neurol Surg* 5:15–151, 1973.

Yaşargil MG: From the microsurgical laboratory to the human operative theater, *Acta Neurochir (Wien)* 147(5):465–468, 2005.

Yaşargil MG: *Microneurosurgery,* St Louis, 1984–1996, G. Thieme: Vol I-II Aneurysms, Vol III A-B AVM Cavernomas, Vol IV A-B Tumors, Cavernous.

Yaşargil MG: The history of optical instruments and microneurosurgery. In Barrow DL, Traynelis VC, Laws ER, Kondziolka DS, eds: *Fifty years of neurosurgery*, Philadelphia, 2000, Lippincott, Williams & Wilkins.

Zhu X-H, Zhang N, Zhang Y, et al: In vivo ^{17}O NMR approaches for brain study at high field, *NMR Biomed* 18:83–103, 2005.

Zwaveling A: Anastomoses in small-calibre arteries, *Arch Chir Neerl* 15:237, 1963.

The field of cerebral revascularization is currently experiencing a major renaissance. We feel the time is appropriate for a textbook dedicated to exploring this subject in great detail, including its historical roots, anatomophysiological underpinnings, current microsurgical and endovascular techniques, and future possibilities.

Since the early days of Professor Yaşargil's pioneering work in the late 1960s, extracranial-to-intracranial (EC-IC) bypass techniques have continued to evolve. Today, they encompass several variations developed to address different pathologies, including cerebral ischemia, Moyamoya disease, skull base tumors, and complex aneurysms. The latter, complex/giant cerebral aneurysms, are the main pathology for which these techniques are utilized at this point. The indications for EC-IC bypass for large-vessel intracranial or extracranial occlusive disease remains unclear. We await the publication of the Carotid Occlusion Surgery Study subgroup analysis, as well as the Japanese EC-IC trial, to shed light on the possible surgical indications for ischemic disease.

In this monograph, evolving techniques in EC-IC bypass surgery are described. The image-guided STA-MCA bypass through a burr hole is elucidated. We also introduce our initial experience with a minimally invasive high-flow bypass technique using the internal maxillary artery that avoids a long cervical incision while providing a short interposition high-flow graft. The technique of excimer laser-assisted non-occlusive anastomosis (ELANA), as developed by Professor Tulleken, is delineated. Evolving endovascular techniques including the use of stents for giant aneurysms as well as reopening of an occluded internal carotid artery are described.

The contributors to this monograph represent some of the key pioneers in cerebrovascular surgery over the past three decades. Their contributions and the composite of their experience within this text allows for a unique understanding of cerebrovascular hemodynamics, natural history of giant aneurysms, evolving microsurgical and endovascular techniques, and a decision-making process for the management of these pathologies. The future of cerebral revascularization will undoubtedly rest on the evolving techniques and technologies of both the microsurgical and the endovascular arenas.

I would like to express my gratitude to my faculty, fellows, residents, and students at Saint Louis University who have tirelessly helped me in putting this monograph together: Jeroen Coppens, Aneela Darbar, Jorge Eller, Deanna Sasaki-Adams, Justin Sweeney, Jonathan Lebovitz, and Sheri Palejwala.

Saleem I. Abdulrauf
St. Louis, MO
October 2010

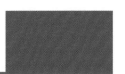
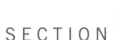

SECTION

CEREBRAL HEMODYNAMICS AND CEREBROVASCULAR IMAGING   1

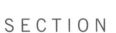

SECTION

EC-IC BYPASS SURGICAL TECHNIQUES   63

S E C T I O N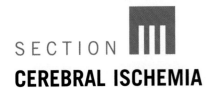

CEREBRAL ISCHEMIA
165

S E C T I O N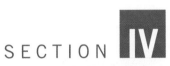

GIANT CEREBRAL ANEURYSMS 223

SECTION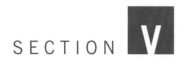

SKULL BASE TUMORS

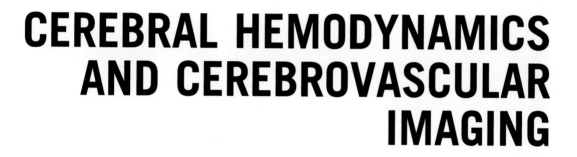

CEREBRAL HEMODYNAMICS AND CEREBROVASCULAR IMAGING

AUTOREGULATION AND HEMODYNAMICS IN HUMAN CEREBROVASCULAR DISEASE

1

WILLIAM J. POWERS

NORMAL CEREBRAL HEMODYNAMICS AND ENERGY METABOLISM

Introduction

Energy in the brain is required for maintenance of membrane potentials, ionic transport, and the biosynthesis and transport of neurotransmitters and cellular elements. Energy for these functions is supplied via adenosine triphosphate (ATP) from metabolism of exogenous compounds with a high-energy content (primarily glucose) to simpler compounds with less energy content (lactate, CO_2, and H_2O). Since storage of substrates for energy metabolism in the brain is minimal, the brain is highly dependent on a continuous supply of oxygen and glucose from the blood for its functional and structural integrity. It is exquisitely sensitive to even brief disturbances in this supply.

Normal Values of CBF and CMR

Healthy young adults have an average whole-brain cerebral blood flow (CBF) of approximately 46 ml $100g^{-1}$ min^{-1}, cerebral metabolic rate of oxygen (CMRO$_2$) of 3.0 ml $100g^{-1}$ min^{-1} (134 μmol $100g^{-1}$ min^{-1}), and cerebral metabolic rate of glucose (CMRglc) of 25 μmol $100g^{-1}$ min^{-1}.[1-4] The CMRO$_2$/CMRglc molar ratio of 5.4 is lower than the value of 6.0 expected for complete glucose oxidation due to the production of a small amount of lactate by glycolysis that occurs even with abundant oxygen supply.[1,3,5] CBF in gray matter (80 ml $100g^{-1}$ min^{-1}) is approximately four times higher than in white matter (20 ml $100g^{-1}$ min^{-1}).[6] Under normal physiological conditions, regional CBF is closely matched to the resting regional metabolic rate of the tissue.[7,8] Thus CMRO$_2$ and CMRglc are also higher in gray matter than in white matter. Because of this relationship between regional flow and metabolism, the fraction of blood-borne glucose and oxygen extracted is relatively constant throughout the brain (Figure 1–1). The oxygen extraction fraction (OEF) is normally 30% to 40%, indicating that oxygen supply is two to three times greater than oxygen demand. The glucose extraction fraction (GEF) is normally about 10%.[8,9]

Many studies report that CBF declines from the third decade onward.[10-13] The change in metabolic rate for oxygen and glucose with age is less clear, with several studies showing a decrease [10,12,14-16] and others showing no change.[17-19] Studies that have corrected for brain atrophy show lesser or absent changes in CBF, CMRO$_2$, and CMRglc in the remaining tissue with increasing age.[15,20-22] Our own data corrected for brain atrophy from 23 normal subjects, ages 23 to 71 years, show no significant change in CBF or CMRO$_2$, but a significant decline in CMRglc of 4% to 5% per decade.

Control of CBF

Cerebral perfusion pressure (CPP) is equal to the difference between the arterial pressure driving blood into the brain and the venous backpressure. Venous backpressure is negligible unless there is elevated intracranial pressure (ICP) or obstruction of venous outflow. Thus, under most circumstances, regional CPP (rCPP) is equal to the regional mean arterial pressure (rMAP). The rMAP will be equal to the systemic MAP when there is no arterial obstruction, but may be substantially lower in the setting of acute or chronic arterial stenosis or occlusion.

Regional CBF (rCBF) is regulated by rCPP and the regional cerebrovascular resistance (rCVR):

$$rCBF = \frac{rCPP}{rCVR}$$

Under conditions of constant rCPP, any changes in rCBF must occur as a result of changes in rCVR. CVR is affected by blood viscosity and vessel length but is primarily determined by vessel radius. Arterial resistance vessels (primarily arterioles) dilate and constrict in response to a variety of stimuli causing changes in rCVR that produce changes in rCBF.

When there is a primary reduction in the metabolic demand of brain cells, such as that caused by hypothermia or barbiturates, arterial resistance vessels constrict to produce a comparable decline in CBF and thus little or no change in OEF or GEF.[23-25] With normal physiological increases in neuronal activity, vessels dilate, producing an increase in regional CBF that is accompanied by an increase in regional CMRglc of

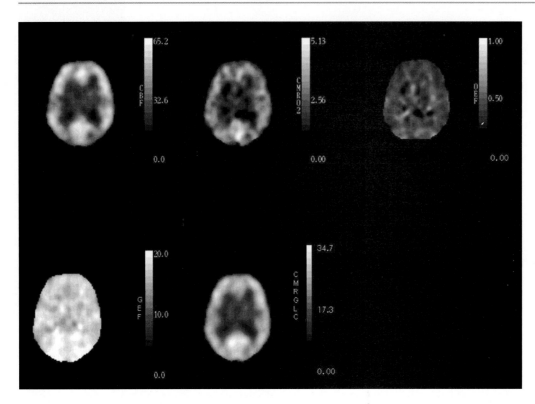

Figure 1–1. Cerebral blood flow and metabolism in a 70-year-old female normal volunteer. Note that cerebral blood flow (top left), cerebral oxygen metabolism (top middle), and cerebral glucose metabolism (bottom right) all show higher values in cortical gray matter than in white matter, whereas oxygen extraction fraction (top right) and glucose extraction fraction (bottom left) are uniform.
(From Powers WJ, Zazulia AR. The use of positron emission tomography in cerebrovascular disease. Neuroimaging Clin N Am 2003;13: 741–758; with permission.)

similar magnitude, but with little or no increase in regional $CMRO_2$.[26–28] Acute changes in arterial pCO_2 cause proportional changes in CBF. The mechanism for the change in CBF is a change in CVR produced by vasodilation with increased pCO_2 and vasoconstriction with decreased pCO_2.[29] With prolonged hyperventilation, CBF returns toward normal values over a period of several hours.[30] The effects of changes in arterial pO_2 on the cerebral circulation show a threshold effect, different from the proportional changes seen with changes in pCO_2. CBF does not increase until arterial pO_2 is below about 30 to 50 mm Hg.[31,32] A significant reduction in hemoglobin saturation and hence in arterial oxygen content (CaO_2) does not occur until arterial pO_2 falls to about 50 to 60 mm Hg, indicating that it is primarily CaO_2 and not pO_2 that determines CBF.[31,33,34] Reductions in CaO_2 due to anemia cause vasodilation and compensatory increases in CBF, whereas the increase in CaO_2 with polycythemia is associated with a decrease in CBF.[34] Acute changes in CaO_2 produce less of an increase in CBF than do chronic changes.[35,36] Hematocrit is an important determinant of viscosity, and thus viscosity and CaO_2 often vary together. It is unlikely that viscosity is an important determinant of CBF under most circumstances, however. Increases in blood viscosity induce compensatory vasodilation to maintain cerebral oxygen delivery (CBF x CaO_2).[37–39] When pre-existing vasodilation impairs the ability of vessels to dilate further to changes in viscosity, this compensatory mechanism may be exhausted.[40] Thus increases in CBF brought about by hemodilution, if they are simply reciprocal responses to changes in arterial oxygen content, will not increase cerebral oxygen delivery and may even decrease it.[41]

In contrast to the relationship of CBF to oxygen supply and demand, the balance between glucose supply and demand has little effect on CBF. Severe reductions in blood glucose down to 1.1 to 2.2 mmol/L produced modest but significant increases in CBF of 12% to 23%.[42–46] This CBF response to severe hypoglycemia likely does not represent a compensatory mechanism to maintain glucose delivery to the brain since a blood glucose level of 2 mmol/L is well below the level at which brain dysfunction and counter-regulatory hormone response occur.[47] Furthermore, increases in CBF do not increase blood:brain glucose transport.[48,49]

All of these responses of the cerebral vasculature occur at normal CPP. When CPP changes, a different set of cerebrovascular and brain metabolic responses occur.

Response of CBF to Changes in Cerebral Perfusion Pressure

Changes in CPP over a wide range have little effect on CBF.[50] When CPP decreases, vasodilation of the small arteries or arterioles reduces CVR. When CPP increases, vasoconstriction of the small arteries or arterioles increases CVR.[51,52] This compensatory mechanism is known as autoregulation.[50] In most studies, the limits of autoregulation in normal normotensive subjects are from approximately 70 to 150 mm Hg.[50,53] Strandgaard determined that the lower limit of autoregulation was 25 mm Hg below the resting BP in normotensive subjects.[54] A contrasting viewpoint has been offered by Schmidt et al., who proposed a new computer method for assessing the lower limit of autoregulation.[55] In this study, the lower limit in normotensive volunteers was only 85 mm Hg (11 mm Hg higher than that calculated from the conventional method) and at times was virtually identical to the baseline blood pressure. Within the limits of autoregulation, a 10% decrease in mean arterial pressure produces only a slight (2% to 7%) decrease in regional CBF.[56,57] When CPP is reduced below the lower limit of autoregulation, more marked reductions in CBF occur. When the cerebral blood vessels are already dilated in response to some other stimulus, they are less able to dilate in response to reduced CPP. Therefore, the autoregulatory response is attenuated or lost in the setting of pre-existing hypercapnia, anemia, or hypoxemia.[58,59]

Chronic hypertension shifts both the lower and upper limits of autoregulation to higher levels. The average value of the lower limit of autoregulation in 13 poorly controlled hypertensive patients, ages 49 to 64, (113 ± 17 mm Hg) and 9 well-controlled hypertensives, ages 42 to 66, (96 ± 17 mm Hg) was elevated compared to 10 normotensive controls, ages 41 to 81 (73 ± 9 mm Hg).[54] For all three groups combined, the lower limit of autoregulation was 70% to 80% of the resting MAP ($r = 0.80$). In another study, the lower limit was 88% to 89% of resting MAP ($r = 0.81$) for 19 normotensive and hypertensive subjects.[55] Prolonged effective antihypertensive treatment may lead to a re-adaptation of autoregulation towards normal in some cases, but there are almost no data on this subject.[54] Because of this upward shift of the lower limit, acute reductions in MAP or CPP that would be safe in normotensive subjects may precipitate cerebral ischemia in patients with chronic hypertension.[60]

These observations of the effect of changes in CPP on CBF were made by changing MAP or ICP over minutes, then measuring CBF at the new stable pressure. Recently, these responses have been termed "static cerebral autoregulation" to differentiate them from measurements of cerebral blood flow velocity with Doppler in response to more rapid and less marked fluctuations in MAP or ICP, termed "dynamic cerebral autoregulation."[61] The relationship between static and dynamic autoregulation is not clear. Abnormalities of dynamic cerebral autoregulation may be associated with normal or abnormal static autoregulation.[62,63]

When CPP falls below the autoregulatory limit and the maximum compensatory vasodilatory capacity of the cerebral circulation has been exceeded, CBF will decline markedly with further reductions in CPP. A progressive increase in OEF occurs as CBF falls and oxygen metabolism is maintained (Figure 1–2).[64–66] OEF may increase by a factor of 2 or even more from its normal value of 30% to 40%.[65] When the increase in OEF is maximal and is no longer adequate to supply the energy needs of the brain, further reductions in CPP disrupt normal cellular metabolism, produce clinical evidence of brain dysfunction, and, if prolonged, will cause permanent damage.

Cerebral blood volume (CBV) is the volume of circulating blood in cerebral vessels. CBV is composed of arterial,

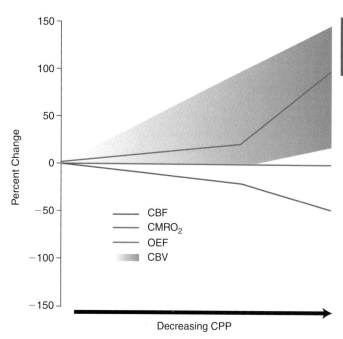

Figure 1–2. Compensatory responses to reduced cerebral perfusion pressure (CPP). As CPP falls, cerebral blood flow (CBF) changes very little due to arteriolar dilation, which reduces cerebrovascular resistance. This vasodilation may be seen as an increase in cerebral blood volume (CBV), but this response is variable, ranging from a steady rise (of as much as 150%) to only a modest increase beginning at the point of autoregulatory failure. When vasodilatory capacity has been exhausted, cerebral autoregulation fails and CBF begins to decrease rapidly. A progressive increase in oxygen extraction (OEF) preserves cerebral oxygen metabolism (CMRO$_2$).

(Redrawn from Powers WJ, Zazulia AR. The use of positron emission tomography in cerebrovascular disease. Neuroimaging Clin N Am 2003;13: 741–758; with permission.)

capillary, and venous segments. Veins account for some 80% to 85% of CBV, arteries 10% to 15%, and capillaries less than 5%.[67,68] Arteries are the most responsive to autoregulatory changes in CPP, veins respond less and capillaries even less.[69,70] During experimental reductions in CPP, it is often possible to measure an increase in CBV that is presumed to be due to autoregulatory vasodilation.[71–73] However, this increase in CBV to reduced CPP is not always evident (Figure 1–2),[66,74] and a decrease in CBV in response to severe reductions in CPP has even been observed.[75] Failure to demonstrate increased CBV in the setting of reduced CPP has been attributed to various possible mechanisms, including differential vasodilatory capacity of different vascular beds, passive collapse of vessels due to low intraluminal pressures, small vessel vasospasm, and re-setting of vascular tone in response to reduced metabolic demands.[76] The CBF/CBV ratio (or its reciprocal, the vascular mean vascular transit time, MTT) has been proposed to be a more sensitive indicator of reduced CPP than CBV alone.[66,77] Although it may be more sensitive, it is not reliable because it may decrease in conditions with low CBF and normal CPP, such as hypocapnia.[78,79]

CEREBRAL HEMODYNAMIC EFFECTS OF ARTERIAL OCCLUSIVE DISEASE

Hemodynamic Effect of Arterial Stenosis

Stenosis of the carotid artery produces no hemodynamic effect until a critical reduction of 60% to 70% in vessel lumen occurs. Even with this or greater degrees of stenosis, distal CPP is variable and may even remain normal with stenosis exceeding 90%.[80] This is because hemodynamic effect of carotid artery stenosis depends not only on the degree of stenosis but also on the adequacy of the collateral circulation. Vascular imaging techniques such as angiography or Doppler ultrasonography can identify the presence of these collateral vessels, but not necessarily the adequacy of the blood supply they provide.[81]

In patients with cerebrovascular disease, determining the hemodynamic effects of arterial stenosis or occlusion is of potential value in predicting the subsequent stroke risk or for choosing preventative therapy. Measurement of rCBF alone is inadequate for this purpose. Normal rCBF may be found when rCPP is reduced but rCBF is maintained by autoregulatory vasodilation of distal resistance vessels. Second, rCBF may be low when rCPP is normal, such as when the metabolic demands of the tissue are reduced by previous ischemic damage or by the destruction of afferent or efferent fibers by a remote lesion (Figure 1–3).[65]

Methods to Measure the Hemodynamic Effects of Large Artery Occlusive Disease

Three strategies are commonly used clinically to determine the local cerebral hemodynamic status. The first relies on measurement of rCBF at baseline and again after a vasodilatory stimulus, such as CO_2 inhalation, breath holding, acetazolamide administration, or physiological activity (e.g., hand movement). An impairment in the normal increase of rCBF or Doppler blood flow velocity in response to the vasodilatory stimulus is assumed to reflect existing autoregulatory vasodilation due to reduced rCPP. Responses to vasodilatory stimuli have been categorized into three grades of hemodynamic impairment: (1) reduced augmentation (relative to contralateral hemisphere or normal controls), (2) absent augmentation (same value as baseline), and (3) paradoxical reduction in regional blood flow compared with baseline measurement. This last category, also known as the "steal" phenomenon, can only be identified with quantitative CBF techniques.[82]

The second strategy entails the quantitative measurement of regional CBV either alone or in combination with measurement of rCBF at rest to detect the presence of autoregulatory vasodilation. Increases in rCBV or the rCBV/rCBF ratio relative to the range observed in normal control subjects is assumed to indicate hemodynamic compromise.

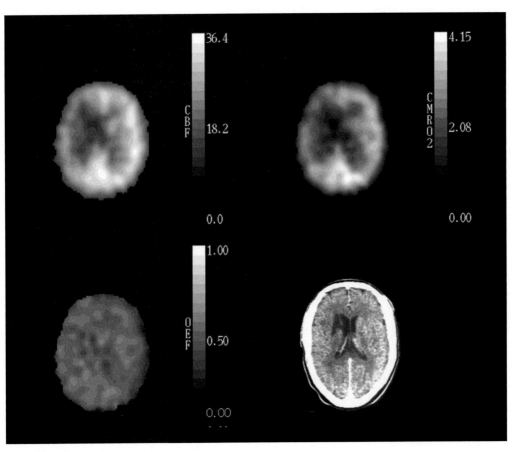

Figure 1–3. Primary metabolic depression in structurally normal brain overlying a subcortical infarct. Two months following a left subcortical infarct shown by CT (bottom right), PET shows reduced cerebral blood flow (top left) and oxygen metabolism (top right) with normal oxygen extraction (bottom left). *(From Powers WJ, Zazulia AR. The use of positron emission tomography in cerebrovascular disease. Neuroimaging Clin N Am 2003;13: 741–758; with permission.)*

Table 1–1. ARTERIOGRAPHIC COLLATERAL PATTERNS IN PATIENTS FROM ST. LOUIS CAROTID OCCLUSION STUDY.

	High OEF	Normal OEF
Acomm	27/32	26/30
Pcomm	6/13	13/18
ECA-OA	19/31	10/28
ECA-Other	3/29	6/28
Cortical	2/29	5/23

The third strategy involves direct measurement of regional OEF as an indicator of a reduction in rCPP below the lower autoregulatory limit.

The pattern of arteriographic collateral circulation to the MCA distal to an occluded carotid artery does not consistently differentiate those patients with poor cerebral hemodynamics (Table 1–1).[74,81,83,84]

Three-Stage Classification System of Cerebral Hemodynamics

Based on the known physiological responses of CBF, CBV, and OEF to reductions in CPP, we proposed a three-stage sequential classification system for the regional cerebral hemodynamic status in patients with cerebrovascular disease.[85] Stage 0 is normal with normal rCPP and normally matched regional CBF and CMRO$_2$, such that rOEF is normal, rCBV and rMTT are not elevated and the rCBF response to vasodilatory stimuli is normal. Stage I hemodynamic compromise represents reduced rCPP, but is still above the lower autoregulatory limit. It is manifested by autoregulatory vasodilation of arterioles to maintain rCBF matched to rCMRO$_2$. Consequently, rCBV and rMTT are increased and the rCBF response to vasodilatory stimuli is decreased, but rOEF remains normal. In Stage II hemodynamic failure, rCPP is below the lower autoregulatory limit. There is a decrease in CBF relative to rCMRO$_2$ with increased OEF (Figure 1–4). This stage has also been termed "misery perfusion" by Baron et al.[86,87] In all of these stages, rCMRO$_2$ is preserved at a level that reflects the underlying energy demands of the tissue, but may be lower than normal due to the effects of previous tissue damage or deafferentation (Figure 1–3).[65,88]

Although the three-stage classification scheme is conceptually and practically useful, it is overly simplistic. First, as discussed above, increases in rCBV and rMTT are not reliable indices of reduced rCPP. Second, rCBF responses to different vasodilatory agents may be impaired or normal in the same patient.[89–91] A normal vasodilatory response may occur in the setting of increased rCBV.[92,93] Finally, according to the three-stage system, all patients with increased rOEF should have increased rCBV and poor response to vasoactive stimuli. However, this increase in rCBV is not always evident.[76]

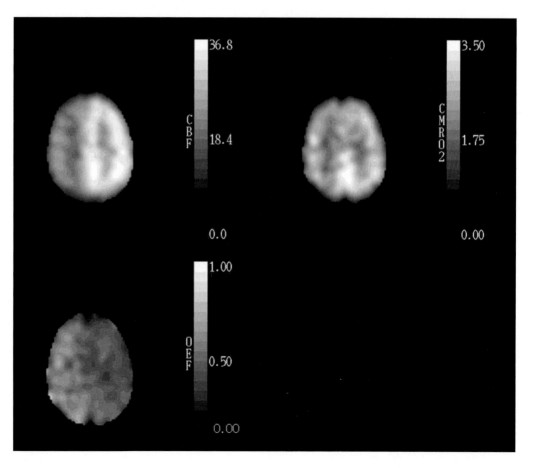

Figure 1–4. Chronically elevated oxygen extraction fraction in a patient with carotid occlusion. In this 56-year-old man with left hemispheric transient attacks, PET show reduced cerebral blood flow (top left), symmetrical oxygen metabolism (top right) and increased oxygen extraction (bottom left) in the left hemisphere (left portion).

(From Powers WJ, Zazulia AR. The use of positron emission tomography in cerebrovascular disease. Neuroimaging Clin N Am 2003;13: 741-758; with permission.)

Correlation of Large Artery Cerebral Hemodynamics with Stroke Risk

Stage I Hemodynamic compromise

Data on vasomotor reactivity to acetazolamide or hypercapnia (Stage I hemodynamic compromise) in predicting subsequent stroke have been inconsistent.[83,94–101]

Yonas and colleagues tested cerebrovascular reserve by paired rCBF measurements with the stable Xenon/CT and acetazolamide in 68 patients with carotid artery disease followed for a mean of 24 months.[99] Patients were placed into two groups based on criteria for hemodynamic compromise of initial rCBF values less than 45 ml 100 g^{-1} min^{-1} and rCBF reduction after acetazolamide of more than 5%. This categorization was done retrospectively based on assessment of the characteristics of the patients who went on to develop stroke. There were two contralateral strokes in 27 patients with normal hemodynamics and eight ipsilateral strokes in 41 patients with hemodynamic compromise. In a subsequent report by these authors, 27 additional patients were included in an analysis of 95 patients with either stenosis of 70% or carotid artery occlusion.[95] The patients were followed for a mean of 19.6 months. These patients were classified into two groups based only on a rCBF reduction of more than 5% to acetazolamide, different criteria than those used in the first study. From the data presented it is possible to determine that three of the five strokes that occurred in the additional 27 patients did so in patients who would not have met criteria for hemodynamic compromise in the first study. Only two of these five new strokes were in the hemodynamically compromised territory of the occluded vessel. Thus the previously retrospectively derived criteria for identifying patients at high risk failed when subjected to a prospective test on a new group of 27 patients.

Kleiser and Widder tested the cerebrovascular reserve capacity in 85 patients with internal carotid artery (ICA) occlusion using transcranial Doppler during normocapnia, hypercapnia, and hypocapnia.[102] At the time of entry into the study, 46 patients were asymptomatic on the ipsilateral side of the occlusion. The patients were followed for a mean of 38 months. In the group with normal CO_2 reactivity, four of 48 patients had an ipsilateral TIA or prolonged reversible ischemic neurological deficit, but none had a stroke. Six of 26 patients with diminished CO_2 reactivity had an ipsilateral ischemic event (three [12%] strokes, three TIAs), and three patients had a contralateral event (two strokes, one TIA). In the group with exhausted CO_2 reactivity, five of 11 patients (45%) had an ipsilateral stroke and one patient had an ipsilateral TIA. Two patients had a contralateral hemisphere stroke. Although this study found a significant association between CO_2 reactivity of the cerebral circulation and ischemic events ipsilateral to an ICA occlusion, there was no significant relationship between prior symptoms and subsequent stroke risk. This is puzzling since the prognosis of asymptomatic carotid occlusion is relatively benign.[103,104] The increased risk of contralateral stroke in the patients with a diminished or exhausted

CO_2 reactivity suggests that the groups were not matched for other stroke risk factors, and this may explain the differences observed. In a subsequent report by these authors, 86 patients with carotid artery occlusion were followed for variable periods of time.[105] A stroke ipsilateral to an occluded ICA occurred in three of 26 patients with an exhausted CO_2 reactivity, corresponding to an annual stroke rate of only 8% (mean follow-up time of 19 months), much lower in the first study. In 37 patients with diminished CO_2 reactivity and 48 patients with normal CO_2 reactivity, only one patient in each group developed an ipsilateral stroke (mean follow-up time of 31.7 months). In this second study, the number of asymptomatic patients is not given. The 86 patients in the second study were selected from 452 patients with ICA occlusion studied with transcranial Doppler cerebrovascular resistance studies. The criteria for selecting these 86 patients were not given.

Vernieri et al. have published a well-designed and well-executed prospective study of 65 patients with both symptomatic and asymptomatic carotid occlusion.[97] Hemodynamic compromise was assessed by using transcranial Doppler measurement of middle cerebral artery (MCA) blood flow velocity during breath holding. Multivariate analysis found only older age and impaired Doppler velocity increase during breath holding to be associated with the subsequent risk of ipsilateral ischemic events (TIA and stroke). No separate analysis of symptomatic patients and no separate analysis of predictive value for stroke only was reported nor was any data on subsequent medical treatment.

Kuroda and colleagues enrolled 77 symptomatic patients in a prospective, longitudinal cohort study. All patients met inclusion criteria of cerebral angiography, no or localized cerebral infarction on MRI or CT, and no or minimal neurological deficit. Regional rCBF and regional cerebrovascular reactivity to CVR to acetazolamide were quantitatively determined by ^{133}Xe SEPCT. During an average follow-up period of 42.7 months, 16 total and seven ipsilateral ischemic strokes occurred. Decreased cerebrovascular reactivity to acetazolamide alone did not predict the subsequent occurrence of stroke. Only the combination of decreased rCBF and decreased cerebrovascular reactivity identified those with a high annual risk for both total and ipsilateral stroke (35.6% and 23.7%, respectively). Kaplan-Meier analysis revealed that the risks of total and ipsilateral stroke in the 11 patients with this combination were significantly higher than in the 66 without (P < 0.0001 and P = 0.0001, respectively, log-rank test). Relative risk was 8.0 (95% confidence interval [CI], 1.9 to 34.4) for ipsilateral stroke and 3.6 (95% CI, 1.4 to 9.3) for total stroke.[94]

In addition to these reported positive associations, other studies with prospectively defined criteria have failed to demonstrate a relationship between the risk of subsequent stroke and Stage I hemodynamic compromise.[96,106] We reported a longitudinal study of stroke risk in 21 medically treated patients with increased CBV/CBF ratios distal to a stenotic or occluded artery. No ipsilateral ischemic strokes occurred during the 1-year follow-up period.[106] Yokota et al. derived criteria for abnormal acetazolamide SPECT CBF responses from a comparison of paired studies of PET OEF in 14 subjects and then used the SPECT criteria to study 105 patients with ischemic cerebrovascular events, minimal infarct on a CT scan, and unilateral occlusion or severe stenosis of the ICA or proximal MCA.[96] Fifty-five patients had abnormal cerebral vasoreactivity response to acetazolamide and 50 patients had a normal response. Risk factors for stroke at entry were recorded and included in the final data analysis. The median follow-up period in the study was 32.5 months. During the follow-up period, 13 patients had a stroke, 11 died, 16 had surgical cerebral revascularization procedures (nine EC-IC bypasses and seven carotid endarterectomies), and 11 were lost to follow-up. There was no significant difference in the rate of subsequent stroke in the two groups. This was generally a well-planned, well-executed prospective study that addressed the possible impact of other risk factors in the largest study reported to date. A relatively large number of patients were censored from the study because of subsequent cerebrovascular surgery and loss to follow-up. Since the criteria used for separating patients into those with normal and abnormal cerebrovascular reactivity were based on a previous study that demonstrated complete congruence with PET measurements of OEF,[92] the negative results of this study are puzzling in the light of two PET studies that both demonstrated a strong association between increased OEF and subsequent stroke (see following). As opposed to other studies comparing CBF response to vasodilatory stimuli and PET OEF, these investigators were able to identify a threshold that was 100% sensitive and 100% specific based on a study of both modalities in 14 patients. It is likely that this small sample of patients was not sufficient to really determine the relationship between the two modalities and the threshold chosen did not reliably correlate with PET OEF in the larger sample of 105 patients followed prospectively.

In 2002, Ogasawara and colleagues published a well-designed, well-executed prospective study of cerebrovascular reactivity (CVR) to acetazolamide using quantitative measurements of CBF with ^{133}Xe inhalation and single-photon emission computed tomography.[101] Seventy patients less than 70 years old with unilateral ICA or MCA occlusion were divided into two groups based on the regional CVR (rCVR) in the territory of the occluded artery. They were prospectively followed for a period of 24 months. Recurrent strokes occurred in eight of the 23 patients with reduced rCVR at entry and in three of 47 patients with normal rCVR ($p = 0.0030$ by Kaplan-Meier analysis). In a companion paper, these same authors directly compared two different methodologies: cerebral blood flow (CBF) percent change obtained quantitatively from xenon-133 (133Xe) SPECT as used in the initial report and asymmetry index (AI) percent change obtained qualitatively from N-isopropyl-p-[123I]-iodoamphetamine (IMP) SPECT. There was no significant difference in cumulative recurrence-free survival rates between patients with decreased AI percent change and those with normal AI percent change. This study demonstrated that, while decreased cerebrovascular reactivity

to acetazolamide determined quantitatively by 133Xe SPECT is an independent predictor of the 5-year risk of subsequent stroke in patients with symptomatic major cerebral artery occlusion, the qualitative method using 123I-IMP SPECT was a poor predictor of the risk of subsequent stroke in this type of patient.[100]

Thus data indicating a relationship between measurements of Stage I hemodynamic impairment and subsequent stroke risk in symptomatic patients remain equivocal at this time. While such a relationship may exist for some measurements of Stage I hemodynamic impairment, it has not been demonstrated with consistency. Since CBF responses may be different to different vasodilatory agents within the same patient, this inconsistency is understandable. Evidence that hemodynamic impairment by one method of assessment predicts subsequent stroke risk does not prove the predictive value of a similar method. Different techniques rely on different physiologic mechanisms from which the presence of reduced perfusion pressure is inferred.

Stage II Hemodynamic compromise ("misery perfusion")

In contrast to the inconsistent data for Stage I hemodynamic impairment, two independent studies have demonstrated that Stage II hemodynamic failure, defined as increased OEF, is a powerful independent predictor of subsequent ipsilateral ischemic stroke.[74,107,108]

Yamauchi and colleagues from Kyoto, Japan reported a strong relationship between absolute measurements of increased cerebral OEF and the subsequent risk of recurrent stroke in a small longitudinal study.[107] PET measurements were performed in 40 medically treated patients with symptomatic occlusion or intracranial stenosis of the internal carotid or middle cerebral arterial system treated medically. Patients were divided into two categories based on the mean hemispheric value of OEF in the symptomatic cerebral hemisphere: patients with normal OEF and those with increased OEF. At 1 year following the PET studies, five of seven patients with increased OEF had developed a stroke; four strokes were ipsilateral and one was contralateral. Four of 33 patients with normal OEF had developed a stroke. Two strokes were ipsilateral and two were contralateral. After the first year of follow-up, one ipsilateral stroke and one contralateral stroke occurred, both occurring in patients with normal OEF. This corresponds to a 2-year ipsilateral stroke rate of 57% in the high OEF group and 15% in the normal OEF group.[108]

The St. Louis Carotid Occlusion Study (STLCOS) was designed to test the hypothesis that increased OEF (Stage II hemodynamic failure) in the cerebral hemisphere distal to symptomatic carotid artery occlusion is an independent predictor of the subsequent risk of stroke in medically treated patients.[74] This study was prospective and blinded, and addressed the possible effect of treatment and other risk factors for stroke. Fifteen hospitals within the St. Louis area collaborated to assist with recruitment for this study. Inclusion criteria were (1) occlusion of one or both common or internal carotid arteries demonstrated by contrast angiography, MR angiography, or carotid ultrasound; and (2) transient ischemic neurological deficits (including transient monocular blindness) or mild to moderate permanent ischemic neurological deficits (stroke) in the appropriate carotid artery territory. Exclusion criteria were (1) inability to give informed consent; (2) not legally an adult; (3) failure to meet the following functional standards—self-care for most activities of daily living (may require some assistance), some useful residual function in the affected arm or leg, language comprehension intact, motor aphasia mild or absent, able to handle own oropharyngeal secretions; (4) nonatherosclerotic conditions causing or likely to cause cerebral ischemia—carotid dissection, fibromuscular dysplasia, arteritis, blood dyscrasia, or heart disease as a source of cerebral emboli; (5) any morbid condition likely to lead to death within 5 years; (6) pregnancy; and (7) subsequent cerebrovascular surgery planned that might alter cerebral hemodynamics. Any subsequent cerebrovascular surgery after the initial PET caused the patient to be censored from the study at the time of surgery.

Just prior to PET, each subject underwent neurological evaluation and assessment of the following baseline risk factors: age, gender, hypertension, previous myocardial infarction, diabetes mellitus, smoking, alcohol consumption, and parental death from stroke. The degree of contralateral carotid stenosis and collateral arterial circulation to the ipsilateral MCA was determined from intra-arterial angiograms, if available. Blood samples were collected for determination of hemoglobin, fasting lipid levels (triglyceride, HDL-cholesterol, LDL-cholesterol), and fibrinogen levels. A non-contrast CT scan of the brain was performed if a CT done as part of usual clinical care did not permit accurate definition of infarct location. This CT was used only to determine the site of tissue infarction so as to exclude these regions from subsequent PET analysis (see below). Eighteen normal control subjects aged 19 to 77 (mean $\pm$ standard deviation [SD] = 45 $\pm$ 18) years were recruited by public advertisement.

Regional OEF was measured by PET with the method of Mintun et al. using $H_2^{15}O$, $C^{15}O$, and $O^{15}O$.[109,110] When technical difficulties precluded collection of arterial time activity curves necessary to determine quantitative OEF, the ratio image of the counts in the unprocessed images of $H_2^{15}O$ and $O^{15}O$ was normalized to a whole brain mean of 0.40 and substituted for the quantitative OEF image. All images were then filtered with a three dimensional Gaussian filter to a uniform resolution of 16-mm, full-width, half maximum. For each subject, seven spherical regions of interest 19 mm in diameter were placed in the cortical territory of the MCA in each hemisphere using stereotactic coordinates based on skull X-ray measurements.[85,111] If any portion of a region overlapped a well-demarcated area of reduced oxygen metabolism that corresponded to areas of infarction by CT or MRI, that region and the homologous contralateral region were excluded. The mean OEF for each MCA territory was calculated from the remaining regions and a left/right MCA OEF ratio was calculated. The maximum and minimum ratios from the 18 normal

control subjects were used to define the normal range (0.914–1.082). A separate range of normal for $H_2^{15}O/O^{15}O$ images was determined (0.934–1.062). Patients with left/right OEF ratios outside the normal range were categorized as having Stage II hemodynamic failure in the hemisphere with higher OEF. These categorizations were made without knowledge of the side of the carotid occlusion or of the clinical course of the patients since the initial PET study.

The primary endpoint was subsequent ischemic stroke defined clinically as a neurological deficit of presumed ischemic cerebrovascular cause lasting more than 24 hours in any cerebrovascular territory. Secondary endpoints were ipsilateral ischemic stroke and death. Patients were followed by the study coordinator for the duration of the study through telephone contact every 6 months with the patient or next of kin. Interval medical treatment on a monthly basis was recorded. No information regarding the PET results was provided to the patients, treating physicians, or the investigator responsible for determining endpoints. The occurrence of any symptoms suggesting a stroke was thoroughly evaluated by the designated blinded investigator based on history from the patient or eyewitness and review of medical records ordered by the patient's physician. If necessary, follow-up examination and brain imaging were arranged. All living patients were followed for the duration of the study.

From May 5, 1992, to November 30, 1996, a total of 419 subjects were referred for screening. Eighty-seven subjects were enrolled in the study. Approximately four fifths of the remaining subjects refused to participate and the other one fifth were willing to participate, but were ineligible. Of 87 patients who consented to participate, 81 successfully underwent initial data collection and PET measurements and were enrolled in the study. The diagnosis of carotid artery occlusion was made by intra-arterial contrast angiography in 75 of the 81 subjects.

Of the 81 patients, 39 had Stage II hemodynamic failure (increased OEF) in one hemisphere and 42 did not. The two groups were well matched for most baseline risk factors, except that retinal symptoms were less common in Stage II subjects (3/39 vs 13/26). Arteriographic collateral circulation pattern did not permit distinction between the two groups (Table 1–1). Mean follow-up duration was 31.5 months. Twelve deaths occurred, six in each group. In the 39 Stage II subjects, 12 total and 11 ipsilateral strokes occurred. In the 42 subjects with normal OEF, there were three total and two ipsilateral strokes. The Kaplan-Meier estimates for the rates of subsequent stroke at 1 and 2 years are given in Table 1–2.

The rate of all stroke and ipsilateral ischemic stroke in Stage II subjects was significantly higher than in those with normal OEF ($p = 0.005$ and $p = 0.004$, respectively). After adjustment for 17 baseline patient characteristics and interval medical treatment, the relative risk conferred by Stage II hemodynamic failure was 6.0 (95% CI, 1.7–21.6) for all stroke and 7.3 (95% CI, 1.6–33.4) for ipsilateral stroke. No ipsilateral strokes occurred in those subjects whose most recent symptoms were more than 120 days or who had had retinal

Table 1–2. STROKE RATES IN ST. LOUIS CAROTID OCCLUSION STUDY.

All Stroke	Total Sample (81)	Stage II (39)	Normal OEF (42)
1 year	7.7%	13.2%	2.4%
2 years	19.0%	29.2%	9.0%
Ipsilateral Stroke			
1 year	6.4%	10.6%	2.4%
2 years	15.8%	26.5%	5.3%

symptoms only. The results of medical treatment of Stage II patients were poor and comparable to those reported for medically treated patients with symptomatic severe carotid stenosis.[112]

In the STLCOS, 13 subjects were categorized based on a count-based method of OEF measurement because arterial blood samples could not be obtained. This method used a simple ratio of the counts in the $H_2^{15}O/O^{15}O$ PET images. The ability of the count-based OEF ratio to predict subsequent stroke was examined. The 81 patients were divided into those with count-based OEF ratios outside the normal range and those with normal count-based OEF ratios. Fifty of the 81 patients with symptomatic carotid occlusion were identified as abnormal. All 13 ipsilateral ischemic strokes occurred in the 50 patients with increased count-based OEF ($p = 0.002$, sensitivity 100%, specificity 45.6%). Second, the count-based technique was compared directly to the quantitative method for predicting ipsilateral stroke. In this analysis, the image data of the 68 patients with arterial time activity curves was processed using both count-based and quantitative methods. Using the normal range of values, 31 of the 68 patients were identified as abnormal using quantitative OEF ratios. Seven ipsilateral ischemic strokes occurred in this group of 31 patients, compared to two strokes in the 37 patients with quantitative OEF ratios within the range of normal ($p = 0.025$, sensitivity 77.8%, specificity 59.3%). The count-based OEF ratio was less specific (specificity 45.7%) and more sensitive (sensitivity 100%) than the quantitative method. Forty-one patients were categorized as abnormal and all strokes occurred in this group ($p = 0.0048$). Comparison of the count-based OEF ratio to the quantitative OEF ratio for each of the 68 patients demonstrated no significant difference by paired t-test analysis ($p = 0.299$). The average absolute difference between count-based OEF and OEF ratios was 0.0345 (95% confidence limit $= \pm0.0091$). Receiver operating curves were generated for both methods. The area under the receiver operating curve for the count-based OEF method (0.815) was greater than the quantitative OEF method (0.737), indicating superior accuracy.[113] A subsequent analysis compared these two techniques that rely on asymmetries of OEF to the technique based on absolute OEF values used in the Kyoto study. All three methods were predictive of stroke risk in univariate analysis. Only the count-based method remained significant in multivariate analysis. The area under the ROC curve was greatest

for the count-based ratio: 0.815 versus 0.769 (absolute) and 0.737 (ratios of absolute).[114]

At this time, it is not possible to identify a non-PET method for assessing OEF that has sufficient proven sensitivity and specificity to substitute for PET. The correlation between the CBF response to vasodilatory agents and increased OEF has been somewhat variable and inconsistent.[92,93,115–124] In general, these studies have shown that measurements of vascular reactivity have high sensitivity but poor positive predictive value for identifying increased OEF.[123] Certain MR pulse sequences are sensitive to the amount of deoxyhemoglobin in blood (blood oxygen level dependent [BOLD]).[125–127] They are commonly used to identify changes in the regional blood flow:metabolism ratio with physiologic brain activation, but their application to static measurements of brain oxygenation has proven more difficult. The signal contribution from non-vascular tissue and the effect of variation in CBV have made quantitative measurement of OEF difficult, although research in this area is being actively pursued.[128–130] BOLD MRI measurements did not correlate well with PET measurements of OEF in patients with carotid occlusion in a previous study.[131]

Other Hemodynamic Classification Schemes

Nemoto and colleagues have postulated that patients who initially have CPP below the autoregulatory limit with increased OEF (Stage II hemodynamic failure) may suffer subsequent ischemic neuronal damage that reduces $CMRO_2$ and normalizes OEF, but without any improvement in CPP. They refer to this as Stage III.[121] The plausibility of this scenario is supported by PET studies that show evidence for selective neuronal necrosis in brain regions with low $CMRO_2$ and normal OEF and the progressive development of selective neuronal necrosis in areas with initially high OEF.[88,132] Nemoto and colleagues propose that, while these patients would look like Stage I hemodynamic compromise (impaired response to vasodilatory stimuli, normal OEF), their stroke risk would in fact be similar to that of Stage II patients due to the persistently low CPP.[121] Thus according to this construct, there should be a group of patients with normal OEF and impaired vasoreactivity who are at high risk for stroke. This does not appear to be the case. In the STLCOS, none of the 13 ipsilateral strokes that occurred in follow-up of 3.1 years occurred in patients with increased CBV and normal OEF.[76] The two patients with normal OEF who had ipsilateral strokes were among the eight patients with the highest OEF values in the normal OEF group of 41 subjects. Furthermore, in this cohort of patients, OEF was predictive of subsequent ipsilateral stroke as a continuous variable, indicating that the higher the OEF the higher the risk of stroke.[114]

Kuroda and colleagues have proposed a four-stage classification based on quantitative SPECT measurements of baseline CBF and cerebrovascular reactivity to acetazolamide or CO_2: Type 1—normal baseline CBF and normal cerebrovascular reactivity; Type 2—normal baseline CBF and reduced cerebrovascular reactivity; Type 3—reduced baseline CBF and reduced cerebrovascular reactivity; and Type 4—reduced baseline CBF and normal cerebrovascular reactivity.[88] Type 1 patients are considered to have a normal CPP because of a well-developed collateral circulation corresponding to Stage 0. Type 2 patients are believed to have moderately reduced CPP corresponding to Stage I. Type 3 patients are believed to have inadequate CPP to maintain a normal resting CBF corresponding to Stage II. Type 4 have reduced oxygen metabolism probably due to ischemia-related neuronal loss with normal hemodynamics corresponding to Stage 0.[88,94] The value of this scheme lies in the identification of the high risk of stroke in Type 3 patients. This is based on a small study of only 11 subjects,[94] and runs counter to the data from Yonas and colleagues who did not find that low baseline CBF in combination with reduced cerebrovascular reactivity was sensitive indicator of stroke risk.[95,99] It also is at odds with the study by Ogasawara et al., who found that quantitative reduced cerebrovascular reactivity alone was sufficient to identify a high-risk group.[101] Thus the value of a four-stage classification based on quantitative SPECT measurements of both baseline CBF and cerebrovascular reactivity instead of a two-stage system based on quantitative cerebrovascular reactivity alone remains to be established.

RANDOMIZED SURGICAL REVASCULARIZATION TRIALS BASED ON HEMODYNAMIC CRITERIA

The findings of the Kyoto and St. Louis studies reawakened interest in extracranial-to-intracranial (EC-IC) bypass for stroke prevention, an approach that had largely been abandoned after the publication of the negative EC-IC Bypass Trial in 1985.[133] The Kyoto and St. Louis studies demonstrated that Stage II hemodynamic failure (increased OEF) distal to a symptomatic occluded carotid artery is an independent predictor of subsequent ischemic stroke. As first demonstrated by Baron in 1981, EC-IC bypass surgery will return hemispheric OEF ratios to normal in patients with increased OEF distal to an occluded carotid artery (Figure 1–5).[87,134–136] The implication of these data is that EC-IC bypass is the logical treatment for these patients with high OEF and high stroke risk on medical therapy. Why does this evidence suggest that EC-IC bypass should be effective in reducing stroke in patients with symptomatic carotid occlusion when the EC-IC Bypass Trial, a large, prospective, and randomized trial of EC-IC bypass versus aspirin in similar patients, failed to demonstrate a benefit? A mathematical simulation using the data from the STLCOS provides the

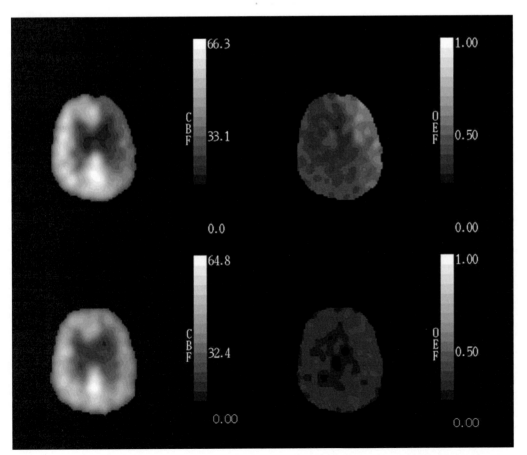

Figure 1–5. Improved oxygen extraction (OEF) after extracranial-intracranial (EC-IC) bypass surgery in a 69-year-old man with symptomatic occlusion of the right carotid artery. The baseline PET images (top row) demonstrate reduced cerebral blood flow (CBF, left) and increased OEF in the right hemisphere (right portion). A second study performed 35 days after EC-IC bypass shows that ipsilateral CBF has improved and OEF has normalized (bottom row).

(From Powers WJ, Zazulia AR. The use of positron emission tomography in cerebrovascular disease. Neuroimaging Clin N Am 2003;13: 741–758; with permission.)

explanation. In STLCOS, the 2-year rate for all stroke was 19% for this entire sample of medically treated patients. If surgery has the same 12.2% morbidity/mortality as in the EC-IC Bypass Trial and reduces the stroke rate in the high OEF patients to that of low OEF patients (9.0%), but does not change the stroke rate in low OEF patients, then the overall stroke rate in the operated group at 2 years will be 9.0% + 12.2% = 21.2%, slightly worse than the medical group. These simulated results at 2 years are remarkably similar to the 5-year results for carotid occlusion in the EC-IC Bypass Trial of 29% for the medical groups and 31% for the surgical group.[133] This analysis underscores the importance of identifying a subgroup of patients at high risk who are likely to benefit and restricting surgery to them.

Two new randomized trials of EC-IC bypass surgery were begun, one in Japan and one in the United States, with patient selection based on hemodynamic criteria.

The Japanese EC-IC Bypass Trial (JET)

The Japanese EC-IC Bypass Trial (JET) uses the combination of reduced baseline CBF and reduced acetazolamide cerebrovascular reactivity measured with quantitative SPECT as eligibility criteria. This trial enrolled 196 patients with major cerebral artery occlusive disease from 1998 to 2002. A second interim analysis with data through January 2002 reported primary endpoints in 14 of 98 medically treated patients and five of 98 surgically treated patients ($p = 0.046$ by Kaplan-Meier analysis).[137] Final results of the 2-year follow-up were due in 2004. However, to date, there has been no publication of the final results.

The Carotid Occlusion Surgery Study (COSS)

This is a randomized, controlled clinical trial that tests the hypothesis that EC-IC bypass when added to best medical therapy can reduce subsequent ipsilateral ischemic stroke at 2 years in patients with recently symptomatic ICA occlusion and increased OEF. The participating centers and data management center are unblinded and the primary clinical coordinating center personnel (principal investigator and project manager) are blinded. This study is funded by the National Institutes of Health.

Final eligibility for randomization is based on fulfilling three different eligibility categories:

1. Clinical
2. PET
3. Arteriographic

Participants who fulfill clinical entry criteria and who have carotid occlusion by vascular imaging (Doppler ultrasound, magnetic resonance angiography, CT angiography, or intra-arterial catheter arteriography) are eligible for enrollment and proceed to PET. If PET meets criteria for ipsilateral increased oxygen extraction, then arteriographic criteria must be met for a participant to be eligible for randomization. Intra-arterial catheter arteriography is required prior to randomization to document carotid occlusion and both extracranial and intracranial arteries suitable for anastomosis.

Initial clinical and vascular imaging criteria to determine PET eligibility

Inclusion criteria

1. Vascular imaging demonstrating occlusion of an ICA.
2. (Criterion eliminated.)
3. Transient ischemic attack (TIA) or ischemic stroke in the hemispheric carotid territory of an occluded ICA.
4. Most recent qualifying TIA or stroke occurring within 120 days prior to performance date of PET.
5. Modified Barthel Index $\geq 12/20$.
6. Language comprehension intact, motor aphasia mild or absent such that effective communication with the participant is possible.
7. Age 18 to 85 years inclusive.
8. Competent to give informed consent.
9. Legally an adult.
10. Geographically accessible and reliable for follow-up.

Exclusion criteria

1. Nonatherosclerotic carotid vascular disease.
2. Blood dyscrasias: *only* polycythemia vera, essential thrombocytosis, and sickle cell disease (SS or SC).
3. Known cardioembolic heart disease: *only* prosthetic valve(s), infective endocarditis, left atrial or ventricular thrombus, sick sinus syndrome, myxoma, or cardiomyopathy with ejection fraction <25%.
4. Other nonatherosclerotic condition likely to cause focal cerebral ischemia.
5. (Criterion eliminated.)
6. Any condition likely to lead to death within 2 years.
7. Other neurological disease that would confound follow-up assessment.
8. Pregnancy.
9. Subsequent cerebrovascular surgery planned that might alter cerebral hemodynamics or stroke risk.
10. Any condition that the participating surgeon's judgment makes the participant an unsuitable surgical candidate.
11. Concurrent participation in any other experimental treatment trial.
12. Participation within the previous 12 months in any experimental study that included exposure to ionizing radiation.

13. Acute, progressing, or unstable neurological deficit.

14. If supplemental arteriography is required, allergy to iodine or X-ray contrast media, serum creatinine >3.0 mg/dl or other contraindication to arteriography.

15. If aspirin is to be used as antithrombotic therapy in the perioperative period, those with allergy or contra-indication to aspirin are ineligible.

16. Medical indication for treatment with anticoagulant drugs, ticlopidine, clopidogrel, or other antithrombotic medications such that these medications cannot be replaced with aspirin in the perioperative period as deemed necessary by the COSS neurosurgeon if the participant is randomized to surgical treatment.

17. Uncontrolled diabetes mellitus (FBS > 300 mg%/16.7 mmol/L).

18. Uncontrolled hypertension (systolic BP > 180, diastolic BP > 110).

19. Uncontrolled hypotension (diastolic BP < 65).

20. Unstable angina.

PET criteria

Ipsilateral: contralateral OEF ratio in the MCA territory > 1.130 determined from the ratio image of $O^{15}O/H_2^{15}O$ counts.

Arteriographic criteria

Intra-arterial catheter contrast arteriography documenting the following:

1. Occlusion of the symptomatic ICA.

2. Intracranial and extracranial arteries suitable for anastomosis in the opinion of the participating surgeon.

Randomized treatment assignments are based on a permuted block strategy stratified by center. For participants who were receiving antithrombotic drugs other than aspirin prior to randomization, surgery is performed as soon as the participating neurosurgeon considers the bleeding risk to be acceptable. Participants randomized to surgery undergo microsurgical end-to-side anastomosis of the optimal branch (frontal or parietal) of the superficial temporal branch to the largest most easily exposed cortical branch of the middle cerebral artery as it emerges from the posterior one-third of the Sylvian fissure. Participating surgeons must (1) demonstrate proficiency in performing EC-IC bypass surgery (STA-MCA cortical branch anastomosis and/or extracranial carotid artery to middle cerebral artery vein graft anastomosis) by demonstrating at least 80% graft patency and less than or equal to 10% stroke and death at 1 month in at least 10 consecutive EC-IC bypass surgeries, *or* (2) have attended the January 2002 training workshop, *or* (3) have been observed during the performance of at least one STA-MCA operation by the surgical principal investigator or his designate. A provisional certification may be issued such that this first STA-MCA operation under the observation may be performed on a patient

enrolled in the trial. All surgical patients are seen 30 days post-operatively. All surgical patients receive Doppler studies to ensure graft patency, and PET to document reversal of hemodynamic abnormalities at 30 days.

All patients are seen 30 days after randomization and at 3-month intervals after randomization for 2 years. At each follow-up examination a neurological history and exam tailored to identifying new stroke is performed. Current medications are recorded. NIHSS, Barthel Index, Rankin Scale, and Stroke Specific Quality of Life assessment are performed at every visit.[138–141] Doppler examination to ensure graft patency is performed for all surgical patients.

Choice of long-term antithrombotic treatment is at the discretion of the participant's personal physician. When deemed appropriate by the surgeon, participants randomized to surgical therapy will return to the antithrombotic treatment preferred by their physicians. Recommendations for antithrombotic treatment follow recommendations for antiplatelet treatment of atherothrombotic TIA of the Ad Hoc Committee on Guidelines for the Management of Transient Ischemic Attacks, Stroke Council, American Heart Association.[142] Efficacy of risk factor intervention is measured at each return visit in the following ways:

1. Smoking: question. Target: not smoking

2. Hypertension: cuff blood pressure. Target systolic < 130 mm Hg, diastolic < 85 mm Hg

3. Hypercholesterolemia: fasting blood cholesterol and triglyceride measurements. Target: low-density lipoprotein < 100 mg/dl, triglycerides < 150 mg/dl

4. Diabetes mellitus: hemoglobin A1C levels. Target < 7.0%

The primary endpoint in the surgical group is the combination of the following: (1) the occurrence of ipsilateral ischemic stroke from randomization to surgery, (2) the occurrence of all stroke and death from surgery through 30 days postoperation, and (3) the occurrence of ipsilateral ischemic stroke within 2 years of randomization. Those in the surgery group who are never operated on by the end of the trial would be evaluated in the same way as the nonsurgical group. The primary endpoint in the nonsurgical group is the combination of the following: (1) the occurrence of all stroke and death from randomization through 30 days post randomization, and (2) the occurrence of ipsilateral ischemic stroke within 2 years of randomization. The primary analysis will be intent-to-treat. A two-sample comparison for the 2-year stroke rate between the surgical and nonsurgical groups will be conducted to test the two-sided hypothesis at a significance level of 5.0%.

Secondary endpoints are all stroke, disabling stroke, fatal stroke, death, Rankin Scale, NIHSS, Barthel Index, and Stroke Specific Quality of Life assessment. Ipsilateral ischemic stroke is defined as the clinical diagnosis of a focal neurological deficit due to cerebral ischemia clinically localizable within the ICA territory distally to the symptomatic occluded ICA that lasts for more than 24 hours. Final adjudication of stroke endpoints (ipsilateral stroke, nonipsilateral stroke, fatal stroke) is by a three-person blinded adjudication panel supplied with information that has been sanitized to remove all information regarding treatment assignment. Information regarding each possible endpoint is sent to two adjudicators. If they agree, the decision is final. If the original two adjudicators do not agree, the third member serves as a tie-breaker.

Adjusting for anticipated 2-year mortality, 372 patients (186 in each group) will provide 90% power to detect the anticipated difference (40% vs 24.2%). Assuming 25% to 30% of PET scans will demonstrate increased OEF, this will require enrolling a total of 1400 clinically eligible subjects for PET. COSS is currently under way in 40 centers in the United States and Canada. The first patient was randomized in 2002. Results are expected in 2015.

CONCLUSIONS

Since the publication of the negative results of the EC-IC Bypass Trial, advances in neuroimaging, especially PET, have greatly increased our understanding of cerebral hemodynamics in human cerebrovascular disease. In turn, this has led to several studies that have shown a significant association between measurements of cerebral hemodynamics and the risk for recurrent stroke. These findings, especially those for PET measurements of OEF, have led to two new clinical trials of EC-IC bypass for stroke prevention, each using different neuroimaging eligibility criteria to identify patients at high risk for recurrent stroke due to hemodynamic mechanisms. The results of these studies will determine whether these types of hemodynamic measurements have clinical value in selecting patients for cerebrovascular revascularization.

ACKNOWLEDGMENTS

This work was supported by U.S. Public Health Service grants NS42167 and NS35966, and the H. Houston Merritt Professorship of Neurology at the University of North Carolina, Chapel Hill.

REFERENCES

1. Cohen PJ, Alexander SC, Smith TC, et al: Effects of hypoxia and normocarbia on cerebral blood flow and metabolism in conscious man, *J Appl Physiol* 23(2):183–189, 1967.
2. Madsen PL, Holm S, Herning M, et al: Average blood flow and oxygen uptake in the human brain during resting wakefulness: A critical appraisal of the Kety-Schmidt technique, *J Cereb Blood Flow Metab* 13:646–655, 1993.
3. Gottstein U, Bernsmeier A, Sedlmeyer I: Der Kohlenhydratstoffwechsel des menschlichen Gehirns bei Schlafmittelvergiftung, *Klin Wschr* 41:943–948, 1963.
4. Scheinberg P, Stead EA: The cerebral blood flow in male subjects as measured by the nitrous oxide technique: normal values for blood flow, oxygen utilization, glucose utilization and peripheral resistance, with observations on the effect of tilting and anxiety, *J Clin Invest* 28:1163–1171, 1949.
5. Glenn TC, Kelly DF, Boscardin WJ, et al: Energy dysfunction as a predictor of outcome after moderate or severe head injury: indices of oxygen, glucose, and lactate metabolism, *J Cereb Blood Flow Metab* 23(10):1239–1250, 2003.
6. McHenry LC Jr, Merory J, Bass E, et al: Xenon-133 inhalation method for regional cerebral blood flow measurements: normal values and test-retest results, *Stroke* 9(4):396–399, 1978.
7. Sette G, Baron JC, Mazoyer B, et al: Local brain haemodynamics and oxygen metabolism in cerebrovascular disease. Positron emission tomography, *Brain* 112(Pt 4):931–951, 1989.
8. Baron JC, Rougemont D, Soussaline F, et al: Local interrelationships of cerebral oxygen consumption and glucose utilization in normal subjects and in ischemic stroke patients: a positron tomography study, *J Cereb Blood Flow Metab* 4(2):140–149, 1984.
9. Lebrun-Grandie P, Baron JC, Soussaline F, et al: Coupling between regional blood flow and oxygen utilization in the normal human brain. A study with positron tomography and oxygen 15, *Arch Neurol* 40(4):230–236, 1983.
10. Leenders KL, Perani D, Lammertsma AA, et al: Cerebral blood flow, blood volume and oxygen utilization. Normal values and effect of age, *Brain* 113(Pt 1):27–47, 1990.
11. Kety SS: Human cerebral blood flow and oxygen consumption as related to aging, *J Chron Dis* 3:478–486, 1956.
12. Pantano P, Baron JC, Lebrun-Grandie P, et al: Regional cerebral blood flow and oxygen consumption in human aging, *Stroke* 15(4):635–641, 1984.
13. Dastur DK: Cerebral blood flow and metabolism in normal human aging, pathological aging, and senile dementia, *J Cereb Blood Flow Metab* 5(1):1–9, 1985.
14. Kuhl DE, Metter EJ, Riege WH, et al: The effect of normal aging on patterns of local cerebral glucose utilization, *Ann Neurol* 15(Suppl):S133–2137, 1984.
15. Marchal G, Rioux P, Petit-Taboue MC, et al: Regional cerebral oxygen consumption, blood flow, and blood volume in healthy human aging, *Arch Neurol* 49(10):1013–1020, 1992.
16. Yamaguchi T, Kanno I, Uemura K, et al: Reduction in regional cerebral metabolic rate of oxygen during human aging, *Stroke* 17(6):1220–1228, 1986.
17. de Leon MJ, George AE, Ferris SH, et al: Positron emission tomography and computed tomography assessments of the aging human brain, *J Comput Assist Tomogr* 8(1):88–94, 1984.
18. Duara R, Margolin RA, Robertson-Tchabo EA, et al: Cerebral glucose utilization, as measured with positron emission tomography in 21 resting healthy men between the ages of 21 and 83 years, *Brain* 106(Pt 3):761–775, 1983.
19. Duara R, Grady C, Haxby J, et al: Human brain glucose utilization and cognitive function in relation to age, *Ann Neurol* 16(6):703–713, 1984.
20. Yoshii F, Barker WW, Chang JY, et al: Sensitivity of cerebral glucose metabolism to age, gender, brain volume, brain atrophy, and cerebrovascular risk factors, *J Cereb Blood Flow Metab* 8(5):654–661, 1988.
21. Meltzer CC, Cantwell MN, Greer PJ, et al: Does cerebral blood flow decline in healthy aging? A PET study with partial-volume correction, *J Nucl Med* 41(11):1842–1848, 2000.
22. Ibanez V, Pietrini P, Furey ML, et al: Resting state brain glucose metabolism is not reduced in normotensive healthy men during aging, after correction for brain atrophy, *Brain Res Bull* 63(2):147–154, 2004.
23. Astrup J, Sorensen PM, Sorensen HR: Oxygen and glucose consumption related to Na+-K+ transport in canine brain, *Stroke* 12(6):726–730, 1981.
24. Bering EAJ, Taren JA, McMurrey JD, et al: Studies on hypothermia in monkeys, II. The effect of hypothermia on the general physiology and cerebral metabolism of monkeys in the hypothermic state, *Surg Gynecol Obstet* 102:134–138, 1956.
25. Nilsson L, Siesjo BK: The effect of phenobarbitone anaesthesia on blood flow and oxygen consumption in the rat brain, *Acta Anaesthesiol Scand Suppl* 57:18–24, 1975.

26. Sokoloff L: Relationships among local functional activity, energy metabolism, and blood flow in the central nervous system, *Fed Proc* 40(8):2311–2316, 1981.

27. Fox PT, Raichle ME: Focal physiological uncoupling of cerebral blood flow and oxidative metabolism during somatosensory stimulation in human subjects, *Proc Natl Acad Sci U S A* 83(4):1140–1144, 1986.

28. Fox PT, Raichle ME, Mintun MA, et al: Nonoxidative glucose consumption during focal physiologic neural activity, *Science* 241 (4864):462–464, 1988.

29. Kety SS, Schmidt CF: The effects of altered arterial tensions of carbon dioxide and oxygen on cerebral blood flow and cerebral oxygen consumption of normal young men, *J Clin Invest* 27:484–492, 1948.

30. Raichle ME, Posner JB, Plum F: Cerebral blood flow during and after hyperventilation, *Arch Neurol* 23(5):394–403, 1970.

31. Shimojyo S, Scheinberg P, Kogure K, et al: The effects of graded hypoxia upon transient cerebral blood flow and oxygen consumption, *Neurology* 18(2):127–133, 1968.

32. Buck A, Schirlo C, Jasinsky V, et al: Changes of cerebral blood flow during short-term exposure to normobaric hypoxia, *J Cereb Blood Flow Metab* 18(8):906–910, 1998.

33. Lassen NA: Cerebral blood flow and oxygen consumption in man, *Physiol Rev* 39:183–238, 1959.

34. Brown MM, Wade JP, Marshall J: Fundamental importance of arterial oxygen content in the regulation of cerebral blood flow in man, *Brain* 108(Pt 1):81–93, 1985.

35. Todd MM, Wu B, Maktabi M, et al: Cerebral blood flow and oxygen delivery during hypoxemia and hemodilution: role of arterial oxygen content, *Am J Physiol* 267(5 Pt 2):H2025–H2031, 1994.

36. Mintun MA, Lundstrom BN, Snyder AZ, et al: Blood flow and oxygen delivery to human brain during functional activity: theoretical modeling and experimental data, *Proc Natl Acad Sci U S A* 98 (12):6859–6864, 2001.

37. Brown MM, Marshall J: Regulation of cerebral blood flow in response to changes in blood viscosity, *Lancet* 1(8429):604–609, 1985.

38. Brown MM, Marshall J: Effect of plasma exchange on blood viscosity and cerebral blood flow, *Br Med J (Clin Res Ed)* 284(6331): 1733–1736, 1982.

39. Paulson OB, Parving HH, Olesen J, et al: Influence of carbon monoxide and of hemodilution on cerebral blood flow and blood gases in man, *J Appl Physiol* 35(1):111–116, 1973.

40. Rebel A, Lenz C, Krieter H, et al: Oxygen delivery at high blood viscosity and decreased arterial oxygen content to brains of conscious rats, *Am J Physiol Heart Circ Physiol* 280(6):H2591–H2597, 2001.

41. Hino A, Ueda S, Mizukawa N, et al: Effect of hemodilution on cerebral hemodynamics and oxygen metabolism, *Stroke* 23(3):423–426, 1992.

42. Tallroth G, Ryding E, Agardh CD: Regional cerebral blood flow in normal man during insulin-induced hypoglycemia and in the recovery period following glucose infusion, *Metabolism* 41(7): 717–721, 1992.

43. Tallroth G, Ryding E, Agardh CD: The influence of hypoglycaemia on regional cerebral blood flow and cerebral volume in type 1 (insulin-dependent) diabetes mellitus, *Diabetologia* 36(6):530–535, 1993.

44. Neil HA, Gale EA, Hamilton SJ, et al: Cerebral blood flow increases during insulin-induced hypoglycaemia in type 1 (insulin-dependent) diabetic patients and control subjects, *Diabetologia* 30(5):305–309, 1987.

45. Kerr D, Stanley JC, Barron M, et al: Symmetry of cerebral blood flow and cognitive responses to hypoglycaemia in humans, *Diabetologia* 36(1):73–78, 1993.

46. Eckert B, Ryding E, Agardh CD: Sustained elevation of cerebral blood flow after hypoglycaemia in normal man, *Diabetes Res Clin Pract* 40 (2):91–100, 1998.

47. Boyle PJ, Nagy RJ, O'Connor AM, et al: Adaptation in brain glucose uptake following recurrent hypoglycemia, *Proc Natl Acad Sci U S A* 91(20):9352–9356, 1994.

48. Chen JL, Wei L, Acuff V, et al: Slightly altered permeability-surface area products imply some cerebral capillary recruitment during hypercapnia, *Microvasc Res* 48(2):190–211, 1994.

49. Chen JL, Wei L, Bereczki D, et al: Nicotine raises the influx of permeable solutes across the rat blood-brain barrier with little or no capillary recruitment, *J Cereb Blood Flow Metab* 15(4):687–698, 1995.

50. Paulson OB, Strandgaard S, Edvinsson L: Cerebral autoregulation, *Cerebrovasc Brain Metab Rev* 2(2):161–192, 1990.

51. MacKenzie ET, Farrar JK, Fitch W, et al: Effects of hemorrhagic hypotension on the cerebral circulation. I. Cerebral blood flow and pial arteriolar caliber, *Stroke* 10(6):711–718, 1979.

52. Symon L, Pasztor E, Dorsch NW, et al: Physiological responses of local areas of the cerebral circulation in experimental primates determined by the method of hydrogen clearance, *Stroke* 4(4):632–642, 1973.

53. Strandgaard S, Olesen J, Skinhoj E, et al: Autoregulation of brain circulation in severe arterial hypertension, *Br Med J* 1(852):507–510, 1973.

54. Strandgaard S: Autoregulation of cerebral blood flow in hypertensive patients. The modifying influence of prolonged antihypertensive treatment on the tolerance to acute, drug-induced hypotension, *Circulation* 53(4):720–727, 1976.

55. Schmidt JF, Waldemar G, Vorstrup S, et al: Computerized analysis of cerebral blood flow autoregulation in humans: validation of a method for pharmacologic studies, *J Cardiovasc Pharmacol* 15(6):983–988, 1990.

56. Dirnagl U, Pulsinelli W: Autoregulation of cerebral blood flow in experimental focal brain ischemia, *J Cereb Blood Flow Metab* 10:327–336, 1990.

57. Heistad DD, Kontos HE: Cerebral circulation. In Shepherd JT, Aboud FM, editors: *Handbook of physiology, Section 2*, Vol. 3, Pt. 1, Bethesda, MD, 1983, American Physiological Society, pp 137–182.

58. Maruyama M, Shimoji K, Ichikawa T, et al: The effects of extreme hemodilutions on the autoregulation of cerebral blood flow, electroencephalogram and cerebral metabolic rate of oxygen in the dog, *Stroke* 16(4):675–679, 1985.

59. Haggendal E, Johansson B: Effect of arterial carbon dioxide tension and oxygen saturation on cerebral blood flow autoregulation in dogs, *Acta Physiol Scand* 66:27–53, 1965.

60. Ledingham JG, Rajagopalan B: Cerebral complications in the treatment of accelerated hypertension, *Q J Med* 48(189):25–41, 1979.

61. van Beek AH, Claassen JA, Rikkert MG, et al: Cerebral autoregulation: an overview of current concepts and methodology with special focus on the elderly, *J Cereb Blood Flow Metab* 28(6):1071–1085, 2008.

62. Dawson SL, Panerai RB, Potter JF: Serial changes in static and dynamic cerebral autoregulation after acute ischaemic stroke, *Cerebrovasc Dis* 16(1):69–75, 2003.

63. Steiner LA, Coles JP, Johnston AJ, et al: Assessment of cerebrovascular autoregulation in head-injured patients: a validation study, *Stroke* 34(10):2404–2409, 2003.

64. Boysen G: Cerebral hemodynamics in carotid surgery, *Acta Neurol Scand Suppl* 52:3–86, 1973.

65. Powers WJ: Cerebral hemodynamics in ischemic cerebrovascular disease, *Ann Neurol* 29(3):231–240, 1991.

66. Schumann P, Touzani O, Young AR, et al: Evaluation of the ratio of cerebral blood flow to cerebral blood volume as an index of local cerebral perfusion pressure, *Brain* 121(Pt 7):1369–1379, 1998.

67. Wiedeman MP: Dimensions of blood vessels from distributing artery to collecting vein, *Circ Res* 12:375–378, 1963.

68. Hilal SK: Cerebral hemodynamics assessed by angiography. In Newton TH, Potts DG, editors: *Radiology of the skull and brain. Angiography*, vol. 2, Book 1, St. Louis, 1974, CV Mosby Company, pp 1049–1085.

69. Auer LM, Ishiyama N, Pucher R: Cerebrovascular response to intracranial hypertension, *Acta Neurochir (Wien)* 84(3–4):124–128, 1987.

70. Kato Y, Auer LM: Cerebrovascular response to elevation of ventricular pressure, *Acta Neurochir (Wien)* 98(3–4):184–188, 1989.

71. Grubb RL Jr, Phelps ME, Raichle ME, et al: The effects of arterial blood pressure on the regional cerebral blood volume by x-ray fluorescence, *Stroke* 4(3):390–399, 1973.

72. Grubb RL Jr, Raichle ME, Phelps ME, et al: Effects of increased intracranial pressure on cerebral blood volume, blood flow, and oxygen utilization in monkeys, *J Neurosurg* 43(4):385–398, 1975.

73. Ferrari M, Wilson DA, Hanley DF, et al: Effects of graded hypotension on cerebral blood flow, blood volume, and mean transit time in dogs, *Am J Physiol* 262(6 Pt 2):H1908–H1914, 1992.

74. Grubb RL Jr, Derdeyn CP, Fritsch SM, et al: Importance of hemodynamic factors in the prognosis of symptomatic carotid occlusion, *JAMA* 280(12):1055–1060, 1998.

75. Zaharchuk G, Mandeville JB, Bogdanov AA Jr, et al: Cerebrovascular dynamics of autoregulation and hypoperfusion. An MRI study of CBF and changes in total and microvascular cerebral blood volume during hemorrhagic hypotension, *Stroke* 30(10):2197–2204, 1999.

76. Derdeyn CP, Videen TO, Yundt KD, et al: Variability of cerebral blood volume and oxygen extraction: stages of cerebral hemodynamic impairment revisited, *Brain* 125:595–607, 2002.

77. Gibbs JM, Wise RJ, Leenders KL, et al: Evaluation of cerebral perfusion reserve in patients with carotid-artery occlusion, *Lancet* 1 (8372):310–314, 1984.

78. Powers WJ: Is the ratio of cerebral blood volume to cerebral blood flow a reliable indicator of cerebral perfusion pressure, *J Cereb Blood Flow Metab* 13(Suppl 1):S325, 1993.

79. Grubb RL Jr, Raichle ME, Eichling JO, et al: The effects of changes in $PaCO_2$ on cerebral blood volume, blood flow, and vascular mean transit time, *Stroke* 5(5):630–639, 1974.

80. Sillesen H, Schroeder T, Steenberg HJ, et al: Doppler examination of the periorbital arteries adds valuable hemodynamic information in carotid artery disease, *Ultrasound Med Biol* 13(4):177–181, 1987.

81. Derdeyn CP, Shaibani A, Moran CJ, et al: Lack of correlation between pattern of collateralization and misery perfusion in patients with carotid occlusion, *Stroke* 30(5):1025–1032, 1999.

82. Lassen NA, Palvolgyi R: Cerebral steal during hypercapnia and the inverse reaction during hypocapnia observed with the 133 xenon technique in man, *Scand J Clin Lab Invest* 22(Suppl 102):13D, 1968.

83. Vernieri F, Pasqualetti P, Matteis M, et al: Effect of collateral blood flow and cerebral vasomotor reactivity on the outcome of carotid artery occlusion, *Stroke* 32(7):1552–1558, 2001.

84. Yamauchi H, Kudoh T, Sugimoto K, et al: Pattern of collaterals, type of infarcts, and haemodynamic impairment in carotid artery occlusion, *J Neurol Neurosurg Psychiatry* 75(12):1697–1701, 2004.

85. Powers WJ, Press GA, Grubb RL Jr, et al: The effect of hemodynamically significant carotid artery disease on the hemodynamic status of the cerebral circulation, *Ann Intern Med* 106(1):27–34, 1987.

86. Baron JC, Bousser MG, Comar D, et al: Human hemispheric infarction studied by positron emission tomography and the 15O continuous inhalation technique. In Caille JM, Salamon G, editors: *Computerized Tomography*, New York, 1980, Springer-Verlag, pp 231–237.

87. Baron JC, Bousser MG, Rey A, et al: Reversal of focal "misery-perfusion syndrome" by extra-intracranial arterial bypass in hemodynamic cerebral ischemia. A case study with 15O positron emission tomography, *Stroke* 12(4):454–459, 1981.

88. Kuroda S, Shiga T, Ishikawa T, et al: Reduced blood flow and preserved vasoreactivity characterize oxygen hypometabolism due to incomplete infarction in occlusive carotid artery diseases, *J Nucl Med* 45(6):943–949, 2004.

89. Kazumata K, Tanaka N, Ishikawa T, et al: Dissociation of vasoreactivity to acetazolamide and hypercapnia. Comparative study in patients with chronic occlusive major cerebral artery disease, *Stroke* 27 (11):2052–2058, 1996.

90. Inao S, Tadokoro M, Nishino M, et al: Neural activation of the brain with hemodynamic insufficiency, *J Cereb Blood Flow Metab* 18 (9):960–967, 1998.

91. Pindzola RR, Balzer JR, Nemoto EM, et al: Cerebrovascular reserve in patients with carotid occlusive disease assessed by stable xenon-enhanced ct cerebral blood flow and transcranial Doppler, *Stroke* 32(8):1811–1817, 2001.

92. Hirano T, Minematsu K, Hasegawa Y, et al: Acetazolamide reactivity on 123I-IMP single photon emission computed tomography in patients with major cerebral artery occlusive disease: correlation with positron emission tomography parameters, *J Cereb Blood Flow Metab* 14(5):763–770, 1994.

93. Nariai T, Suzuki R, Hirakawa K, et al: Vascular reserve in chronic cerebral ischemia measured by the acetazolamide challenge test: comparison with positron emission tomography, *AJNR Am J Neuroradiol* 16(3):563–570, 1995.

94. Kuroda S, Houkin K, Kamiyama H, et al: Long-term prognosis of medically treated patients with internal carotid or middle cerebral artery occlusion: can acetazolamide test predict it? *Stroke* 32 (9):2110–2116, 2001.

95. Webster MW, Makaroun MS, Steed DL, et al: Compromised cerebral blood flow reactivity is a predictor of stroke in patients with symptomatic carotid artery occlusive disease, *J Vasc Surg* 21(2):338–344, 1995.

96. Yokota C, Hasegawa Y, Minematsu K, et al: Effect of acetazolamide reactivity on long-term outcome in patients with major cerebral artery occlusive diseases, *Stroke* 29(3):640–644, 1998.

97. Vernieri F, Pasqualetti P, Passarelli F, et al: Outcome of carotid artery occlusion is predicted by cerebrovascular reactivity, *Stroke* 30 (3):593–598, 1999.

98. Klijn CJ, Kappelle LJ, van Huffelen AC, et al: Recurrent ischemia in symptomatic carotid occlusion: prognostic value of hemodynamic factors, *Neurology* 55(12):1806–1812, 2000.

99. Yonas H, Smith HA, Durham SR, et al: Increased stroke risk predicted by compromised cerebral blood flow reactivity, *J Neurosurg* 79(4):483–489, 1993.

100. Ogasawara K, Ogawa A, Terasaki K, et al: Use of cerebrovascular reactivity in patients with symptomatic major cerebral artery occlusion to predict 5-year outcome: comparison of xenon-133 and iodine-123-IMP single-photon emission computed tomography, *J Cereb Blood Flow Metab* 22(9):1142–1148, 2002.

101. Ogasawara K, Ogawa A, Yoshimoto T: Cerebrovascular reactivity to acetazolamide and outcome in patients with symptomatic internal carotid or middle cerebral artery occlusion: a xenon-133 single-photon emission computed tomography study, *Stroke* 33 (7):1857–1862, 2002.

102. Kleiser B, Widder B: Course of carotid artery occlusions with impaired cerebrovascular reactivity, *Stroke* 23(2):171–174, 1992.

103. Powers WJ, Derdeyn CP, Fritsch SM, et al: Benign prognosis of never-symptomatic carotid occlusion, *Neurology* 54(4):878–882, 2000.

104. Bornstein NM, Norris JW: Benign outcome of carotid occlusion, *Neurology* 39(1):6–8, 1989.

105. Widder B, Kleiser B, Krapf H: Course of cerebrovascular reactivity in patients with carotid artery occlusions, *Stroke* 25(10):1963–1967, 1994.

106. Powers WJ, Tempel LW, Grubb RL Jr, : Influence of cerebral hemodynamics on stroke risk: one-year follow-up of 30 medically treated patients, *Ann Neurol* 25(4):325–330, 1989.

107. Yamauchi H, Fukuyama H, Nagahama Y, et al: Evidence of misery perfusion and risk for recurrent stroke in major cerebral arterial occlusive diseases from PET, *J Neurol Neurosurg Psychiatry* 61 (1):18–25, 1996.

108. Yamauchi H, Fukuyama H, Nagahama Y, et al: Significance of increased oxygen extraction fraction in five-year prognosis of major cerebral arterial occlusive diseases, *J Nucl Med* 40(12):1992–1998, 1999.

109. Mintun MA, Raichle ME, Martin WR, et al: Brain oxygen utilization measured with O-15 radiotracers and positron emission tomography, *J Nucl Med* 25(2):177–187, 1984.

110. Videen TO, Perlmutter JS, Herscovitch P, et al: Brain blood volume, flow, and oxygen utilization measured with 15O radiotracers and positron emission tomography: revised metabolic computations, *J Cereb Blood Flow Metab* 7(4):513–516, 1987.

111. Powers WJ, Grubb RL Jr, Darriet D, et al: Cerebral blood flow and cerebral metabolic rate of oxygen requirements for cerebral function and viability in humans, *J Cereb Blood Flow Metab* 5(4):600–608, 1985.

112. Rothwell PM, Eliasziw M, Gutnikov SA, et al: Analysis of pooled data from the randomised controlled trials of endarterectomy for symptomatic carotid stenosis, *Lancet* 361(9352):107–116, 2003.

113. Derdeyn CP, Videen TO, Simmons NR, et al: Count-based PET method for predicting ischemic stroke in patients with symptomatic carotid arterial occlusion, *Radiology* 212(2):499–506, 1999.

114. Derdeyn CP, Videen TO, Grubb RL Jr, et al: Comparison of PET oxygen extraction fraction methods for the prediction of stroke risk, *J Nucl Med* 42(8):1195–1197, 2001.

115. Hayashida K, Hirose Y, Tanaka Y: Stratification of severity by cerebral blood flow, oxygen metabolism and acetazolamide reactivity in patients with cerebrovascular disease. In Ishii K, editor: *Recent advances in biomedical imaging*, Amsterdam, 1997, Elsevier, pp 113–119.

116. Herold S, Brown MM, Frackowiak RS, et al: Assessment of cerebral haemodynamic reserve: correlation between PET parameters and CO_2 reactivity measured by the intravenous 133 xenon injection technique, *J Neurol Neurosurg Psychiatry* 51(8):1045–1050, 1988.

117. Kanno I, Uemura K, Higano S, et al: Oxygen extraction fraction at maximally vasodilated tissue in the ischemic brain estimated from the regional CO_2 responsiveness measured by positron emission tomography, *J Cereb Blood Flow Metab* 8(2):227–235, 1988.

118. Sugimori H, Ibayashi S, Fujii K, et al: Can transcranial Doppler really detect reduced cerebral perfusion states? *Stroke* 26(11):2053–2060, 1995.

119. Hasegawa Y, Minematsu K, Matsuoka H, et al: CBF Responses to Acetazolamide and CO_2 for the Prediction of Hemodynamic Failure: A PET Study, *Stroke* 28(1):242, 1997.

120. Nemoto EM, Yonas H, Chang Y: Stages and thresholds of hemodynamic failure, *Stroke* 34(1):2–3, 2003.

121. Nemoto EM, Yonas H, Kuwabara H, et al: Identification of hemodynamic compromise by cerebrovascular reserve and oxygen extraction fraction in occlusive vascular disease, *J Cereb Blood Flow Metab* 24(10):1081–1089, 2004.

122. Imaizumi M, Kitagawa K, Oku N, et al: Clinical significance of cerebrovascular reserve in acetazolamide challenge -comparison with acetazolamide challenge H2O-PET and Gas-PET, *Ann Nucl Med* 18(5):369–374, 2004.

123. Yamauchi H, Okazawa H, Kishibe Y, et al: Oxygen extraction fraction and acetazolamide reactivity in symptomatic carotid artery disease, *J Neurol Neurosurg Psychiatry* 75(1):33–37, 2004.

124. Okazawa H, Tsuchida T, Kobayashi M, et al: Can the detection of misery perfusion in chronic cerebrovascular disease be based on reductions in baseline CBF and vasoreactivity? *Eur J Nucl Med Mol Imaging* 34(1):121–129, 2007.

125. Ogawa S, Lee TM, Kay AR, et al: Brain magnetic resonance imaging with contrast dependent on blood oxygenation, *Proc Natl Acad Sci* 87:9868–9872, 1990.

126. Ogawa S, Menon RS, Tank DW, et al: Functional brain mapping by blood oxygenation level-dependent contrast magnetic resonance imaging, *Biophysical J* 64:803–812, 1993.

127. Kwong K, Belliveau JW, Chesler DA, et al: Dynamic magnetic resonance imaging of human brain activity during primary sensory stimulation, *Proc Natl Acad Sci U S A* 89:5675–5679, 1992.

128. Fernandez-Seara MA, Techawiboonwong A, Detre JA, et al: MR susceptometry for measuring global brain oxygen extraction, *Magn Reson Med* 55(5):967–973, 2006.

129. He X, Yablonskiy DA: Quantitative BOLD: mapping of human cerebral deoxygenated blood volume and oxygen extraction fraction: default state, *Magn Reson Med* 57(1):115–126, 2007.

130. An H, Lin W, Celik A, et al: Quantitative measurements of cerebral metabolic rate of oxygen utilization using MRI: a volunteer study, *NMR Biomed* 14:441–447, 2001.

131. Lin W, Derdeyn CP, Celik A, et al: A Comparison of BOLD MRI and PET OEF Measurements on Patients with Carotid Artery Occlusion, *Annual Meeting Society of Magnetic Resonance in Medicine* 1155:1998, 1998.

132. Yamauchi H, Kudoh T, Kishibe Y, et al: Selective neuronal damage and chronic hemodynamic cerebral ischemia, *Ann Neurol* 61(5):454–465, 2007.

133. EC-IC Bypass Study Group: Failure of extracranial-intracranial arterial bypass to reduce the risk of ischemic stroke. Results of an international randomized trial, *N Engl J Med* 313(19):1191–1200, 1985.

134. Gibbs JM, Wise RJ, Thomas DJ, et al: Cerebral haemodynamic changes after extracranial-intracranial bypass surgery, *J Neurol Neurosurg Psychiatry* 50(2):140–150, 1987.

135. Powers WJ, Martin WR, Herscovitch P, et al: Extracranial-intracranial bypass surgery: hemodynamic and metabolic effects, *Neurology* 34(9):1168–1174, 1984.

136. Samson Y, Baron JC, Bousser MG, et al: Effects of extra-intracranial arterial bypass on cerebral blood flow and oxygen metabolism in humans, *Stroke* 16(4):609–616, 1985.

137. JET Study Group: Japanese EC-IC Bypass Trial (JET Study), *Surg Cereb Stroke* 30:434–437, 2002.

138. Brott T, Adams HP Jr, Olinger CP, et al: Measurements of acute cerebral infarction: a clinical examination scale, *Stroke* 20(7):864–870, 1989.

139. Sulter G, Steen C, De Keyser J: Use of the Barthel index and modified Rankin scale in acute stroke trials, *Stroke* 30(8):1538–1541, 1999.

140. Williams LS, Weinberger M, Harris LE, et al: Development of a stroke-specific quality of life scale, *Stroke* 30(7):1362–1369, 1999.

141. Williams LS, Weinberger M, Harris LE, et al: Measuring quality of life in a way that is meaningful to stroke patients, *Neurology* 53(8):1839–1843, 1999.

142. Albers GW, Hart RG, Lutsep HL, et al: AHA Scientific Statement. Supplement to the guidelines for the management of transient ischemic attacks: A statement from the Ad Hoc Committee on Guidelines for the Management of Transient Ischemic Attacks, Stroke Council, American Heart Association, *Stroke* 30(11):2502–2511, 1999.

USING CEREBRAL VASO-REACTIVITY IN THE SELECTION OF CANDIDATES FOR EC-IC BYPASS SURGERY

ANDREW P. CARLSON; HOWARD YONAS

INTRODUCTION

Since the failure of the EC-IC (extracranial-intracranial) bypass study in showing decreased risk of stroke after bypass,[1] the utility of this procedure, particularly in chronic occlusive vascular disease (OVD), has come into serious question. Despite that failure in an unselected group of patients, anecdotal and clinical experience has lead clinicians who treat patients with occlusive vascular disease to conclude that there must be a subgroup of patients who are at a much higher risk of stroke than the general population who would still benefit from this procedure. This has lead to a great deal of research into the underlying pathophysiology in OVD and subsequently the development of a number of physiology-based techniques that are able to predict patients at increased risk of stroke. Once a technique has been established to identify a high-risk group, it then remains to be proven to decrease subsequent stroke risk when used as a selection tool for bypass. In order to understand the rationale for using cerebral vaso-reactivity (CVR) studies as a rational tool for the selection of candidates for flow augmentation surgery, a review of the pathophysiology is first necessary.

PHYSIOLOGY OF OCCLUSIVE VASCULAR DISEASE

Central to the physiology in carotid occlusion is the concept of cerebral autoregulation and its interrelationship with chemoregulation. Cerebral autoregulation is an intrinsic property of the cerebral vasculature that allows for maintaining consistency of CBF (cerebral blood flow) over a wide range of cerebral perfusion pressures (CPPs). This property is not unique to the cerebral vasculature, and involves very tight molecular regulation, allowing very precise, second-to-second adaptation to changing stresses. It is important to emphasize that this is an intrinsic property of the vessels, and is separate from other chemical or neural mediators of CBF adaptation. The molecular mechanisms are signaled by stretch of the vasculature, which initiates a phospholipase C mediated cascade,

resulting in inhibition of calcium-activated potassium channels in smooth muscle, leading to smooth muscle contraction. The opposing forces are likely related to the cellular metabolic activity within neural and glial cells leading to activation of the same potassium channels and vasodilatation.[2]

As the CPP drops, the CBF is maintained within the range of autoregulation by this compensatory vasodilatation up to a point of maximal dilation. One can hypothesize a number of approaches to evaluate that state of vessel dilation. Direct measurement of vessel diameter seems intuitive, but due to the varying sizes of vessels in the arterial tree and the primary location of autoregulation being in the arteriolar region, this approach is impractical. An alternate measurement might be the cerebral blood volume (CBV). If the CBV is increased, it may be a reflection of increasing arteriolar diameter. This technique relies on the above noted assumptions, and provides one snapshot into the underlying physiologic state.

An alternate method of testing the state of autoregulation involves testing vascular reactivity. This approach involves performing a baseline study to assess CBF, followed by a vasodilatory challenge and repeat of the study. The challenge can be as simple as breath holding to increase pCO_2 or inhalation of CO_2 gas—both relying on the principle that increasing brain CO_2 acidifies the tissue and leads to vasodilatation (called *chemoregulation*). Alternatively, a cerebral vasodilatory agent such as acetazolamide that blocks carbonic anhydrase can be administered to induce tissue acidification and vasodilatation. These methods do not alter the underlying state of intrinsic autoregulation or metabolism, but they are able to determine to what degree the vessels can respond to such a challenge. In normal brain vasculature, a vasodilatory agent should lead to an increase in CBF by a certain percentage over the baseline level (typically 15% to 40%). If the vasodilatory agent does not cause an increase in CBF, one can conclude that the vessels have reached a maximal level of autoregulatory vasodilatation. In some cases, one may even see in one or more vascular territories a paradoxical drop in CBF in response to a vasodilatory challenge. This has been referred to as a "steal" phenomenon, where the portion of the vasculature that has a normal blood supply dilates normally in response to the challenge while the vascular territory that is already maximally dilated, and most often dependent upon leptomeningeal collaterals, experiences a loss of collateral supply.[3] This approach thereby identifies a vascular territory that has experienced a failure of autoregulation with a reduction of CBF and a state of maximal vasodilation, and potentially the tissue most at risk for infarction due to a progression of hemodynamic compromise.

The cerebral vasculature has other adaptive mechanisms for compensating for decreasing perfusion pressure. Once the vessels are maximally dilated and the CPP continues to fall, the normally excessive levels of tissue nutrients (i.e., glucose and oxygen) carried within the blood supply begin to fall. A common measurement is the oxygen extraction fraction (OEF), which normally is less than 50% and rises with a progressive fall of CPP. With a fall of CBF below about 20cc/100 g/min, the oxygen reserves become exhausted and metabolism becomes compromised. The increase in OEF can be measured using positron emission tomography (PET), although there remains controversy regarding the most accurate method.[4,5] This physiology underlies the now well accepted stages of hemodynamic insufficiency described by Powers et al.[6,7] that with the progressive fall of CPP, CBF is maintained by vasodilatation with the rise of CBV. This is referred to as Stage I insufficiency. Stage II insufficiency involves the failure of autoregulation with a fall of CBF and a state of maximal vasodilatation and an increasing OEF. With a continued fall of CPP the brain enters Stage III, with progressive cellular death. This metabolic decline can be directly measured by the CMRO2 (cerebral metabolic rate of oxygen use) as a single PET study. A vasodilatory challenge study done in Stage III will show a loss of positive reactivity or a "steal" as described previously. Because OEF is a ratio of CBF and CMRO$_2$, with progressive cellular injury the CMRO$_2$ will fall and the OEF can potentially return to "normal" with an equally reduced CBF and CMRO$_2$. This stage has been referred to as a progression of Stage III with "matched hypoperfusion"[8–12,70] (Figure 2–1).

Measurement of OEF is a predictive tool in determining patients at an elevated risk of hemodynamic infarction and who will most likely benefit from carotid bypass surgery, and is discussed in depth elsewhere. The concept of measuring vasoreactivity to assess the state of Stages I to III hemodynamic failure offers some practical and theoretical advantages, and will be covered in detail in this section. It is important to understand this physiological background to place various techniques into perspective, and more importantly, to understand that techniques that may seem disparate with differing endpoints may be evaluating the same concept and paradigm of cerebral physiology from different perspectives.

TECHNIQUES USED FOR TESTING CVR

The bulk of work trying to incorporate the concept of CVR was born out of the Pittsburg group in the 1980s and 1990s as it relates to carotid occlusion using [133]Xenon and Xenon/CT (computed tomography). Since that time, the utilization of

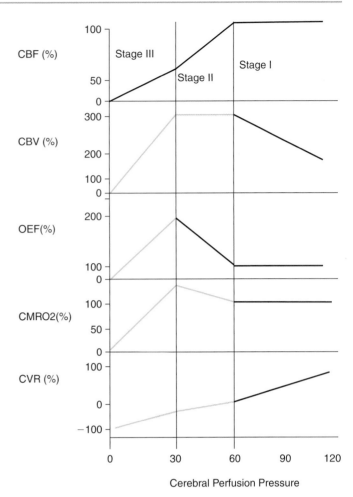

Figure 2–1. Stages of hemodynamic failure, showing the parallel response of variables to decreasing cerebral perfusion pressure. CBF, cerebral blood flow; CBV, cerebral blood volume; OEF, oxygen extraction fraction; CMRO2, cerebral metabolic rate for oxygen; CVR, cerebrovascular reserve. The stages are referenced to the changes in OEF. Stage I, OEF is unchanged. Stage II, OEF begins to increase. Whether the increase is linear is unknown. Stage III, OEF declines again. Solid lines show changes that are known, and dashed lines, those that are postulated.
(Redrawn from Nemoto EM, Yonas H, Chang Y. Stages and thresholds of hemodynamic failure. Stroke 2003;34:2-3.)

Xenon/CT techniques has expanded across the world, and still continues in the United States at several institutions as part of a Food and Drug Administration (FDA) Investigational New Drug (IND) exemption. Despite the current limitations in access, data from the ongoing centers as well as the hundreds of centers in Japan and Europe give promise to the future of the technique. In addition, multiple other modalities are beginning to utilize the concept of assessment of CVR and stroke risk, and may offer some more widely accessible options in the future.

Xenon/CT

Xenon has been thought to be an ideal technique for CBF determination due to its ability to provide quantitative data safely. [133]Xenon may utilize individual gamma counters or an array that integrates information. Regional or tomographic SPECT (single photon emission tomography) techniques are utilized to record the washout of Xenon from the brain tissue with end tidal values being utilized to obtain an assessment of arterial content. A vast amount of information about CBF has been gained with this approach that is, however, limited by the need for precautions with radioactive Xenon and the inability to resolve information below the surface of the brain. Xenon/CT offers the advantage of providing high-resolution CBF information with equal validity in the center as well as the surface of the brain. Stable Xenon, which is radiodense and similar to iodine, is also a noble gas, thus not requiring any concerns about environmental contamination. The technique involves the measurement of both the arterial concentration and tissue arrival of Xenon on CT, allowing for solving of the Kety-Schmidt equation by integral math for each of the $\sim$24,000 CT pixels. The validity of the technique has been confirmed by cross-correlation with destructive (microspheres,[13] iodoantipyrine[14]), and in vivo ([133]Xenon,[15] PET,[16] thermal dilution flow probes[17]) CBF technologies. No permanent morbidity or death has been reported despite its wide use for over 25 years, and Xenon gas is generally considered safe.[18]

Xenon techniques including [133]Xenon SPECT and Xenon/CT have been used for examining CBF in carotid occlusion even before the failure of the EC-IC bypass trial.[19] It was clearly recognized, even at that time, that physiological methods must have some role in selecting these patients. One observational study noted that only a small minority of patients (two of 20) showed increased CBF after bypass compared to the test done before bypass.[20] Initially, decreased baseline CBF alone was used to select potential candidates for bypass and of 25 patients with normal baseline CBF, no early strokes were seen with no bypass, while bypass was shown to normalize decreased CBF levels in seven of eight patients. At the same time, other clinicians, mainly in Scandinavia, began to explore the concept of testing the CVR by administration of acetazolamide, as described previously, in selecting patients using regional [133]Xenon who might benefit from bypass.[21]

The failure of the EC-IC bypass trial, however, meant that the financial and practical ability to perform bypass surgery for OVD was relegated to a primarily research role. As the group in St. Louis began a natural history study to define the stroke risk associated with increased OEF,[22] similar work was being done with regard to CVR. Rogg[23] first demonstrated that patients with symptomatic carotid occlusion or stenosis can have very different patterns of response to acetazolamide challenge. Forty-five percent of patients showed normal baseline CBF that augmented with acetazolamide ipsilateral to the occlusion. Thirty-one percent started with low baseline flow, but still augmented appropriately with acetazolamide, while 24% showed either no response or decreased response to acetazolamide, regardless of baseline CBF. Later, the same Pittsburg group, in a prospective trial, showed that patients with symptomatic carotid stenosis or occlusion can be divided more specifically to better predict subsequent stroke. Patients with normal baseline CBF and normal CVR had a stroke risk of

4.4% (2/46) in the mean 24-month follow-up period compared to 36% (8/22) patients with baseline CBF < 45 cc/100 g/min in any territory on the affected side as well as CVR showing negative reactivity (steal) of >5%. This translated to a 12.6 times increased risk of stroke in the group with a severe compromise of CVR. Furthermore, the two strokes in the normal reactivity group were contralateral to the affected carotid side, and were both in patients with carotid stenosis rather than occlusion.[24] This represented some of the first data clearly linking the importance of poor CVR to subsequent stroke. Further data from this group confirmed this association further, especially in carotid occlusion, where the stroke rate in the 19.6-month mean follow-up period was 10% (2/26) in patients with normal CVR compared to 26% (10/38) in the patients with steal.[25]

This data has been cross-validated in other institutions as well, where the stroke rate was found to be 0.5% to 2.4% annually with normal CVR (measured by [133]Xenon SPECT) compared to a 21.8% annual stroke rate if CVR was impaired in patients with carotid or MCA (middle cerebral artery) occlusion.[26] Another group from Japan found a 6% (3/47) stroke rate in patients with normal CVR compared to 35% (8/23) with poor CVR. Decreased CVR was also found to be the only factor that the group measured that was associated with an increased stroke rate.[27] There are some limitations in all of these data, particularly with regard to sampling error. None of these are long-term prospective observational studies, and the inclusion varies in terms of methodology, specific definition of impaired CVR, stenosis versus occlusion, intracranial versus extracranial disease, and clinical status of the patient. That said, there seems to be very convincing evidence from several sources that in patients with OVD there is a dramatic, statistically significant increase in risk of stroke predicted by impaired CVR.

Despite the fact that there is no randomized, controlled data to support the use of CVR, there has been nonrandomized data accruing over many years. As mentioned, the use of CVR in assessing patients with OVD began in the mid-1980s concurrent with the publication of the bypass trial. Vorstrup[21] showed some of the first physiological data supporting the use of CVR in bypass selection. Adequate reactivity was defined as at least 13% flow augmentation from normal control data. Eighteen patients were bypassed for clinical reasons, nine of whom showed decreased CVR on acetazolamide testing, two of whom showed negative reactivity. Postoperatively, all of these patients showed improved CVR, but the two with negative reactivity were the only two whose baseline CBF increased. None of the remaining nine patients who were bypassed with normal CVR showed increased CBF postop, likely suggesting the lack of hemodynamic stress. The authors concluded that a randomized controlled trial was needed to assess this technique.[21] Groups in Japan have also been using the technique in evaluating patients for bypass. In one study, 15 patients were studied before and after bypass. Three showed decreased CVR (again defined by normal controls), which improved after bypass. Furthermore, six patients had decreased baseline CBF and CVR pre-operatively. In three of these, the baseline CBF improved, and in four, the CVR improved postop.[28] These early studies showed that in patients with impaired CVR, bypass can improve these physiologic parameters.

The next important step is to link whether bypass can decrease stroke risk in selected patients, and there have been some preliminary studies addressing this question. Kuroda[29] first used CVR as a selection criterion for bypass in patients with OVD. Out of 32 patients, six who showed normal CBF and CVR were not bypassed, and there were no ischemic events in the mean 24-month follow-up. Of the nine patients with normal CBF but impaired CVR, eight were bypassed, and they showed no ischemic event and return of normal CVR on follow-up imaging. The one patient with poor CVR and without bypass suffered a CVA. Of the 11 patients with decreased baseline CBF and poor CVR, nine had bypass—of these, one suffered a perioperative CVA, one died of pneumonia, and CVR normalized in the rest with no further ischemic events. Of the two not bypassed, one suffered a CVA, and one had progressive deterioration followed by a basal ganglia hemorrhage. The final group consisted of patients with decreased baseline CBF, but normal CVR. Five of six were bypassed and none had subsequent CVA. The authors suggested that this may not, in fact, have represented a high-risk group, and that metabolic data may have shown decreased tissue metabolic demand.[29] This study, although somewhat complicated and clearly limited due to the nonrandomized nature, seems to offer supportive evidence that normal CVR is protective, decreased CVR has a high rate of stroke when untreated (all three patients in this series), and bypass seems to offer significant protection from CVA with some risk of significant perioperative complications (two of 22 in this series).

A larger series looking specifically at this at-risk group based on decreased CVR followed again from the Pittsburg group.[30] Forty-two patients with hemodynamic insufficiency were examined (baseline CBF < 45 cc/100 g/min and >5% negative reactivity). Thirty were treated medically and there were nine (30%) CVAs within 12 months (mean of 5 months). Twelve were bypassed only after developing an ischemic stroke and showed normalization of CVR in all, and there was no CVA in the 18-month follow-up with one asymptomatic hemorrhage. This was further strong evidence for both the dangerous natural history of these patients and the ability of bypass to not only reverse the hemodynamic findings, but decrease CVA risk with a very low risk of morbidity.[30]

Xenon techniques have provided the backbone of the data with regard to providing the ability to determine patients at risk for hemodynamic infarction and to be able to test response to bypass. It is the most widely utilized approach for selection of bypass candidates for Moya Moya in Asia. That said, current limitations in terms of availability have led researchers to attempt to glean similar physiologic data in terms of CVR from other techniques; however, they must be viewed with caution and must be subject to the same

paradigm, where the technique must be predictive of increased CVA risk and be able to demonstrate improvement with surgical intervention. That is certainly not to discredit any of the following techniques, but merely to stress the importance of each technique to prove that the data it provided truly is prognostic as has been seen with Xenon techniques.

SPECT

Qualitative SPECT-based techniques have an instructive history in emphasizing the importance of quantitative measurements. With qualitative techniques, an index must be assigned based on the asymmetry, usually between the two hemispheres. These asymmetry indices have shown poor correlation with CBF patterns.[31] The other practical limitation is that since these techniques assess the accumulation of the isotope in tissue over time, rather than the direct wash-in (as with Xenon/CT), an immediate acetazolamide or other challenge study cannot be done. Typically, to test response to acetazolamide, the SPECT study is repeated 3 days after the first, allowing for many potentially confounding variables. Given this, it does not seem surprising that Yokota was unable to determine a difference in stroke rates in patients with normal and "impaired" CVR by [123I] IMP(N-isopropyl-p-[123I] iodoamphetamine) SPECT.[32] Another study using the tracer 99mTc-HMPAO also showed the ability to detect the increasing asymmetry and reported that one patient predicted to be at risk did subsequently have a stroke.[33] A very interesting confirmation of the limitations of the qualitative tracer rather than simply the SPECT technique was reported by Ogasawara,[34] who showed that in the same group of patients, CVR as measured by 133Xenon SPECT was strongly predictive of 5-year stroke risk, whereas CVR measured by [123I] IMP SPECT was not predictive. This study strongly refutes the conclusion drawn by Yokota that "reduced vasodilatory capacity does not play a major role in stroke recurrence."[32] For this reason, we strongly would discourage any extrapolation of data from quantitative techniques to qualitative techniques in the future. Qualitative CBF techniques cannot predict patients with OVD at risk for subsequent CVA and should not be used as criteria for bypass.

Perfusion CT

With the ready availability of perfusion CT techniques at most institutions with modern CT scanners, a push has begun to find prognostic utility in these techniques, although definitive evidence is currently lacking. There are some very promising potential uses for this technique; however, there are also several limitations. First, the technique measures only intravascular contrast rather than tissue contrast as with Xenon. CT perfusion measures the arrival time of the intravascular contrast with about 50 scans at the same level within 1 minute as it is rapidly infused intravenously. There is no arterial input function, and so several assumptions are made in terms of calculating the resultant values. The CBF is calculated based on the MTT (mean transit time) or TTP (time to peak) and CBV values. In addition, there are serious risks of iodinated contrast as well as of radiation exposure for multiple studies that should not be overlooked.[35,36] That said, one recent study demonstrated that after acetazolamide challenge in 15 patients with OVD, decreases in CBF and increases in MTT were noted.[37] Another very small study also showed that there was increased MTT seen in three patients with OVD compared to one control with acetazolamide challenge.[38] These preliminary data should suggest that perfusion CT may offer some insight into physiology in OVD, but at this point there are insufficient data to suggest that it is able to predict stroke or determine selection for bypass.

Perfusion MRI

Perfusion MRI is based on similar techniques as perfusion CT, and offers the same potential insights and limitations. Schreiber demonstrated the potential ability to detect a group of patients with impaired hemodynamics, showing that in five of eight patients with carotid occlusion, impaired CBF reactivity to acetazolamide was observed.[39] Newer MR techniques may allow for some quantification of these values as well. In order to assess the validity of these measurements, perfusion MRI values were cross-correlated with Xenon/CT values. Since the MTT and the Tmax (maximum arrival time) are the only variables that are directly measured, these were thought to likely be the most accurate. It was found that the Tmax was slightly more accurate than MTT. The authors found that a Tmax of >4 sec showed 68% sensitivity, 80% specificity, and 77% accuracy for detecting a CBF of <20 sec by Xenon/CT.[40] Although the authors demonstrated that Tmax and MTT were strongly associated with Xenon/CT values, it is unclear whether these moderately sensitive and specific values will translate into the ability to predict stroke or select patients for bypass.

TCD

TCD (transcranial Doppler) is a simple, noninvasive test that can be performed in a variety of situations, and for practical reasons, is a very attractive modality for assessing cerebral hemodynamics. The technique relies on measurement of the flow velocity in large proximal vessels such as the MCA. Although flow velocity alone has been shown to be poorly correlated with quantitative CBF,[41,42] performing a vasodilatory challenge to assess CVR likely is closely correlated with CVR as tested with a CBF study.[41,43] This is likely explained by the fact that large vessel morphology may be variable, and several factors including diameter and length will affect velocity besides CBF. When these are controlled for by testing the same vessel with a vasodilatory challenge, the velocity should then be reflective of the change in flow in the distal

vasculature. It is clear that there is correlation of TCD CVR and Xenon-based CVR,[41,43,44] although this is clearly not absolute. The correlation coefficient ranges from 0.45[41] in asymptomatic patients (22.5% correlation) to 0.59[41] and 0.63[43] in symptomatic patients (35% to 40% correlation). For the average of the MCA territory by Xenon/CT, CVR measured by TCD of the MCA showed only 33% sensitivity, with 90.6% specificity.[44]

TCD-based CVR measurement is also limited in terms of the fact that there can be a great deal of interobserver variability. The reliability of the test is dependent on the TCD operator's experience and consistency. In addition, a number of different techniques have been developed to measure CVR. Though an acetazolamide challenge is frequently used, just as with other techniques described above, attempts have been made to use even less invasive techniques such as breath-holding index (measured as a rise in end-tidal CO_2 after breath holding), hyper- and hypo-ventilation, and breathing various concentrations of CO_2 gas.[45–47] All of these techniques rely on tissue acidification and cerebral chemoregulation, whether by varying the pCO_2 or administering acetazolamide as described previously, but the variability in measurement techniques makes cross-comparison more difficult. It is clear that these various methods are closely correlated,[45–47] although acetazolamide likely offers a slight advantage in distinguishing the degree of impairment.[46,47]

Despite the somewhat limited sensitivity and variety of vasodilatory stimuli, TCD has been shown to have utility in assessment of hemodynamics in patients with carotid occlusive vascular disease. Overall, worsened CVR compared to normal controls has been documented in patients with higher-grade carotid stenosis and occlusion.[48,49] In addition, it is clear that worsened CVR is related to some surrogate measures of hemodynamic insufficiency including symptomatic patients, signs of ipsilateral low-flow infarction on CT,[50] and neuropsychiatric testing.[51] CVR testing of patients with high-grade stenosis has been used to determine if there is increased stroke risk in some patients with hemodynamic factors, and in fact, poor CVR is clearly associated with increased stroke risk.[52–54] Although these studies seem to show that there is a flow-related component in some patients with carotid stenosis in addition to the well-known thromboembolic risk, it does not significantly change treatment strategies in these patients. It has been clearly shown that carotid endarterectomy (CEA) decreases stroke risk in patients with high-grade stenosis.[55,56] It is interesting, however, that in patients with impaired CVR who undergo CEA, that these values normalize postoperatively.[54] Furthermore, in patients with carotid occlusion and contralateral stenosis with poor CVR, the values often normalize on the occluded side after contralateral CEA.[57]

The value of CVR measured by TCD has been established in patients with carotid occlusion as well. In one group using inhaled CO_2 gas, only four of 48 (8%) patients with normal CVR suffered ipsilateral ischemic events compared to 12 of 33 (32%) with impaired reactivity in the mean 38-month follow-up.[58] Another group showed that breath holding index of <0.69 was the only factor of their measured variables associated with subsequent stroke.[59] This group later showed that this impaired CVR was also associated with a lack of angiographic collaterals, with a 32.7% stroke rate with no major collateral vessels. All of these patients had impaired CVR. If patients have one or two collateral vessels, the CVR pattern was variable, and impaired CVR was associated with subsequent stroke risk, pointing out the utility of physiologic assessment in these patients. Furthermore, none of their patients with normal CVR had ischemic events in the mean 24-month follow-up.[60] The concentration of inhaled CO_2 may affect the sensitivity of measurement as well, and 8% CO_2 seemed to show the best predictive value, with a Kaplan-Meyer log rank statistic of 7.81 ($p = 0.0052$) and annual ischemic event rate of 8.53%.[61]

These data have yet to be carried forward to be used to predict patients in need of bypass, although likely offer an attractive possibility for many reasons. It is easily assessable and noninvasive, although it does require a skilled operator. The results of correlation studies show fairly good correlation with quantitative techniques, but with lower sensitivity. The technique has been shown to be predictive of stroke risk in patients with carotid occlusion as well, so ongoing studies will be needed to clarify the role of the technique in predicting patients for bypass.

PET

The power of PET data is, that in addition to quantitative CBF data, it also provides metabolic data. Unfortunately, access to the oxygen isotope needed for the cerebral studies requires an on-site cyclotron, and is limited at many institutions. That said, the technique offers powerful, quantitative insight into cerebral hemodynamics. Quantitative CBF can be obtained using PET by injection of ^{15}O [H_2O]. The tissue arrival time is calculated by the PET detectors, and the arterial concentration (input function) is calculated by measuring the arterial concentration of the radioactive tracer either continuously or by frequent sampling.[62] Although this is slightly more labor intensive than measuring the end tidal Xenon with Xenon/CT, a repeat study can be performed to determine the response to an intervention. By administering acetazolamide as described previously, the CVR can be determined tomographically.[63]

The majority of data using PET in predicting patients at hemodynamic risk in carotid occlusion has focused on the ability to detect Stage II hemodynamic insufficiency by measuring an increased OEF. This is the basis of a study funded by the National Institutes of Health (Carotid Occlusion Surgery Study [COSS]) to use increased OEF as the entry criteria in symptomatic patients with carotid occlusion followed by randomization to bypass surgery or medical management.[64,65] It is clear that increased OEF has been shown to be predictive of subsequent stroke risk.[5,6,22,66] In 2001, Derdeyn[5] proposed using qualitative OEF data rather than quantitative data and that became the model for the COSS trial as of 2003.[64]

It has come into question as to why there is discordance between the patients detected to be at risk by CVR-based techniques and OEF. Yamauchi using quantitative OEF found a 50% PPV of increased OEF in detecting patients with impaired CVR as measured by PET.[67] Likewise, Nemoto found 37.5% of patients with poor CVR by Xenon/CT but normal OEF,[8] and Kuroda found 57%.[11] These data then beg the question as to whether CVR techniques detect some patients without hemodynamic impairment or whether OEF is missing some patients with hemodynamic impairment. To address this question, surrogate markers of severe impairment have been used. Nemoto showed that in the patients with impaired CVR but normal OEF, there remained a highly significant association with a subcortical, low-flow related pattern of infarction on MRI.[8] Likewise, Kuroda found that OEF did not correlate with subcortical white matter changes,[11] suggesting that many patients with normal OEF may still have signs of hemodynamic insufficiency.

These data lend support to an addition to the concept of stages of hemodynamic failure, in that there is likely a stage after Stage II, where CBF continues to fall, reactivity continues to worsen or even become negative (steal), and OEF falls along with baseline cellular metabolism[8] (see Figures 2–1 and 2–2). This clarifies the seeming discordant physiology conceptually, and explains why patients who seem to have some of the most impaired hemodynamics, as measured by CVR and confirmed with presence of white matter changes, may in fact show "normal" OEF.

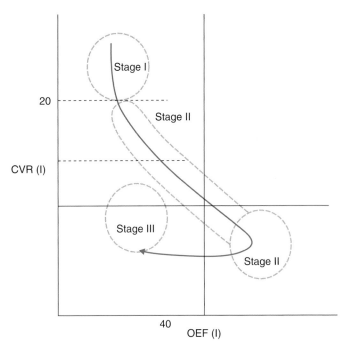

Figure 2–2. Proposed changes through stages of hemodynamic failure. Initially OEF increases as CVR decreases into the negative (steal) range. At some point, the stage of matched hypometabolism is reached and OEF falls again, while CVR remains negative.

(Redrawn from Nemoto EM, Yonas H, Kuwabara H, et al. Identification of hemodynamic compromise by cerebrovascular reserve and oxygen extraction fraction in occlusive vascular disease. J Cereb Blood Flow Metab 2004;24:1081-1089.)

In order to measure these physiologic discrepancies, the change in OEF after acetazolamide challenge can be determined. The OEF should decrease if there is an increase in CBF (normal reactivity) with acetazolamide. The OEF reactivity (OEFR) has been found to correlate with CVR much better than OEF alone,[10,68,69] likely identifying patients with severe hemodynamic compromise despite normal baseline OEF values. In these preliminary studies, two patients with the poorest CVR values and severe white matter changes were found to have normal baseline OEF, but were identified as compromised using OEFR.[68] Furthermore, based on these data it has been proposed that demonstration of positive OEFR definitively indicates a state of hemodynamic impairment, where as a negative OEFR demonstrates a state of hemodynamic reserve.[69] This may offer an alternative to the difficulty with assigning threshold values for OEF.[7]

Despite the evidence that patients with poor CVR and normal OEF may still have hemodynamic insufficiency, it is unclear if this is predictive of future stroke. This question was recently addressed by Hokari in a small preliminary study that showed a stroke rate in mean 45.6-month follow-up of three of nine patients with poor CVR and increased OEF compared to 0/11 with poor CVR and normal OEF.[69] One may surmise based on these data that when this group of patients enters the state of matched hypometabolism, where OEF begins to fall along with metabolism, that the decreased metabolic demand may be protective in terms of hemodynamic stroke. That is to say that as the tissue enters a state of severe hemodynamic insufficiency, decreased CBF is needed to maintain tissue viability. Clearly, further studies are needed to assess stroke risk and therapeutic interventions in this group.

CONCLUSIONS

Testing CVR or OEF reactivity allows for a dynamic insight into cerebrovascular physiology that is not afforded by static tests. Quantitative measurement of CVR by Xenon/CT is the gold standard, and poor reactivity has been proven to be associated with future stroke risk. Furthermore, preliminary data suggest the utility in using quantitative CVR techniques to assess patients need for EC-IC bypass, although a randomized clinical trial is still lacking. Other techniques, particularly TCD reactivity, may offer some important physiological information as well. The apparent discrepancies between patients selected by OEF as hemodynamically at risk may be explained by a false normalization of OEF in the state of matched hypometabolism. This state can be detected using a challenge study of OEF reactivity. A clear understanding of the advantages and limitations of various physiologic assessment tools will be of critical importance for a rational approach to selecting patients in need of bypass in the future.

REFERENCES

1. The EC/IC Bypass Study Group: Failure of extracranial-intracranial arterial bypass to reduce the risk of ischemic stroke. Results of an international randomized trial, N Engl J Med 313:1191–1200, 1985.
2. Harder DR, Roman RJ, Gebremedhin D, et al: A common pathway for regulation of nutritive blood flow to the brain: arterial muscle membrane potential and cytochrome P450 metabolites, Acta Physiol Scand 164:527–532, 1998.
3. Yonas H, Kromer H, Jungreis C: Compromised vascular reserves does predict subgroups with carotid occlusion and an increased stroke risk, J Stroke Cereb Dis 6:458, 1997.
4. Lin R, Uchino K, Zaidi S, et al: Quantitative versus qualitative OEF identification of hemodynamic compromise in stroke patients with large artery occlusion, J Cereb Blood Flow Metab 29:S593, 2009.
5. Derdeyn CP, Videen TO, Grubb RL Jr, et al: Comparison of PET oxygen extraction fraction methods for the prediction of stroke risk, J Nucl Med 42:1195–1197, 2001.
6. Grubb RL Jr, Derdeyn CP, Fritsch SM, et al: Importance of hemodynamic factors in the prognosis of symptomatic carotid occlusion, JAMA 280:1055–1060, 1998.
7. Derdeyn CP, Grubb RL Jr, Powers WJ: Re: Stages and thresholds of hemodynamic failure, Stroke 34:589, 2003.
8. Nemoto EM, Yonas H, Kuwabara H, et al: Identification of hemodynamic compromise by cerebrovascular reserve and oxygen extraction fraction in occlusive vascular disease, J Cereb Blood Flow Metab 24:1081–1089, 2004.
9. Nemoto EM, Yonas H, Kuwabara H, et al: Hemodynamic compromise in occlusive vascular disease by PET OEF with acetazolamide, Stroke 35:269–270, 2004.
10. Nemoto EM, Yonas H, Kuwabara H, et al: Differentiating hemodynamic compromise by the OEF response to acetazolamide in occlusive vascular disease, Oxygen Trans Tissue 26(566):135–141, 2005.
11. Kuroda S, Shiga T, Houkin K, et al: Cerebral oxygen metabolism and neuronal integrity in patients with impaired vasoreactivity attributable to occlusive carotid artery disease, Stroke 37:393–398, 2006.
12. Pindzola RR, Sashin D, Nemoto EM, et al: Identifying regions of compromised hemodynamics in symptomatic carotid occlusion by cerebrovascular reactivity and oxygen extraction fraction, Neurol Res 28: 149–154, 2006.
13. Gur D, Yonas H, Jackson DL, et al: Simultaneous measurements of cerebral blood flow by the Xenon/CT method and the microsphere method: a comparison, Invest Radiol 20:672–677, 1985.
14. Wolfson SK Jr, Clark J, Greenberg JH, et al: Xenon-enhanced computed tomography compared with [14C]iodoantipyrine for normal and low cerebral blood flow states in baboons, Stroke 21:751–757, 1990.
15. Matsuda M, Lee H, Kuribayashi K, et al: Comparative study of regional cerebral blood flow values measured by Xe CT and Xe SPECT, Acta Neurol Scand Suppl 166:13–16, 1996.
16. Nariai T: Comparison of measurement between Xe/CT CBF and PET in cerebrovascular disease and brain tumor, Acta Neurol Scand Suppl 166:10–12, 1996.
17. Valadka AB, Hlatky R, Furuya Y, et al: Brain tissue PO2: correlation with cerebral blood flow, Acta Neurochir Suppl 81:299–301, 2002.
18. Latchaw RE, Yonas H, Pentheny SL, et al: Adverse reactions to Xenon-enhanced CT cerebral blood flow determination, Radiology 163: 251–254, 1987.
19. Yonas H, Gur D, Good BC, et al: Stable Xenon CT blood flow mapping for evaluation of patients with extracranial-intracranial bypass surgery, J Neurosurg 62:324–333, 1985.
20. Vorstrup S, Lassen NA, Henriksen L, et al: CBF before and after extracranial-intracranial bypass surgery in patients with ischemic cerebrovascular disease studied with 133Xe-inhalation tomography, Stroke 16:616–626, 1985.
21. Vorstrup S, Brun B, Lassen NA: Evaluation of the cerebral vasodilatory capacity by the acetazolamide test before EC-IC bypass surgery in

patients with occlusion of the internal carotid artery, *Stroke* 17: 1291–1298, 1986.

22. Powers WJ, Tempel LW, Grubb RL Jr: Influence of cerebral hemodynamics on stroke risk: one-year follow-up of 30 medically treated patients, *Ann Neurol* 25:325–330, 1989.

23. Rogg J, Rutigliano M, Yonas H, et al: The acetazolamide challenge: imaging techniques designed to evaluate cerebral blood flow reserve, *Am J Roentgenol* 153:605–612, 1989.

24. Yonas H, Smith HA, Durham SR, et al: Increased stroke risk predicted by compromised cerebral blood flow reactivity, *J Neurosurg* 79: 483–489, 1993.

25. Webster MW, Makaroun MS, Steed DL, et al: Compromised cerebral blood flow reactivity is a predictor of stroke in patients with symptomatic carotid artery occlusive disease, *J Vasc Surg* 21:338–344, 1995; discussion 44–5.

26. Kuroda S, Houkin K, Kamiyama H, et al: Long-term prognosis of medically treated patients with internal carotid or middle cerebral artery occlusion: can acetazolamide test predict it? *Stroke* 32:2110–2116, 2001.

27. Ogasawara K, Ogawa A, Yoshimoto T: Cerebrovascular reactivity to acetazolamide and outcome in patients with symptomatic internal carotid or middle cerebral artery occlusion: a Xenon-133 single-photon emission computed tomography study, *Stroke* 33: 1857–1862, 2002.

28. Yamashita T, Kashiwagi S, Nakano S, et al: The effect of EC-IC bypass surgery on resting cerebral blood flow and cerebrovascular reserve capacity studied with stable XE-CT and acetazolamide test, *Neuroradiology* 33:217–222, 1991.

29. Kuroda S, Kamiyama H, Abe H, et al: Acetazolamide test in detecting reduced cerebral perfusion reserve and predicting long-term prognosis in patients with internal carotid artery occlusion, *Neurosurgery* 32:912–918, 1993; discussion 8–9.

30. Przybylski GJ, Yonas H, Smith HA: Reduced stroke risk in patients with compromised cerebral blood flow reactivity treated with superficial temporal artery to distal middle cerebral artery bypass surgery, *J Stroke Cerebrovasc Dis* 7:302–309, 1998.

31. Witt JP, Yonas H, Jungreis C: Cerebral blood flow response pattern during balloon test occlusion of the internal carotid artery, *Am J Neuroradiol* 15:847–856, 1994.

32. Yokota C, Hasegawa Y, Minematsu K, et al: Effect of acetazolamide reactivity on long-term outcome in patients with major cerebral artery occlusive diseases, *Stroke* 29:640–644, 1998.

33. Knop J, Thie A, Fuchs C, et al: 99mTc-HMPAO-SPECT with acetazolamide challenge to detect hemodynamic compromise in occlusive cerebrovascular disease, *Stroke* 23:1733–1742, 1992.

34. Ogasawara K, Ogawa A, Terasaki K, et al: Use of cerebrovascular reactivity in patients with symptomatic major cerebral artery occlusion to predict 5-year outcome: comparison of Xenon-133 and iodine-123-IMP single-photon emission computed tomography, *J Cereb Blood Flow Metab* 22:1142–1148, 2002.

35. Krol AL, Dzialowski I, Roy J, et al: Incidence of radiocontrast nephropathy in patients undergoing acute stroke computed tomography angiography, *Stroke* 38:2364–2366, 2007.

36. Wang CL, Cohan RH, Ellis JH, et al: Frequency, outcome, and appropriateness of treatment of nonionic iodinated contrast media reactions, *AJR Am J Roentgenol* 191:409–415, 2008.

37. Chen A, Shyr MH, Chen TY, et al: perfusion imaging with acetazolamide challenge for evaluation of patients with unilateral cerebrovascular steno-occlusive disease, *AJNR Am J Neuroradiol* 27: 1876–1881, 2006.

38. Smith LM, Elkins JS, Dillon WP, et al: Perfusion-CT assessment of the cerebrovascular reserve: a revisit to the acetazolamide challenges, *J Neuroradiol* 35:157–164, 2008.

39. Schreiber WG, Guckel F, Stritzke P, et al: Cerebral blood flow and cerebrovascular reserve capacity: estimation by dynamic magnetic resonance imaging, *J Cereb Blood Flow Metab* 18:1143–1156, 1998.

40. Olivot JM, Mlynash M, Zaharchuk G, et al: Perfusion MRI (Tmax and MTT) correlation with Xenon CT cerebral blood flow in stroke patients, *Neurology* 72:1140–1145, 2009.

41. Piepgras A, Schmiedek P, Leinsinger G, et al: A simple test to assess cerebrovascular reserve capacity using transcranial Doppler sonography and acetazolamide, *Stroke* 21:1306–1311, 1990.

42. Sekhar LN, Wechsler LR, Yonas H, et al: Value of transcranial Doppler examination in the diagnosis of cerebral vasospasm after subarachnoid hemorrhage, *Neurosurgery* 22:813–821, 1988.

43. Dahl A, Lindegaard KF, Russell D, et al: A comparison of transcranial Doppler and cerebral blood flow studies to assess cerebral vasoreactivity, *Stroke* 23:15–19, 1992.

44. Pindzola RR, Balzer JR, Nemoto EM, et al: Cerebrovascular reserve in patients with carotid occlusive disease assessed by stable Xenon-enhanced CT cerebral blood flow and transcranial Doppler, *Stroke* 32:1811–1817, 2001.

45. Markus HS, Harrison MJG: Estimation of cerebrovascular reactivity using transcranial Doppler, including the use of breath-holding as the vasodilatory stimulus, *Stroke* 23:668–673, 1992.

46. Muller M, Voges M, Piepgras U, et al: Assessment of cerebral vasomotor reactivity by transcranial Doppler ultrasound and breath-holding: a comparison with acetazolamide as vasodilatory stimulus, *Stroke* 26: 96–100, 1995.

47. Ringelstein EB, Vaneyck S, Mertens I: Evaluation of cerebral vasomotor reactivity by various vasodilating stimuli: comparison of CO2 to acetazolamide, *J Cereb Flow Metab* 12:162–168, 1992.

48. Chimowitz MI, Furlan AJ, Jones SC, et al: Transcranial Doppler assessment of cerebral perfusion reserve in patients with carotid occlusive disease and no evidence of cerebral infarction, *Neurology* 43: 353–357, 1993.

49. Orosz L, Fulesdi B, Hoksbergen A, et al: Assessment of cerebrovascular reserve capacity in asymptomatic and symptomatic hemodynamically significant carotid stenoses and occlusions, *Surg Neurol* 57: 333–339, 2002.

50. Ringelstein EB, Sievers C, Ecker S, et al: Noninvasive assessment of CO2-induced cerebral vasomotor response in normal individuals and patients with internal carotid artery occlusions, *Stroke* 19:963–969, 1988.

51. Silvestrini M, Paolino I, Vernieri F, et al: Cerebral hemodynamics and cognitive performance in patients with asymptomatic carotid stenosis, *Neurology* 72:1062–1068, 2009.

52. Silvestrini M, Vernieri F, Pasqualetti P, et al: Impaired cerebral vasoreactivity and risk of stroke in patients with asymptomatic carotid artery stenosis, *JAMA* 283:2122–2127, 2000.

53. Gur AY, Bova I, Bornstein NM: Is impaired cerebral vasomotor reactivity a predictive factor of stroke in asymptomatic patients? *Stroke* 27:2188–2190, 1996.

54. Widder B, Paulat K, Hackspacher J, et al: Transcranial Doppler CO2 test for the detection of hemodynamically critical carotid artery stenoses and occlusions, *Eur Arch Psychiatry Neurol Sci* 236:162–168, 1986.

55. Barnett HJ, Taylor DW, Eliasziw M, et al: Benefit of carotid endarterectomy in patients with symptomatic moderate or severe stenosis. North American Symptomatic Carotid Endarterectomy Trial Collaborators, *N Engl J Med* 339:1415–1425, 1998.

56. Randomised trial of endarterectomy for recently symptomatic carotid stenosis: final results of the MRC European Carotid Surgery Trial (ECST), *Lancet* 351:1379–1387, 1998.

57. Vernieri F, Pasqualetti P, Diomedi M, et al: Cerebral hemodynamics in patients with carotid artery occlusion and contralateral moderate or severe internal carotid artery stenosis, *J Neurosurg* 94:559–564, 2001.

58. Kleiser B, Widder B: Course of carotid artery occlusions with impaired cerebrovascular reactivity, *Stroke* 23:171–174, 1992.

59. Vernieri F, Pasqualetti P, Passarelli F, et al: Outcome of carotid artery occlusion is predicted by cerebrovascular reactivity, *Stroke* 30: 593–598, 1999.

60. Vernieri F, Pasqualetti P, Matteis M, et al: Effect of collateral blood flow and cerebral vasomotor reactivity on the outcome of carotid artery occlusion, *Stroke* 32:1552–1558, 2001.

61. Markus H, Cullinane M: Severely impaired cerebrovascular reactivity predicts stroke and TIA risk in patients with carotid artery stenosis and occlusion, *Brain* 124:457–467, 2001.

62. Huang SC, Carson RE, Hoffman EJ, et al: Quantitative measurement of local cerebral blood-flow in humans by positron computed-tomography and O-15-water, *J Cereb Blood Flow Metab* 3:141–153, 1983.

63. Kuwabara Y, Ichiya Y, Sasaki M, et al: Time dependency of the acet-azolamide effect on cerebral hemodynamics in patients with chronic occlusive cerebral arteries. Early steal phenomenon demonstrated by [15O]H2O positron emission tomography, *Stroke* 26:1825–1829, 1995.

64. Grubb RL Jr, Powers WJ, Derdeyn CP, et al: The carotid occlusion surgery study, *Neurosurg Focus* 14:e9, 2003.

65. Adams HP Jr, Powers WJ, Grubb RL Jr, et al: Preview of a new trial of extracranial-to-intracranial arterial anastomosis: the carotid occlusion surgery study, *Neurosurg Clin N Am* 12:613–624, ix–x, 2001.

66. Derdeyn CP, Grubb RL Jr, Powers WJ: Cerebral hemodynamic impairment: methods of measurement and association with stroke risk, *Neurology* 53:251–259, 1999.

67. Yamauchi H, Okazawa H, Kishibe Y, et al: Oxygen extraction fraction and acetazolamide reactivity in symptomatic carotid artery disease, *J Neurol Neurosurg Psychiatry* 75:33–37, 2004.

68. Nemoto EM, Yonas H, Pindzola RR, et al: PET OEF reactivity for hemo-dynamic compromise in occlusive vascular disease, *J Neuroimaging* 17:54–60, 2007.

69. Jumaa M, Hammer M, Uchino K, et al: Hemodynamic compromise identified by oxygen extraction fraction response (OEFR) to acetazol-amide in stroke patients with large artery occlusion, *J Cereb Blood Flow Metab* 29:S592, 2009.

70. Nemoto EM, Yonas H, Chang Y: Stages and thresholds of hemody-namic failure, *Stroke* 34:2–3, 2003.

PET MEASUREMENTS OF OEF FOR CEREBRAL REVASCULARIZATION

3

COLIN DERDEYN

INTRODUCTION

Positron emission tomography (PET) provides regional, quantitative measurements of important parameters such as cerebral blood flow (CBF) and oxygen metabolism, as well as molecular imaging using specific physiologic and pathologic chemical compounds (molecular imaging), in living humans. The ability to quantitatively measure regional oxygen metabolism and oxygen extraction fraction (OEF) remains unique to PET imaging. OEF increases in response to a reduction in the delivery of oxygen to normal brain tissue. In patients with atherosclerotic occlusive disease, this occurs when collateral channels are insufficient to maintain normal blood flow. Increased OEF is a powerful and independent predictor of future stroke in patients with atherosclerotic carotid artery occlusion and there is an ongoing clinical trial of surgical bypass in this population.

PET IMAGING PHYSICS

PET imaging requires three components: a positron-emitting isotope (radiotracer), a tomographic imaging system to detect the location and to measure the quantity of radiation, and a mathematical model relating the physiological process under study to the detected radiation.[1,2] For example, the method used in our laboratory for the measurement of cerebral blood flow uses a bolus injection of O-15 labeled water ($H_2^{15}O$, the radiotracer).[3] The PET camera system records the location and number of counts during the circulation of the water through the brain. Finally, the tomographic PET images of raw counts are converted into maps of regional quantitative CBF using computer algorithms. This processing requires measurement of arterial blood counts and incorporates models and assumptions regarding the transit of water through the cerebral circulation.

Radiotracers are radioactive molecules administered in such small quantities that they do not affect the physiologic process under study. PET radiotracers decay by positron emission and may be separated into two broad categories:

normal biological molecules, such as ^{15}O-labeled water, or non-biologic elements attached to organic molecules as radiolabels, such as ^{18}F-labeled deoxy-glucose (FDG). PET imaging detection systems use the phenomenon of annihilation radiation to both localize and to measure physiologic processes in the brain. In the body, the positron (a positively charged electron emitted by the radionuclide) travels up to a few millimeters before encountering an electron. This encounter results in the annihilation of both the positron and electron and the consequent generation of two gamma photons of equal energy. These two photons are emitted in characteristic 180-degree opposite directions. A pair of detectors positioned on either side of the source of the annihilation photons detects them simultaneously. This allows localization of the point source of the radiation.

The most important limitations of PET imaging of physiologic processes relate to the phenomenon of full-width, half-maximum (FWHM) and a related phenomenon of partial-volume averaging. Detected radiation is observed over a larger area than the actual source. The spread or distribution of activity is approximately Gaussian for a point source of radiation, with the maximum located at the original point. The FWHM describes the degree of smearing of radioactivity in a reconstructed image. The ability of a PET scanner to discriminate between two small adjacent structures or accurately measure the activity in a small region will depend on the FWHM of the system as well as the amount and distribution of activity within the region of interest and the surrounding areas. Because of the smearing or redistribution of detected radioactivity, any given region in the reconstructed image will not contain all the activity actually within the region. Some of the activity will spill over into adjacent areas. This phenomenon is known as the partial volume effect. An important consequence of this principle is that PET will always measure a gradual change in activity where an abrupt change actually exists, such as in an infarct or hemorrhage, or at the border of different structures like brain and CSF or gray and white matter.[4]

Finally, the externally measured tissue concentration of the positron emitting radiotracer (PET counts) is quantitatively related to the physiologic variable under study by a mathematical model. The PET scanner measures the total counts in a volume of tissue over time. The model then calculates how that measured activity reflects the physiologic parameter under study. These calculations account for several factors related to the tracer biomechanics and metabolism. These factors include the mode of tracer delivery to the tissue, the distribution and metabolism of the tracer within the tissue, the egress of the tracer and metabolites from the tissue, the recirculation of both the tracer and its labeled metabolites, and the amount of tracer and metabolites remaining in the blood.

NORMAL CEREBRAL HEMODYNAMICS AND METABOLISM

A brief introduction and definition of the common physiologic parameters measured with PET is useful prior to the discussion of normal hemodynamics and metabolism. *Cerebral blood flow* (CBF) the volume of blood delivered to a defined mass of tissue per unit time, generally in milliliters of blood per 100 g of brain per minute (ml/100g/min) (Figure 3–1). ^{15}O-labeled water is the most commonly used tracer for measurements of CBF and the method used in our laboratory.[3] *Cerebral blood volume* (CBV) is the volume of blood within a given mass of tissue and is expressed as milliliters of blood per 100 g of brain tissue. Regional CBV measurements may serve as an indicator of the degree of cerebrovascular vasodilatation, as discussed further in this chapter. CBV can be measured by PET with either trace amounts of ^{15}O-labeled carbon monoxide or ^{11}CO.[5] Both carbon monoxide tracers label the red blood cells. Blood volume is then calculated using a correction factor for

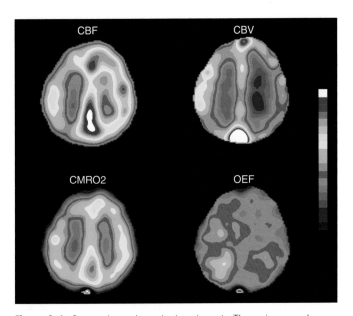

Figure 3–1. Severe hemodynamic impairment. These images show a unilateral reduction in CBF distal to a complete atherosclerotic right carotid artery occlusion. This patient was a 70-year-old male presenting with TIA. Brain CT showed no evidence of stroke. CBV is elevated owing to autoregulatory vasodilation. CMRO$_2$ is relatively preserved owing to the increase in OEF.

the difference between peripheral vessel and cerebral vessel hematocrit. *Mean transit time* (MTT) is usually calculated as the ratio of CBV/CBF. By the central volume theorem, this ratio yields mean transit time, the hypothetical mean time for a particle to pass through the cerebral circulation. Increased MTT is used as an indicator of autoregulatory vasodilation. Some PET groups have advocated the use of the inverse of this ratio instead.[6]

Oxygen extraction fraction (OEF) is the proportion of oxygen delivered that is extracted by tissue for metabolism. In the brain, OEF normally varies between 0.25 and 0.5, with values over 0.5 signifying increased extraction. It is measured in our laboratory by an O^{15}O inhalation scan and independent measurements of CBF and CBV[7] (Figure 3–1). The CBF accounts for the amount of oxygen delivered to the brain. The CBV corrects for oxygen in the blood that is not extracted. An alternative count based method uses the ratio of the counts after an O^{15}O inhalation scan to the counts from an O^{15}O water scan, without CBV correction.[8-11] Other similar methods are also in common use. *Cerebral metabolic rate of oxygen* (CMRO$_2$) is the amount of oxygen consumed by tissue metabolism, measured in milliliters of oxygen per 100 g of brain tissue per minute[7] (Figure 3–1). CMRO$_2$ is equal to the CBF multiplied by OEF and the CaO$_2$ (delivery of oxygen times the fraction extracted times the amount of available oxygen).

Whole-brain, mean CBF of the adult human brain is approximately 50 ml per 100 g per minute. Functional activation increases local or regional CBF, but global CBF generally remains unchanged. Under normal conditions any change in regional CBF must be caused by a change in regional vascular resistance. Vascular resistance is mediated by alterations in the diameter of small arteries or arterioles. In the resting brain with normal perfusion pressure, CBF is closely matched to the metabolic rate of the tissue. Regions with higher metabolic rates have higher levels of CBF. For example, gray matter has a higher CBF than white matter. While there is wide variation in levels of flow and metabolism, the ratio between regional CBF (rCBF) and metabolism is nearly constant in all areas of the brain. Consequently, the maps of OEF from the blood show little regional variation.[12] One exception to this is seen with physiological activation, where blood flow increases well beyond the metabolic needs of the tissue. This leads to a relative decrease of OEF and a reduction in local venous deoxyhemoglobin.[13] This phenomenon is the basis for the use of magnetic resonance imaging (MRI) as a means to map brain function.

Responses to Reductions in Cerebral Perfusion Pressure: Oligemia and Ischemia

Cerebral perfusion pressure (CPP) is the difference between mean arterial pressure and venous back pressure (or intracranial pressure). An arterial stenosis or occlusion may cause a reduction in perfusion pressure if collateral sources of flow are not adequate.[14] The presence of arterial stenosis or occlusion does not equate with hemodynamic impairment: up to

50% of patients with complete carotid artery occlusion and prior ischemic symptoms have no evidence of reduced CPP.[15] The adequacy of collateral sources of flow determines whether an occlusive lesion will cause a reduction in perfusion pressure. When perfusion pressure falls owing to an occlusive lesion and an inadequate collateral system, the brain and its vasculature will maintain the normal delivery of oxygen and glucose through two mechanisms—autoregulatory vasodilation and increased OEF.[16] The presence of these mechanisms has been extensively studied, primarily in animal models employing acute reductions in perfusion pressure. The extent to which these models are applicable to humans with chronic regional reductions in perfusion pressure is not completely known. Autoregulatory vasodilation and increased OEF may also occur in response to reduced cerebral perfusion pressure owing to increases in venous back pressure.[17-20]

Changes in perfusion pressure have little effect on CBF over a wide range of pressure owing to vascular autoregulation. Increases in mean arterial pressure produce vasoconstriction of the pial arterioles, serving to increase vascular resistance and maintain CBF at a constant level.[21] Conversely, when the pressure falls, reflex vasodilation will maintain CBF at near normal levels.[22,23] Two measurable parameters that indicate autoregulatory vasodilation are increases in mean transit time and CBV (Figure 3–2). Despite vasodilation, there is some slight reduction in CBF through the autoregulatory range as perfusion falls, leading to a slight increase in oxygen extraction to compensate for the reduced delivery of oxygen.[16,24]

At some point the capacity for autoregulatory vasodilation can be exceeded. The threshold value for autoregulatory failure is variable between patients and can be shifted higher or lower by prior ischemic injury or longstanding hypertension. Beyond this point, CBF falls linearly as a function of pressure. Direct measurements of arteriovenous oxygen differences ($CaO_2 \times OEF$) using jugular venous oximetry have demonstrated the brain's capacity to increase OEF and maintain normal $CMRO_2$ in circumstances where oxygen delivery diminishes due to decreasing CBF[25] (Figure 3–1). The precise mechanism by which OEF increases is not completely understood. Oxygen passively diffuses from the blood to the tissue. The best current hypothesis is that more of the oxygen that diffuses into the tissue is used for oxidative metabolism, thus reducing the amount of oxygen available to diffuse back to the capillaries.[26]

If the perfusion pressure of the brain continues to fall beyond the capacity for increases in OEF to compensate for the reduced delivery of oxygen, oxygen extraction will become insufficient to meet the energy requirements of the brain and true ischemia ensues.[27] $CMRO_2$ begins to fall and neurological dysfunction occurs. This may be reversible if oxygen delivery is rapidly restored. Persistent or further declines in flow can lead to permanent tissue damage, depending on the duration and degree of ischemia.[28]

Once tissue damage has occurred, the normal mechanisms of cerebrovascular control may no longer operate.[29] Therefore, in some patients who have had transient ischemic attacks (TIA) or mild ischemic strokes with subsequent recanalization, autoregulation or the normal cerebrovascular response to partial pressure of carbon dioxide ($PaCO_2$) may be abnormal for up to several weeks.[30] Over time, flow will fall to match the metabolic needs of the tissue and autoregulatory capacity will be regained. Following reperfusion, the biochemical and ionic abnormalities resolve to a degree dependent on the severity of the initial ischemic insult. The acidosis of anaerobic glycolysis may be replaced by alkalosis.

Chronic oligemia may lead to other compensatory mechanisms, in addition to autoregulatory vasodilation and increased OEF. These include possible reversible metabolic downregulation, accompanied by a reversible cognitive impairment.[31,32] This phenomenon remains an unproven hypothesis and is being evaluated in ongoing trials.

PET STUDIES OF OEF IN CHRONIC ARTERIAL OCCLUSIVE DISEASE (OLIGEMIA)

The identification of compensatory responses to reduced perfusion pressure, or hemodynamic impairment as it is frequently called, may play an important role in medical decision making in a number of subacute or chronic arterial occlusive disorders. These conditions include atherosclerotic carotid occlusion, arterial dissection, Moyamoya disease, and possibly asymptomatic atherosclerotic carotid stenosis.

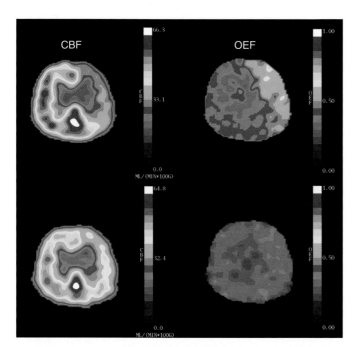

Figure 3–2. Improvement in OEF after extracranial to intracranial bypass. This patient presented with a small left frontal infarction. Baseline PET measurements of CBF and OEF (top row) show reduction in CBF and increased OEF in the hemisphere distal to the carotid occlusion. Seven days after successful superficial temporal to middle cerebral artery bypass (bottom row), CBF has improved and OEF is now normal.

PET and other hemodynamic studies in these patient populations have been aimed primarily at establishing if the presence of these compensatory mechanisms is associated with future stroke risk (natural history studies), if particular medical or surgical interventions can improve cerebral hemodynamics (i.e., using imaging as a secondary endpoint), and finally, pivotal intervention studies of efficacy based on hemodynamic criteria. In this section we will first review PET methods for identification of increased OEF, and then clinical studies in different patient populations.

Identification of Compensatory Reponses to Reduced Perfusion Pressure with PET

As discussed previously, the hemodynamic effect of an arterial stenosis or occlusion depends on the adequacy of collateral circulation as well as the degree of stenosis. An occluded carotid artery, for example, often has no measurable effect on the distal CPP because the collateral flow through the circle of Willis is adequate. Many imaging techniques, such as arteriography, MRI, computed tomography angiography (CTA), and Doppler ultrasound, can identify the presence of these collaterals. These tools show us the highways for blood flow, but not the traffic on them.

Atherosclerotic Carotid Occlusion

The patient population that has been the focus of the most investigation has been atherosclerotic carotid artery occlusion. The presence of increased OEF as measured by PET has been established as a powerful and independent risk factor for future stroke in these patients.[15] Based on this information, a clinical trial of surgical revascularization is underway—the Carotid Occlusion Surgery Study (COSS).[33] The details of these natural history studies and the design and rationale for the current trial will be described in this section.

Patients with complete atherosclerotic occlusion of the carotid artery are at high risk for future stroke.[34] A randomized trial of extracranial to intracranial arterial bypass (the EC-IC Bypass Trial) failed to show a benefit of surgical revascularization in over 800 patients randomized to surgery or aspirin.[35] One possible reason for the failure of this study to show a benefit was the lack of an effective tool to establish whether flow was normal or impaired. A procedure intended to improve flow is unlikely to provide any benefit if flow at baseline is normal. It is possible that a benefit of bypass was missed for a subgroup at particularly high risk due to hemodynamic impairment.

The St. Louis Carotid Occlusion Study was designed to determine if such a subgroup existed.[15] This was a blinded, prospective study of stroke risk designed to test the hypothesis that increased OEF in patients with symptomatic atherosclerotic carotid occlusion predicted future stroke risk. Eighty-one patients with complete carotid occlusion and ipsilateral ischemic symptoms were enrolled. At baseline, 17 clinical, epidemiologic, and laboratory stroke risk factors were recorded. PET measurements of oxygen extraction were obtained.[36] Thirty-nine of the 81 patients had increased OEF. All 81 patients were followed for a mean duration of 3.1 years. Fifteen total and 13 ipsilateral ischemic strokes occurred during this period. Eleven of the 13 ipsilateral strokes occurred in the 39 patients with increased OEF. Multivariate analysis found only age and OEF as predictors of stroke risk. Log rank analysis demonstrated increased OEF to be a powerful predictor of subsequent stroke ($p = 0.004$). Similar results were found by Yamauchi and coworkers.[37]

Prior studies with PET have shown that the superficial temporal artery to middle cerebral artery bypass procedure is capable of reversing the OEF abnormality[29,38] (Figure 3–2). Based on these facts, the COSS was funded by the National Institutes of Health and is underway.[33] Patients with complete atherosclerotic carotid artery occlusion and recent (120 days) ipsilateral cerebral ischemic symptoms are eligible for enrollment. PET studies are obtained on enrollment to identify patients with increased OEF for randomization to surgery or best medical therapy. The primary hypothesis is that bypass surgery will prevent stroke in this high-risk group.

Border-zone hemodynamics

Acute reductions in perfusion pressure can cause ischemic infarction of the cortex and adjacent subcortical white matter located at the border zones between major cerebral arterial territories, such as the middle and anterior cerebral arteries.[39,40] Severe systemic hypotension is a well-recognized cause of multiple bilateral discrete cortical border-zone infarctions.[39] However, the mechanism of cortical border-zone infarction in most patients with carotid atherosclerotic disease is likely embolic and not purely hemodynamic.[41–44]

In addition to this cortical arterial border zone, there is good evidence for an arterial border zone within the white matter of the centrum semiovale and corona radiata.[45,46] This has been called the internal arterial border zone (between lenticulostriate perforators and deep penetrating branches of the distal middle cerebral artery).[45] There is a strong association between hemodynamic impairment of the hemisphere and prior stroke in the white matter, but not cortical border zone.[42] Interestingly, the degree of oligemia as indicated by increased OEF is not higher in noninfarcted white matter regions than the overlying cortex in patients with chronic carotid disease.[47] This suggests that these white matter infarctions may occur at the time of occlusion or soon after (when some selective increase in OEF is present) and not in the chronic situation.

Improvement in hemodynamics over time

In some patients with atherosclerotic carotid occlusion, hemodynamic impairment can improve over time, as collateral flow increases.[48] We repeated PET measurements in 10 patients with complete atherosclerotic carotid artery occlusion who exhibited increased OEF by PET and had no interval stroke 12 to 59 months after the initial examination. Quantitative regional measurements of CBF, CBV, $CMRO_2$, and OEF were obtained. Regional measurements of the cerebral rate of glucose metabolism (CMRGlc) were also made on follow-up in five patients. As a group, the ratio of ipsilateral to contralateral OEF declined from a mean of 1.16 to 1.08 ($p = 0.022$). Greater reductions were seen with longer duration of follow-up ($p = 0.023$, $r = 0.707$). The CBF ratio improved from 0.81 to 0.85 ($p = 0.021$). No change in CBV or $CMRO_2$ was observed. CMRGlc was reduced in the ipsilateral hemisphere ($p = 0.001$ compared with normal), but the $CMRO_2$/CMRGlc ratio was normal. These findings allowed us to conclude that increased glucose transport was not a compensatory response to chronic hemodynamic impairment.

This improvement in collateral sources of flow over time may be a factor that accounts for the reduction in stroke risk over time in all the major cerebral revascularization trials. The greatest risk for stroke in medically treated patients in the North American Symptomatic Carotid Stenosis Trial, the EC-IC Bypass Trial, the European Carotid Stenosis Trial, as well as the St. Louis Carotid Occlusion Study was in the first 2 years after stroke.[35,49,50]

Moyamoya disease

Moyamoya disease is an obliterative vasculopathy of unknown etiology affecting the anterior circulation at the circle of Willis. In North America, it most frequently affects women in their third and fourth decades. Ischemic symptoms of stroke or TIAs are the most common presentation.[51] It is highly likely that hemodynamic mechanisms play a role in the pathogenesis of stroke in these patients. Hemodynamic assessment may be able to provide prognostic information regarding stroke risk in this patient population, analogous to the atherosclerotic carotid occlusion.

We have used PET to study 42 patients with Moyamoya disease and found the frequency of hemodynamic impairment to be quite variable despite uniformly severe vasculopathy: 29 had normal OEF, eight had elevated unilateral OEF, and five had elevated bilateral OEF. Interval improvement in CBF and OEF was observed in one patient with increased OEF at baseline who underwent surgical revascularization. Whether increased OEF predicts stroke risk in this patient population (as it does in atherosclerotic carotid occlusion) is an area of ongoing study.[52]

SUMMARY

In conclusion, the identification of increased OEF has been shown to be a powerful and independent predictor of future stroke in patients with atherosclerotic carotid occlusion. This is the basis for the ongoing randomized trial of surgical bypass for patients with increased OEF (COSS).

ACKNOWLEDGMENTS

This work is supported by the National Institutes of Health grants NINDS P50 55977 and R01 NS051631.

REFERENCES

1. Derdeyn CP: Positron emission tomography imaging of cerebral ischemia, *Neuroimaging Clin N Am* 15:341–350, x–xi, 2005.
2. Derdeyn CP, Powers WJ: *Positron emission tomography: experimental and clinical applications*, Philadelphia, 1997, Lippincott-Raven, pp 239–253.
3. Raichle ME, Martin WR, Herscovitch P, et al: Brain blood flow measured with intravenous H2(15)O. II. Implementation and validation, *J Nucl Med* 24:790–798, 1983.
4. Videen TO, Dunford-Shore JE, Diringer MN, et al: Correction for partial volume effects in regional blood flow measurements adjacent to hematomas in humans with intracerebral hemorrhage: implementation and validation, *J Comput Assist Tomogr* 23:248–256, 1999.
5. Martin WRW, Powers WJ, Raichle ME: Cerebral blood volume measured with inhaled C15O and positron emission tomography, *J Cereb Blood Flow Metab* 7:421–426, 1987.
6. Sette G, Baron JC, Mazoyer B, et al: Local brain haemodynamics and oxygen metabolism in cerebrovascular disease, *Brain* 113:931–951, 1989.
7. Mintun MA, Raichle ME, Martin WRW, et al: Brain oxygen utilization measured with O-15 radiotracers and positron emission tomography, *J Nucl Med* 25:177–187, 1984.
8. Jones T, Chesler DA, Ter-Pogossian MM: The continuous inhalation of oxygen-15 for assessing regional oxygen extraction in the brain of man, *Br J Radiol* 49:339–343, 1976.
9. Derdeyn CP, Videen TO, Simmons NR, et al: Count-based PET method for predicting ischemic stroke in patients with symptomatic carotid arterial occlusion, *Radiology* 212:499–506, 1999.
10. Derdeyn CP, Videen TO, Grubb RL Jr, et al: Comparison of PET oxygen extraction fraction methods for the prediction of stroke risk, *J Nucl Med* 42:1195–1197, 2001.
11. Kobayashi M, Okazawa H, Tsuchida T, et al: Diagnosis of misery perfusion using noninvasive 15O-gas PET, *J Nucl Med* 47:1581–1586, 2006.
12. Baron JC, Rougemont D, Soussaline F, et al: Local interrelationships of cerebral oxygen consumption and glucose utilization in normal subjects and in ischemic stroke patients: a positron tomography study, *J Cereb Blood Flow Metab* 4:140–149, 1984.
13. Fox PT, Raichle ME: Focal physiological uncoupling of cerebral blood flow and oxidative metabolism during somatosensory stimulation in human subjects, *Proc Natl Acad Sci U S A* 83:1140–1144, 1986.
14. Powers WJ, Tempel LW, Grubb RL Jr, et al: Clinical correlates of cerebral hemodynamics, *Stroke* 18:284, 1987.
15. Grubb RL Jr, Derdeyn CP, Fritsch SM, et al: The importance of hemodynamic factors in the prognosis of carotid artery occlusion, *J Am Med Association* 280:1055–1060, 1998.
16. Derdeyn CP, Videen TO, Yundt KD, et al: Variability of cerebral blood volume and oxygen extraction: stages of cerebral haemodynamic impairment revisited, *Brain* 125:595–607, 2002.
17. Wei EP, Kontos HA: Increased venous pressure causes myogenic constriction of cerebral arterioles during local hyperoxia, *Circ Res* 55:249–252, 1984.
18. Ekstrom-Jodal B: On the relation between blood pressure and blood flow in the canine brain with particular regard to the mechanism responsible for cerebral blood flow autoregulation, *Acta Physiol Scand Suppl* 350:1–61, 1970.
19. Iwama T, Hashimoto N, Takagi Y, et al: Hemodynamic and metabolic disturbances in patients with intracranial dural arteriovenous fistulas: positron emission tomography evaluation before and after treatment, *J Neurosurg* 86:806–811, 1997.

20. McPherson RW, Koehler RC, Traystman RJ: Effect of jugular venous pressure on cerebral autoregulation in dogs, *Am J Physiol* 255: H1516–H1524, 1988.

21. Forbes HS: The cerebral circulation, I: observation and measurement of pial vessels, *Arch Neurol Psychiatry* 19:751–761, 1928.

22. Fog M: Cerebral circulation. The reaction of the pial arteries to a fall in blood pressure, *Arch Neurol Psychiatry* 24:351–364, 1937.

23. Rapela CE, Green HD: Autoregulation of canine cerebral blood flow, *Circ Res* 15:I205–211, 1964.

24. Schumann P, Touzani O, Young AR, et al: Evaluation of the ratio of cerebral blood flow to cerebral blood volume as an index of local cerebral perfusion pressure, *Brain* 121:1369–1379, 1998.

25. McHenry LC Jr, Fazekas JF, Sullivan JF: Cerebral hemodynamics of syncope, *Am J Med Sci* 80:173–178, 1961.

26. Mintun MA, Lundstrom BN, Snyder AZ, et al: Blood flow and oxygen delivery to human brain during functional activity: theoretical modeling and experimental data, *Proc Natl Acad Sci U S A* 98:6859–6864, 2001.

27. Marshall RS, Lazar RM, Mohr JP, et al: Higher cerebral function and hemispheric blood flow during awake carotid artery balloon test occlusions, *J Neurol Neurosurg Psychiatry* 66:734–738, 1999.

28. Heiss WD, Rosner G: Functional recovery of cortical neurons as related to degree and duration of ischemia, *Ann Neurol* 14:294–301, 1983.

29. Powers WJ, Martin WR, Herscovitch P, et al: Extracranial-intracranial bypass surgery: hemodynamic and metabolic effects, *Neurology* 34:1168–1174, 1984.

30. Powers WJ: Cerebral hemodynamics in ischemic cerebrovascular disease, *Ann Neurol* 29:231–240, 1991.

31. Sasoh M, Ogasawara K, Kuroda K, et al: Effects of EC-IC bypass surgery on cognitive impairment in patients with hemodynamic cerebral ischemia, *Surg Neurol* 59:455–460, 2003; discussion 460–463.

32. Chmayssani M, Festa JR, Marshall RS: Chronic Ischemia and Neurocognition, *Neuroimaging Clin N Am* 17:313–324, 2007.

33. Grubb RL Jr, Powers WJ, Derdeyn CP, et al: The carotid occlusion surgery study, *Neurosurg Focus* 14:e9, 2003.

34. Klijn CJM, Kappelle LJ, Tulleken CAF, et al: Symptomatic carotid artery occlusion: a reappraisal of hemodynamic factors, *Stroke* 28:2084–2093, 1997.

35. The EC/IC Bypass Study Group: Failure of extracranial-intracranial arterial bypass to reduce the risk of ischemic stroke: results of an international randomized trial, *N Engl J Med* 313:1191–2000, 1985.

36. Derdeyn CP, Yundt KD, Videen TO, et al: Increased oxygen extraction fraction is associated with prior ischemic events in patients with carotid occlusion, *Stroke* 29:754–758, 1998.

37. Yamauchi H, Fukuyama H, Nagahama Y, et al: Significance of increased oxygen extraction fraction in five-year prognosis of major cerebral arterial occlusive disease, *J Nucl Med* 40:1992–1998, 1999.

38. Baron JC, Bousser MG, Rey A, et al: Reversal of focal "misery perfusion syndrome" by extra-intracranial artery bypass in hemodynamic cerebral ischemia. A case study with 0-15 positron emission tomography, *Stroke* 12:454–459, 1981.

39. Adams J, Brierley J, Connor R, et al: The effects of systemic hypotension upon the human brain. Clinical and neuropathological observations in 11 cases, *Brain* 89:235–268, 1966.

40. Brierley JB, Excell BJ: The effects of profound systemic hypotension upon the brain of M. Rhesus: physiological and pathological observations, *Brain* 89:269–298, 1966.

41. De Reuck JL: Pathophysiology of carotid artery disease and related clinical syndromes, *Acta Chir Belg* 104:30–34, 2004.

42. Derdeyn CP, Khosla A, Videen TO, et al: Severe hemodynamic impairment and border zone—region infarction, *Radiology* 220:195–201, 2001.

43. Torvik A, Skellerud K: Watershed infarcts in the brain caused by microemboli, *Clin Neuropath* 1:99–105, 1982.

44. Torvik A: The pathogenesis of watershed infarctions in the brain, *Stroke* 15:221–223, 1984.

45. Zulch KJ: Uber die entstehung und lokalization der hirn-infarkte, *Zentralbl Neurochir* 21:158–178, 1961.

46. Wodarz R: Watershed infarctions and computed tomography. A topographical study in cases with stenosis or occlusion of the carotid artery, *Neuroradiol* 19:245–248, 1980.

47. Derdeyn CP, Simmons NR, Videen TO, et al: Absence of selective deep white matter ischemia in chronic carotid disease: a positron emission tomographic study of regional oxygen extraction, *Am J Neuroradiol* 21:631–638, 2000.

48. Derdeyn CP, Videen TO, Fritsch SM, et al: Compensatory mechanisms for chronic cerebral hypoperfusion in patients with carotid occlusion, *Stroke* 30:1019–1024, 1999.

49. North American Symptomatic Carotid Endarterectomy Trial (NASCET) Collaborators: Beneficial effect of carotid endarterectomy in symptomatic patients with high-grade carotid stenosis, *N Engl J Med* 325:445–453, 1991.

50. European Carotid Surgery Trialists' Collaborative Group: MRC European Carotid Surgery Trial: interim results for symptomatic patients with severe (70%–99%) or with mild (0%–29%) carotid stenosis, *Lancet* 337:1235–1243, 1991.

51. Chiu D, Shedden P, Bratina P, et al: Clinical features of Moyamoya disease in the United States, *Stroke* 29:1347–1351, 1998.

52. Zipfel GJ, Sagar J, Miller JP, et al: Cerebral hemodynamics as a predictor of stroke in adult patients with moyamoya disease: a prospective observational study, *Neurosurg Focus* 26:E6, 2009.

ASSESSMENT OF CEREBROVASCULAR REACTIVITY USING EMERGING MR TECHNOLOGIES

4

DANIEL M. MANDELL; DAVID J. MIKULIS

Extracranial-intracranial (EC-IC) arterial bypass is a potential therapy for the prevention of ischemic stroke in patients with high internal carotid or middle cerebral artery (MCA) steno-occlusive disease. This procedure was popular until the EC-IC Bypass Study[1] was published in 1985. This study of patients with ischemic symptoms and atherosclerotic stenosis or occlusion of the high internal carotid artery or MCA found no difference in stroke incidence between patients randomized to medical therapy versus surgical bypass. A critique of the EC-IC Bypass Study was that patients were included based on angiographic stenosis, without specifically selecting the subset of patients who had cerebral hemodynamic compromise. Subsequent advances in brain imaging have made it possible to better identify this subset.

The most widely studied imaging markers of cerebral hemodynamic compromise are increased oxygen extraction fraction (OEF) and decreased cerebrovascular reactivity (CVR). A major trial currently under way, the North American Carotid Occlusion Surgery Study (COSS),[2] uses increased OEF on positron emission tomography (PET) to select patients for EC-IC bypass. PET measurement of OEF is accurate and the results of this trial are highly anticipated, yet clinical translation of PET OEF may remain a challenge due to limited availability, high cost, and the requirement for an on-site cyclotron to produce the very short-lived radiopharmaceutical oxygen-15 (half-life 2 minutes). This chapter will focus on CVR measurement using MRI.

CEREBROVASCULAR REACTIVITY

Severe stenosis or occlusion of a major cerebral artery does not usually result in a blood flow deficit. The cerebral autoregulatory mechanism maintains flow by compensatory dilatation of downstream arterial vessels and corresponding reduction of flow resistance. The presence of collateral flow pathways, including the circle of Willis and pial collaterals, also play an important compensatory role. However, increasing severity of steno-occlusive disease, with limited collateral flow, can lead to exhaustion of vasodilatory capacity. In this setting, blood flow becomes dependent on systemic blood pressure. One can assess cerebrovascular reserve by applying a vasodilatory stimulus, and measuring the resulting augmentation of cerebral blood flow (CBF). *Cerebrovascular reactivity* (CVR) is defined as the change in CBF per unit change in vasodilatory stimulus.

EXISTING TECHNIQUES FOR MEASURING CVR

Assessment of CVR requires a vasodilatory stimulus and a technique for measuring the resulting change in CBF. The commonly used vasodilatory stimuli used are intravenous administration of acetazolamide and induction of hypercapnia through breath holding or inhalation of carbon dioxide (CO_2). Acetazolamide is widely available and administration does not require special equipment, but the technique does have limitations. After baseline CBF measurement and then acetazolamide injection, one must wait 10 to 15 minutes for peak change in CBF before imaging again. Differences in pharmacokinetics and pharmacodynamics between sessions for a given patient, and among patients, result in unmeasured variation in magnitude of the vasodilatory stimulus. Induction of hypercapnia through breath holding suffers from a constantly changing blood CO_2 level and it is therefore extremely difficult to quantify the magnitude of vasodilatory stimulus. Our preferred technique uses a re-breathing device called the RespirAct™ developed by one of our collaborators. This device is capable of controlling end-tidal CO_2 and O_2 precisely and independently with transitions between a stable baseline state and stable hypercapnic state occurring within three breaths.[3] End-tidal PCO_2 measured with this device is as accurate a measurement of arterial PCO_2 as actual arterial blood sampling.[4]

Techniques for measuring the acetazolamide or hypercapnia-induced changes in CBF have traditionally included transcranial Doppler ultrasound (TCD), single-photon emission tomography (SPECT), and stable-xenon inhalation computed tomography (Xe-CT). TCD is inexpensive, noninvasive, and free of ionizing radiation. However, the technique yields only a single measurement of CVR for each MCA territory rather than a spatial map of reactivity for the brain, it is technically not feasible in about 10% of patients due to lack of an acoustic window, and it is highly operator dependent. SPECT has had relatively widespread use for mapping CVR. A major limitation of SPECT is that the study is typically performed over 2 days due to radiopharmaceutical kinetics. It is possible to perform the study over a single day, but this requires much higher activity for the second scan, increasing the radiation dose to the patient.[5] Xe-CT is an excellent imaging technique, but it not widely available and inhalation of stable xenon can have undesirable side effects.

CLINICAL SIGNIFICANCE OF IMPAIRED CVR

CVR is typically categorized into three patterns: normal, reduced, and paradoxical (negative). The paradoxical pattern refers to vasodilatory stimulus–induced reduction of CBF. This "steal phenomenon"[6] develops because flow is diverted away from tissue that can no longer vasodilate toward tissues that retain this ability. Blood simply follows the path of least resistance. Consider a patient with severe stenosis of the right middle cerebral artery (MCA), and a normal right internal carotid artery (ICA) and right anterior cerebral artery (ACA). A vasodilatory stimulus will result in dilatation of the arterial vessels of the right ACA territory, and a corresponding decrease in vascular resistance in this territory. The right MCA territory arterial vessels are already maximally dilated at rest, and will not dilate any further. Following application of a vasodilatory stimulus, the decrease in vascular resistance in the ACA territory relative to the MCA territory results in redistribution of blood flow from the MCA to the ACA. In this way, the ACA territory "steals" from the MCA territory. Reduced CVR indicates impairment of cerebral hemodynamics, and paradoxical CVR indicates particularly severe impairment.[7,8]

CVR Impairment is a strong and independent predictor of future ischemic events. Ogasawara et al.[9] studied 70 patients with symptomatic unilateral ICA or MCA occlusion. Patients were categorized as having normal versus impaired CVR using acetazolamide and Xe-133 SPECT, and were followed prospectively for 2 years. The recurrent stroke rate was 6% in patients with normal CVR at entry, compared with 35% in patients with impaired CVR (significant difference, $p = 0.03$). Silvestrini et al.[10] studied 94 patients with asymptomatic carotid artery stenosis of at least 70%. Patients were categorized as having normal versus impaired CVR using CO_2 and TCD, and were followed prospectively for a median of 2.4 years. The annual rate of ipsilateral ischemic events was 4% in patients with normal CVR at entry, compared with 14% in patients with impaired CVR. Markus et al.[11] studied 107 patients with symptomatic carotid artery stenosis or carotid occlusion. Patients were categorized as having normal versus impaired CVR using CO_2 and TCD, and were prospectively followed for a mean of 4.4 years. Controlling for patient demographics, vascular risk factors, prior infarct, and

degree of stenosis, impaired reactivity was an independent predictor of ipsilateral TIA or stroke (odds ratio 14.4, 95% CI 2.63–78.74, $p = 0.002$). From these studies, and others with similar results,[12,13] it is well known that CVR can identify a subgroup of steno-occlusive disease patients at higher risk of stroke. The Japanese Extracranial to Intracranial Bypass Trial (JET),[14] is an ongoing surgical study using acetazolamide SPECT CVR and acetazolamide Xe-CT CVR to identify this high-risk subgroup.

Other important uses of CVR in the context of EC-IC bypass are follow-up of those patients who do not initially meet criteria for bypass, and long-term follow-up of patients who do undergo bypass. A recent acetazolamide SPECT CVR study[15] of 77 patients with Moyamoya disease demonstrated that CVR performed 6 to 12 months following bypass is a strong predictor of long-term post-operative clinical course.

EMERGING MR TECHNIQUES FOR MEASURING CVR

Emerging MRI techniques for measuring CVR offer major advantages over the traditional techniques. We have had particular success applying blood oxygen level–dependent (BOLD) MRI measurement of CVR in a clinical cerebrovascular disease population. We will also briefly discuss dynamic susceptibility contrast (DSC) and arterial spin–labeling (ASL) MRI techniques for measuring CVR.

I. BOLD CO_2 MR Measurement of CVR

Blood oxygen level–dependent (BOLD) MRI refers to a MRI acquisition that is sensitive to the concentration of deoxyhemoglobin in blood. Arterial blood is normally 95% to 100% saturated with oxygen, and venous blood is approximately 60% to 70% saturated. An increase in CBF during stable neuronal activity (i.e., a stable number of deoxyhemoglobin molecules produced per unit time) results in dilution or "wash-out" of deoxyhemoglobin in the cerebral microcirculation. Deoxyhemoglobin is a paramagnetic substance. Paramagnetic substances constrained by boundaries such as red cell membranes or blood vessel walls yield magnetic field inhomogeneities that act to reduce the MRI signal. Therefore, an increase in CBF in the setting of constant neural activity results in a decrease in deoxyhemoglobin concentration in the microcirculation, yielding an increase in MR signal. Furthermore, %△ BOLD MRI signal is linearly related to %△ CBF over the range of CBF changes that occur in a CVR study,[16] enabling the use BOLD MRI to measure CVR.

Advantages of the BOLD MRI technique are the use of an MR pulse sequence that is standard on modern clinical MR systems, short duration of study (acquisition time less than 10 minutes, and real-time data analysis), no requirement for intravenous injection, no ionizing radiation, and the ability to acquire routine MRI and magnetic resonance angiography (MRA) of the brain in the same imaging session. This technique has particular potential when one uses CO_2 as the vasodilatory stimulus: unlike the sustained effect of acetazolamide, arterial pCO_2 is rapidly responsive to changes in the inhaled concentration of CO_2. The BOLD MRI pulse sequence, which is based on rapid echoplanar imaging, can acquire a complete data set covering the entire brain in 2 seconds. The sequence is repeated several hundred times over the course of several minutes in order to provide statistical power for the data analysis while correcting for imaging system instabilities.

The greatest concern with BOLD CVR has been that BOLD MRI signal depends on CBF, but also (and to an unknown extent) on other factors: cerebral blood volume (CBV), cerebral metabolic rate of oxygen consumption ($CMRO_2$), arterial partial pressure of oxygen (PaO_2), and hematocrit. However, we now have empirical evidence that these other factors are not major issues. Goode et al.[17] and Kassner et al.[18] have demonstrated between-session reproducibility of BOLD CO_2 CVR, and Shiino et al.[19] and our group[20] have demonstrated the accuracy of BOLD CO_2 CVR in patients with severe cerebrovascular disease. Shiino et al. compared BOLD CO_2 CVR with SPECT acetazolamide CVR in 10 patients with severe carotid stenosis or occlusion. They found that the degree of impairment and distribution of impaired areas detected by BOLD MRI correlated with the results of SPECT. Our group studied 38 patients with steno-occlusive disease by both BOLD CO_2 CVR and arterial spin labeling (ASL) MRI. The latter technique does not have the CBV and $CMRO_2$ dependencies of BOLD MRI. Hemispheric CVR measured by BOLD MRI was significantly correlated with that measured by ASL MRI for both gray matter ($r = 0.83$, $p < 0.0001$) and white matter ($r = 0.80$, $p < 0.0001$). Diagnostic accuracy (area under receiver operating characteristic curve) for BOLD MRI discrimination between normal and abnormal hemispheric CVR was 0.90 (95% CI = 0.81 to 0.98; $p < 0.001$) for gray matter and 0.82 (95% CI = 0.70 to 0.94; $P<0.001$) for white matter. Regions of paradoxical CVR on BOLD MRI had a moderate predictive value (14 of 19 hemispheres) for spatially corresponding paradoxical CVR on ASL MRI. Complete absence of paradoxical CVR on BOLD MRI had a high predictive value (31 of 31 hemispheres) for corresponding nonparadoxical CVR on ASL MRI.

The BOLD CO$_2$ CVR examination

There are a variety of ways to perform a BOLD CO_2 CVR study. Our technique has evolved over time, and we will discuss our current technique in detail.

Patient Preparation: We have performed BOLD CO_2 CVR studies in over 400 patients with the most severe forms of cerebrovascular disease. pCO_2 levels are used that are similar to the range of pCO_2 that occurs during daily living. Fewer than 5% of patients have not been able to complete the examination. Outside the MR scan room, we place a soft plastic facemask on the patient, and use plastic tape (3M Tegaderm™) to ensure an air-tight seal to the face. The patient is then taken

into the MR scan room, and positioned supine on the scanner table with head inside the head coil.

Vasodilatory Stimulus: Patients' expiratory gas concentrations are controlled by providing a series of gas flows with variable CO_2, O_2, and N_2 concentrations to a sequential re-breathing manifold[21] (Thornhill Research Inc., Toronto, Canada) attached to the facemask. Gas flows to the manifold are controlled by a computer-controlled gas blender (RespirAct™, Thornhill Research, Toronto, Canada) programmed to provide the flow and proportion of O_2, N_2, and CO_2 needed to attain the target end-tidal partial pressures of CO_2 (PETCO$_2$) and O_2 (PETO$_2$). Our target gas sequence is 8 minutes and 20 seconds in duration, with target PETO$_2$ of 100 mm Hg throughout, and target PETCO$_2$ alternating between normocapnia (40 mm Hg) and hypercapnia (50 mm Hg) (Figure 4–1). Tidal pCO_2 and pO_2 are monitored continuously (RespirAct™), digitized, and recorded using data acquisition software (LabView, National Instruments Corporation, Austin, TX). The apparatus and technique are described in greater detail elsewhere.[3,4]

MRI: Although imaging can be performed at 1.5 Tesla (50% longer data acquisition time to compensate for reduced signal at this field strength), we currently use a 3.0 Tesla system (Signa HDx; GE Healthcare, Milwaukee, WI) with an eight-channel, phased-array head coil. A T1-weighted three-dimensional spoiled gradient echo sequence is used to acquire anatomical images for co-registration (matrix: 256 × 256; slice thickness: 2.2 mm; no interslice gap). During the controlled changes in PETCO$_2$, BOLD MR acquisitions are obtained. Twenty-six slices are acquired every 2 seconds over a total acquisition time of 8 minutes and 20 seconds. The BOLD sequences is a T2*-weighted single-shot gradient echo echoplanar acquisition (field of view: 24 × 24 cm; matrix: 64 × 64; TR: 2000 ms; TE: 30 ms; flip angle: 85 degrees; slice thickness: 5.0 mm; no interslice gap; number of frames: 254).

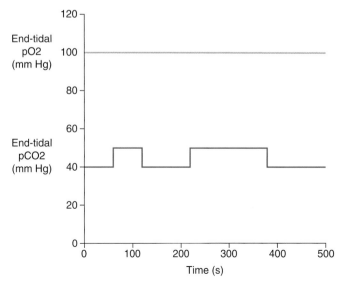

Figure 4–1. Target gas sequence for PETO$_2$ (black line) and PETCO$_2$ (gray waveform).

Data Processing: MRI and $P_{ET}CO_2$ data are imported into AFNI,[22] a functional neuroimaging software package available for download at http://afni.nimh.nih.gov/afni/. Total MR signal is calculated for each whole-brain acquisition (i.e., for every set of images covering the entire brain), yielding a whole-brain BOLD MR signal waveform of 500 seconds duration. This whole-brain BOLD MR signal waveform is temporally shifted to the point of maximum statistical correlation with the $P_{ET}CO_2$ waveform (output from the RespirAct). Figure 4–2 shows $P_{ET}CO_2$ (in red) and whole-brain BOLD MR signal (in blue) as a function of time for a normal subject. Note how each increase in $P_{ET}CO_2$ is accompanied by a corresponding increase in BOLD MR signal.

The BOLD MRI signal time course is then regressed (least squares) against the $P_{ET}CO_2$ waveform on a voxel-by-voxel basis. The slope of the regression, expressed as %ΔBOLD MR signal per mm Hg $\Delta P_{ET}CO_2$, is CVR. The CVR map is color-coded using a two-color continuous spectrum ranging from red for positive CVR to blue for negative CVR, and then overlaid voxel by voxel on the anatomical images (Figure 4–3).

BOLD MR measurement of CVR in the EC-IC bypass population

We routinely use BOLD CO_2 CVR to evaluate possible candidates for EC-IC bypass. The majority of these patients have Moyamoya disease or Moyamoya syndrome, and a smaller number have intracranial steno-occlusive disease of atherosclerotic or other etiology. We map CVR in patients for whom surgical revascularization is contemplated, but also to follow those patients who are not surgical candidates, and to postoperatively evaluate those who undergo bypass. The following cases illustrate the technique:

- Case 1: Paradoxical reactivity on BOLD CO_2 CVR (Figure 4–4 through 4–6)

- Case 2: Bilateral disease and BOLD CO_2 CVR evidence of bypass failure (Figure 4–7 through 4–9)

- Case 3: Quantitative BOLD CO_2 CVR (Figure 4–10)

Qualitatively, BOLD CO_2 CVR maps convey important information. They demarcate a clear difference between positive CVR and paradoxical CVR, and we know that paradoxical CVR indicates significant hemodynamic compromise.

The term "quantitative" can have many meanings in the context of CVR. Some groups conducting CVR studies use the contralateral hemisphere as an internal standard and report "quantitative" interhemispheric asymmetry indices, typically a ratio of right-hemisphere CVR to left-hemisphere CVR. Other groups have used cerebellar CVR as an internal standard. The disadvantage of these approaches is that they are only valid in patients with unilateral disease or lack of posterior circulation involvement, respectively. This is a major limitation. The major advantage of our approach is that it is independent of the number and degree of vascular stenoses.

In addition to patient factors (CBV, $CMRO_2$, pO_2, hematocrit) discussed earlier, BOLD MR signal depends on both MR hardware (most notably magnetic field strength) and MR pulse sequence specifics (sequence type, echo time, voxel size, etc.). When performing CVR studies using one MR scanner with consistent sequence parameters, CVR measured as %ΔBOLD MR signal per mm Hg $\Delta P_{ET}CO_2$ is highly reproducible. This does not provide a measure of CVR in the gold-standard CBF units of ml/100 g/min, but it does enable quantitative comparisons within individual patients over time, and among patients. The ability to quantitatively compare BOLD CO_2 CVR values across institutes using different MR scanners and MR sequences will require further development, but interinstitute reproducibility studies[23,24] of myocardial T2* measurements suggest that this is feasible.

We are currently studying the ability of preoperative CVR to predict the degree of hemodynamic improvement postbypass. To date we have studied 16 consecutive patients with arterial steno-occlusive disease undergoing EC-IC bypass surgery. Preliminary results[25] show that ipsilateral MCA territory BOLD CO_2 CVR (%ΔBOLD MR signal per mm Hg $\Delta P_{ET}CO_2$) improves significantly following revascularization (0.07% ± 0.08% prebypass to 0.24% ± 0.07% postbypass [two-sided

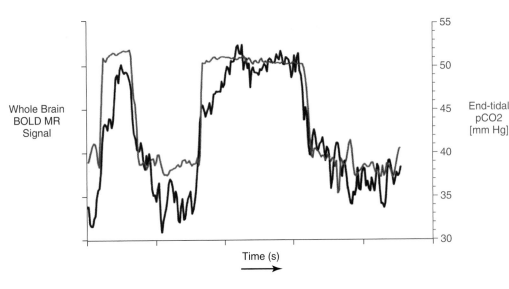

Figure 4–2. $P_{ET}CO_2$ (in red) and whole-brain BOLD MR signal (in blue) as a function of time for a normal subject. This was an 8-minute, 20-second CVR acquisition.

4

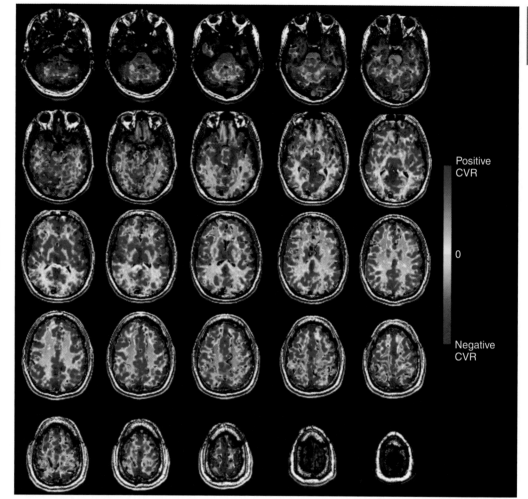

Figure 4–3. BOLD CO_2 CVR map (%ΔBOLD MR signal per mm Hg $\Delta P_{ET}CO_2$) overlaid on T1-weighted anatomical images in a young healthy subject.

Positive CVR

0

Negative CVR

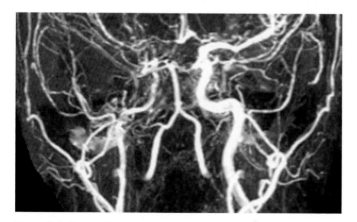

Figure 4–4. Twenty-three-year-old man with neurofibromatosis type 1 and secondary Moyamoya syndrome. Contrast-enhanced MR angiogram shows stenosis of the terminal right ICA and right MCA, and Moyamoya-type collateral vessels about the circle of Willis bilaterally.

$p < 0.01$]). Greater impairment of CVR preoperatively correlates with greater improvement in that territory following bypass ($r = 0.73$, $p < 0.01$). Figure 4–10 illustrates a case from this series.

II. DSC MR Measurement of CVR

Whereas BOLD MRI exploits the magnetic properties of endogenous deoxyhemoglobin, dynamic susceptibility contrast (DSC) MRI is based on imaging following intravenous injection of a gadolinium chelate. Both deoxyhemoglobin and gadolinium possess a property called "magnetic susceptibility" that enables their detection on MRI, and this is reflected in the name of this technique. Both operate on the same principle of contained or bounded paramagnetic substances reducing the MRI signal. In the case of DSC, it is gadolinium that is contained by the walls of the microvessels. Methods of DSC MRI measurement of cerebral perfusion have been described in detail elsewhere. A typical approach follows.

A T2*-weighted echo-planar MR pulse sequence (which is sensitive to the susceptibility effects of gadolinium) is used to repeatedly image the whole brain every 1 to 2 seconds. This records the baseline signal intensity of each voxel prior to the gadolinium bolus. After several whole-brain acquisitions, a tight bolus of intravenous contrast is infused using a power injection of gadolinium chelate at 5 ml/s through an 18-gauge intravenous catheter in the antecubital fossa. Brain imaging continues during and after contrast injection, for a total of

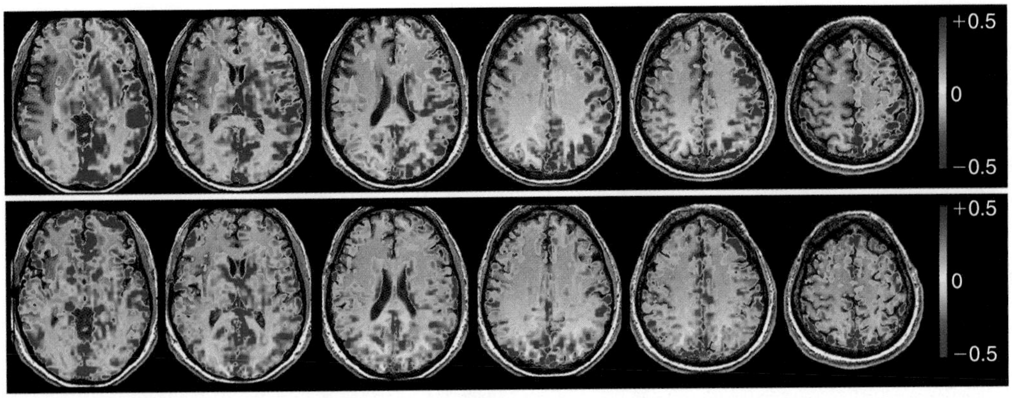

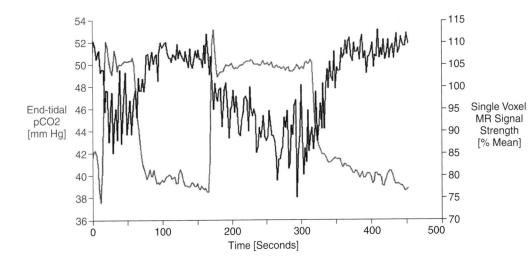

Figure 4–5. Initial BOLD CO₂ CVR study (top row) demonstrates paradoxical reactivity in the right anterior and middle cerebral artery territories. The patient underwent right-sided superficial temporal artery (STA) to MCA bypass 3 months later, and a follow-up CVR study 5 months postbypass (bottom row) demonstrates near normalization of CVR. Units are %ΔBOLD MR signal per mm Hg ΔPₑₜCO₂.

Figure 4–6. A plot of BOLD MR signal (blue) versus PₑₜCO₂ (red) for a single voxel with paradoxical reactivity shows that each increase in PₑₜCO₂ is accompanied by a decrease in BOLD MR signal.

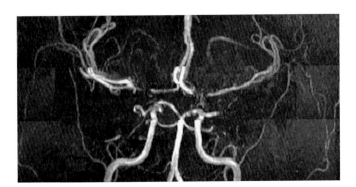

Figure 4–7. Thirty-eight–year-old women with Moyamoya syndrome. Time-of-flight MR angiogram shows severe stenosis of the distal ICAs and proximal MCA M1 segments.

90 seconds, capturing the first pass of gadolinium through the microcirculation. It has been shown that the signal change in a voxel is directly related to the amount of gadolinium in that voxel,[26] and thus the signal-time curve for each voxel is converted into a tissue concentration–time curve. Calculation of CBF requires one additional parameter: an arterial input function (AIF). The AIF describes the concentration-time curve of the contrast bolus on the arterial side, before it passes through the tissue (capillaries). There are a variety of methods for determining the AIF, but most often it is measured as the concentration-time curve for a single region of interest drawn near a major artery supplying the brain. CBF is then calculated based on indicator-dilution theory for a nondiffusible tracer. There are commercial software packages that perform this postprocessing, generating maps of perfusion including relative blood flow, blood volume, and transit time. The extension of DSC MRI perfusion to DSC MRI CVR simply involves performing DSC MRI before and after a vasodilatory stimulus, and then calculating the percent change in CBF per unit vasodilatory stimulus on a voxel-by-voxel basis.

DSC MRI CVR shares some of the advantages of BOLD CO₂ CVR: wide availability, lack of ionizing radiation, relatively high spatial resolution, and ability to obtain anatomical MRI and MRA in the same imaging session. A potential advantage of DSC MRI over BOLD CO₂ MRI is the ability to measure CVR using the standard units of milliliters per 100 g per minute. However, a major disadvantage compared with BOLD MRI is the requirement for an arterial input function. The choice of a reference artery is critical for accurate CBF measurement; this remains non-straightforward and there is no general consensus on how this should be done. This is a particular challenge in patients with severe steno-occlusive

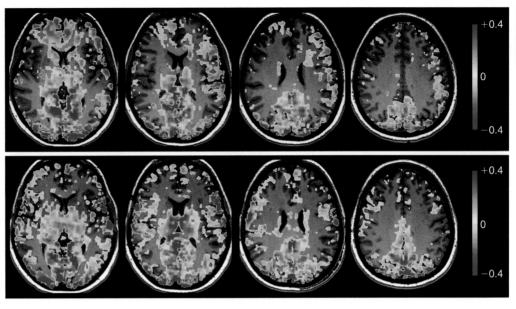

Figure 4–8. Initial BOLD CO_2 CVR study (top row) demonstrates paradoxical reactivity in the ACA and MCA territories bilaterally with preservation of CVR in the posterior cerebral artery (PCA) territories. The patient underwent left-sided STA-MCA bypass 2 months later, and 1 month following that, right-sided direct STA-MCA bypass in addition to right-sided indirect bypass. A follow-up CVR study (bottom row) 6 months postsurgery demonstrates moderate improvement in CVR in the anterior circulation bilaterally, although somewhat less than is typical following bypass. The right side has improved more than the left. Units are %Δ BOLD MR signal per mm Hg $\Delta P_{ET}CO_2$.

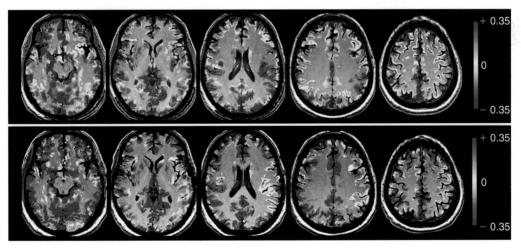

Right EC-IC Bypass   Left EC-IC Bypass

Figure 4–9. Maximum intensity projections from 3D time-of-flight MR angiogram show stenosis at the STA (white arrows) to MCA (black arrows) anastomoses bilaterally, explaining the moderately improved CVR following bypass.

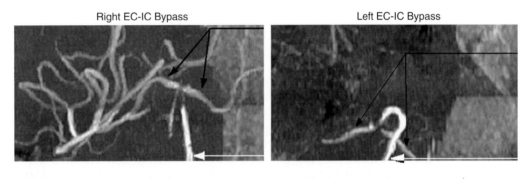

Figure 4–10. Twenty-two-year-old woman with Moyamoya disease involving the anterior circulation bilaterally. A BOLD CO_2 CVR study was performed (top row), the patient underwent left-sided STA-MCA bypass 14 weeks later, and repeat BOLD CO_2 CVR study (bottom row) was performed 13 weeks following bypass. CVR in the MCA gray matter ipsilateral to EC-IC bypass increased from 0.02% ΔBOLD MR signal per mm Hg $\Delta P_{ET}CO_2$ before bypass to 0.25% after bypass. The contralateral side demonstrated a milder increase from 0.12% ΔBOLD MR signal per mm Hg $\Delta P_{ET}CO_2$ before bypass to 0.21% after bypass.

disease, as large artery involvement can preclude use of the arteries typically used for the AIF. It is even more problematic when there are bilateral vascular occlusions. Current research in this area is focused on deriving input functions at the tissue level rather than at large feeding arteries.

There is a wealth of literature on DSC for measuring perfusion, but only a few reports of DSC CVR. Schreiber et al.[27] studied 13 normal subjects and eight patients with steno-occlusive disease using DSC acetazolamide CVR and found reduced CVR in disease patients compared with normals. Similarly,

Guckel et al.[28] studied 21 symptomatic patients with occlusive cerebrovascular disease using DSC acetazolamide CVR, and demonstrated significantly reduced CVR in the affected hemisphere compared with the contralateral side. Ma et al.[29] studied 12 patients with symptomatic unilateral ICA occlusion using DSC acetazolamide CVR and Tc-99m ECD SPECT acetazolamide CVR in each patient. Statistical conclusions were limited given the small sample size: seven of nine patients with impaired CVR on SPECT had impaired CVR on DSC MRI, and two of three patients with normal CVR on SPECT had normal CVR on DSC.

III. ASL MR Mapping of CVR

In its most basic form, ASL MRI uses radiofrequency pulses to magnetically label water protons that then flow into a selected imaging slice in the brain. These modified protons then act as an endogenous contrast agent causing an MRI signal change that is directly proportional to CBF. There are many technical variations on this basic approach.

ASL MRI CVR shares some of the advantages of BOLD CO_2 CVR: lack of ionizing radiation, no need for intravenous injection, and ability to obtain anatomical MRI and MRA in the same imaging session. A potential advantage over BOLD CO_2 CVR is the ability to quantify CVR in standard units; however, quantitative ASL analysis is complex and currently not widely available for clinical use. A major disadvantage of ASL is lower signal-noise ratio than BOLD. Another disadvantage is that delayed arterial transit can cause a significant overestimation of the CVR deficit due to loss of the water proton label through T1 relaxation mechanisms.

ASL MRI CVR in a cerebrovascular disease population has been demonstrated by Detre et al.,[30] Arbab et al.,[31] and our group,[18] but further validation and dissemination of the MR pulse sequences are still needed before this can become a routine clinical technique.

REFERENCES

1. The EC/IC Bypass Study Group: Failure of extracranial-intracranial arterial bypass to reduce the risk of ischemic stroke. Results of an international randomized trial, N Engl J Med 313:1191–1200, 1985.
2. Grubb RL Jr, Powers WJ, Derdeyn CP, et al: The Carotid Occlusion Surgery Study, Neurosurg Focus 14:e9, 2003.
3. Slessarev M, Prisman E, Han J, et al: Prospective targeting and control of end-tidal CO_2 and O_2 concentrations, J Physiol 581(Pt3): 1207–1219, 2007.
4. Ito S, Mardimae A, Han J, et al: Non-invasive prospective targeting of arterial P(CO2) in subjects at rest, J Physiol 586(Pt 15):3675–3682, 2008.
5. Vagal AS, Leach JL, Fernandez-Ulloa M, et al: The acetazolamide challenge: techniques and applications in the evaluation of chronic cerebral ischemia, AJNR Am J Neuroradiol 30(5):876–884, 2009.
6. Nariai T, Senda M, Ishii K, et al: Posthyperventilatory steal response in chronic cerebral hemodynamic stress: a positron emission tomography study, Stroke 29(7):1281–1292, 1998.
7. Webster MW, Makaroun MS, Steed DL, et al: Compromised cerebral blood flow reactivity is a predictor of stroke in patients with symptomatic carotid artery occlusive disease, J Vasc Surg 21(2): 338–344, 1995; discussion 44–45.
8. Yonas H, Smith HA, Durham SR, et al: Increased stroke risk predicted by compromised cerebral blood flow reactivity, J Neurosurg 79(4): 483–489, 1993.
9. Ogasawara K, Ogawa A, Yoshimoto T: Cerebrovascular reactivity to acetazolamide and outcome in patients with symptomatic internal carotid or middle cerebral artery occlusion: a xenon-133 single-photon emission computed tomography study, Stroke 33(7):1857–1862, 2002.
10. Silvestrini M, Vernieri F, Pasqualetti P, et al: Impaired cerebral vasoreactivity and risk of stroke in patients with asymptomatic carotid artery stenosis [see comment], JAMA 283(16):2122–2127, 2000.
11. Markus H, Cullinane M: Severely impaired cerebrovascular reactivity predicts stroke and TIA risk in patients with carotid artery stenosis and occlusion, Brain 124(Pt 3):457–467, 2001.
12. Kleiser B, Widder B, Kleiser B, et al: Course of carotid artery occlusions with impaired cerebrovascular reactivity, Stroke 23(2):171–174, 1992.
13. Blaser T, Hofmann K, Buerger T, et al: Risk of stroke, transient ischemic attack, and vessel occlusion before endarterectomy in patients with symptomatic severe carotid stenosis, Stroke 33(4):1057–1062, 2002.
14. Hayden MG, Lee M, Guzman R, et al: The evolution of cerebral revascularization surgery, Neurosurg Focus 26(5):E17, 2009.
15. So Y, Lee H-Y, Kim S-K, et al: Prediction of the clinical outcome of pediatric moyamoya disease with postoperative basal/acetazolamide stress brain perfusion SPECT after revascularization surgery, Stroke 36(7):1485–1489, 2005.
16. Hoge RD, Atkinson J, Gill B, et al: Investigation of BOLD signal dependence on cerebral blood flow and oxygen consumption: the deoxyhemoglobin dilution model, Magn Reson Med 42(5):849–863, 1999.
17. Goode SD, Krishan S, Alexakis C, et al: Precision of cerebrovascular reactivity assessment with use of different quantification methods for hypercapnia functional MR imaging, AJNR Am J Neuroradiol 30 (5):972–977, 2009.
18. Kassner A, Winter JD, Poublanc J, et al: Blood-oxygen level dependent MRI measures of cerebrovascular reactivity using a controlled respiratory challenge: reproducibility and gender differences, J Magn Reson Imaging 31(2):298–304, 2010.
19. Shiino A, Morita Y, Tsuji A, et al: Estimation of cerebral perfusion reserve by blood oxygenation level-dependent imaging: comparison with single-photon emission computed tomography, J Cereb Blood Flow Metab 23(1):121–135, 2003.
20. Mandell DM, Han JS, Poublanc J, et al: Mapping cerebrovascular reactivity using blood oxygen level–dependent MRI in patients with arterial steno-occlusive disease: comparison with arterial spin labeling MRI, Stroke 39(7):2021–2028, 2008.
21. Somogyi RB, Vesely AE, Preiss D, et al: Precise control of end-tidal carbon dioxide levels using sequential rebreathing circuits, Anaesth Intensive Care 33(6):726–732, 2005.
22. Cox RW, AFNI: Software for analysis and visualization of functional magnetic resonance neuroimages, Comput Biomed Res 29:162–173, 1996.
23. Westwood MA, Firmin DN, Gildo M, et al: Intercentre reproducibility of magnetic resonance T2* measurements of myocardial iron in thalassaemia, Int J Cardiovasc Imaging 21(5):531–538, 2005.
24. Westwood MA, Anderson LJ, Firmin DN, et al: Interscanner reproducibility of cardiovascular magnetic resonance T2* measurements of tissue iron in thalassemia, J Magn Reson Imaging 18(5):616–620, 2003.
25. Mandell DM, Han JS, Poublanc J, et al: Absolute measurement of cerebrovascular reactivity on BOLD MRI predicts response to surgical revascularization, Abstract in press. Proc American Society of Neuroradiology, 2010.
26. Rosen BR, Belliveau JW, Vevea JM, et al: Perfusion imaging with NMR contrast agents, Magn Reson Med 14(2):249–265, 1990.

27. Schreiber WG, Guckel F, Stritzke P, et al: Cerebral blood flow and cerebrovascular reserve capacity: estimation by dynamic magnetic resonance imaging, *J Cereb Blood Flow Metab* 18(10):1143–1156, 1998.

28. Guckel FJ, Brix G, Schmiedek P, et al: Cerebrovascular reserve capacity in patients with occlusive cerebrovascular disease: assessment with dynamic susceptibility contrast-enhanced MR imaging and the acetazolamide stimulation test, *Radiology* 201(2):405–412, 1996.

29. Ma J, Mehrkens JH, Holtmannspoetter M, et al: Perfusion MRI before and after acetazolamide administration for assessment of cerebrovascular reserve capacity in patients with symptomatic internal carotid artery (ICA) occlusion: comparison with 99mTc-ECD SPECT, *Neuroradiology* 49(4):317–326, 2007.

30. Wray DW, Nishiyama SK, Monnet A, et al: Antioxidants and aging: NMR-based evidence of improved skeletal muscle perfusion and energetics, *Am J Physiol Heart Circ Physiol* 297(5):H1870–H1885, 2009.

31. Arbab AS, Aoki S, Toyama K, et al: Quantitative measurement of regional CBF with flow-sensitive alternating inversion recovery imaging: comparison with [iodine 123]-iodoamphetamin single photon emission CT, *AJNR Am J Neuroradiol* 23(3):381–388, 2002.

4

DECISION MAKING IN CEREBRAL REVASCULARIZATION SURGERY USING INTRAOPERATIVE CBF MEASUREMENTS

5

FADY T. CHARBEL; SEPIDEH AMIN-HANJANI

INTRODUCTION

Surgical cerebral revascularization can be performed through various extracranial-intracranial (EC-IC) bypass approaches, using a variety of different donor and recipient vessels, interposition grafts and anastomotic techniques. The specific choice of the type of bypass is dependent on several factors, incusing the ultimate goal of the operation, as well as the availability and suitability of particular donor and recipient vessels. The indications for EC-IC bypass fall into two broad categories:[1]

1. Flow augmentation bypass for treatment of cerebral ischemia.

2. Flow replacement bypass for treatment of complex aneurysms or skull base tumors requiring parent vessel sacrifice.

Intraoperative blood flow measurements can provide a useful adjunct to optimizing decision making and outcomes during both flow augmentation and flow replacement bypass.

INTRAOPERATIVE BLOOD FLOW MEASUREMENT

Intraoperative blood flow measurements can be easily and repeatedly performed using an ultrasonic flow probe (Charbel Micro-Flowprobe; Transonics Systems Inc., Ithaca, NY) that provides flow quantification in millimeters per minute, and is available in a variety of sizes to accommodate vessels ranging from 1 to 3 mm in width. The flow probe uses the principle of ultrasonic transit time to measure flow in vessels independent of the flow velocity profile, turbulence, or hematocrit.[2,3] The body of the probe consists of two ultrasonic transducers and a fixed acoustic reflector. Once the probe is placed around a vessel, a wave of ultrasound is alternately emitted from the two ultrasonic transducers, intersects the vessel, bounces off the acoustic reflector, is received by the other transducer, and converted into an electrical signal. The flow detection unit derives from these signals an accurate measure of the transit time, namely the time it has taken for the wave of ultrasound to travel from one transducer to the other. The transit time of the ultrasound is determined by the motion of blood flowing through the vessel, and the difference between the upstream and downstream transit time is used to derive the flow in millimeters per minute through the blood vessel. The accuracy of the device has been established with in vitro and in vivo studies.[3]

It is important when measuring intraoperative vessel flow to keep blood pressure and end-tidal carbon dioxide (CO_2) constant, as changes in these parameters will create alterations in blood flow; decrease in blood pressure and/or arterial (CO_2) will physiologically decrease the flow and vice versa. In addition, if burst suppression is used for brain protection during surgery, physiological reduction in blood flows will occur in response to the reduced metabolic demand induced by burst suppression. Therefore, flow measurements should be performed once a steady state of burst suppression has been achieved.

BYPASS FOR FLOW AUGMENTATION

EC-IC bypass for cerebral ischemia remains controversial. Superficial temporal artery (STA)–middle cerebral artery (MCA) bypass is the mainstay of cerebral revascularization surgery in the setting of anterior circulation ischemia. The goal of the surgery is to augment flow to the ischemic hemisphere. The use of the procedure decreased markedly after the randomized EC-IC bypass study published in 1985 failed to demonstrate the efficacy of bypass over medical management for carotid occlusive disease.[4] However, subsequent analysis of the EC-IC bypass trial methodology and results have identified shortcomings in the study design and implementation, and suggested that universal abandonment of cerebral revascularization for cerebral ischemia is likely not warranted.[5,6] One of the primary drawbacks of the trial was the lack of hemodynamic evaluation in the selection criteria for patients enrolled in the study. No objective physiological criteria were utilized to assess cerebral blood flow, and enrolled patients may have presented with ischemic events due to embolic phenomenon or small vessel disease, which would not be expected to respond to the flow augmentation provided by bypass surgery. Subsequent studies have demonstrated that careful evaluation of patients with occlusive cerebrovascular disease can identify a subgroup with severe compromise in cerebrovascular reserve capacity, who are at higher risk for stroke,[7–12] and who may be reasonable candidates for surgical revascularization. Recently, the Japanese EC-IC Bypass Trial (JET) has reported favorable results for bypass in patients with internal carotid or MCA occlusive disease with hemodynamic compromise.[13] In the United States, the role of STA-MCA bypass for recently symptomatic carotid occlusion is being re-evaluated by the Carotid Occlusion Surgery Study (COSS), which selects patients as candidates only if they demonstrate hemodynamic impairment on positron emission tomography (PET).[14]

In patients with ischemia who are selected to undergo flow augmentation bypass surgery, intraoperative blood flow measurements can be helpful in decision making and predicting graft patency and success. The techniques and principles for flow measurement can be similarly applied to those undergoing STA-MCA bypass for anterior circulation ischemia, as to those undergoing bypass for posterior circulation ischemia, such as occipital artery–posterior inferior cerebellar artery (OA-PICA) or STA–superior cerebellar artery (STA-SCA) bypass.

Bypass Technique

Standard surgical technique is applied to performing the bypass.[15,16] Briefly, for STA-MCA bypass surgery, a linear incision is placed along the course of the STA branch, and the vessel is dissected for a distance of approximately 8 cm. The temporalis fascia and muscle are divided and a craniotomy is performed. A recipient cortical MCA vessel is freed of its arachnoid attachments in preparation for anastomosis. The STA vessel is cleared of its connective tissue distally, cut at an oblique angle, and fish-mouthed. An end-to-side anastomosis is performed to the recipient cortical MCA branch under temporary occlusion, utilizing interrupted or continuous 10-0 nylon sutures. The dural opening is covered with gelfoam, and the bone flap replaced, removing any portion of the flap that may lead to pressure on the STA. The muscle is loosely re-approximated and the skin closed. For OA-PICA bypass, the occipital artery is dissected from beneath the skin and muscle flap after creating a posterior hockey-shaped suboccipital incision; a lateral suboccipital craniotomy extending across midline is performed. An anastomosis is created between the OA and the tonsillomedullary loop of the PICA, running below the edge of the cerebellar tonsil. For the STA-SCA bypass, or its variant, the STA–posterior cerebral artery (PCA) bypass, the recipient vessel is exposed via a subtemporal approach, as it courses around the midbrain. Anastomosis is performed under temporary vessel occlusion along a perforator-free segment of the SCA or PCA.

Intraoperative blood flow measurement technique

Application of intraoperative flow measurements to flow augmentation bypass entails making flow measurements at two points during the surgery. The first flow measurement needed is the cut flow (Figure 5–1A). The cut flow refers to the maximal potential flow capacity of the in situ donor vessel (STA or OA) once it has been dissected and cut open. The flow in the intact STA or OA in situ is generally very low, less than 5 to 10 ml/min, because of the small caliber of the vessel and the high resistance of the distal scalp tissue bed. However, once the vessel is dissected free from its surrounding tissue, and its distal end is cut, the full carrying capacity of the vessel in the absence of downstream resistance can be determined. This constitutes

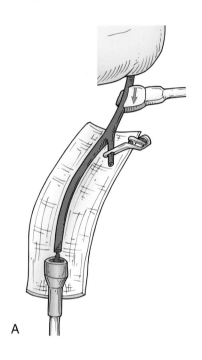

A

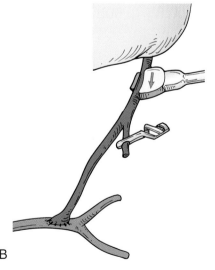

B

Figure 5–1. Intraoperative flow measurement performed in flow augmentation bypass. **A,** Cut flow of donor vessel. **B,** Bypass flow following completion of anastomosis.

the cut flow of the vessel. Prior to flow measurement, the vessel is wrapped in papaverine-soaked cottonoids following dissection to prevent any reductions in flow related to spasm induced by vessel manipulation.

The second flow measurement of importance is the "bypass flow" (Figure 5–1B). Following the anastomosis, the flow in the STA or OA graft is re-measured, which constitutes the flow in the bypass. If the resistance in the cortical recipient bed is sufficiently low, as would be expected in patients with hemodynamic compromise due to cerebrovascular occlusive disease, the bypass flow would be expected to approximate the cut flow of the donor vessel. This can be quantified as a cut flow index (CFI):

$$\text{Cut Flow Index} = \text{Bypass Flow (ml/min)} / \text{Cut Flow (ml/min)}$$

This simple index provides insight into the success of the bypass operation, with a CFI of 1.0 indicating a highly successful bypass. It is important to maintain blood pressure, end-tidal CO_2, and anesthetic technique (such as burst suppression) stable during measurements to avoid spurious physiologic changes in the blood flow measurements.

Interpretation of intraoperative blood flow measurements

The CFI serves as a useful indicator of bypass function and long-term success. In a series of 51 bypass operations performed for flow augmentation in 47 patients, CFI was found to be a significant predictor of bypass patency ($p < 0.01$).[17] Using a CFI of 0.5 as a threshold, the bypass patency rate was 92% in cases when CFI > 0.5, compared with 50% in cases when the CFI < 0.5. Critical examination of the cases with poor CFI revealed that a logical interpretation of bypass function can be performed intraoperatively. A low CFI can be a result of varying forms of intrinsic or extrinsic errors, which can be classified as follows:

Type 1 error: Signifies that the hemodynamic status of the patient may not have been compromised to a significant degree, resulting in lack of demand on the graft. Although recognition of this type of error does not assist in altering the operative plan, information gained in this manner can help to modify the future indications for performing the procedure.

Type 2 error: Signifies a technical problem with the graft relating to the donor, the anastomosis, or the recipient vessel/bed. These fall into categories as below:

- Type 2A error is the result of donor vessel problems, such as atheromatous or calcific changes in the STA, or iatrogenic injury to the vessel during dissection.

- Type 2B error results from an anastomotic problem, such as thrombosis at the suture line.

- Type 2C error signifies a problem with graft outflow, either due to a poor recipient vessel or abnormal recipient vascular bed; this can result from a very diminutive cortical vessel that may not be able to

carry the full flow of the donor, and become the limiting factor in the ultimate bypass flow; other factors such as diffuse atherosclerosis or vessel stenosis/occlusion proximal to the anastomosis may also limit the outflow from the bypass into the recipient bed (Figure 5–2).

Recognition of these errors may direct intraoperative actions, such as reopening and revising an anastomosis for a Type 2B error, or considering a second bypass to a separate

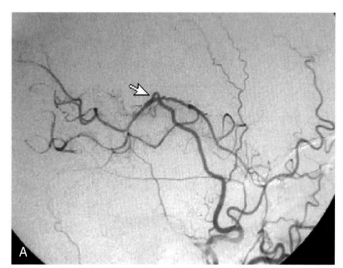

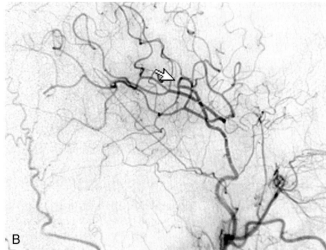

Figure 5–2. Angiographic images following STA-MCA bypass to demonstrate a Type 2C error. **A,** Lateral view of carotid injection after STA-MCA bypass in a 59-year-old male with carotid occlusion. The CFI at time of surgery was only 0.27. The graft (*arrow*) is patent but filling only the temporal branches of the MCA distribution, secondary to a pre-existing proximal disease of the MCA that prohibits retrograde flow into the full MCA territory. **B,** In comparison, lateral view of carotid injection after STA-MCA bypass in a 48-year-old male with a carotid occlusion and CFI of 1.0 at the time of surgery. The bypass (*arrow*) fills the entire MCA distribution.
(From Amin-Hanjani S, Du X, Mlinarevich N, et al.: The cut flow index: an intraoperative predictor of the success of extracranial-intracranial bypass for occlusive cerebrovascular disease, Neurosurgery 2005;56:75–85, with permission.)

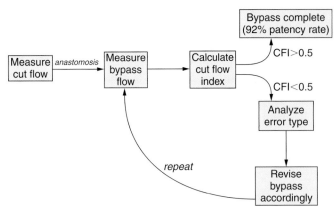

Figure 5–3. Flow measurement algorithm for flow augmentation bypass. *(Adapted from Ashley WW, Amin-Hanjani S, Alaraj A, et al: Flow-assisted surgical cerebral revascularization, Neurosurg Focus 24:E20, 2008.)*

recipient using the anterior STA branch for a Type 2C error (as could have been performed for the case demonstrated in Figure 5–2).

Overall, intraoperative flow measurements allow immediate verification of bypass patency. Additionally, in flow augmentation bypass, the CFI provides a sensitive predictor of postoperative bypass patency. CFI > 0.5 predicts high rates of postoperative bypass patency, whereas a poor CFI can alert surgeons to potential difficulties with the donor vessel, anastomosis, or recipient vessel intraoperatively, allowing the opportunity to rectify the problem (Figure 5–3). Furthermore, a CFI closely approximating 1.0 provides physiologic confirmation of impaired cerebrovascular reserve in the recipient bed. Mere bypass patency can be judged intraoperatively with other techniques including intraoperative micro-Doppler, indocyanine green (ICG) angiography, or conventional angiography. However, given that bypasses with a low CFI are often patent at the time of surgery, the predictive value of CFI highlights the notion that mere anatomic patency may not be as useful in predicting a successful bypass procedure as the assessment of quantitative intraoperative bypass flow.

BYPASS FOR FLOW REPLACEMENT

Definitive management of giant or complex aneurysms may require sacrifice of the parent vessel. Permanent occlusion of the ICA has been successfully used to treat inoperable intracranial aneurysms, and similarly, complete excision of skull base tumors occasionally requires resection of a major vessel.[18,19]

Although carotid sacrifice may be tolerated, ischemia and subsequent stroke can occur in up to 30% of patients.[18] In young patients with a risk of de novo aneurysms over time, or in patients with existing contralateral aneurysm, bypass

may be routinely warranted. Otherwise, tolerance to carotid sacrifice is most frequently evaluated using endovascular balloon occlusion testing (BOT), during which the response to temporary carotid occlusion is evaluated. Tolerance to occlusion is based upon several criteria including neurologic, radiographic, electrophysiological, perfusion, and provocative testing. Neurological criteria are the primary modality of evaluation, consisting of continuous monitoring of the patient for symptoms or signs of cerebral ischemia during a period of 20 to 30 minutes. This can be supplemented with electrophysiological monitoring with the use of electroencephalography (EEG) or evoked potentials.[20] Radiographic features such as the degree of cross-filling from the communicating arteries and the speed of venous filling in the affected hemisphere can also be used to assess adequacy of collaterals.[21,22] Perfusion imaging with modalities such as Xenon computed tomography (CT) and single-photon emission tomography (SPECT) can be used to further assess collateral reserve during test occlusion.[23–25] Provocative testing can be added for those patients who tolerate the initial segment of BOT, by providing an additional hypotensive challenge. Patients who fail BOT require revascularization prior to carotid sacrifice to avert ischemia.[26] The results of BOT in addition to intraoperative assessment using flow measurements can help to determine the best strategy for revascularization.

For management of fusiform or complex aneurysms of distal vessels, such as the MCA or its branches, revascularization using bypass techniques is typically required, as collaterals to such terminal vessels are generally inadequate in the acute setting to avert stroke.

Bypass Technique

The STA for anterior circulation aneurysms, or the OA for PICA/vertebral aneurysms, are carefully preserved in these cases. The general technique for STA or OA for bypass has been described previously. For interposition grafts, saphenous vein grafts or radial artery can be used. A vein can be harvested in the calf or thigh following preoperative mapping to determine the suitability (size and length) of the vein. The radial artery is generally harvested from the non-dominant arm after ensuring adequate ulnar artery collaterals to the hand with the Allen test. The graft is typically subjected to pressure distention with heparinized saline utilizing the Shiley balloon distention kit, and sutured to the appropriate recipient branch with 9-0 or 8-0 nylon using the running suture technique for the distal anastomosis. The graft is tunneled preauricular through a 28 French chest tube to the neck for proximal anastomosis to the external carotid artery or common carotid in end-to-side fashion after creating an arteriotomy with an appropriately sized aortic punch device. Running suture technique using 7-0 prolene is utilized. Typically, 2000 units of intravenous heparin is administered prior to temporary occlusion for the distal anastomosis, and an additional 1000 units prior the proximal anastomosis. The proximal anastomosis is occasionally created in an end-to-end fashion to the stump of the STA as the donor vessel.

Intraoperative blood flow measurement technique

The relevant flow measurements for intraoperative decision making during flow replacement bypass include the following:

- Flows through the distal vessel(s) associated with the aneurysm
- In situ donor vessel (STA or OA when available) cut flow
- The bypass conduit after completion of the anastomosis, and after proximal occlusion or trapping of the aneurysm

Terminal aneurysm flow measurements

For fusiform or complex terminal artery aneurysms located on arteries beyond the anastomotic connections of the Circle of Willis such as the ICA terminus, MCA, PCA, PICA, and ICA terminus, the standard cranial approaches are utilized. Once the aneurysm and associated vessels are exposed using standard microdissection, flow measurements are obtained in all distal vessels that could be compromised by trapping of the aneurysm. For example, the M2 branches would represent the distal vessels in the case of an M1 aneurysm (Figure 5–4), or the PICA trunk would represent the distal vessel in a PICA origin aneurysm. The cumulative flow in the distal vasculature reflects the *distal territory flow* requiring replacement via the bypass.

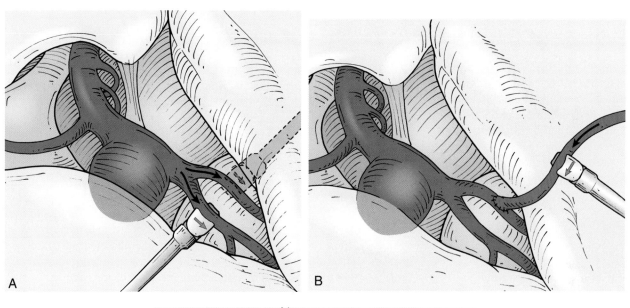

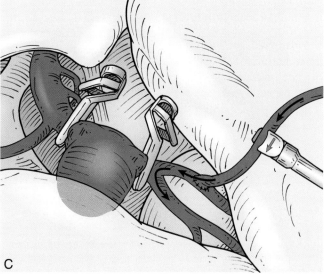

Figure 5–4. Intraoperative flow measurements performed in flow replacement bypass for a terminal aneurysm requiring trapping located at the M1 segment of the MCA. **A,** Flow is measured in the branches distal to the aneurysm to establish the distal territory flow in need of replacement after trapping of the M1 aneurysm. **B,** If the cut flow of the STA is confirmed to match or exceed the distal territory flow, anastomosis is performed; immediate bypass flow is checked but is expected to be low since the parent vessel is still open. **C,** The M1 aneurysm is trapped, and the bypass flow is re-measured to confirm that the bypass adequately replaces the originally measured distal territory flow, verifying both patency and function.

Proximal ICA aneurysm flow measurements

For proximal ICA aneurysms (Figure 5–5), including cavernous segment, ophthalmic, and paraclinoid aneurysms, the operation is performed with simultaneous exposure of the cervical ICA in the neck, while performing a standard pterional craniotomy on the ipsilateral side. Following craniotomy, the sylvian fissure is routinely opened with microdissection, exposing the M1 and A1 segments. Flow in the M1 and A1 (if the ACA territory is at risk) is measured and recorded at baseline, and then repeated following temporary occlusion of the ICA. Temporary occlusion is performed on the cervical ICA when the planned surgical intervention is to be proximal occlusion or on the supraclinoid ICA distal to the aneurysm if the surgical plan is to be trapping of the lesion. The decrement in M1 flow, and A1 flow if relevant, during temporary vessel occlusion is designated as the *flow deficit.*

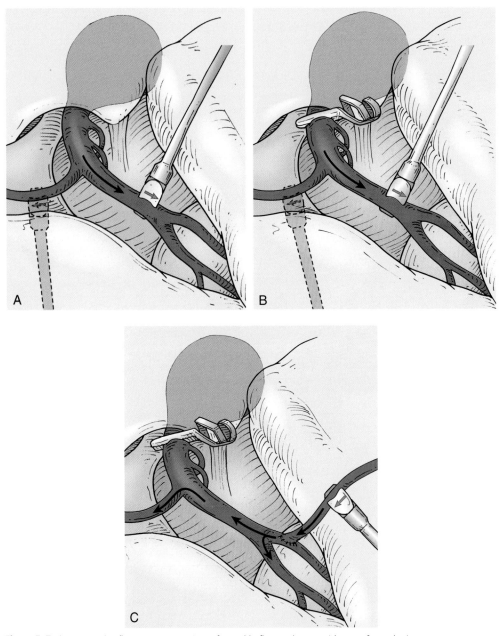

Figure 5–5. Intraoperative flow measurements performed in flow replacement bypass for a giant cavernous aneurysm in a case where BOT resulted in failure, and demonstrated absent anterior communicating artery (both ACA and MCA territory at risk). **A,** Flow is measured at baseline both in the A1 and M1 as a reflection of hemispheric flow. **B,** After temporary clipping the ICA below the posterior communicating artery, flows in the A1 and M1 are re-measured; the drop in flow constitutes the flow deficit that will need to be replaced by a bypass to avert ischemia in the affected hemisphere. **C,** If the cut flow of the STA is confirmed to match or exceed the flow deficit, anastomosis is performed. If the STA flow is inadequate, an interposition graft is placed. Permanent carotid occlusion bypass flow is re-measured to confirm that it adequately replaces the originally measured flow deficit, verifying both patency and function of the graft.

Donor vessel flow measurement

The flow capacity of in situ pedicle grafts (STA or OA) is directly measured to determine their adequacy for replacing the *distal territory flow* in terminal aneurysms or the *flow deficit* in proximal ICA aneurysms. This is performed by determining the *cut flow* of the donor graft,[17] as described earlier, as this reflects the maximal potential flow capacity of the vessel. Once the vessel has been dissected free from surrounding tissues, it is wrapped in papaverine-soaked cottonoids for 20 to 30 minutes during the time that the craniotomy is performed, to relieve any spasm induced by vessel manipulation. The flow is then measured shortly prior to planned bypass.

Interpretation of intraoperative blood flow measurements

Once the *distal territory flow* for terminal aneurysms, or *flow deficit* in proximal ICA aneurysms, has been determined, the selection of bypass can then be tailored to the flow replacement needed (Figure 5–6). If the cut flow of the in situ STA or OA approaches or exceeds the flow required for adequate flow replacement, the in situ graft can be utilized for the bypass. Existing data regarding blood flow and perfusion assessment during vessel occlusion indicate that a 20% to 25% or greater reduction in distal flow is correlated with ischemia.[27–29] Therefore, to avoid risk of ischemia, only a cut flow within at least 20% of the recipient territory flow can be accepted as adequate. It is also important to note that the cut flow is generally measured prior to cutting the graft to its final length in order to allow heparin flushing of the vessel distal to the ultimate anastomosis site (in order to prevent risk of endothelial injury from the flushing needle). For vessels of small diameter such as the STA, the reduction in length of the graft

with final trimming will inevitably result in some increase in carrying capacity. If the in situ donor vessel flow is inadequate, an interposition graft is necessary to ensure adequate flow replacement. In such cases, the choice of a long interposition graft to the cervical ICA or common carotid artery (CCA) versus a short interposition graft to the stump of the STA can also be determined by measuring the flow in the STA stump once the vessel has been truncated.

At the completion of the bypass, whether utilizing the STA/OA as an in situ pedicle graft, or a vein/artery interposition graft, the flow in the bypass is measured to confirm adequate flow replacement following parent vessel occlusion. This provides quantitative confirmation regarding the success of the bypass, superior to the purely anatomic information provided by video indocyanine green angiography or conventional intraoperative angiography.

Intraoperative flow measurements can also be particularly valuable in cases when the need for carotid sacrifice is unanticipated at the time of surgery or when BOT cannot be performed safely preoperatively (as in patients with ruptured aneurysms, or in poor neurological condition). The need for bypass can be tested by temporary clipping of the carotid to determine whether a flow deficit is present. A deficit of >20% would be the cut-off correlated with ischemia, and would indicate the need for bypass for flow replacement. If no significant flow deficit is encountered, suggesting adequate collaterals, a confirmatory vasodilatory challenge can be performed intraoperatively. This is accomplished by increasing the end-tidal CO_2 by 10 Torr, and determining whether there is an appropriate increase in flow to confirm cerebrovascular reserve via the collaterals.[30] This intraoperative version of a carotid occlusion test, if passed, would provide assurance that vessel sacrifice without the need for bypass can be undertaken.

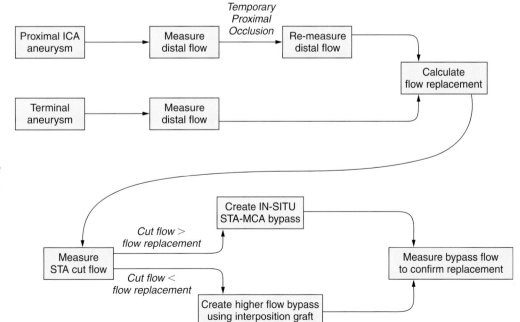

Figure 5–6. Flow measurement algorithm for flow replacement bypass.
(Adapted from Ashley WW, Amin-Hanjani S, Alaraj A, et al: Flow-assisted surgical cerebral revascularization, Neurosurg Focus 24:E20, 2008.)

PERIOPERATIVE FLOW MEASUREMENT

Direct vessel flow measurement prior to and after EC-IC bypass can also provide useful information for surgical planning and for postoperative follow-up. Noninvasive flow measurements can be performed with quantitative MRA (QMRA), which provides the ability to measure flow in millimeters per minute directly in vessels of interest[27,31–34] using phase-contrast MR (PCMR) techniques. QMRA can be readily performed using commercially available software called NOVA (Non-invasive Optimal Vessel Analysis) system (VasSol, Inc., Chicago, IL): an axial three-dimensional (3-D) time-of-flight MRA is first performed to create a 3-D surface rendering of the vasculature, including the circle of Willis, generated using a marching cube algorithm. Vessels including bypass grafts can then be easily identified via the rotating 3-D image. A cut perpendicular to the axis of the vessel is automatically generated when picked in the 3-D image. A double-oblique cine PCMR scan is then performed based on the prescription values of the perpendicular cut from the NOVA system, and a flow value in millimeters per minute obtained.

Preoperative Planning

In patients under consideration for flow augmentation bypass, preoperative QMRA provides a measure of intracranial large vessel flows and can be used as an indicator of reduced flow to a vascular territory (Figure 5–7). These measurements can also provide an indication of the presence, quantity, and pattern of collateral flow through other vessels to the affected territory. When combined with challenge testing, cerebrovascular reserve can be evaluated by determining whether the primary arterial vessel supplying a given territory has the appropriate increase in flow in response to a vasodilatory agent such as acetazolamide. In conjunction with tissue level perfusion imaging, the large vessel flows obtained with QMRA can be utilized to assess hemodynamic compromise.[35]

When flow replacement bypass with parent vessel sacrifice is planned, QMRA provides measures of blood flow in the distal vessels (Figure 5–8). This serves as a baseline measure that can be used for postoperative comparison. The flows can also provide some indication of the flow replacement that will be required, although in our experience, it is expected that vessel flows measured intraoperatively will be ≥40% lower under anesthesia than when measured by QMRA in the awake state.

Postoperative Surveillance

Although postoperative assessment of EC-IC bypass patency has traditionally been documented with catheter angiography, less invasive modalities, both for early assessment and long-term follow-up, are desirable. Although CT angiography and standard MRA can be used for visualization of a graft, QMRA

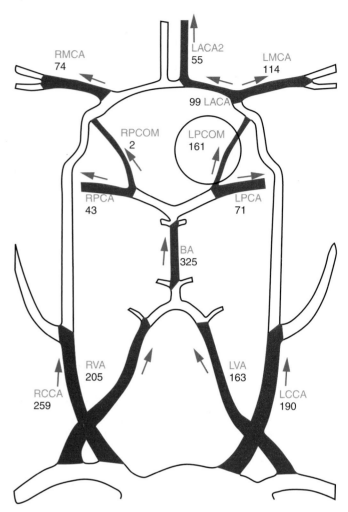

Figure 5–7. Flow map of QMRA performed using NOVA technique in a 71-year-old with bilateral carotid occlusion and recent right frontal and watershed territory strokes. Despite the carotid occlusion on the left, the flow to the left hemisphere is relatively maintained primarily through collateral flow from the posterior communicating artery (*circled*), with well-maintained MCA flow of 114 ml/min. In the right hemisphere, however, there are poor Circle of Willis collaterals, and the MCA flow is low at 74 ml/min.

allows graft function to be measured and followed longitudinally, not merely on the basis of its structural appearance, but on the basis of its flow.

In flow replacement bypass, postoperative QMRA measurement of flow within the graft and within the revascularized vessels can be compared to baseline to confirm the ultimate success of the bypass strategy (Figure 5–8). In flow augmentation bypass, the graft flow provides a quantitative indication of the graft's ability to provide additional flow to the ischemic territory. Furthermore, flow measurements provide a reliable method for assessing long-term patency and function of bypass grafts. Bypass function can worsen over time, with failure occurring at an average of 2.7 years for STA-MCA grafts, and 1.4 years for vein grafts in one series of 47 patients treated for ICA occlusion.[36] Serial follow-up is therefore an important aspect in judging the long-term success of the bypass.

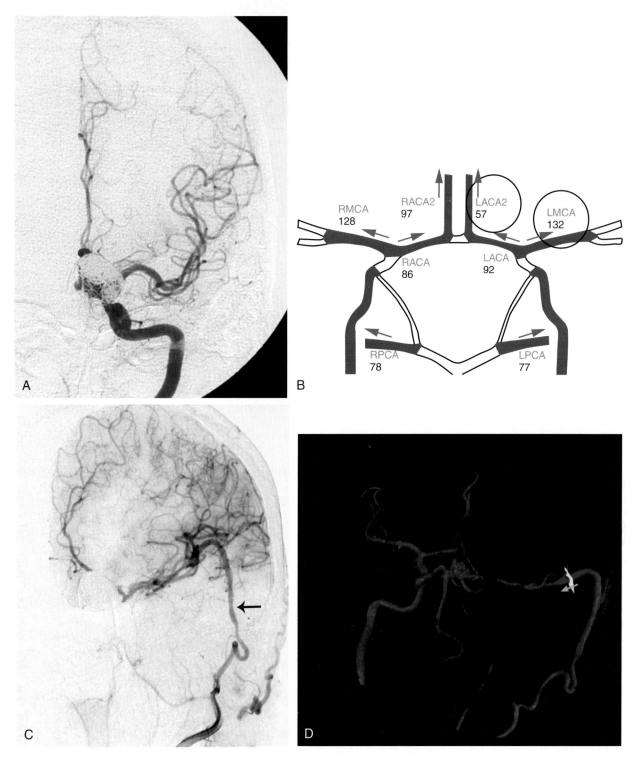

Figure 5–8. Flow measurements in a 53-year-old female with progressive visual loss treated with carotid occlusion and bypass for a giant previously coiled and stented ophthalmic aneurysm. Patient failed BOT clinically with no posterior or anterior communicating artery collateral to the left hemisphere. Intraoperatively, the M1 and A1 flows were measured to be 42 ml/min and 20 ml/min, respectively, while under burst suppression. With a temporary clip on the carotid, the flow dropped to 2 ml/min and 0 ml/min in the measured vessels, respectively, indicating a near complete flow deficit of 60 ml/min. The STA branch flow was inadequate, but the STA stump flow was measured to be 120 ml/min. Therefore an interposition vein graft was performed between the STA stump and an M2 branch. After completion of the bypass and carotid occlusion, the final bypass flow measured 62 ml/min while still under burst suppression, matching the original flow deficit. Final bypass flow intraoperatively out of burst suppression measured 125 ml/min. **A,** Preoperative AP angiogram demonstrating the aneurysm. **B,** Preoperative NOVA flow map showing a baseline flow of 132 ml/min in the left MCA and 57 ml/min in the left ACA for a total flow of 191 ml/min. **C,** Postoperative AP angiogram demonstrating the STA-vein-MCA bypass (*arrow*) and exclusion of the aneurysm from the circulation. **D,** Postoperative NOVA 3D image with flow measurement.

Continued

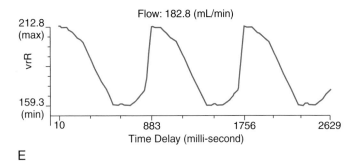

Figure 5-8—cont'd E, in the bypass graft of 182 ml/min (*arrow*), closely matching the total preoperative flow of 189 ml/min for the MCA and ACA.

In a series of 62 bypass cases comparing conventional angiography and QMRA for postoperative bypass evaluation and surveillance, excellent correlation was found between the modalities.[37] Occluded bypasses ($n = 4$) were consistently not visualized on QMRA. Flow rates were found to be significantly lower in bypasses that were stenotic or diminutive in caliber over time, compared to those that remained fully patent on angiography. All angiographically poor bypasses were identifiable by flow rates of <20 ml/min or a reduction in bypass flow of >30% within 3 months, indicating that a low or rapidly declining flow is an indicator of a failing graft.

CONCLUSION

In flow augmentation bypass for ischemia, intraoperative flow measurements provide an indication of bypass patency, as well as the success of the bypass in revascularizing the ischemic territory. In flow replacement bypass for planned vessel sacrifice, intraoperative flow measurements provide a mechanism for guiding graft selection to provide the optimal revascularization strategy, as well as verifying the function and adequacy of the bypass. Pre- and post-operative flow measurements can be used in surgical planning and long-term surveillance after EC-IC bypass surgery.

REFERENCES

1. Charbel FT, Guppy KH, Ausman JI: Cerebral revascularization: Superficial temporal middle cerebral artery anastomosis. In Sekhar LN, Fessler RG, editors: *Atlas of Neurosurgical Techniques*, New York, 2006, Thieme, pp 370–378.
2. Charbel FT, Hoffman WE, Misra M, et al: Ultrasonic perivascular flow probe: technique and application in neurosurgery, *Neurol Res* 20:439–442, 1998.
3. Lundell A, Bergqvist D, Mattsson E, et al: Volume blood flow measurements with a transit time flowmeter: an in vivo and in vitro variability and validation study, *Clin Physiol* 13:547–557, 1993.
4. The EC/IC Bypass Study Group: Failure of extracranial-intracranial arterial bypass to reduce the risk of ischemic stroke. Results of an international randomized trial, *N Engl J Med* 313:1191–1200, 1985.
5. Goldring S, Zervas N, Langfitt T: The Extracranial-Intracranial Bypass Study. A report of the committee appointed by the American Association of Neurological Surgeons to examine the study, *N Engl J Med* 316:817–820, 1987.
6. Sundt TM Jr: Was the international randomized trial of extracranial-intracranial arterial bypass representative of the population at risk? *N Engl J Med* 316:814–816, 1987.
7. Grubb RL Jr, Derdeyn CP, Fritsch SM, et al: Importance of hemodynamic factors in the prognosis of symptomatic carotid occlusion, *JAMA* 280:1055–1060, 1998.
8. Kleiser B, Widder B: Course of carotid artery occlusions with impaired cerebrovascular reactivity, *Stroke* 23:171–174, 1992.
9. Kuroda S, Houkin K, Kamiyama H, et al: Long-term prognosis of medically treated patients with internal carotid or middle cerebral artery occlusion: can acetazolamide test predict it? *Stroke* 32:2110–2116, 2001.
10. Ogasawara K, Ogawa A, Yoshimoto T: Cerebrovascular reactivity to acetazolamide and outcome in patients with symptomatic internal carotid or middle cerebral artery occlusion: a xenon-133 single-photon emission computed tomography study, *Stroke* 33:1857–1862, 2002.
11. Vernieri F, Pasqualetti P, Passarelli F, et al: Outcome of carotid artery occlusion is predicted by cerebrovascular reactivity [see comment], *Stroke* 30:593–598, 1999.
12. Webster MW, Makaroun MS, Steed DL, et al: Compromised cerebral blood flow reactivity is a predictor of stroke in patients with symptomatic carotid artery occlusive disease, *J Vasc Surg* 21:338–344, 1995; discussion 344–345.
13. JET Study Group: Japanese EC-IC bypass Trial (JET Study): The second interim analysis, *Surg Cereb Stroke (Jpn)* 30:434–437, 2002.
14. Grubb RL Jr, Powers WJ, Derdeyn CP, et al: The carotid occlusion surgery study, *Neurosurg Focus* 14:e9, 2003.
15. Charbel FT, Meglio G, Amin-Hanjani S: Superficial temporal artery-to-middle cerebral artery bypass, *Neurosurgery* 56:186–190, 2005.
16. Ausman JI, Diaz FG, Vacca DF, et al: Superficial temporal and occipital artery bypass pedicles to superior, anterior inferior, and posterior inferior cerebellar arteries for vertebrobasilar insufficiency, *J Neurosurg* 72:554–558, 1990.
17. Amin-Hanjani S, Du X, Mlinarevich N, et al: The cut flow index: an intraoperative predictor of the success of extracranial-intracranial bypass for occlusive cerebrovascular disease, *Neurosurgery* 56:75–85, 2005.
18. Nishioka H: Results of the treatment of intracranial aneurysms by occlusion of the carotid artery in the neck, *J Neurosurg* 25:660–704, 1966.
19. Drake CG, Peerless SJ, Ferguson GG: Hunterian proximal arterial occlusion for giant aneurysms of the carotid circulation, *J Neurosurg* 81:656–665, 1994.
20. Liu AY, Lopez JR, Do HM, et al: Neurophysiological monitoring in the endovascular therapy of aneurysms, *AJNR Am J Neuroradiol* 24:1520–1527, 2003.
21. Abud DG, Spelle L, Piotin M, et al: Venous phase timing during balloon test occlusion as a criterion for permanent internal carotid artery sacrifice, *AJNR Am J Neuroradiol* 26:2602–2609, 2005.
22. van Rooij WJ, Sluzewski M, Slob MJ, et al: Predictive value of angiographic testing for tolerance to therapeutic occlusion of the carotid artery, *AJNR Am J Neuroradiol* 26:175–178, 2005.
23. Lorberboym M, Pandit N, Machac J, et al: Brain perfusion imaging during preoperative temporary balloon occlusion of the internal carotid artery, *J Nucl Med* 37:415–419, 1996.
24. Witt JP, Yonas H, Jungreis C: Cerebral blood flow response pattern during balloon test occlusion of the internal carotid artery, *AJNR Am J Neuroradiol* 15:847–856, 1994.
25. Eckard DA, Purdy PD, Bonte FJ: Temporary balloon occlusion of the carotid artery combined with brain blood flow imaging as a test to predict tolerance prior to permanent carotid sacrifice, *AJNR Am J Neuroradiol* 13:1565–1569, 1992.
26. Amin-Hanjani S, Charbel FT: Is extracranial-intracranial bypass surgery effective in certain patients? *Neurol Clin* 24:729–743, 2006.

27. Charbel FT, Zhao M, Amin-Hanjani S, et al: A patient-specific computer model to predict outcomes of the balloon occlusion test, *J Neurosurg* 101:977–988, 2004.

28. Eckert B, Thie A, Carvajal M, et al: Predicting hemodynamic ischemia by transcranial Doppler monitoring during therapeutic balloon occlusion of the internal carotid artery, *AJNR Am J Neuroradiol* 19:577–582, 1998.

29. Jawad K, Miller D, Wyper DJ, et al: Measurement of CBF and carotid artery pressure compared with cerebral angiography in assessing collateral blood supply after carotid ligation, *J Neurosurg* 46:185–196, 1977.

30. Ashley WW, Amin-Hanjani S, Alaraj A, et al: Flow-assisted surgical cerebral revascularization, *Neurosurg Focus* 24:E20, 2008.

31. Neff KW, Horn P, Dinter D, et al: Extracranial-intracranial arterial bypass surgery improves total brain blood supply in selected symptomatic patients with unilateral internal carotid artery occlusion and insufficient collateralization, *Neuroradiology* 46:730–737, 2004.

32. van Everdingen KJ, Klijn CJ, Kappelle LJ, et al: MRA flow quantification in patients with a symptomatic internal carotid artery occlusion. The Dutch EC-IC Bypass Study Group, *Stroke* 28:1595–1600, 1997.

33. Guppy KH, Charbel FT, Corsten LA, et al: Hemodynamic evaluation of basilar and vertebral artery angioplasty, *Neurosurgery* 51:327–333, 2002; discussion 333–334.

34. Zhao M, Charbel FT, Alperin N, et al: Improved phase-contrast flow quantification by three-dimensional vessel localization, *Magn Reson Imaging* 18:697–706, 2000.

35. Thulborn KR: MRI in the management of cerebrovascular disease to prevent stroke, *Neurol Clin* 26:897–921, vii–viii, 2008.

36. Schick U, Zimmermann M, Stolke D: Long-term evaluation of EC-IC bypass patency, Acta *Neurochir (Wien)* 138:938–942, 1996; discussion 942–943.

37. Amin-Hanjani S, Shin J, Zhao M, et al: Evaluation of extracranial-intracranial bypass using quantitative magnetic resonance angiography, *J Neurosurg* 106:291–298, 2007.

5

NEW DAYS FOR OLD WAYS IN TREATING GIANT ANEURYSMS—FROM HUNTERIAN LIGATION TO HUNTERIAN CLOSURE?

6

MIIKKA KORJA; MIKA NIEMELÄ; LEENA KIVIPELTO;
MARTIN LEHECKA; ROSSANA ROMANI; JOUKE VAN POPTA;
HANNA LEHTO; HIDEKI OKA; JUHA HERNESNIEMI

HUNTERIAN LIGATION

Hunterian ligation (i.e., proximal artery ligation) was the first surgical method for treating intracranial aneurysms. At the end of 18th century, a Scottish surgeon and scientist, John Hunter, established the procedure more or less in its current fashion by ligating certain peripheral arteries.[2,8,12] However, the first planned ICA ligation for the treatment of a preoperatively diagnosed nontraumatic saccular aneurysm was apparently performed in 1928,[16] and in subsequent decades several papers reported inconsistent mortality rates of the procedure. In 1966, a highly detailed and one-of-a-kind analysis of nearly 800 cases of Hunterian ligation for aneurysm patients reported an ischemic complication rate of 30% and a mortality rate of 24%.[11] However, 89% of the occlusions were CCA occlusions, and they were mainly performed in the acute phase of subarachnoid hemorrhage (SAH). Following Hunterian ligation, only 16 (12%) and three (2%) out of 129 patients with unruptured aneurysms experienced ischemic deficits or died, respectively. Hunterian ligation of the ICA had almost a double risk of ischemic complications in comparison to CCA occlusion, even though severely ill and high-risk patients were more frequently selected for CCA rather than ICA occlusion.

The series of Drake and Peerless, which the senior author (JH) has scrutinized, represents the largest and most experienced data of the procedure for giant aneurysms to date; it consists of 732 giant aneurysms, 396 of which were treated with Hunterian ligation before December 1992. Due to their special referral policy, posterior circulation aneurysms outnumbered anterior circulation aneurysms in the series.[21] Excluding infraclinoid aneurysms (five petrous and 77 intracavernous carotid aneurysms), more than two thirds (69%) of the 253 giant anterior circulation aneurysms were treated with direct clipping, whereas only one third (32%) of the 397 giant posterior circulation aneurysms were directly clipped. For the remainder, Hunterian ligation was used in the treatment of 48% and 60% of the anterior and posterior circulation aneurysms, respectively.

In general, Hunterian ligation has been used on every major intracranial artery, mostly as the only reasonable treatment option for impractical giant aneurysms, but occasionally as the safest and most simple alternative of all possible options. In our own literature survey of more than 2000 giant aneurysms, which were treated between 1970 and 1994 (i.e., microsurgery era) at various institutions all over the world, Hunterian ligation was used as the only treatment method in one third of the cases. However, the method does not seem to be very widespread; many of the reported cases come from London, Ontario, Canada. In our own database, which contains all intracranial aneurysms treated between 1977 and 2000 in eastern Finland, 128 (5.5%) of the 2330 treated aneurysms were giant. The same incidence rate has also been seen in southern Finland in the last 13 years (during which Professor Hernesniemi has been working in Helsinki), where roughly 15 giant aneurysms are treated every year. Of these 15 giant aneurysms, Hunterian ligation without other treatment modalities was involved in only one or two desperate cases.

Today, even though most saccular aneurysms at any site can technically be considered as clippable, especially fusiform, dissecting highly atherosclerotic and giant aneurysms remains cumbersome. Since giant aneurysms often have a very slow or stagnant intra-aneurysmal blood flow, resulting in asymptomatic or symptomatic distal perfusion changes, Hunterian ligation can provide better than expected surgical results in these otherwise inoperable and unfavorable cases. For the aforementioned reasons, Hunterian ligation has remained a useful adjunct to tackle giant aneurysms, often combined with a bypass procedure. Therefore, the number of Hunterian ligation procedures performed at our institution has continued to be more or less the same throughout the years. Disappointing results in using Hunterian ligation for patients with ruptured giant aneurysms have made us cautious in attempting Hunterian ligation in the week following SAH.[11,13]

After the early years of Hunterian ligation, the field of neurovascular treatments was revolutionized by endovascular approaches. Proximal closure of any intracranial vessel, in principle, can be achieved by endovascular means as well. Thus, instead of *Hunterian ligation*, it would perhaps make more sense to use the term *Hunterian closure*, which is not tied to any particular occlusion technique, when any kind of proximal occlusion of an intracranial artery is performed. The following surgical views represent our simplified perspective of using Hunterian closure in the treatment of giant aneurysms at different locations.

ANTERIOR CIRCULATION

Giant ICA Aneurysms

Permanent occlusion of the ICA with or without a prior test occlusion leads to a high cumulative stroke rate and mortality of 26% and 12%, respectively.[9] Therefore, a preoperative evaluation of collateral potential of the circle of Willis is necessary. After a diagnostic angiography, we typically perform a test occlusion for a minimum of 30 minutes using an inflated endovascular balloon in the high cervical ICA (at the C1-2 level of the ICA) of a conscious patient. If the patient tolerates the test occlusion without neurological symptoms, and the angiographic architecture of the venous phase does not show substantial asymmetry, Hunterian closure of the ICA can be considered as a treatment option. The venous phase is symmetrical if the venous phase of both cerebral hemispheres is synchronous (venous filling delay is less than 0.5 seconds) after collateral filling via the anterior communicating artery, or if the venous phase of the posterior circulation on vertebral angiography is simultaneous (venous filling delay is less than 0.5 seconds) after collateral filling via the posterior communicating artery.[18] We do not routinely use blood flow or perfusion analyses (e.g., MRI-NOVA, perfusion CT, perfusion MRI) during or after the balloon test occlusion. At present, we do not perform Hunterian closure of the CCA, because we have seen retrograde recanalization of the ICA, which increases the risk of aneurysm rupture.[11] In addition, we have not found test occlusions of the CCA reliable, and permanent occlusion of the CCA evidently affects EC-IC collateral flow. Whatever the clinical preoperative evaluation of the collateral flow potential of the ICA territory, unexpected ischemic events are always possible after Hunterian closure of the ICA. Even though today it is also possible to measure the blood flow intraoperatively, current flow probes and intraoperative monitoring modalities cannot be used to reliably estimate the circulatory changes after Hunterian closure.

If any doubts or objective signs of insufficient collateral flow of the ICA territory exist, it is advisable to do a bypass instead of sole Hunterian closure or a direct attack to the aneurysm. Depending on the degree of the patient's collateral circulation, either a low-flow or a high-flow replacement or protective bypass is constructed, prior to occlusion of the ICA or direct aneurysm clipping. When a high-flow bypass is needed, we usually construct a nonocclusive, high-flow, laser-assisted Excimer Laser-Assisted Nonocclusive Anastomosis (ELANA) bypass.[17] Hunterian closure, trapping, or direct clipping of the giant aneurysm is performed either immediately after the bypass procedure in the same session or later. Giant ICA aneurysms located in the supraclinoid segment of the ICA are usually the most difficult to treat. The most difficult ones are located at the bifurcation, where direct clipping may easily occlude anterolateral central arteries in addition to A1 or M1 origins. Unfortunately, bypass requirements for giant ICA bifurcation aneurysms are also very demanding, since sometimes even a Y-shaped or dual bypass to both A1 and to distal M1 segments is needed in order to treat the lesion. Flow reduction with Hunterian closure without bypass may in rare cases be the only reasonable treatment option, but whether this procedure provides any benefit for patients is unknown.

Currently, improved microsurgery techniques and instruments allow many of the giant ophthalmic and posterior communicating artery aneurysms to be treated by direct surgery. In these cases, the finishing touch with Drake's ring clips after a tandem clipping method can be used with or without the Dallas technique, where the aneurysm sac is collapsed in order to achieve a more complete exposure of the neck.

Giant ACA and MCA Aneurysms

The incidence of giant anterior cerebral artery (ACA) aneurysms, especially of ruptured ones, is very low. Before the microsurgery era, Hunterian closure of the dominant/only A1 was a frequently used surgical alternative even when small-size anterior communicating artery aneurysms were to be treated. Sudden occlusion of the dominant A1 causes ischemic complications almost without exception. A giant A1 aneurysm can be rather safely clipped or sometimes even trapped if the contralateral A1 is filling both A2s. According to Drake, leptomeningeal collaterals from the middle cerebral artery (MCA) and posterior cerebral artery (PCA) may fill A2 segments sufficiently, even in a retrograde fashion when both A1s are occluded. Drake used Hunterian closure of the A1 segment in some cases to treat giant aneurysms of the ACA,[7] and also a so-called tourniquet occlusion of the A1 segments in conscious patients when direct clipping was not possible. Giant ACA aneurysms are very difficult to treat with direct clipping, but after temporary clipping of both A1s and one or two A2s, it is often possible to dissect the aneurysm sac, evacuate the thrombus, and finally, clip the aneurysm. The problem is how to keep the medial lenticulostriate arteries patent even if blood supply to the A2s is provided by the contralateral A1.

Giant MCA aneurysms are the most common giant aneurysms in Finland, and they represent about 4% of all MCA aneurysms.[3] Most of these aneurysms are MCA bifurcation aneurysms, and approximately half of all giant MCA

New Days for Old Ways in Treating Giant Aneurysms—from Hunterian Ligation to Hunterian Closure?

6

aneurysms can be surgically resected. After the resection, the diseased MCA segment is reconstructed by clipping the aneurysm base—for example, in tandem fashion—and sometimes suturing of the resected aneurysm wall is necessary. A vascular clamp may sometimes be helpful in assisting direct clipping of thick-walled and calcified giant aneurysms.[10] For patients whose aneurysms cannot be directly resected and clipped, one option is to revascularize the distal-to-aneurysm branches with a bypass and then induce a flow change and thrombosis of the aneurysm by Hunterian closure.

POSTERIOR CIRCULATION

Giant VA Aneurysms

Saccular giant vertebral artery (VA) aneurysms are a rarity, and can rarely be clipped. This is mainly due to the fact that these aneurysms involve the posterior inferior cerebral artery (PICA) origin. After a test occlusion, Hunterian closure of the VA is an alternative for clipping, as there is almost always sufficient collateral flow from the contralateral VA to the ipsilateral PICA. Surgical Hunterian closure of the VA can be performed just proximal to the sulcus arteriosus extracranially, but the vessel ligation can also be performed intracranially. If dissection and decompression of the aneurysm are necessary, trapping of the giant VA aneurysm is needed prior to the decompression. Today, EC-IC or IC-IC bypasses are increasingly used as adjuncts to Hunterian closure of one or both VAs.

Giant Vertebrobasilar Junction, Basilar Trunk, and Basilar Tip Aneurysms

Vertebrobasilar junction aneurysms, which very often associate with proximal basilar fenestration,[14] as well as saccular basilar trunk aneurysms, are extremely rare (<0.1% of all saccular aneurysms). Most of the large and giant vertebrobasilar junction and basilar trunk aneurysms are fusiform or dissecting in nature. We have been successful in treating these aneurysms with direct surgery, which, in practice, is a technically demanding high-risk treatment option. In the presence of a good posterior communicating artery/arteries (>1 mm), unilateral or bilateral Hunterian closure of the VA or direct Hunterian closure of the basilar artery (BA) may be applied to induce thrombosis of the aneurysm due to flow diversion. Therefore if the patient tolerates a unilateral VA test occlusion time of 30 minutes and has symmetrical venous phases, one VA can be sacrificed relatively safely. After 2 to 4 weeks, when natural adaptation of the collateral vasculature has already occurred to some extent, another test occlusion and hopefully permanent occlusion of the remaining patent VA can be performed. Our experience indicates that this "tandem occlusion" strategy may facilitate occlusion of both VAs in cases where this seemed too risky in the first place.

If collateral flow through posterior communicating arteries is insufficient, a bypass has to be constructed, such as to the P1 segment prior to occlusion of the BA or VAs. Since most of the giant BA tip aneurysms can less often be safely clipped, and endovascular surgery offers unsatisfactory results, Hunterian closure of the BA in the treatment of giant basilar tip saccular aneurysms is a good option when functioning posterior communication arteries are present. Unfortunately, sometimes the giant aneurysm remains open and growing even after Hunterian closure due to this vivid collateral flow through posterior communicating arteries. In brief, giant BA tip aneurysms are very difficult to treat both surgically and endovascularly, and poor outcome is often observed using either modality.

Giant PCA Aneurysms

Saccular aneurysms of the PCA are rare. The most common location for PCA aneurysms, also for giant ones, is the P2 segment. Distal PCA aneurysms are very rare. Only approximately 10% of all PCA aneurysms are located distal to the P3 segment. Even though small, medium, large, and even giant saccular aneurysms of the PCA segments can be successfully treated with direct clipping, Hunterian closure should be considered as a treatment option for giant aneurysms of the PCA. Due to usually robust collateral flow up to the P1/P2 junction, Hunterian closure of the P1 segment can often be used safely to treat P1/P2 junction aneurysms, and Hunterian closure of the P2 segment in order to treat P2-P4 aneurysms has even more favorable outcomes. From the surgical point of view, it may be surprisingly difficult to place even a very small narrow clip on the P1 segment between the giant aneurysm and the perforating arteries (often only 1 or 2 mm), which usually arise from the proximal segment of the P1. Balloon test occlusions are difficult to perform in the vessels around the BA tip, because even the smallest balloon occludes several BA tip and P1 perforators. Therefore, endovascular assessment of collateral flow prior to occlusion of any PCA segment is not very reliable and reproducible. A bypass procedure should be planned, if possible, as one of the adjunctive options to treat the aneurysm. In these cases, intraoperative flow measurements may relatively reliably suggest when collateral flow is inadequate. In any case, PCA region bypasses are technically very difficult to perform.

In the Drake's series of 31 PCA aneurysms, 13 were giant aneurysms.[5,6] In the series of 174 giant intracranial aneurysms, 13 (7.5%) were giant PCA aneurysms, of which nine P1 and P2 aneurysms were treated with Hunterian closure or trapping.[5] According to Drake, only one patient (trapped P2 segment giant aneurysm) developed a visual field defect, and it was speculated that good collateral circulation was the main reason for the lack of serious neurological sequelae.[5] Yasargil has also reported good results after trapping five nonclippable fusiform and giant aneurysms in the P1 and P2 segments.[20] There are several reports on giant PCA aneurysms treated with Hunterian closure or trapping, without any serious neurological deficits. The decision between trapping and Hunterian closure is ultimately based on the intraoperative evaluation of the presence of perforators originating from the diseased segment. If there is any danger of causing iatrogenic thalamic syndrome (occlusion of the thalamogeniculate artery), it is advisable to do Hunterian closure alone instead of trapping.

DISCUSSION

Based on the International Study of Unruptured Intracranial Aneurysms (ISUIA) data, the lifetime rupture risk of giant aneurysms has been estimated to exceed 87% in a 30-year-old patient and 71% in a 50-year-old patient.[1] Thus, it is evident that most of the giant intradural ICA aneurysms should be treated. Except for the ICA bifurcation aneurysms, giant ICA aneurysms are very satisfactorily and safely treated with Hunterian closure of the ICA, if the patient tolerates the occlusion. Only a minority of giant ICA aneurysms remain unchanged in size after ICA occlusion,[4] and symptoms of mass effect are cured or improved in more than 90% of patients.[4] Since Hunterian closure of the ICA is a simple, safe, and effective therapy for these patients,[4] it is fair to say that there are still some scientific grounds for Hunterian closure in the treatment of giant ICA aneurysms. However, because ICA occlusion may cause progressive degenerative processes in the brain due to changes in cerebral oxygen metabolism,[19] we try to avoid ICA occlusion in patients aged <50 years. Furthermore, ICA occlusion is far from optimal for intracranial aneurysms due to its ischemic and embolic complication risks. In recent years, new endovascular techniques capable of sparing vessel patency have become available. Indeed, these new microcatheter-delivered, self-expanding, and stent-like endovascular constructs (i.e., flow-diverting stents) are engineered specifically for the treatment of intracranial aneurysms, and they completely exclude the aneurysm from circulation. These devices represent a revolutionary remodeling tool for aneurysm treatment, especially for the treatment of symptomatic cavernous sinus aneurysms. However, these devices are not yet established widely enough, and objective reports of complication rates and long-term results have yet to be published.

In common neurosurgical practice, Hunterian ligation is equivalent to proximal ligation of the ICA. However, the term is originally defined as "surgical occlusion of any artery in its proximal segment." Despite increasing advances in endovascular surgery, we believe that when proximal occlusion of an intracerebral artery is considered, surgical Hunterian closure is a better option than endovascular occlusion, especially when occluding P1, A1, or M1 segments. This is mainly due to the fact that crucial perforators originate from these segments, and at least in our institution, there are no reliable endovascular means to visualize all small perforators and to perform reliable test occlusions. We also need better methodology and instruments to measure blood flow and collateral potential

during surgery in order to select the best possible operative approaches (e.g., bypass, partial clipping, Hunterian closure, trapping, no treatment). In surgery, it is essential to plan all possible (even anecdotal) surgical nuances prior to operating giant aneurysms.

In contrast to the P1, A1, and M1 segments, microsurgery in the treatment of giant P2, basilar trunk, vertebrobasilar junction, and VA aneurysms has become a secondary option in a number of institutions. This also applies to surgical Hunterian closure. Despite the giant steps of the ongoing endovascular revolution, "aneurysm surgeons should maintain technical proficiency with difficult lesions."[15] Indeed, we believe that in very experienced hands, the procedural risk of surgery of giant aneurysms in any location is acceptable and comparable to that of endovascular treatments. Unorthodox ideas, innovative applications, and imagination are required to revolutionize neurovascular surgery again, such as in the 1960s.

Since the principle of proximal vessel occlusion does not change depending on the maneuver itself, in honor of John Hunter, we could start using the term *Hunterian closure* instead of *Hunterian ligation*, whenever a proximal vessel is occluded by endovascular or surgical means. Hunterian closure is an option in situations where very demanding surgical procedures (e.g., bypasses and direct clipping) are not considered feasible (lack of competence or facilities). It is our belief that the treatment of all unruptured and perhaps ruptured giant aneurysms be nationally centralized in high-quality neurovascular centers.

REFERENCES

1. Chang HS: Simulation of the natural history of cerebral aneurysms based on data from the International Study of Unruptured Intracranial Aneurysms, *J Neurosurg* 104:188–194, 2006.
2. Cooper BB: *Lectures on the Principles and Practice of Surgery*, Philadelphia, 1852, Blanchard and Lee.
3. Dashti R, Hernesniemi J, Niemela M, et al: Microneurosurgical management of middle cerebral artery bifurcation aneurysms, *Surg Neurol* 67:441–456, 2007.
4. de Gast AN, Sprengers ME, van Rooij WJ, et al: Midterm clinical and magnetic resonance imaging follow-up of large and giant carotid artery aneurysms after therapeutic carotid artery occlusion, *Neurosurgery* 60:1025–1029, 2007; discussion 1029–1031.
5. Drake CG: Giant intracranial aneurysms: experience with surgical treatment in 174 patients, *Clin Neurosurg* 26:12–95, 1979.
6. Drake CG: The treatment of aneurysms of the posterior circulation, *Clin Neurosurg* 26:96–144, 1979.
7. Drake CG, Peerless SJ, Ferguson GG: Hunterian proximal arterial occlusion for giant aneurysms of the carotid circulation, *J Neurosurg* 81:656–665, 1994.
8. Hunter J: *Some Observations on Digestion*, London, 1935, Longman et al.
9. Linskey ME, Jungreis CA, Yonas H, et al: Stroke risk after abrupt internal carotid artery sacrifice: accuracy of preoperative assessment with balloon test occlusion and stable xenon-enhanced CT, *AJNR Am J Neuroradiol* 15:829–843, 1994.
10. Navratil O, Lehecka M, Lehto H, et al: Vascular clamp-assisted clipping of thick-walled giant aneurysms, *Neurosurgery* 64:113–120, 2009; discussion 120–121.

11. Nishioka H: Results of the treatment of intracranial aneurysms by occlusion of the carotid artery in the neck, *J Neurosurg* 25:660–704, 1966.

12. Paget S: *John Hunter, Man of Science and Surgeon*, London, 1897, T. Fisher Unwin.

13. Peerless SJ, Hernesniemi JA, Gutman FB, et al: Early surgery for ruptured vertebrobasilar aneurysms, *J Neurosurg* 80:643–649, 1994.

14. Peluso JP, van Rooij WJ, Sluzewski M, et al: Aneurysms of the vertebrobasilar junction: incidence, clinical presentation, and outcome of endovascular treatment, *AJNR Am J Neuroradiol* 28:1747–1751, 2007.

15. Sanai N, Tarapore P, Lee AC, et al: The current role of microsurgery for posterior circulation aneurysms: a selective approach in the endovascular era, *Neurosurgery* 62:1236–1249, 2008; discussion 1249–1253.

16. Schorstein J: Carotid ligation in saccular intracranial aneurysms, *Br J Surg* 28:50–70, 1940.

17. Tulleken CA, Verdaasdonk RM, Beck RJ, et al: The modified excimer laser-assisted high-flow bypass operation, *Surg Neurol* 46:424–429, 1996.

18. van Rooij WJ, Sluzewski M, Metz NH, et al: Carotid balloon occlusion for large and giant aneurysms: evaluation of a new test occlusion protocol, *Neurosurgery* 47:116–121, 2000; discussion 122.

19. Yamauchi H, Pagani M, Fukuyama H, et al: Progression of atrophy of the corpus callosum with deterioration of cerebral cortical oxygen metabolism after carotid artery occlusion: a follow-up study with MRI and PET, *J Neurol Neurosurg Psychiatry* 59:420–426, 1995.

20. Yasargil MG: *Microneurosurgery*, George Thieme Verlag, 1984, Stuttgart.

21. Drake CG, Peerless SJ, Hernesniemi J: *Surgery of vertebrobasilar aneurysms,* Springer-Verlag, 1996, Wien.

6

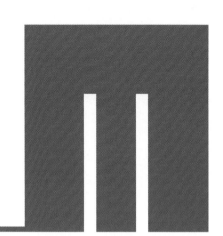

EC-IC BYPASS SURGICAL TECHNIQUES

SURGICAL ANATOMY OF EC-IC BYPASS PROCEDURES

MASATOU KAWASHIMA; ALBERT L. RHOTON, JR

7

INTRODUCTION

The number of cerebral revascularization procedures performed by neurosurgeons has declined after the Cooperative Study of Extracranial-Intracranial Arterial Anastomosis[1] failed to demonstrate that this procedure reduced the risk of stroke in patients with cerebral ischemia. However, cerebral revascularization is now well recognized as an important element in the treatment of complex intracranial aneurysms, cranial base tumors, and certain kinds of ischemic diseases.

In this study, we examined microsurgical anatomy for cerebral revascularization in the anterior and posterior circulations and demonstrated various procedures for bypass surgery.

METHODS

Microsurgical anatomy of cerebral revascularization, including the donor and recipient vessels, and the techniques, including the superficial temporal artery (STA)–middle carotid artery, middle meningeal artery (MMA)–middle cerebral artery (MCA), STA–posterior carotid artery (PCA), STA–superior cerebellar artery (SCA), occipital artery (OA)–anterior inferior carotid artery (AICA), and OA–posterior inferior cerebellar artery (PICA), and side-to-side anastomoses, short arterial and venous interposition grafting, and external carotid artery (ECA)/internal carotid artery (ICA)–M2, ICA-ICA, and ECA-PCA bypasses, were examined, using 22 adult cadaveric specimens and 3x to 40x magnification. Depending on the thickness of the vessel wall, 10-0, 8-0, 7-0, or 6-0 nylon sutures (Ethicon, Inc., Somerville, NJ) were used for suturing. The saphenous vein and the radial artery were used as grafts for bypass procedures. The arteries and veins were perfused with colored silicone. The bone dissections were performed with the Midas Rex drill (Fort Worth, TX).

RESULTS

Arterial Relationships

The diameters of vessels measured, which are frequently used for cerebral revascularization procedures, are shown in Tables 7–1 and 7–2.

Internal carotid artery

The common carotid artery divides into the internal (ICA) and external carotid artery (ECA) at the level of C2-C3 below the mandibular angle. The cervical, petrous, and supraclinoid ICAs are the sites of cerebral revascularization procedures. The average diameters of the cervical, petrous, and supraclinoid ICAs were 8.57, 5.42, and 3.95 mm, respectively (Table 7–1). The cervical portion of the ICA is covered by the skin, superficial cervical fascia, platysma, deep fascia, anterior margin of the sternocleidomastoid muscle, and internal jugular vein. Dissecting these anatomic structures exposes the carotid triangle, which is formed by the posterior belly of the digastric, omohyoid, and sternocleidomastoid muscles. In the carotid triangle, the ICA begins at the bifurcation of the common carotid, opposite the upper border of the thyroid cartilage, and runs perpendicularly upward, in front of the transverse processes of the upper three cervical vertebrae, to the carotid canal in the petrous portion of the temporal bone (Figures 7–1A and 7–1B).

The petrous portion of the ICA courses within the carotid canal and ends where the artery enters the cavernous sinus. The carotid artery, at the point where it enters the carotid canal, is surrounded by a strong layer of connective tissue that makes it difficult to mobilize the artery. The roof of the carotid canal opens below the trigeminal ganglion near the distal end of the carotid canal. The greater petrosal nerve runs beneath the dura of the middle fossa, immediately superior and anterolateral to the horizontal segment of the petrous carotid. The cochlea lies below the floor of the middle fossa, just

Table 7–1. DIAMETER OF VESSELS FOR CEREBRAL REVASCULARIZATION IN ANTERIOR CIRCULATION (MM).

ICA

Cervical segment: 8.57 ± 1.34
Petrous segment: 5.42 ± 0.68
Supraclinoid segment: 3.95 ± 0.56

ECA

Cervical portion: 5.75 ± 0.94

STA

At the level of zygoma: 1.93 ± 0.48

MCA

M2 (largest branch near the central sulcus): 1.76 ± 0.36
M4 (largest branch in the area)
Frontal branch: 1.19 ± 0.32
Temporal branch: 1.22 ± 0.23
Parietal branch: 1.36 ± 0.24

ACA

A2: 2.35 ± 0.60
A3: 1.98 ± 0.35
A4: 1.94 ± 0.40
A5: 1.55 ± 0.12

Table 7–2. DIAMETER OF VESSELS FOR CEREBRAL REVASCULARIZATION IN POSTERIOR CIRCULATION (MM).

PCA

P2A: 2.13 ± 0.38
P2P: 1.73 ± 0.33
P3: 1.67 ± 0.16

SCA

Anterior pontomesencephalic segment: 1.67 ± 0.16
Lateral pontomesencephalic segment
Single trunk: 1.51 ± 0.12
Rostral trunk: 1.25 ± 0.17
Caudal trunk: 1.15 ± 0.30

AICA

Anterior pontomesencephalic segment: 1.34 ± 0.28
Cortical segment: 1.07 ± 0.29

PICA

Anterior medullary segment: 1.84 ± 0.45
Tonsillomedullary segment (caudal loop): 1.68 ± 0.38

OA

At the digastric groove: 2.05 ± 0.48
At the level of the superior nuchal line: 2.01 ± 0.45

posterosuperior to the lateral genu of the petrous carotid artery. The Eustachian tube and the tensor tympani muscle are located parallel to and along the anterior margin of the horizontal segment, where they are separated from the artery by a thin layer of bone (Figure 7–1C).

The supraclinoid segment of the ICA begins where the artery emerges from the dura mater and enters the cranial cavity by passing along the medial side of the anterior clinoid process and below the optic nerve. It reaches the lateral side of the optic chiasm and bifurcates below the anterior perforated substance at the medial end of the sylvian fissure to give rise to the anterior cerebral artery (ACA) and middle cerebral artery (MCA). The supraclinoid segment of the ICA gives rise to three branches: the ophthalmic, posterior communicating, and anterior choroidal arteries. In addition, this segment gives off perforating branches including the superior hypophyseal artery (Figure 7–1D).

External carotid artery

The external carotid artery (ECA) begins at the bifurcation of the common carotid in front of the ICA and ascends backward to the space behind the neck of the mandible, where it divides into the superficial temporal and maxillary arteries. The average diameter of the ECA was 5.75 mm (Table 7–1). The ECA is crossed by the hypoglossal nerve, common facial and superior thyroid veins, and the digastric and stylohyoid muscles. The superior thyroid artery arises from the external carotid artery just below the level of the greater cornu of the hyoid bone and ends in the thyroid gland. The STA, the smaller of the two terminal branches of the ECA, appears, from its direction, to be the continuation of that vessel. The STA plays an important role as a donor vessel in cerebral revascularization. The STA begins in the substance of the parotid gland, behind the neck of the mandible, and crosses over the posterior root of the zygomatic process of the temporal bone. The average diameter of the STA at the level of the zygoma was 1.93 mm (Table 7–1). The STA divides into two branches, frontal and parietal. The frontal branch (anterior temporal) runs tortuously upward and forward to the forehead, supplying the muscles, integument, and pericranium in this region, and anastomosing with the supraorbital and frontal arteries. The parietal branch (posterior temporal), larger than the frontal, curves upward and backward on the side of the head, lying superficial to the temporal fascia and anastomosing with its fellow of the opposite side and with the posterior auricular and occipital arteries (Figure 7–1B).

Middle cerebral artery

M2 and M4 are the sites of cerebral revascularization procedures. The M2 segment includes the trunk that lie on and supply the insula. This segment begins at the genu where the middle cerebral artery (MCA) trunk passes over the limen insulae and terminates at the circular sulcus of the insula. The greatest branching of the MCA occurs distal to the genu as these trunks cross the anterior part of the insula. The M2 branches are used for a bypass procedure, especially for a high-flow bypass. Important factors in selecting an artery for the procedure are its diameter, the length of artery available on the cortical surface, and perforating arteries to the basal ganglia. The average diameter of the largest branch near the central sulcus of the insula was 1.76 mm (Table 7–1).

The M4 is composed of the branches to the lateral convexity. They begin at the surface of the sylvian fissure and extend over the cortical surface of the cerebral hemisphere. The largest cortical artery is the temporo-occipital artery. Nearly two-thirds are 1.5 mm or more in diameter, and 90% are 1 mm or more in diameter. The smallest cortical artery is the orbitofrontal artery; approximately one-quarter are 1 mm or more in diameter. The average diameters of the largest M4 in the parietal, temporal, and frontal area were 1.36, 1.22, and 1.19 mm, respectively (Table 7–1). The central sulcal artery is the largest branch to the frontal lobe, and the angular artery is the largest branch to the parietal lobe. The temporo-occipital and the posterior temporal arteries are the largest branches to the temporal lobe. The minimum length of a cortical artery needed to complete a bypass is 4 mm. The angular, posterior parietal, and temporo-occipital arteries have the longest segments on the cortical surface, and the orbitofrontal and temporopolar arteries have the shortest cortical segment (Figures 7–1E and 7–1F).

Anterior cerebral artery

The anterior cerebral artery (ACA) is divided at the anterior communicating artery (AComA) into two parts, proximal (A1) and distal (A2–5). The A3 segment of the ACA is the dominant site of cerebral revascularization procedures, including side-to-side anastomosis and short arterial and venous interposition grafting. The average diameters of A2, A3, A4, and A5 were 2.35, 1.98, 1.94, and 1.55 mm, respectively (Table 7–1). The pericallosal artery is the portion of the ACA distal to the AComA and is constantly present. The pericallosal artery ascends in front of the lamina terminalis to pass into the interhemispheric fissure (A2). Above the lamina terminalis, the artery makes a smooth curve around the genu of the corpus callosum (A3) and then courses backward above the corpus callosum in the pericallosal cistern (A4 and A5).

The callosomarginal artery is defined as the artery that courses in or near the cingulate sulcus and gives rise to two or more major cortical branches.[2] When the callosomarginal artery is well formed, it lies in the cingulate sulcus above the cingulate gyrus and follows a course roughly parallel to that of the pericallosal artery. Its origin varies from just distal to the AComA to the level of the genu of the corpus callosum. Its frequent origin was from the A3 segment, followed by the A2 segment and AComA. The size of the pericallosal artery distal to the callosomarginal origin varies inversely with the size of the callosomarginal artery (Figures 7–1G and 7–1H).

Posterior cerebral artery

The posterior cerebral artery (PCA) arises at the basilar bifurcation, is joined by the posterior communicating artery (PComA) at the lateral margin of the interpeduncular cistern, encircles the brainstem passing through the crural and ambient cisterns to reach the quadrigeminal cistern, and is distributed to the posterior part of the hemisphere. The PCA supplies not only the posterior part of the cerebral hemispheres, but also sends critical branches to the thalamus, midbrain, and other deep structures, including the choroid plexus and walls of the lateral and third ventricles. Each segment of the PCA is classified according to our already proposed system.[3] The P1 is the segment proximal to the PComA. The P2 segment extends from the PComA to the point at which the PCA enters the quadrigeminal cistern. The P2 segment is subdivided into equal anterior (P2A) and posterior (P2P) halves. The P2A begins at the PComA and courses between the cerebral peduncle and uncus that forms the medial and lateral walls of the crural cistern, and inferior to the optic tract and basal vein that crosses the roof of the cistern, to enter the proximal portion of the ambient cistern. The P2P begins at the posterior edge of the cerebral peduncle at the junction of the crural and ambient cisterns. It courses between the lateral midbrain and the parahippocampal and dentate gyri, which form the medial and lateral walls of the ambient cistern, below the optic tract, basal vein, and geniculate bodies and the inferolateral part of the pulvinar in the roof of the cistern, and superomedial to the trochlear nerve and tentorial edge. The P3 segment begins at the posterior midbrain, courses within the quadrigeminal cistern, and ends at the anterior limit of the calcarine fissure. The P4 segment is the distal branch of the P3 segment. The average diameters of P2A, P2P, and P3 were 2.13, 1.73, and 1.67 mm, respectively (Table 7–2). The PCA gives rise to three types of branches:[1] central perforating branches to the diencephalon and midbrain,[2] ventricular branches to the choroid plexus and walls of the lateral and third ventricles and adjacent structures,[3] and cerebral branches to the cerebral cortex and splenium of the corpus callosum. The central branches include the direct and circumflex perforating arteries, including the thalamoperforating, peduncular perforating, and thalamogeniculate arteries. The ventricular branches are the lateral and medial posterior choroidal arteries. The cerebral branches include the inferior temporal group of branches, which are divided into hippocampal and the anterior, middle, posterior, and common temporal branches, plus the parieto-occipital, calcarine, and splenial branches. The long and short circumflex, thalamoperforating, and medial posterior choroidal arteries arise predominantly from P1, and the other PCA branches most frequently arise from P2 or P3. The hippocampal, anterior temporal, peduncular perforating, and medial posterior choroidal arteries most frequently arise from P2A. The middle temporal, posterior temporal, common temporal, and lateral posterior choroidal arteries most frequently arise from P2P. The thalamogeniculate arteries arise only slightly more frequently from P2P than from P2A. The calcarine and parieto-occipital arteries most frequently arise from P3 (Figure 7–2A).

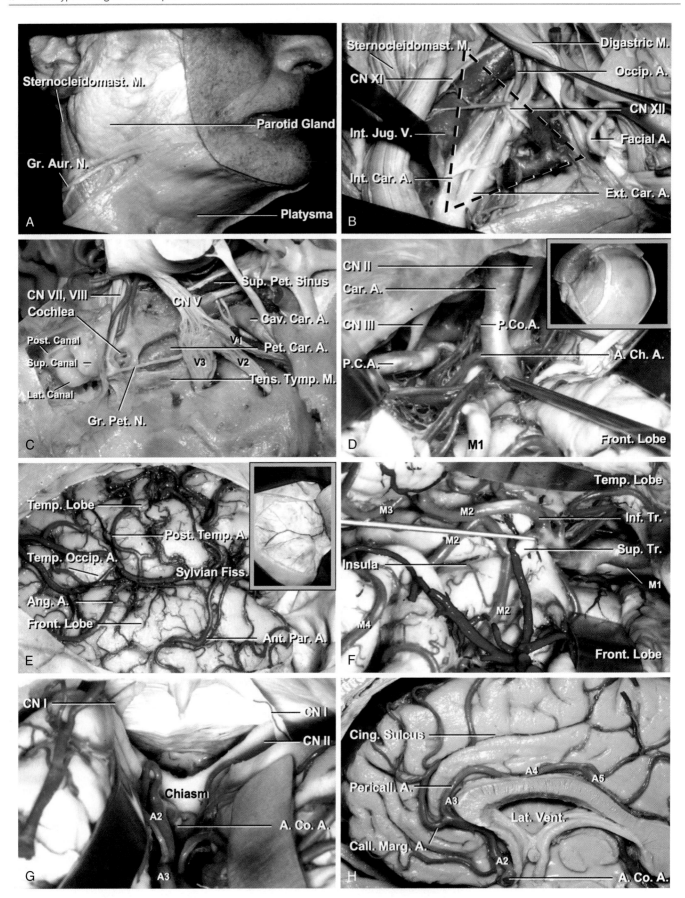

Figure 7–1. For legend see opposite page.

Figure 7–1. Arterial relationships of donor and recipient vessels. **A** and **B.** Anterolateral view, Cervical ICA and ECA. **A.** Cervical portion of ICA and ECA is covered by the skin, superficial cervical fascia, platysma, deep fascia, anterior margin of the sternocleidomastoid muscle, and internal jugular vein. **B.** Dissecting these anatomic structures exposes the carotid triangle (dotted line), which is formed by the posterior belly of the digastric, omohyoid, and sternocleidomastoid muscles. In the carotid triangle the ICA and ECA begin at the bifurcation of the common carotid and run perpendicularly upward. **C.** Petrous segment of the ICA, superior view. The petrous portion of the ICA courses within the carotid canal and ends where the artery enters the cavernous sinus. The roof of the carotid canal opens below the trigeminal ganglion near the distal end of the carotid canal. The third division of the trigeminal nerve, greater petrosal nerve, cochlea, the Eustachian tube, and the tensor tympani muscle are located near the horizontal segment of the petrous carotid artery. **D.** Supraclinoid segment of the ICA, left pterional approach. The anterior clinoid process has been removed. The supraclinoid segment of the ICA begins where the artery emerges from the dura mater and enters the cranial cavity by passing along the medial side of the anterior clinoid process and below the optic nerve. It reaches the lateral side of the optic chiasm and bifurcates to the ACA and MCA. The supraclinoid segment of the ICA gives rise to three branches: the ophthalmic, posterior communicating, and anterior choroidal arteries. **E.** M4 segment of the MCA, left pterional approach. The M4 is composed of the branches to the lateral convexity, which are used for a low-flow bypass. They begin at the surface of the sylvian fissure and extend over the cortical surface of the cerebral hemisphere. The largest cortical artery is the temporo-occipital artery. The central sulcal artery is the largest branch to the frontal lobe, and the angular artery is the largest branch to the parietal lobe. The temporo-occipital and the posterior temporal arteries are the largest branches to the temporal lobe. **F.** M2 segment of the MCA, left pterional approach. The M2 segment includes the trunks that lie on and supply the insula. This segment begins at the genu where the MCA trunk passes over the limen insulae and terminates at the circular sulcus of the insula. The M2 branches are used for a bypass procedure, especially for high-flow bypass. Important factors in selecting an artery for the procedure are its diameter, the length of artery available on the cortical surface, and perforating arteries to the basal ganglia. **G** and **H.** ACA, anterior and lateral views. The ACA is divided at the AComA into two parts, proximal (A1) and distal (A2–5). The A3 segment of the ACA is the dominant site of cerebral revascularization procedures, including side-to-side anastomosis and short arterial and venous interposition grafting. The callosomarginal artery, the largest branch of the pericallosal artery, generally arises at the A3 segment. A., artery; A.Ch.A., anterior choroidal artery; A.Co. A., anterior communicating artery; Ant., anterior; Aur., auricular; Call. Marg., callosomarginal; Car., carotid; Cav., cavernous; Cing., cingulate; CN., cranial nerve; Ext., external; Fiss., fissure; Front., frontal; Gr., greater; Inf., inferior; Int., internal; Jug., jugular; Lat., lateral; M., muscle; N., nerve; Occip., occipital; Par., parietal; P.C.A., posterior cerebral artery; P.Co.A., posterior communicating artery; Pericall., pericallosal; Pet., petrosal, petrous; Post., posterior; Sternocleidomast., sternocleidomastoid; Sup., superior; Temp., temporal; Tens., tensor; Tr., trunk; Tymp., tympani; V., vein; Vent., ventricle.

Superior cerebellar artery

The superior cerebellar artery (SCA) arises in front of the midbrain, usually from the basilar artery near the apex, and passes below the oculomotor nerve. Its proximal portion courses medial to the free edge of the tentorium cerebelli around the brainstem near the pontomesencephalic junction, and its distal part passes below the tentorium, making it the most rostral of the infratentorial arteries. All of the SCAs that arise as a single vessel bifurcate into two major trunks, one rostral and one caudal, most commonly near the point of maximal caudal descent of the artery on the lateral side of the brainstem. The SCA is divided into four segments: anterior pontomesencephalic, lateral pontomesencephalic, cerebellomesencephalic, and cortical. The anterior pontomesencephalic segment begins at the origin of the SCA and extends below the oculomotor nerve to the anterolateral margin of the brainstem. The average diameter of the vessel was 1.67 mm in the segment (Table 7–2). The lateral pontomesencephalic segment begins at the anterolateral margin of the brainstem and frequently dips caudally onto the lateral side of the pons. This segment terminates at the anterior margin of the cerebellomesencephalic fissure. The average diameters of rostral and caudal trunks in this segment were 1.25 and 1.15 mm, respectively. If it is a single trunk, the average diameter was 1.51 mm in the segment (Table 7–2). The cerebellomesencephalic segment courses within the cerebellomesencephalic fissure, giving off branches that penetrate fissure's opposing walls. The cortical segment includes the branches distal to the cerebellomesencephalic fissure that pass under the tentorial edge and are distributed to the tentorial surface (Figures 7–2B through 7–2D).

Anterior inferior cerebellar artery

The anterior inferior cerebellar artery (AICA) originates from the basilar artery, usually as a single trunk, and encircles the pons near the abducent, facial, and vestibulocochlear nerves. After coursing near and sending branches to the nerves entering the acoustic meatus and to the choroid plexus protruding from the foramen Luschka, it passes around the flocculus on the middle cerebellar peduncle to supply the cerebellopontine fissure and the petrosal surface. It commonly bifurcates near the facial-vestibulocochlear nerve complex to form a rostral and a caudal trunk. The AICA is divided into four segments: anterior pontine, lateral pontine, flocculonodular, and cortical. Each segment may include more than one trunk, depending on the level of bifurcation of the artery. The average diameters of the anterior pontine and cortical segments were 1.34 and 1.07 mm, respectively (Table 7–2). The most common pattern is for the AICA to supply the majority of the petrosal surface, but overlap of the SCA onto the upper part of the petrosal surface and the PICA onto the lateral part of the suboccipital surface is not uncommon, depending on the size of the AICA (Figures 7–2C and 7–2D).

Posterior inferior cerebellar artery

The PICA has the most complex, tortuous, and variable course and area of supply of the cerebellar arteries. The PICA arises from the vertebral artery near the inferior olive and passes posteriorly around the medulla. After passing the lateral aspect of the medulla, it courses around the cerebellar tonsil and enters the cerebellomedullary fissure and passes posterior to the lower half of the roof of the fourth ventricle. On exiting the cerebellomedullary fissure, its branches are distributed to

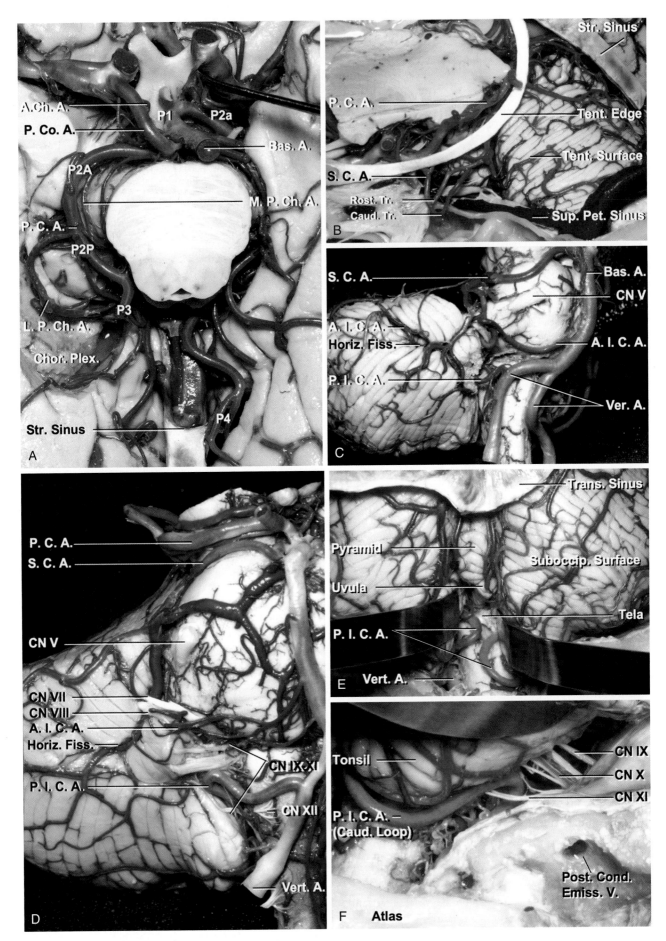

Figure 7–2. For legend see opposite page.

Figure 7–2. Arterial relationships. **A** and **B.** Inferior and anterosuperior views, PCA. The PCA arises at the basilar bifurcation, is joined by the PComA at the lateral margin of the interpeduncular cistern, encircles the brainstem passing through the crural and ambient cisterns to reach the quadrigeminal cistern above the edge of the cerebellar tentorium, and is distributed to the posterior part of the hemisphere. The PCA is divided into P1 to P4. The PCA gives rise to three types of branches:[1] central perforating branches to the diencephalon and midbrain,[2] ventricular branches to the choroid plexus and walls of the lateral and third ventricles and adjacent structures,[3] and cerebral branches to the cerebral cortex and splenium of the corpus callosum. **C** and **D.** Anterolateral and anterior views of the brainstem and the cerebellum, SCA, AICA, and PICA. The SCA arises in front of the midbrain, usually from the basilar artery near the apex, and passes below the oculomotor nerve. Its proximal portion courses medial to the free edge of the tentorium cerebelli around the brainstem near the pontomesencephalic junction, and its distal part passes below the tentorium, making it the most rostral of the infratentorial arteries. All of the SCAs that arise as a single vessel bifurcate into two major trunks, one rostral and one caudal, most commonly near the point of maximal caudal descent of the artery on the lateral side of the brainstem (**B**). The AICA originates from the basilar artery, usually as a single trunk, and encircles the pons near the abducent, facial, and vestibulocochlear nerves. After coursing near and sending branches to the nerves entering the acoustic meatus and to the choroid plexus protruding from the foramen Luschka, it passes around the flocculus on the middle cerebellar peduncle to supply the cerebellopontine fissure and the petrosal surface. The PICA arises from the vertebral artery near the inferior olive and passes posteriorly around the medulla. **E** and **F.** Posterior and posterolateral views of the brainstem and the cerebellum and PICA. After passing the lateral aspect of the medulla, the PICA courses around the cerebellar tonsil and enters the cerebellomedullary fissure and passes posterior to the lower half of the roof of the fourth ventricle. On exiting the cerebellomedullary fissure, its branches are distributed to the vermis and hemisphere of the suboccipital surface. In the tonsillomedullary segment of the PICA, the loop passing near the lower part of the tonsil, referred to as the caudal loop, forms a caudally convex loop that coincides with the caudal pole of the tonsil, but it may also course superior or inferior to the caudal pole of the tonsil without forming a loop. The telovelotonsillar segment commonly forms a loop with a convex rostral curve, called the cranial loop. The apex of the cranial loop usually overlies the central part of the inferior medullary velum. A., artery; A.Ch.A., anterior choroidal artery; A.I.C.A., anterior inferior cerebellar artery; Bas., basilar; Caud., caudal; Chor. Plex., choroid plexus; CN, cranial nerve; Cond., condylar; Emiss., emissary; Fiss., fissure; Horiz., horizontal; L.P.Ch.A., lateral posterior choroidal artery; M.P.Ch.A., medial posterior choroidal artery; P.C.A., posterior cerebral artery; P.Co.A., posterior communicating artery; Pet., petrosal; P.I.C.A., posterior inferior cerebellar artery; Post., posterior; Rost., rostral; S.C.A., superior cerebellar artery; Str., straight; Suboccip., suboccipital; Sup., superior; Tent., tentorial; Tr., trunk; Trans., transverse; V., vein; Vert., vertebral.

the vermis and hemisphere of the suboccipital surface. Most PICAs bifurcate into a medial and a lateral trunk. The medial trunk supplies the vermis and adjacent part of the hemisphere, and the lateral trunk supplies the cortical surface of the tonsil and the hemisphere. The PICA is divided into five segments: anterior medullary, lateral medullary, tonsillomedullary, telovelotonsillar, and cortical. The anterior medullary segment begins at the origin of the PICA anterior to the medulla and extends backward to the inferior olivary prominence, passing near the hypoglossal rootlets. The lateral medullary segment begins where the artery passes the most prominent point of the inferior olive and ends at the level of the origin of the glossopharyngeal, vagus, and accessory rootlets. The tonsillomedullary segment begins where the PICA passes posterior to the glossopharyngeal, vagus, and accessory nerves and extends medially across the posterior aspect of the medulla near the caudal half of the tonsil. It ends where the artery ascends to the midlevel of the medial surface of the tonsil. This segment commonly passes medially between the lower margin of the tonsil and the medulla before turning rostrally along the medial surface of the tonsil. The loop passing near the lower part of the tonsil, referred to as the caudal loop, forms a caudally convex loop that coincides with the caudal pole of the tonsil, but it may also course superior or inferior to the caudal pole of the tonsil without forming a loop. The average diameter of the caudal loop was 1.68 mm, which is one of the largest distal vessels in the cerebellar arteries (Table 7–2). The telovelotonsillar segment begins at the mid-portion of the PICA's ascent along the medial surface of the tonsil toward the roof of the fourth ventricle and ends where it exits the fissures between the vermis, tonsil, and hemisphere to reach the suboccipital surface. This segment commonly forms a loop with

a convex rostral curve, called the cranial loop. The apex of the cranial loop usually overlies the central part of the inferior medullary velum, but its location varies from the superior to the inferior margin and from the medial to the lateral extent of the inferior medullary velum. The cortical segment begins where the trunks and branches leave the groove between the vermis medially and the tonsil and the hemisphere laterally, and includes the terminal cortical branches (Figures 7–2C through 7–2F).

Occipital artery

The occipital artery (OA) arises from the posterior part of the external carotid, opposite the external maxillary, near the lower margin of the posterior belly of the digastric muscle, and ends in the posterior part of the scalp. At its origin, it is covered by the posterior belly of the digastric and the stylohyoid muscles, and the hypoglossal nerve winds around it from behind forward; higher up, it crosses the internal carotid artery, the internal jugular vein, and the vagus and accessory nerves. It ascends to the interval between the transverse process of the atlas and the mastoid process of the temporal bone, and passes horizontally backward, grooving the surface of the mastoid bone, being covered by the sternocleidomastoid, splenius capitis, longissimus capitis, and digastric muscles, and resting upon the rectus capitis lateralis, the superior oblique, and semispinalis capitis muscles. The average diameter of the OA was 2.05 mm in the exit of the digastric groove (Table 7–2). It then changes its course and runs vertically upward, pierces the fascia connecting the cranial attachment of the trapezius with the sternocleidomastoid muscles, and ascends in a tortuous course in the superficial fascia of the scalp, where it divides

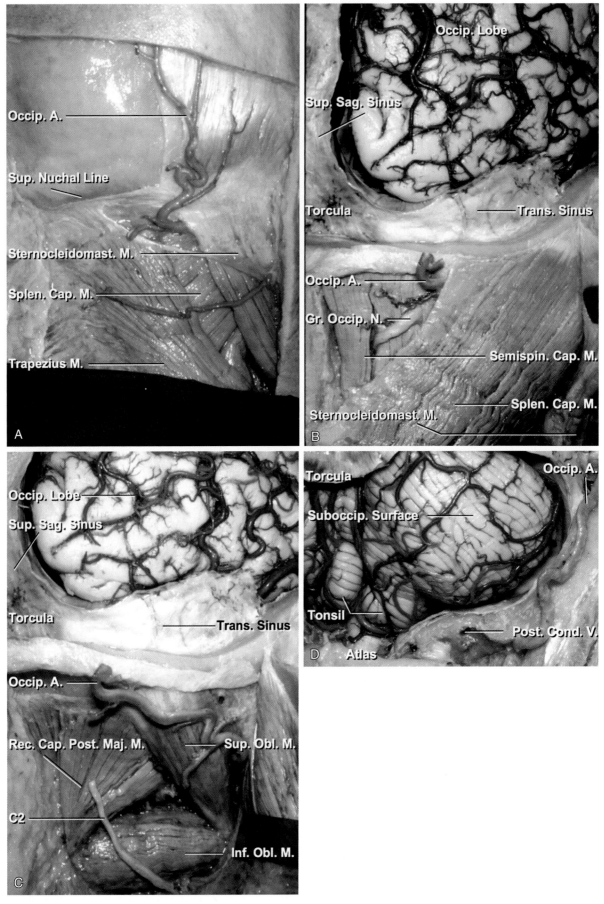

Figure 7–3. For legend see opposite page.

Figure 7–3. Graft extraction. **A** to **D.** Right posterior and posterolateral views, OA. The OA arises from the posterior part of the external carotid and ends in the posterior part of the scalp. The OA ascends to the interval between the transverse process of the atlas and the mastoid process of the temporal bone, and passes horizontally backward, grooving the surface of the mastoid bone, being covered by the sternocleidomastoid, and splenius capitis muscles, and resting upon the superior oblique and semispinalis capitis muscles. It then changes its course and runs vertically upward, pierces the fascia connecting the cranial attachment of the trapezius with the sternocleidomastoid muscles, and ascends in a tortuous course in the superficial fascia of the scalp, where it divides into numerous branches, which reach as high as the vertex of the skull and anastomose with the posterior auricular and superficial temporal arteries. Its terminal portion is accompanied by the greater occipital nerve. A., artery; Cap., capitis; Cond, condylar; Gr., greater; Inf., inferior; M., muscle; Maj., major; N., nerve; Obl., oblique; Occip., occipital; Post., posterior; Rec., rectus; Sag., sagittal; Semispin., semispinalis; Splen., splenius; Sternocleidomast., sternocleidomastoid; Suboccip., suboccipital; Sup., superior; Trans., transverse; V., vein.

into numerous branches, which reach as high as the vertex of the skull and anastomose with the posterior auricular and superficial temporal arteries. The average diameter of the OA was 2.01 mm at the level of the superior nuchal line (see Table 7–2). In three specimens (four sides), length of the OA from the exit of the digastric groove to the level of the superior nuchal line was measured. An average distance between them was 81.9 mm. Its terminal portion is accompanied by the greater occipital nerve (Figures 7–3A through 7–3D).

Graft

Artery graft, radial artery

The radial artery appears, from its direction, to be the continuation of the brachial, but it is smaller in caliber than the ulnar artery. The radial artery begins at the bifurcation of the brachial, just below the bend of the elbow, passes along the radial side of the forearm to the wrist, and then winds backward around the lateral side of the carpus, beneath the tendons of the abductor pollicis longus and extensores pollicis longus. In the upper third of its course in the forearm, the radial artery lies between the brachioradialis and the pronator teres muscles; in the lower two-thirds, between the tendons of the brachioradialis and flexor carpi radialis. The superficial branch of the radial nerve is close to the lateral side of the artery in the middle third of its course.

Before the dissection of the radial artery, an Allen test[4] is necessary to check the collateral circulation to its territory. The radial artery is exposed at the wrist where it is located beneath the skin. The artery is traced proximally in the forearm, between the brachioradialis and the pronator teres muscles, up to the bifurcation of the brachial artery. Branches joining the artery are either ligated or bipolar-cauterized. Heparinized saline solution is used to wash out the blood inside the vessel and to check for leaks. The harvested radial artery graft is placed in heparinized saline (Figures 7–4A and 7–4B).

Vein graft, great saphenous vein

In the superficial veins of the lower extremity, the great saphenous vein has been used as a graft for cerebral revascularization. The great saphenous vein, the longest vein in the body, begins in the medial marginal vein of the dorsum of the foot

and ends in the femoral vein about 3 cm below the inguinal ligament. It ascends along the medial side of the leg in relation with the saphenous nerve. It runs upward behind the medial condyles of the tibia and femur and along the medial side of the thigh and, passing through the fossa ovalis, ends in the femoral vein. The vessel usually becomes somewhat smaller at the level of the knee. This reduction in size helps to reduce the discrepancy between the caliber of the vein graft and that of the intracranial artery recipient. The valves in the great saphenous vein vary from ten to twenty in number; they are more numerous in the leg than in the thigh.

The vein is harvested from the leg or the thigh, depending on the caliber of the graft required, with care to avoid vascular injury and potential thrombosis. The incision is begun 1 cm anterior and 1 cm rostral to the medial malleolus and the vein is located in the subcutaneous tissue. The vein is traced superiorly toward the medial side of the knee for a distance of 15 to 20 cm, as needed. Branches joining the vein are either ligated or occluded with small clips. Before the saphenous vein is dissected, it is marked superficially with a skin marker to avoid later kinking. After complete dissection of the saphenous vein, it is ligated proximally and distally, sectioned, and removed. Heparinized saline solution is used to wash out the blood inside the vessel and to check for leaks. The harvested saphenous graft is placed in heparinized saline (Figures 7–4C and 7–4D).

Procedures for Cerebral Revascularization

STA-MCA anastomosis

An STA to MCA anastomosis is the most common operative procedure performed. The patient is positioned supine, with the head turned so that the side of bypass is easily accessible. The STA courses in the subcutaneous tissue above the galea (Figure 7–5A). The STA is outlined either by palpation of the artery or with a portable Doppler device. The severed end of the STA is stripped of its fascial layer, and the vessel is exposed over 7 to 8 mm (Figure 7–5B). Once dissection of the STA is completed, the temporal muscle and fascia are incised at the site of the craniotomy (Figures 7–5C and 7–5D). Removing the bone flap and dura mater exposes cerebral cortex, where the anastomosis is performed. The frontal branch of the STA courses above the frontotemporal region, whereas the parietal

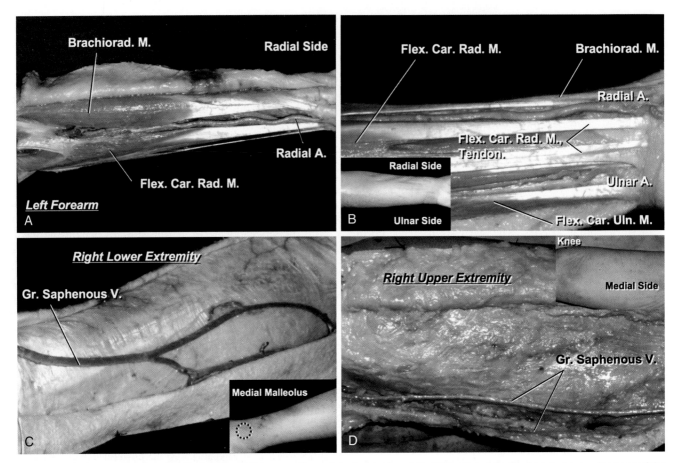

Figure 7–4. Graft extraction. **A** and **B.** Radial artery, left forearm. The radial artery begins at the bifurcation of the brachial, just below the bend of the elbow, passes along the radial side of the forearm to the wrist, and then winds backward around the lateral side of the carpus, beneath the tendons of the abductor pollicis longus and extensores pollicis longus. In the upper third of its course in the forearm, the radial artery lies between the brachioradialis and the pronator teres muscles; in the lower two-thirds, between the tendons of the brachioradialis and flexor carpi radialis. **C** and **D.** Great saphenous vein, right lower extremity. The great saphenous vein, the longest vein in the body, begins in the medial marginal vein of the dorsum of the foot and ends in the femoral vein about 3 cm below the inguinal ligament. It runs upward behind the medial condyles of the tibia and femur and along the medial side of the thigh and, passing through the fossa ovalis, ends in the femoral vein. The vein is harvested from the leg or the thigh, depending on the caliber of the graft required, with care to avoid vascular injury and potential thrombosis. The incision is begun 1 cm anterior and 1 cm rostral to the medial malleolus (dotted circle) and the vein is located in the subcutaneous tissue. A., artery; Brachiorad., brachioradialis; Car., carpi; Flex., flexor; Gr., great; M., muscle; Rad., radialis; Uln., ulnar; V., vein.

branch of the STA passes above the parietotemporal region (Figure 7–5E). The recipient artery, which is over 1 mm in size and have a segment at least 6 to 8 mm for microanastomosis, is chosen according to its supplying area. One or two small branches from the recipient vessel may need to be coagulated and sacrificed. A colored background material is then placed beneath the recipient artery. The tip of the STA is then cut, making the fish-mouthed shape suitable for the anastomosis site. The recipient vessel is prepared by placing the temporary clips across the vessel and performing the small arteriotomy. Placing two stay-sutures, anastomosis of the STA to the recipient vessel is performed using interrupted 10-0 nylon sutures (Figures 7–5F and 7–5G).

MMA-MCA anastomosis

The MMA is anastomosed to the MCA in this procedure. After a frontotemporal craniotomy, the MMA is dissected

from between the dural leaves. The anastomosis is accomplished with interrupted 10-0 nylon sutures (Figures 7–6A through 7–6D).

Side-to-side anastomosis (MCA and ACA)

This procedure is mainly used for cerebral revascularization for MCA branches and distal ACA (A3), combined with occlusion of their proximal branch vessels. Arteriotomies, 4 mm in length, were made on both donor and recipient arteries. Most difficult procedure here is to make a tight suture on a back wall. After two stay-sutures were placed in the distal and caudal edges of the arteriotomies, the back wall was sutured using a continuous running fashion from the intravascular side and then the anterior wall closed with interrupted sutures (10-0 nylon). Then, occlusion of the proximal vessel is completed. The distal part of the artery beyond the occlusion site is supplied by the adjacent artery (Figures 7–7A through 7–7F).

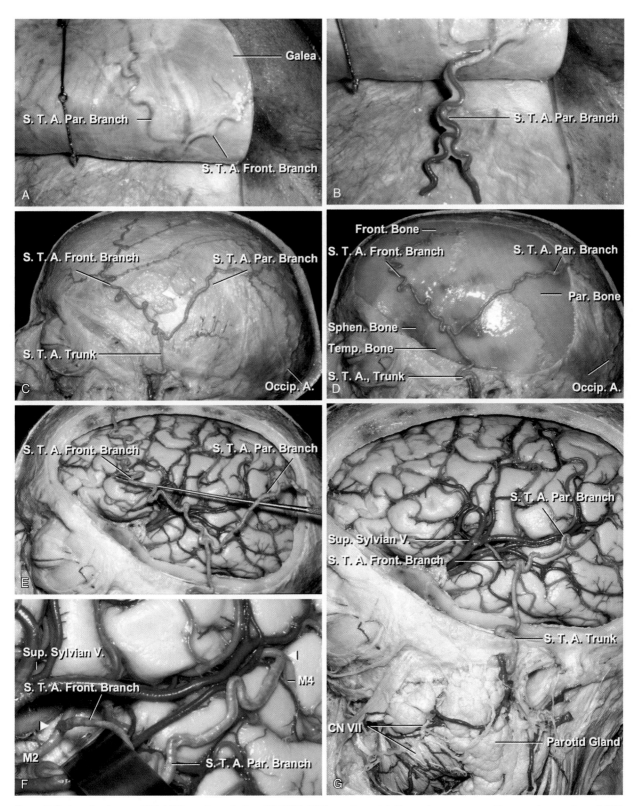

Figure 7–5. Low-flow bypass: STA-MCA anastomosis. **A** and **B,** STA to MCA anastomosis is the most common operative procedure performed. STA is outlined either by palpation of the artery or with a portable Doppler device. Severed end of the STA is stripped of its fascial layer, and the vessel is exposed over 7 to 8 mm. **C** and **D,** STA divides into two branches, frontal and parietal. Once dissection of the STA is completed, the temporal muscle and fascia are incised at the site of the craniotomy. **E,** Removing the bone flap and dura mater exposes cerebral cortex, where the anastomosis is performed. The anterior branch of the STA courses above the frontotemporal region, whereas the posterior branch of the STA passes above the parietotemporal region. **F** and **G,** Recipient artery, which is over 1 mm in size and has a segment at least 6 to 8 mm for microanastomosis, is chosen according to its supplying area. One or two small branches from the recipient vessel may need to be coagulated and sacrificed. The tip of the STA is then cut making the fish-mouthed shape suitable for the anastomosis site. The recipient vessel is prepared by placing the temporary clips across the vessel and performing the small arteriotomy. Placing two stay-sutures, anastomosis of the STA to the recipient vessel is performed using 10-0 nylon interrupted sutures (*arrows* in **F**). A., artery; CN, cranial nerve; Front., frontal; S.T.A., superficial temporal artery; Occip., occipital; Par., parietal; Sphen., sphenoid; Sup., superficial., Temp., temporal; V., Vein.

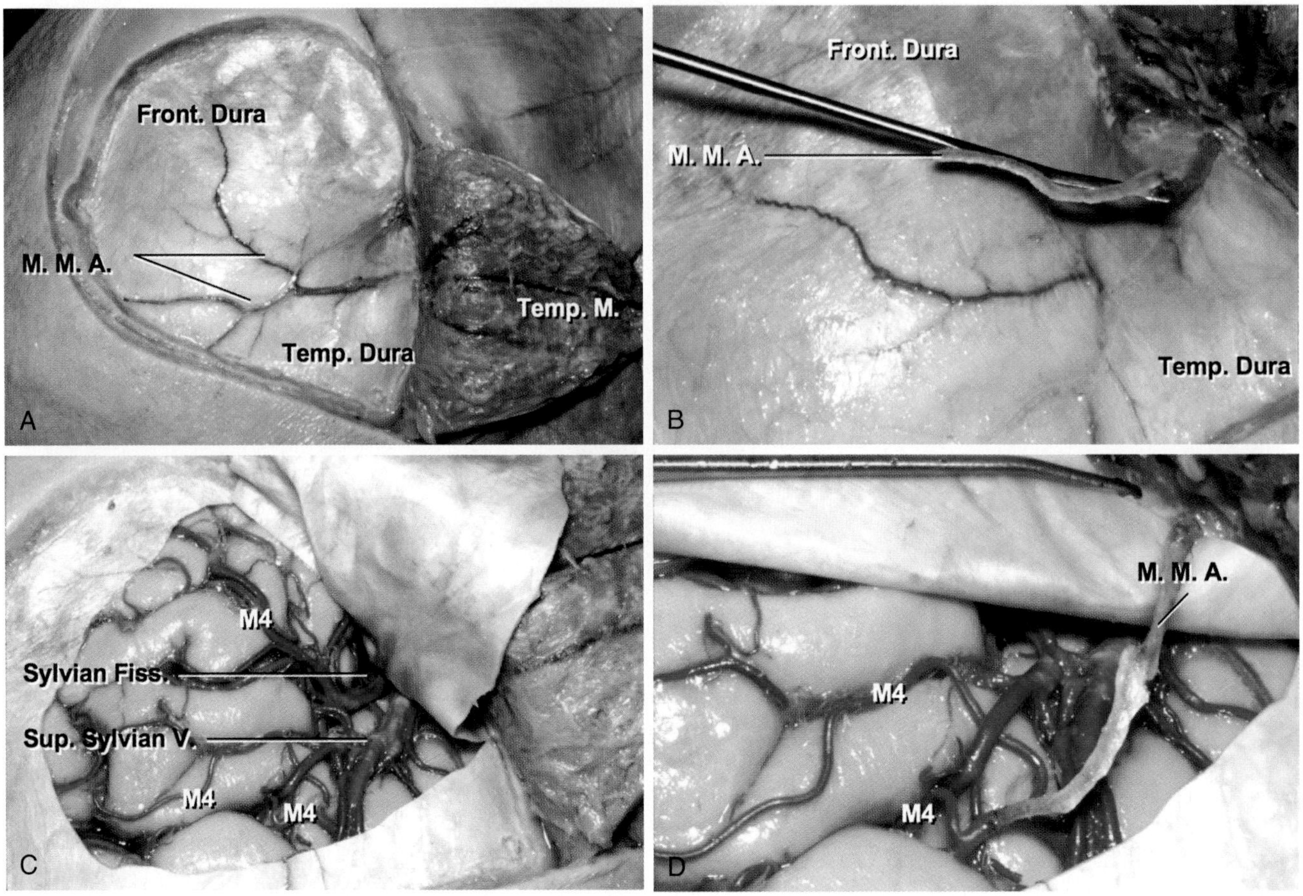

Figure 7–6. Low-flow bypass: MMA-MCA anastomosis. **A** to **D.** The MMA is anastomosed to the MCA. After a frontotemporal craniotomy, the MMA is dissected from between the dural leaves. The anastomosis is performed using interrupted 10-0 nylon sutures. Fiss., fissure; Front., frontal; M., muscle; M.M.A., middle meningeal artery; Sup., superficial; Temp., temporal; V., vein.

Short arterial interposition grafting anastomosis

The STA or occipital artery is used for an arterial graft. A section of STA graft approximately 4 cm in length is dissected from a skin flap and then both severed ends of the STA are stripped of their fascial layer. The graft is anastomosed between bilateral A3s with interrupted sutures (10-0 nylon). Then the right pericallosal and callosomarginal junction is occluded. The distal part of the right pericallosal artery is supplied by the left pericallosal artery (Figures 7–8A and 7–8B).

Short venous interposition grafting anastomosis

In this technique, a short vein graft was used to connect the donor and recipient arteries. Cerebral revascularization was performed using a shot saphenous vein graft or a superior temporal vein graft, 5 to 10 cm in length, extending from the STA trunk anterior to the ear to M2 or M4. An end-to-side anastomosis of the vein to the recipient artery was carried out using 10-0 nylon interrupted sutures. Following completion of the anastomosis at the distal end, an end-to-end

Figure 7–7. Low-flow bypass: Side-to-side anastomosis. **A** to **C.** The M2 segments of the MCA. **A.** Side-to-side anastomosis is performed between distal M2s (dotted area), preparing for proximal occlusion of M2. **B.** Side-to-side anastomosis between distal M2s has been completed (arrowhead), followed by occlusion of the proximal M2 segment using permanent clips (arrow). **C.** Distal part of M2 beyond the occlusion site is supplied by the adjacent M2 (dotted arrows) through anastomotic site (arrowhead). **D-F.** A3 segments of the ACA. **D** and **E.** Side-to-side anastomosis is performed between A3s (arrowhead), preparing for proximal occlusion of right A2. **F.** Distal part of right M2 beyond the occlusion site (arrow) is supplied by left A3 (dotted arrows) through anastomotic site (arrowhead). A., artery; Call. Marg., callosomarginal; Fiss., fissure; Front., frontal; Pericall., pericallosal; Sup., superficial; Temp., temporal; V., vein.

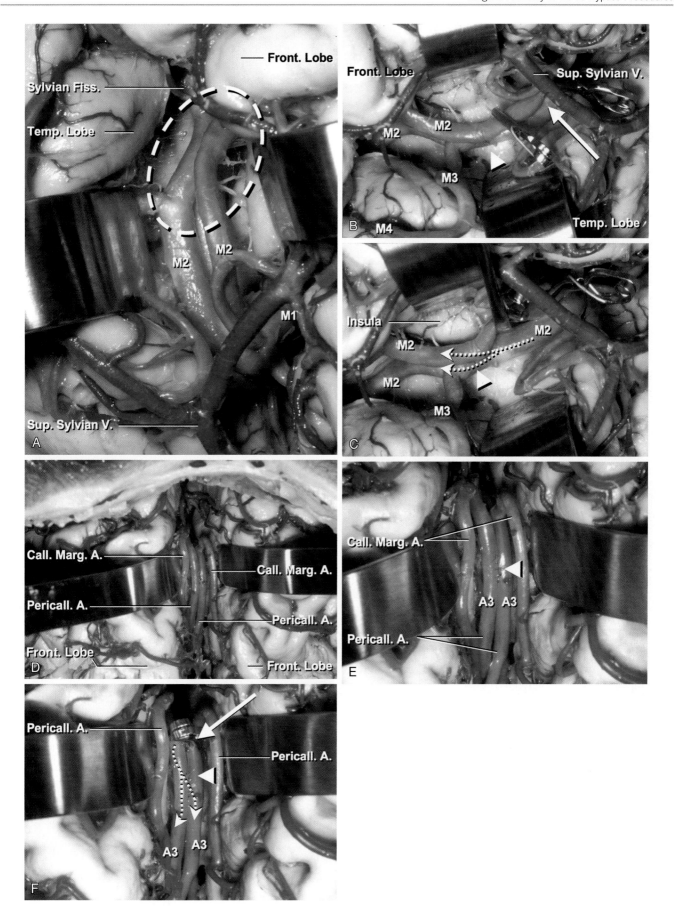

Figure 7–7. For legend see facing page.

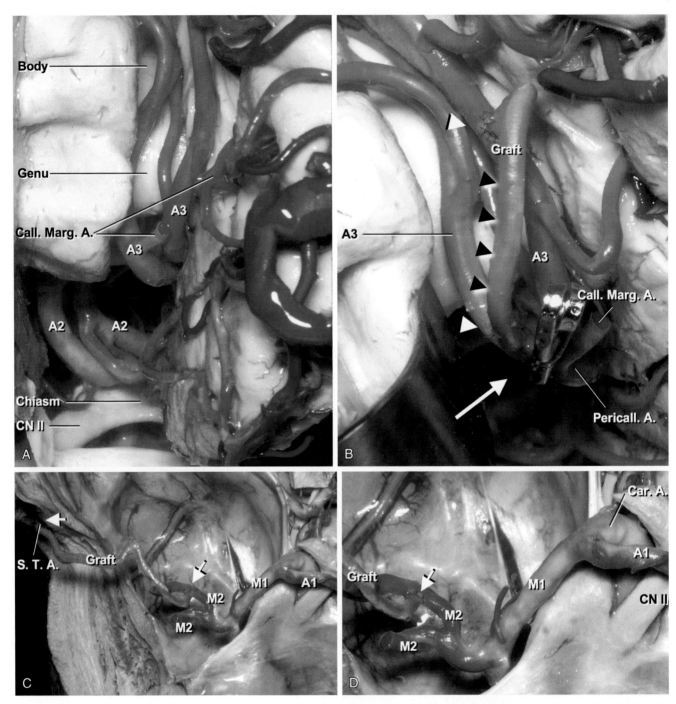

Figure 7–8. Low-flow bypass: Short interposition grafting anastomosis. **A** and **B,** Short arterial interposition grafting anastomosis. A section of STA graft, approximately 5 cm in length, is dissected from a skin flap and then both severed ends of the STA are stripped of their fascial layer. The graft (black arrowheads) is anastomosed between bilateral A3s with interrupted sutures (10-0 nylon). Then the right pericallosal and callosomarginal junction is occluded (arrow). The distal part of the right pericallosal artery is supplied by the left pericallosal artery through the anastomotic sites (white arrowheads). **C** and **D,** Short venous interposition grafting anastomosis. Cerebral revascularization was performed using a short saphenous vein graft or a superior temporal vein graft, 5 to 10 cm in length, extending from the STA trunk anterior to the ear to M2 (arrows). An end-to-side anastomosis of the vein to the recipient artery was carried out using 10-0 nylon interrupted sutures. Following completion of the anastomosis at the distal end, an end-to-end anastomosis of the vein to the STA trunk immediately above the zygoma was carried out in using 8-0 nylon interrupted sutures. A., artery; Car., carotid; CN, cranial nerve; Call. Marg.; callosomarginal; Pericall., pericallosal; S.T.A., superficial temporal artery.

anastomosis of the vein to the STA trunk immediately above the zygoma was carried out in using 8-0 nylon interrupted sutures (Figures 7–8C and 7–8D).

Cervical ECA/ICA–M2 anastomosis

Either a saphenous vein graft or a radial artery graft is used for this bypass procedure. The common carotid artery, ICA, and ECA are exposed in the carotid triangle making a cervical incision along the anterior aspect of the sternocleidomastoid muscle. The zygomatic arch is drilled to fashion a conduit for the graft when it is placed in a preauricular position. After the craniotomy, wide dissection of the sylvian fissure is performed. The MCA trunk is identified and the secondary branches are dissected at their origin. The

secondary vessel, which is thick and with the least number of side branches, is chosen and mobilized for the anastomosis. The diameter of the vessels in the insular area is normally larger than 1 mm. Care should be taken to avoid damaging the lenticulostriate perforators from the M2 branches. The main trunk of the MCA is occluded distal to the lenticulostriate perforators, and its branches are also occluded. The distal anastomosis between M2 and the graft is then performed in an end-to-side fashion with interrupted 10-0 nylon sutures. After completion of the distal anastomosis, the cervical ECA is occluded proximally and distally. The graft is pulled down through the subcutaneous tunnel. An arteriotomy, approximately 6 to 8 mm, is made on the ECA. The graft is anastomosed to the artery in an end-to-side fashion, using 7-0 nylon sutures (Figures 7–9A through 7–9C).

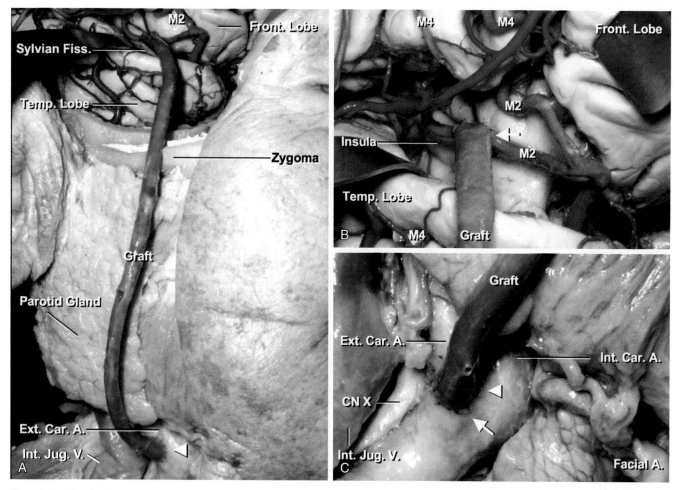

Figure 7–9. High-flow bypass: cervical ECA/ICA–M2 anastomosis. **A** to **C,** Either saphenous vein graft or radial artery graft is used for this procedure. The common carotid artery, ICA, and ECA are exposed in the carotid triangle. The zygomatic arch is drilled to fashion a conduit for the graft when it is placed in a preauricular position. After the craniotomy, wide dissection of the sylvian fissure is performed. The MCA trunk is identified and the secondary branches are dissected at their origin. The secondary vessel, which is thick and with the least number of side branches, is chosen and mobilized for the anastomosis. The main trunk of the MCA is occluded distal to the lenticulostriate perforators, and its branches are also occluded. The distal anastomosis is then performed in an end-to-side fashion with interrupted 10-0 nylon sutures (*arrow* in **B**). After completion of the distal anastomosis, the cervical ECA or ICA is occluded proximally and distally. An arteriotomy, approximately 6 to 8 mm, is made on the arterial surface. The graft is anastomosed to the artery in an end-to-side fashion, using 7-0 nylon sutures (*arrow* in **C**). A., artery; Car, carotid; Ext., external; Fiss., fissure; Front., frontal; Int., internal; Jug., jugular; Temp., temporal; V., vein.

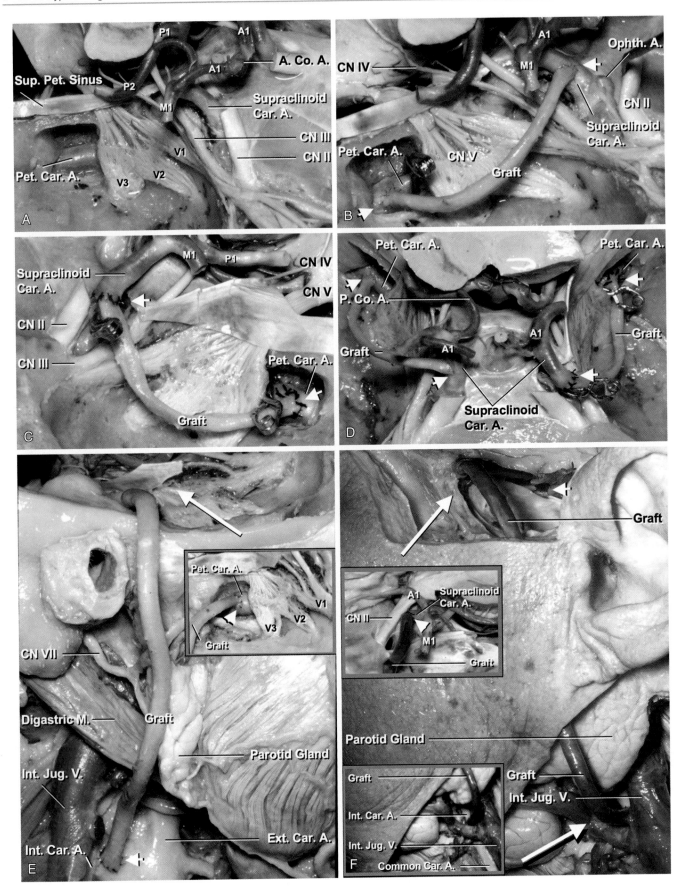

Figure 7–10. For legend see opposite page.

7

Figure 7–10. ICA-ICA high-flow bypasses. **A** to **D,** Petrous ICA–supraclinoid ICA anastomosis. The sphenoid ridge, anterior clinoid, and proximal optic canal are drilled away. The distal dural ring is cut to provide room to place a clip on the ICA proximal to the ophthalmic artery. Sufficient ICA is then available between the ophthalmic and posterior communicating arteries for anastomosing a graft. Exposure of the petrous segment of the ICA is performed extradurally under the middle fossa dura. A small area of the bone posterior to the third branch of the trigeminal nerve and medial to the foramen spinosum is drilled away to expose more than 1-cm length of the petrous ICA. The Eustachian tube and the tensor tympani muscle will be identified with attempted preservation. The saphenous vein is anastomosed to the petrous segment of the ICA in an end-to-side or end-to-end fashion between temporary clips. Interrupted sutures are made using 8-0 nylon. The other end of the saphenous vein graft is then anastomosed to the ICA in an end-to-side (right side) or end-to-end (left side) fashion between the ophthalmic and posterior communicating arteries, using 8-0 or 10-0 nylon. **E,** Cervical ICA–petrous ICA anastomosis. The cervical segment of the ICA in the carotid triangle and the horizontal segment of the petrous ICA are exposed. A radial artery graft is passed from the cervical area toward the petrous ICA. The proximal end of the saphenous vein graft is anastomosed in an end-to-side fashion to the cervical ICA with interrupted sutures (7-0 nylon). The distal end of the saphenous vein graft is then anastomosed in an end-to-side fashion to the petrous ICA with interrupted sutures (8-0 nylon). **F,** Cervical ICA–supraclinoid ICA anastomosis. The supraclinoid segment of the ICA can be used as the recipient vessel when the MCA is not suitable for anastomosis. The cervical and supraclinoid segments of the ICAs are exposed. The proximal end of the saphenous vein graft is anastomosed in an end-to-side or end-to-end fashion to the cervical ICA with interrupted sutures (7-0 nylon). The distal end of the saphenous vein graft is then anastomosed in an end-to-side fashion to the supraclinoid ICA with interrupted sutures (8-0 or 6-0 nylon). Frequently the intima of the ICA in the supraclinoid portion is atherosclerotic. (Arrows indicate anastomotic sites.) A., artery; A.Co.A., anterior communicating artery; Car., carotid; CN, cranial nerve; Ext., external; Int., internal; Jug., jugular; M., muscle; Ophth., ophthalmic; P.Co.A., posterior communicating artery; Pet., petrosal, petrous; Sup., superior; V., vein.

Petrous ICA–supraclinoid ICA anastomosis

After the pterional craniotomy, the sylvian fissure is opened widely. The sphenoid ridge, anterior clinoid, and proximal optic canal are drilled away. The distal dural ring is cut to provide room to place a clip on the ICA proximal to the ophthalmic artery. Sufficient ICA is then available between the ophthalmic and posterior communicating arteries for anastomosing a saphenous vein graft. Exposure of the petrous segment of the ICA is performed extradurally under the middle fossa dura. The dura is elevated along the course of the middle meningeal artery to the foramen spinosum. The middle meningeal artery is divided, and exposure is continued medially and anteriorly to the foramen ovale. A small area of the bone posterior to the third branch of the trigeminal nerve and medial to the foramen spinosum is drilled away to expose approximately a 1-cm length of the petrous ICA. The Eustachian tube and the tensor tympani muscle will be identified with attempted preservation. The saphenous vein is anastomosed to the petrous segment of the ICA in an end-to-side or end-to-end fashion between temporary clips. Interrupted sutures are made using 8-0 nylon. The other end of the saphenous vein graft is then anastomosed to the ICA in an end-to-side or end-to-end fashion between the ophthalmic and posterior communicating arteries, using 8-0 or 10-0 nylon depending on the wall thickness of the ICA and vein graft. The anastomosis on this site is often difficult, because sclerotic change of the arterial wall is frequently observed in the supraclinoid segment of the ICA (Figures 7–10A through 7–10D).

Cervical ICA–petrous ICA anastomosis

The cervical segment of the ICA in the carotid triangle and the horizontal segment of the petrous ICA are exposed as previously described. A radial artery graft is passed from the cervical area through beneath the subcutaneous tissue on the zygomatic arch toward the petrous ICA. The proximal end of the radial artery graft is anastomosed in an end-to-side or end-to-end fashion to the cervical ICA with interrupted sutures (7-0 nylon). The distal end of the radial artery graft is then anastomosed in an end-to-side fashion to the petrous ICA with interrupted sutures (8-0 or 6-0 nylon) (Figure 7–10E).

Cervical ICA–supraclinoid ICA anastomosis

The supraclinoid segment of the ICA can be used as the recipient vessel when the MCA is not suitable for anastomosis. The cervical and supraclinoid segments of the ICAs are exposed as previously described. The proximal end of the saphenous vein graft is anastomosed in an end-to-side or end-to-end fashion to the cervical ICA with interrupted sutures (7-0 nylon). The distal end of the saphenous vein graft is then anastomosed in an end-to-side fashion to the supraclinoid ICA with interrupted sutures (8-0 or 6-0 nylon). Frequently the intima of the ICA in the supraclinoid portion is atherosclerotic (Figure 7–10F).

Bonnet bypass

In the absence of an available ipsilateral donor artery in a patient requiring cerebral revascularization, an anastomosis between the contralateral STA or ICA/ECA and the branch of the MCA (M2 or M4) should be performed using the saphenous vein or radial artery graft. After a left frontotemporal craniotomy, the saphenous vein graft is anastomosed to the contralateral ICA. Then, the graft is placed over the skull through the subcutaneous tunnel and anastomosed to left M2 (Figures 7–11A through 7–11D).

STA–PCA anastomosis

The anastomosis is performed via subtemporal route. After positioning the temple region flat on the table, the STA is outlined either by palpation of the artery or with a portable Doppler device. Once dissection of the STA is completed, the temporal muscle and fascia are incised at the site of the

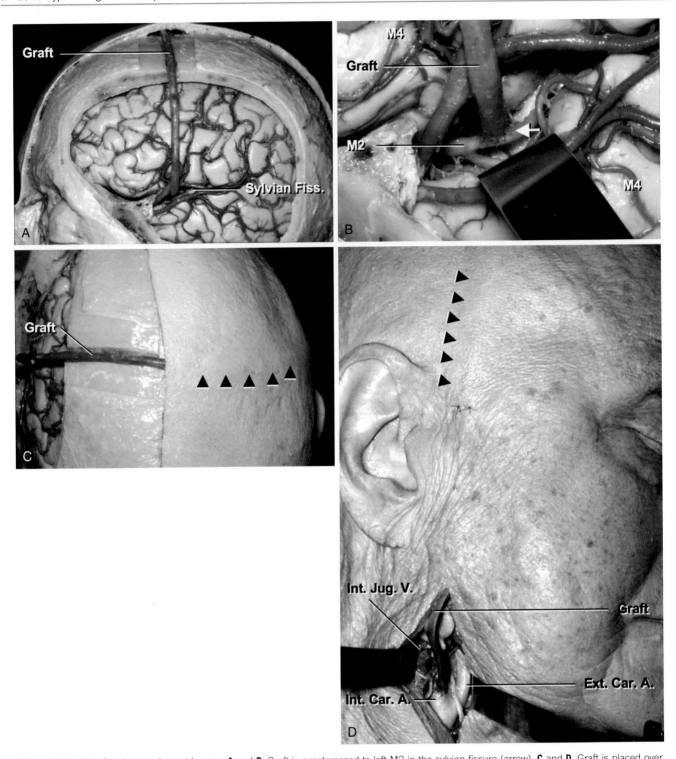

Figure 7–11. High-flow bypass: bonnet bypass. **A** and **B**, Graft is anastomosed to left M2 in the sylvian fissure (arrow). **C** and **D**, Graft is placed over the skull through the subcutaneous tunnel (arrowheads) and anastomosed to the right ICA. A., artery; Car., carotid; Ext., external; Int., internal; Jug., jugular; V., vein.

craniotomy for the subtemporal approach. After the dura has been opened, the temporal lobe is elevated until the tentorial edge is identified. Care should be taken not to damage the vein of Labbé or posterior temporal veins as they enter the transverse sinus. The PCA is dissected free from the arachnoid as it courses around the cerebral peduncle. It is not necessary to expose the P1 segment of the PCA. The portion of the vessel that is isolated for temporary occlusion is the P2A segment of the PCA. A portion of the vessel about 1.5 cm in length, which is free of perforating vessels, is selected for the anastomosis. Care should be taken to avoid damaging these vessels that pass near the anastomotic site, including the long and short circumflex, thalamoperforating, medial and lateral posterior choroidal, hippocampal, anterior temporal, middle temporal, posterior temporal, common temporal, and peduncular perforating arteries. It may be difficult to see the PCA in the center of the operative field when the artery courses the upper part of the cistern around the brainstem. However, excess retraction of the temporal lobe should be avoided to protect the temporal lobe and bridging veins. After the PCA has been exposed, the severed end of the STA is stripped of its fascial layer, and the vessel is exposed over 7 to 8 mm. The tip of the STA is then cut making the shape suitable for the anastomotic site. The recipient vessel is prepared by placing the temporary clips across the vessel and performing the small arteriotomy. Placing two stay-sutures, anastomosis of the STA to the recipient vessel is performed using interrupted 10-0 nylon sutures (Figures 7–12A through 7–12C).

ECA–PCA anastomosis

Either a saphenous vein graft or a radial artery graft is used for this bypass procedure. The common carotid artery, ICA, and ECA are exposed in the carotid triangle, making a cervical incision along the anterior aspect of the sternocleidomastoid muscle. The zygomatic arch is drilled to fashion a conduit for the graft when it is placed in a preauricular position. After the craniotomy for the subtemporal approach, dissection of the P2 segment of the PCA is performed through the subtemporal route. The P2 segment of the PCA, which is thick and with the least number of side branches, is chosen and mobilized for the anastomosis. Care should be taken to avoid damaging the perforators. The distal anastomosis between P2 and the graft is then performed in an end-to-side fashion with interrupted 8-0 nylon sutures. After completion of the distal anastomosis, the cervical ECA is occluded proximally and distally. The graft is pulled down through the subcutaneous tunnel. An arteriotomy, approximately 6 to 8 mm, is made on the ECA. The graft is anastomosed to the artery in an end-to-side fashion, using 6-0 nylon sutures (Figures 7–12D and 7–12E).

STA–SCA anastomosis

The STA-SCA anastomosis is performed in the same operative view described in the STA-PCA anastomosis. After completion of dissecting the STA, the tentorial edge is identified through the subtemporal space. The edge of the tentorium is elevated and sectioned to provide more exposure. The flap of the tentorium is retracted and reflected, and is anchored to a more lateral aspect of the tentorium. Care is taken not to damage the fourth nerve, which courses beneath the tentorial edge. The SCA is then identified in its lateral pontomesencephalic segment. The artery usually has no perforating branches as it travels from the lateral portion of the midbrain to the superior portion of the cerebellum. If there are branches to the brainstem, a portion of the SCA beyond the area within the brainstem branch is selected for the anastomosis. As the SCA frequently divides into rostral and caudal branches in this segment, the larger of the two branches is used for the anastomosis. After the SCA has been exposed, the severed end of the STA is stripped of its fascial layer, and the vessel is exposed over 7 to 8 mm. The tip of the STA is then cut making the shape suitable for the anastomotic site. The recipient vessel is prepared by placing the temporary clips across the vessel and performing the small arteriotomy to equal the length prepared on the SCA. Placing two stay-sutures, anastomosis of the STA to the recipient vessel is performed using interrupted 10-0 nylon sutures (Figures 7–13A through 7–13E).

OA–AICA anastomosis

The course of the OA was outlined the scalp with a portable Doppler device. The OA can be dissected from its point of penetration through the occipital muscle to its most distal extent. It is important to dissect sufficient length of OA to be able to reach the cerebellar arteries; therefore, the dissection may be extended to the level of the mastoid. This dissection is generally difficult because the OA is more tortuous and deeper than the STA. The OA is gently retracted off the field, and a lateral suboccipital craniotomy is completed from the foramen magnum to the transverse sinus and from the edge of the mastoid to the midline. Generally, removal of the arch of C1 is not necessary. After opening the dura mater, the suboccipital surface of the cerebellum can be seen. With careful retraction of the cerebellum laterally, the AICA in the petrous surface is visualized (Figure 7–14A). To perform the anastomosis to the proximal portion of the AICA near the basilar artery would require continuous compression of the cerebellum with compromise of the collateral branches between AICA and PICA or AICA and SCA. Therefore, the flocculonodular (Figures 7–14B and 7–14C) or cortical segment (Figures 7–14D and 7–14E) of the AICA distal to the

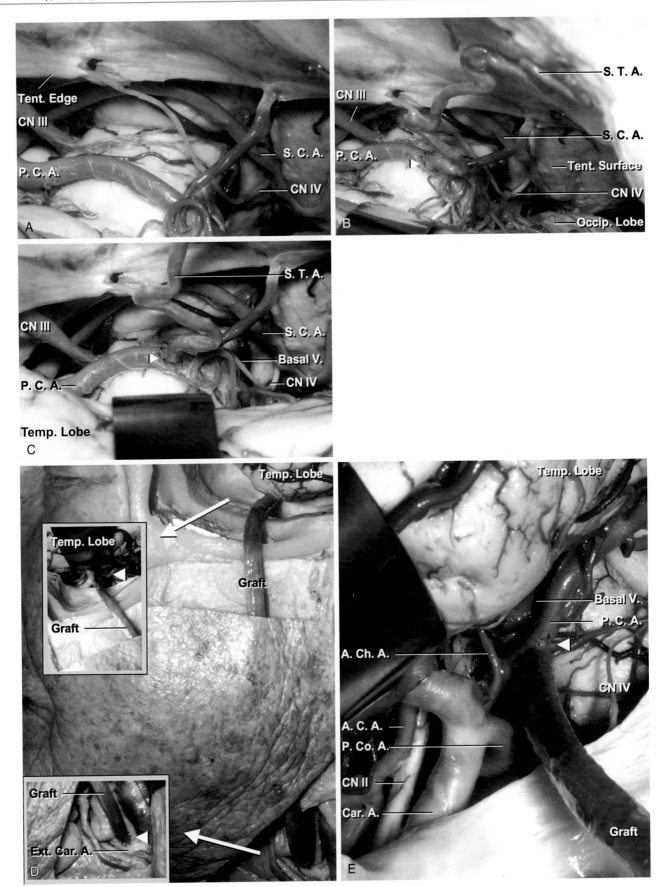

Figure 7–12. For legend see opposite page.

Figure 7–12. Right STA-PCA anastomosis (**A** to **C**) and left ECA-PCA anastomosis using a saphenous vein graft (**D** and **E**). **A,** Anastomosis is performed via subtemporal route. After the dura has been opened, the temporal lobe is elevated until the tentorial edge is identified. Care should be taken not to damage the vein of Labbé or posterior temporal veins as they enter the transverse sinus. The tentorial edge has been removed to expose the SCA and the fourth nerve. The PCA is dissected free from the arachnoid as it courses around the cerebral peduncle. The portion of the vessel that is isolated for temporary occlusion is the P2A segment of the PCA. A portion of the vessel about 1.5 cm in length, which is free of perforating vessels, is selected for the anastomosis. Care should be taken to preserve vessels passing near the anastomotic site, including the long and short circumflex, thalamoperforating, medial and lateral posterior choroidal, hippocampal, anterior temporal, middle temporal, posterior temporal, common temporal, and peduncular perforating arteries. Excess retraction of the temporal lobe should be avoided to protect the temporal lobe and bridging veins. **B** and **C,** After the PCA has been exposed, the severed end of the STA is stripped of its fascial layer, and the vessel is exposed over 7 to 8 mm. The tip of the STA is then cut making the shape suitable for the anastomotic site. The recipient vessel is prepared by placing the temporary clips across the vessel and performing the small arteriotomy. Placing two stay-sutures, anastomosis of the STA to the recipient vessel is performed using interrupted 10-0 nylon sutures (arrowheads). **D,** Either saphenous vein graft or radial artery graft is used for this bypass procedure. After the craniotomy for the subtemporal approach, the P2 segment of the PCA, which is thick and with the least number of side branches, is chosen and mobilized for the anastomosis. The distal anastomosis between P2 and the graft is then performed in an end-to-side fashion with interrupted sutures (upper arrowhead). After completion of the distal anastomosis, the graft is pulled down through the subcutaneous tunnel. An arteriotomy, approximately 6 to 8 mm, is made on the ECA. The graft is anastomosed to the artery in an end-to-side fashion (lower arrowhead). **E,** The graft is anastomosed to P2 (arrowhead). Care should be taken to avoid damaging the perforators. A., artery; A.C.A., anterior cerebral artery; A.Ch.A., anterior choroidal artery; Car., carotid; CN, cranial nerve; Ext., external; Occip., occipital; P.C.A., posterior cerebral artery; P.Co.A., posterior communicating artery; S.C.A., superior cerebellar artery; S.T.A., superficial temporal artery; Temp., temporal; Tent., tentorial; V., vein.

facial-vestibulocochlear nerve complex is selected for the anastomosis. The vessel is freed of the petrous surface of the cerebellum and is isolated. After the AICA has been exposed, the served end of the OA is stripped of its fascial layer, and the vessel is exposed over 7 to 8 mm. The tip of the OA is then cut making the shape suitable for the anastomotic site. The recipient vessel is prepared by placing the temporary clips across the vessel and performing the small arteriotomy to equal the length prepared on the AICA. Placing two stay-sutures, anastomosis of the OA to the recipient vessel is performed using 10-0 nylon interrupted sutures. Generally, the anastomosis procedure for the AICA is more difficult than that for the PICA because of depth of the operative field and smaller diameter of the recipient vessel.

OA–PICA anastomosis

After completion of dissecting the OA, a suboccipital craniotomy is performed described in the OA-AICA anastomosis. The arch of C1 is removed, if needed. After the dura is opened, exposure of the caudal loop of the PICA is obtained. Then, the vessel is freed from the arachnoid. After the PICA has been exposed, the severed end of the OA is stripped of its fascial layer, and the vessel is exposed over 7 to 8 mm. The tip of the OA is then cut making the shape suitable for the anastomotic site. The recipient vessel is prepared by placing the temporary clips across the vessel and performing the small arteriotomy to equal the length prepared on the PICA. Placing two stay-sutures, anastomosis of the OA to the recipient vessel is performed using interrupted 10-0 nylon sutures (Figures 7–15A through 7–15C).

Short arterial interposition grafting anastomosis (OA–PICA)

The STA or OA is used for an arterial graft. OA–AICA, OA–PICA, or vertebral artery to PICA anastomoses can be performed using an interposition graft. A section of STA or OA graft of approximately 8 cm in length is dissected from a skin flap and then both severed ends of the donor vessel are stripped of their fascial layer. The graft is anastomosed between the OA and the caudal loop of the PICA with interrupted 10-0 nylon sutures (Figures 7–15D and 7–15E).

Side-to-side anastomosis (PICA)

This procedure is chiefly used for cerebral revascularization for the distal portion of the PICA after occlusion of its proximal portion. The proximity and parallel courses of the tonsillomedullary and the telovelotonsillar segments of the PICAs permit their side-to-side anastomosis. Arteriotomies, 4 mm in length, were made on both donor and recipient arteries. The most difficult procedure here is to make a tight suture on a back wall. After two stay-sutures are placed, the back wall is sutured using a continuous running fashion from the intravascular side and then the anterior wall closed with interrupted sutures (10-0 nylon). The distal part of the artery beyond the occlusion site is supplied by the adjacent artery (Figures 7–16A through 7–16F).

End-to-end anastomosis (PICA)

The diseased PICA segment that is involved with the tumor or aneurysm can be excised, and the remaining vessel can be directly re-anastomosed in an end-to-end fashion. The proximal

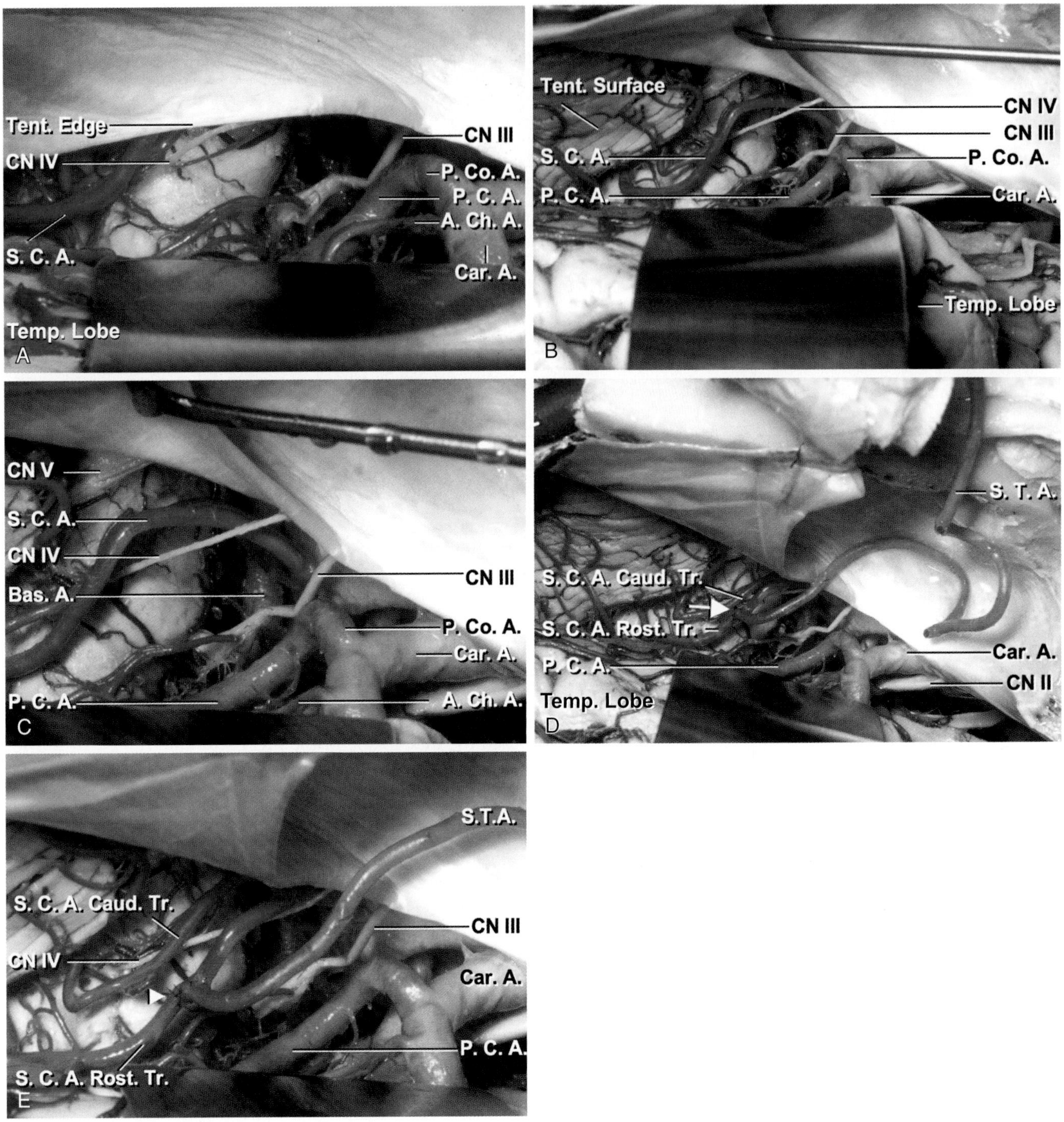

Figure 7–13. Left STA-SCA anastomosis. **A,** Anastomosis is performed via subtemporal route. After the dura has been opened, the temporal lobe is elevated until the tentorial edge is identified. Care should be taken not to damage the vein of Labbé or posterior temporal veins as they enter the transverse sinus. **B** and **C,** Tentorial edge has been removed to expose the SCA and the fourth nerve. As the SCA frequently divides into rostral and caudal branches in this segment, the larger of the two branches is used for the anastomosis. **D** and **E,** After the SCA has been exposed, the severed end of the STA is stripped of its fascial layer, and the vessel is exposed over 7 to 8 mm. The tip of the STA is then cut making the shape suitable for the anastomotic site. The recipient vessel is prepared by placing the temporary clips across the vessel and performing the small arteriotomy to equal the length prepared on the SCA. Placing two stay-sutures, anastomosis of the STA to the recipient vessel is performed using interrupted 10-0 nylon sutures (arrowheads). A., artery; A.Ch.A., anterior choroidal artery; Bas., basilar; Car., carotid; Caud., caudal; CN, cranial nerve; P.C.A., posterior cerebral artery; P.Co.A., posterior communicating artery; Rost., rostral; S.C.A., superior cerebellar artery; S.T.A., superficial temporal artery; Temp., temporal; Tent., tentorial; Tr., trunk.

and distal stumps of the PICA are anastomosed with interrupted sutures (10-0 nylon), unless a gap between the diameters of the stumps are greater than 10 mm.

CONCLUSION

Cerebral revascularization is an important procedure in the treatment of complex intracranial aneurysms, cranial base tumors, and certain ischemic diseases.[5,6] In this study, we examined microsurgical procedures for cerebral revascularization in the anterior and posterior circulation and showed each procedure using cadaveric specimen. It will help not only surgeons, but also neurologists, neuroradiologists, and other physicians to further understand the mechanism of cerebral revascularization.

Cerebral revascularization technique has developed in the last three to four decades. It is still developing, with changes of technique and new indications for operative intervention, such as combination with endovascular procedures. The value of cerebral revascularization surgery as an aid to improve cerebral ischemia differs not only between neurosurgeon and physician, but also among neurosurgeons. It is important to understand the mechanism of each bypass procedure. It is also necessary to understand various microsurgical techniques and their related anatomic structures. Careful consideration, including hemodynamic status of patients and difficulties with techniques, should be taken when a cerebral revascularization procedure is planned.

ACKNOWLEDGMENTS

The authors thank Ronald Smith, PhD, director, and Robin Barry, MS, and David Peace, MS, medical illustrators of the Microneuroanatomy Laboratory, Department of Neurological Surgery, University of Florida, for constant support. We also thank Laura Dickinson for preparation of the manuscript.

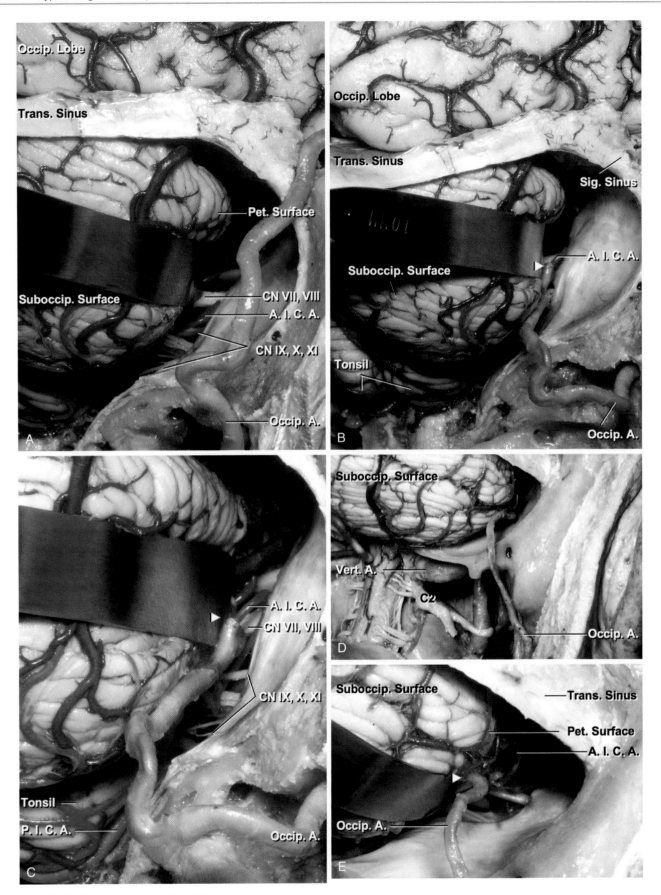

Figure 7–14. For legend see opposite page.

Figure 7–14. OA-AICA anastomosis (right side). **A,** The OA can be dissected from its point of penetration through the occipital muscle to its most distal extent. The OA is gently retracted off the field, and a lateral suboccipital craniotomy is completed. After opening the dura mater, the suboccipital surface of the cerebellum can be seen. With careful retraction of the cerebellum laterally, the AICA in the petrous surface is visualized. The flocculonodular segment (**B** and **C**) and the cortical segment (**D** and **E**) of the AICAs distal to the facial-vestibulocochlear nerve complex are selected for the anastomoses. The vessel is freed of the petrous surface of the cerebellum and is isolated. After the AICA has been exposed, the severed end of the OA is stripped of its fascial layer, and the vessel is exposed over 7 to 8 mm. The tip of the OA is then cut, making the shape suitable for the anastomotic site. The recipient vessel is prepared by placing the temporary clips across the vessel and performing the small arteriotomy to equal the length prepared on the AICA. Placing two stay-sutures, anastomosis of the OA to the recipient vessel is performed using interrupted 10-0 nylon sutures (arrowheads). Generally, the anastomosis procedure for the AICA is more difficult than that for the PICA because of the depth of the operative field and smaller diameter of the recipient vessel. A., artery; A.I.C.A., anterior inferior cerebellar artery; CN, cranial nerve; Occip., occipital; Pet., petrosal; P.I.C.A., posterior inferior cerebellar artery; Sig., sigmoid; Suboccip., suboccipital; Trans., transverse; Vert., vertebral.

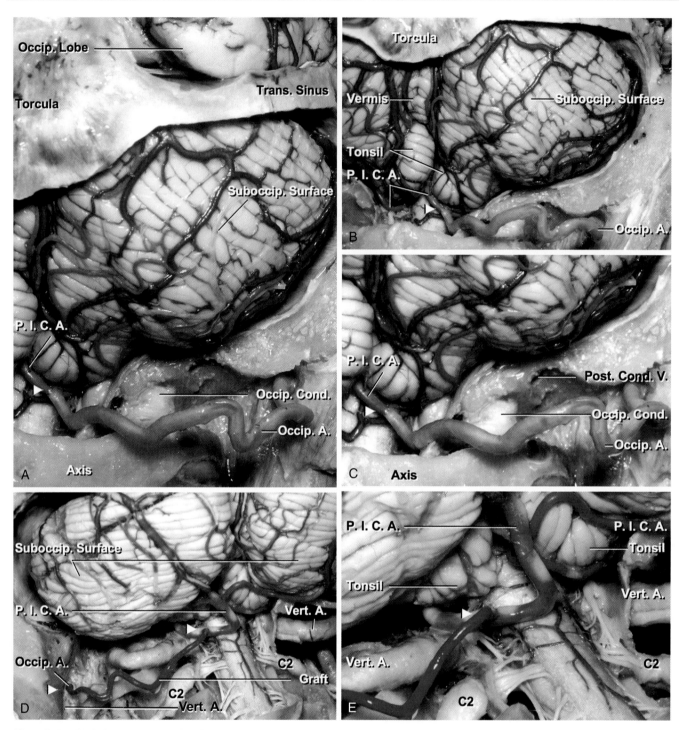

Figure 7–15. OA-PICA anastomosis. **A** to **C.** Pedicled graft (right side). **D** and **E.** Short arterial interposition graft (left side). **A** to **C.** After completion of dissecting the OA, the suboccipital dura is opened to expose the caudal loop of the PICA. Then, the vessel is freed from the arachnoid. After the PICA has been exposed, the severed end of the OA is stripped of its fascial layer, and the vessel is exposed over 7 to 8 mm. The tip of the OA is then cut, making the shape suitable for the anastomotic site. The recipient vessel is prepared by placing the temporary clips across the vessel and performing the small arteriotomy to equal the length prepared on the PICA. Placing two stay-sutures, anastomosis of the OA to the recipient vessel is performed using interrupted 10-0 nylon sutures (arrowheads). **D** and **E.** Free STA or OA is used for an arterial graft. A section of STA or OA graft, approximately 8 cm in length, is dissected from a skin flap and then both severed ends of the donor vessel are stripped of their fascial layer. The graft is anastomosed between the OA and the caudal loop of the PICA with interrupted 10-0 nylon sutures (arrowheads). A., artery; Cond., condyle or condylar; Occip., occipital; P.I.C.A., posterior inferior cerebellar artery; Post., posterior; Suboccip., suboccipital; Trans., transverse; V., vein; Vert., vertebral.

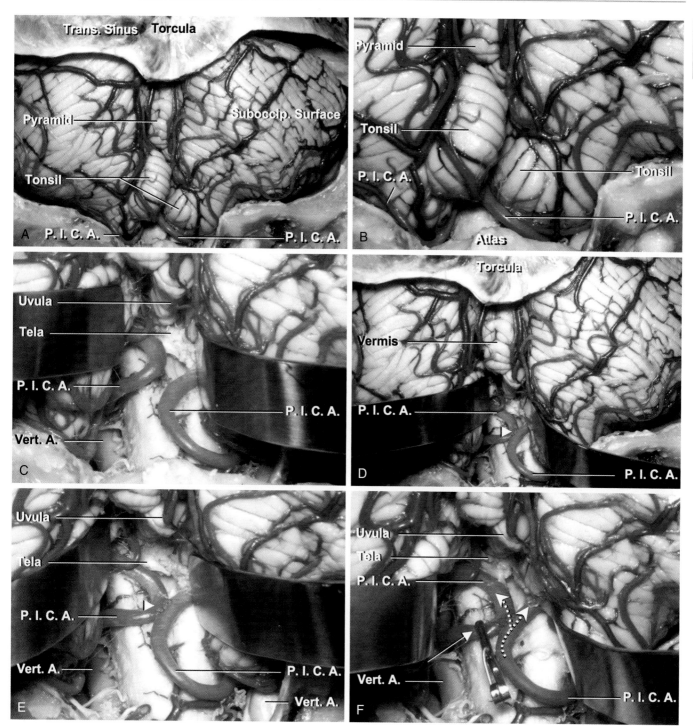

Figure 7–16. A to **F.** Side-to-side anastomosis of PICAs, posterior view. This procedure is mainly used for cerebral revascularization for the distal part of the PICA after occlusion of its proximal portion. The proximity and parallel courses of the tonsillomedullary and the telovelotonsillar segments of the PICAs permit their side-to-side anastomosis. Arteriotomies, 4 mm in length, are made on both donor and recipient arteries. After two stay-sutures are placed, the back wall is sutured using a continuous running fashion from the intravascular side and then the anterior wall closed with interrupted sutures (arrowheads). The distal part of the artery beyond the occlusion site (arrow) is supplied by the adjacent artery (dotted arrows). A., artery; P.I.C.A., posterior inferior cerebellar artery; Suboccip., suboccipital; Trans., transverse; Vert., vertebral.

REFERENCES

1. The EC/IC Bypass Study Group: Failure of extracranial-intracranial arterial bypass to reduce the risk of ischemic stroke. Results of an international randomized trial, *N Engl J Med* 313(19):1191–1200, 1985.
2. Perlmutter D, Rhoton AL Jr: Microsurgical anatomy of the distal anterior cerebral artery, *J Neurosurg* 49(2):204–228, 1978.
3. Zeal AA, Rhoton AL Jr: Microsurgical anatomy of the posterior cerebral artery, *J Neurosurg* 48(4):534–559, 1978.
4. Allen EV: Thromboangitis obliterans: Methods of diagnosis of chronic occlusive arterial lesions distal to the wrist with illustrative cases, *Am J Med Sci* 178:237–243, 1929.
5. Kawashima M, Rhoton AL Jr, Tanriover N, et al: Microsurgical anatomy of cerebral revascularization, Part I: Anterior circulation, *J Neurosurg* 102(1):116–131, 2005.
6. Kawashima M, Rhoton AL Jr, Tanriover N, et al: Microsurgical anatomy of cerebral revascularization, Part II: Posterior circulation, *J Neurosurg* 102(1):132–147, 2005.

STA-MCA MICROANASTOMOSIS: SURGICAL TECHNIQUE

8

NADIA KHAN; LUCA REGLI

INTRODUCTION

The purpose of extracranial to intracranial bypass is always to improve the cerebral blood flow (CBF) by diverting blood flow from the extracranial carotid artery circulation to the intracranial cerebral circulation. There are two main indications for cerebral revascularization procedures: (1) *flow augmentation* to increase CBF in patients with chronic compromised CBF (chronic cerebral ischemia), and (2) *flow preservation* to maintain CBF in patients undergoing acute vessel sacrifice (complex aneurysms, skull base tumors). Revascularization procedures can be divided into *direct* (connecting the donor and recipient vessel directly by microanastomosis) and *indirect* techniques (laying vascularized tissue in contact with the brain to develop delayed collateralization).

The first successful direct extracranial-intracranial (EC-IC) bypass surgery was performed by Yasargil in 1967.[1] Since then, many operative techniques for direct cerebral revascularization have been described (see chapters 7 through 14). The most commonly used EC-IC procedure to revascularize the anterior circulation is the superficial temporay artery (STA)–middle cerebral artery (MCA) bypass between one branch of the STA and a cortical MCA branch (M4). It has the advantage of being a safe, simple, and readily available technique, and the disadvantage of supplying low flow rates. In this chapter we will describe the technical aspects of the STA-MCA bypass as well as the pitfalls and lessons learned by the authors based on their longstanding experience.

PERIOPERATIVE CONSIDERATIONS AND SURGICAL TECHNIQUE

The preoperative as well as the postoperative period and special anesthetic considerations are important general steps of the STA-MCA procedures. The surgical technique of the STA-MCA bypass can be divided into four fundamental steps:

1. Preparation of the donor STA vessel
2. Localization and performance of the craniotomy
3. Preparation of the recipient vessel and completion of the microanastomosis
4. Closure

Preoperative Period

Patients to receive cerebral revascularization must have accurate preoperative systemic assessment especially for cardiovascular risk factors to optimize their medical condition and reduce operative and postoperative morbidity and mortality. Patients presenting with cerebral ischemic disorders frequently have systemic atherosclerotic disease.

Antiplatelet treatment with low-dose anesthetic is begun three days preoperatively and continued daily thereafter in order to optimize microanastomosis patency rates (>95%). Variability in individual response to antiplatelet therapy exists, and 4% to 20% of patients are resistant to low-dose treatment.[2,3]

The STA has two main branches, parietal and frontal, either of which can be used as the donor vessel. The choice is for the branch with the largest diameter as the amount of flow is proportionate to the radius at the power of 4 (Poiseuille's law). The availability of an adequate STA branch is checked on preoperative imaging (six-vessel intra-arterial angiography or computed tomography angiography [CTA]). In patients with chronic ischemia, preoperative cerebrovascular hemodynamic assessment is essential for proper indication.

Anesthesia and Cerebral Protection

Patients are operated under general anesthesia. All the anesthetic interventions that decrease cerebral perfusion pressure (CPP) must be strictly avoided. Therefore hyperventilation is not used and patients are operated under normocapnia (35 to 40 mm Hg). Similarly, hypotension must be avoided and slight (10% to 20%) elevation of mean arterial pressure is aimed at during cross-clamping. There is no clear evidence in the literature that inducing brain protection via decreased metabolism changes outcome, and we do not recommend it for the standard STA-MCA. However, hyperthermia must be avoided.

Surgical Technique

Preparation of the STA

The patient is placed supine and the head is fixed in a three-point Mayfield fixation frame. The head should be elevated above the heart, turned to the contralateral side, keeping the operative field horizontal to the floor. Depending on the suppleness of the cervical spine, a shoulder roll may or may not be required.

The STA and its branches are mapped with a Doppler ultrasound probe and serve as a guideline for the skin incision (Figure 8–1). Using the operative microscope, a linear skin incision is made directly over the course of the parietal branch of the STA all the way to the zygoma and an 8-cm length of the STA is dissected out. In the event that the frontal branch of the STA is to be used, a curvilinear frontotemporal skin flap behind the hairline allows for a clean dissection of the frontal branch from the underside of the scalp flap. This can be tedious since the dissection from under the flap may require additional skin retraction and dissection through the fat plane.

The STA is then dissected out from the galeal tissue, ensuring that a small cuff (2 to 3 mm) of soft tissue surrounding it remains. Bipolar electrocoagulation of the arterial side branches is performed at a distance of several millimeters to avoid thermal injury to the STA. The isolated STA must be long enough so that no traction occurs during the bypass. The distal end of the artery can then be clipped and divided after temporary clamping at the proximal end, or left intact until after the craniotomy and just prior to the anastomosis (Figure 8–2). After the STA is divided, meticulous care must

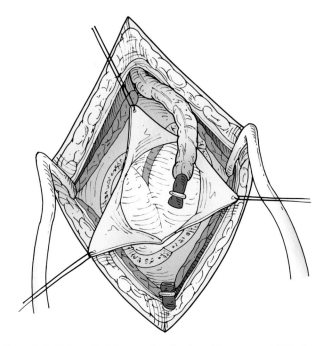

Figure 8–2. Schematic intraoperative drawing of the prepared STA clipped and ready for anastomosis. Underlying craniotomy with dural opening and visualization of a cortical branch.

be taken to irrigate it with heparinized saline and then place it protected in moist gauze at the proximal end of the incision.

Performance of the craniotomy: Location and size

The craniotomy is planned so as to expose at least one adequate recipient cortical MCA branch. Numerous modifications for the identification of the site have been proposed in the literature.[4] Considerations by Chater et al.[5] to locate the craniotomy are recommended: "[P]erform the craniotomy at a point 6 cm above the external auditory meatus on a line perpendicular to the base of the skull." To approximate the base of the skull, "a horizontal line from the external auditory canal to the lateral canthus of the eye" is the most suitable as shown by Pena-Tapia et al.[4] The temporalis muscle is divided in a linear incision and mobilized in order to expose the region of the planned craniotomy. After placing a temporal burr hole, a 3x3-cm craniotomy is performed. The size of craniotomy varies depending on the indication or need for revascularization. For Moyamoya angiopathy, a larger craniotomy is usually preferable, allowing for a wider selection of suitable cortical vessels as well as for a larger surface area for additional indirect revascularization as needed.

Preparation of the recipient vessel and completion of the microanastomosis

The dural opening can be performed in a Y-fashion to allow for three triangular dural flaps, or the opening can be further extended into several flaps, depending on the location of the preferred cortical M4 branch (Figure 8–3). These are retracted

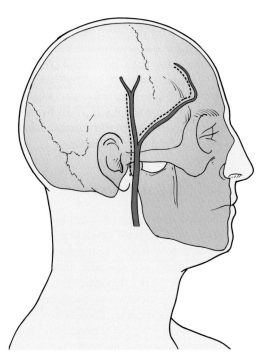

Figure 8–1. The two major STA branches, parietal and frontal. Dotted line indicates line of surgical incision for dissection.

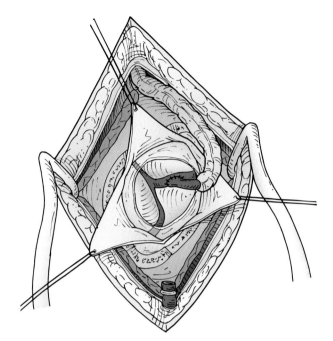

Figure 8–3. Schematic intraoperative drawing of prepared STA-MCA anastomosis.

with tag-up sutures, and the cortex is inspected to locate the most suitable M4 recipient artery. The ideal recipient artery is the one located at the cortical surface, has a straight segment without significant side branches, and usually is the largest in diameter (ideally 1.5 mm). Cortical vessel length of 1 to 1.5 cm is adequate. The M4 recipient cortical vessels that can be used include *suprasylvian*: precentral, central, anterior parietal, posterior parietal, and angular branches; and *infrasylvian*: anterior temporal, middle temporal, and posterior temporal. With extension of the craniotomy in the anterior and posterior directions, the prefrontal branch anteriorly and the temporo-occipital branch posteriorly can also be visualized.

After localizing a recipient cortical artery, the arachnoid over it is opened and dissected with microsurgical instruments. Small side branches (usually not more than two or three) are cauterized and cut. A small rubber high-visibility background is placed under the recipient artery. Papaverine is intermittently instilled over the cortical branch and the predissected STA.

Once preparation to perform the anastomosis is complete, the STA is prepared. The STA is flushed with heparinized saline, and the distance between the donor and recipient artery is measured. It is important to allow for 2 cm of redundancy in order to ease flipping the artery forward and backward while placing the microsutures on both sides of the microanastomosis. The distal end of the STA is cleared of any remaining adventitia over 1 to 2 cm to allow for a clean microanastomosis. The STA is then cut at a sharp angle and fish-mouthed in order to obtain an opening that is at least twice the diameter of the recipient artery. In making the operative field ready for the

microanastomosis, it is essential to keep it clean from cerebrospinal fluid (CSF) and blood. Placing a flexible microsuction system is helpful. The recipient cortical branch is then clamped on both ends with atraumatic clips and an arteriotomy is performed in accordance with the size of the distal end of the STA. The arteriotomy is irrigated and rinsed with heparinized saline. Using 10-0 or 11-0 microsutures (depending on the size and fragility of both the donor and recipient vessels), two anchoring sutures (one on the heel and the other on the toe of the donor vessel) are placed followed by 10 to 14 interrupted sutures to complete the microanastomosis. Alternatively, two running sutures can be used. Whether interrupted or continuous sutures are placed depends on surgeon preference and training. Once suturing is complete, flow is restored by removing first the distal clip, followed by the proximal, and finally the clip on the STA. Minor oozing from the anastomosis site can be controlled by placing small hemostatic sponges locally (surgical or tachosyl) without compressing the anastomosis. More brisk bleeding points may need additional microsutures. The anastomosis is tested for patency either with near-infrared indocyanine green fluorescence angiography or an intraoperative quantitative flow meter (Charbel Micro Flowprobe, Transonic).

Surgical closure

The dura is closed leaving a generous durotomy at the point of entry of the STA. The bone flap is repositioned and fixed with titanium plates. Here again sufficient bone opening at the point of entry of the STA is allowed for. The temporalis muscle is then sutured, leaving a generous space for the artery. Wound drain is not used as standard. Subcutaneous 3-0 vicryl and separate skin sutures are applied while ensuring that a puncture or compression of the donor graft does not occur. It can be advantageous at this point in time to mark the point of penetration of the STA on the skin to allow for ease of detection at the time of postoperative Doppler measurements. Light, noncircumferential postoperative head dressing should be applied. Writing "Attention: Bypass" on the wound dressing helps prevent pressure on the graft in a setting where bypass grafts are not performed routinely.

Postoperative Care

Patients should spend the first night in an intensive or intermediate care bed for close monitoring of neurological and hemodynamic parameters. Blood pressure control is important to prevent hypotension and the risk of graft thrombosis or hypertension and the risk of hyperperfusion. Graft patency can be checked by Doppler ultrasound, while always avoiding compression of the graft. We like to perform an imaging of the bypass (preferably a CTA) between 24 and 48 hours after the surgery as a baseline exam for future follow-up. A six-vessel cerebral angiogram is performed usually at 6 months (Figure 8–4).

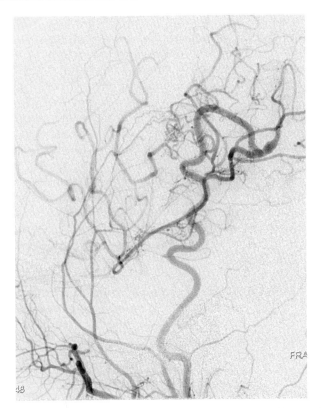

Figure 8–4. Postoperative cerebral angiogram showing lateral external carotid injection demonstrating a patent robust graft with good distal filling of MCA territory.

SPECIAL CONSIDERATIONS AND PITFALLS

Intraoperative Tests for Anastomosis Patency

Patency of the anastomosis can be evaluated using a micro-Doppler probe. However, we prefer to use intraoperative quantitative blood-flow measurements with calculation of the cut flow index (CFI). The CFI is calculated by dividing the bypass flow by the cut STA flow (free flow through the cut STA). This index has been shown to be a predictor of bypass patency: CFI > 0.5, permeability of 92%; CFI < 0.5, permeability 50%.[6]

Near-infrared indocyanine green fluorescence angiography to visualize graft, cortical, and pial filling is also a useful technique, allowing direct visualization of the anastomosis patency and dynamic distribution of flow.[7] Fluorescence angiography does not indicate quantitative blood flow, and we recommend using it in combination with a quantitative measurement.

It is important to remember that graft pulsation is not a reliable indicator of graft patency and one should not rely solely on this indicator.

Complication: Microanastomosis Occlusion

Poor anastomosis flow will normally induce subsequent thrombosis and graft occlusion. It is therefore mandatory to identify these situations perioperatively. Graft occlusion can be attributed to two major causes: poor indication and technical errors.

Poor indication refers to patients undergoing a bypass without cerebral hemodynamic compromise. The blood flow in the MCA territory is strong enough to be competitive with the bypass flow. This cannot be corrected perioperatively.

The most frequent *technical errors* are traumatic handling of the endothelium; inadequate flushing with heparinized saline; misplacement of the microsutures, catching the back wall or irregular stitches; inadequate anastomosis size; twisting or kinking of the donor vessel; and inadequate length of STA resulting in continuous traction and preventing proper suturing of the frontal and back wall. In case of poor flow or occlusion, the microanastomosis has to be inspected and opened and redone to correct the technical error.

Wound Healing

Skin blood flow is reduced because the STA flow has been diverted to the brain. This reduces the natural healing process, sometimes resulting in necrosis, secondary infection, and wound dehiscence. Careful postoperative wound inspection is recommended.

Instrumentation and Training

Choice of microinstruments, microscope, and flow measuring devices all depend on the surgeon's choice, preference, and experience. There is, however, no doubt that successful microanastomosis requires meticulous microsurgical skills and frequent training of microanastomosis techniques in the laboratory.

Less-Invasive Technique for STA-MCA Bypass

Preoperative identification of the STA and a sizable recipient artery on CTA is easy: the larger STA branch is chosen as the donor vessel. The choice of the recipient vessel is based on the size and superficial cortical location. Using 3-D CTA reconstructions, a small craniotomy (2 to 2.5 cm in diameter) can be ideally located to expose the recipient vessel. Using CTA-based neuronavigation, the craniotomy and a short linear incision (5 cm) over the STA can be planned to overlie the recipient and the donor vessel. The precise localization of the target point allows the procedure to be less invasive.[8,9]

REFERENCES

1. Yasargil MG: *Microsurgery Applied to Neurosurgery.* Stuttgart, 1969, Georg Thieme-Verlag.
2. Blais N, et al: Response to aspirin in healthy individuals. Cross-comparison of light transmission aggregometry, VerifyNow system, platelet count drop, thromboelastography (TEG) and urinary 11-dehydrothromboxane B(2) *Thromb Haemost* 102(2):404–411, 2009.
3. Collet JP, Montalescot G: Platelet function testing and implications for clinical practice *J Cardiovasc Pharmacol Ther* 14(3):157–169, 2009.
4. Pena-Tapia PG, et al: Identification of the optimal cortical target point for extracranial-intracranial bypass surgery in patients with hemodynamic cerebrovascular insufficiency, *J Neurosurg* 108(4):655–661, 2008.
5. Chater N, et al: Microvascular bypass surgery. Part 1: anatomical studies, *J Neurosurg* 44(6):712–714, 1976.
6. Amin-Hanjani S, et al: The cut flow index: an intraoperative predictor of the success of extracranial-intracranial bypass for occlusive cerebrovascular disease, *Neurosurgery* 56(Suppl 1):75–85, 2005.
7. Woitzik J, et al: Intraoperative control of extracranial-intracranial bypass patency by near-infrared indocyanine green videoangiography, *J Neurosurg* 102(4):692–698, 2005.
8. Coppens JR, Cantando JD, Abdulrauf SI: Minimally invasive superficial temporal artery to middle cerebral artery bypass through an enlarged bur hole: the use of computed tomography angiography neuronavigation in surgical planning, *J Neurosurg* 109(3):553–558, 2008.
9. Kaku Y, et al: Less invasive technique for EC-IC bypass, *Acta Neurochir Suppl* 103:83–86, 2008.

8

OA-PICA BYPASS

MOHAMED SAMY ELHAMMADY; JACQUES J. MORCOS

INTRODUCTION

Yasargil et al.[1] demonstrated the feasibility of EC-IC bypass surgery in 1967 after performing the first successful superficial temporal artery to middle cerebral artery anastomosis. Ausman and colleagues[2] applied these techniques for vertebral artery (VA) occlusive disease and reported the first intracranial posterior circulation revascularization procedure in 1976 after performing an occipital artery (OA) to posterior inferior cerebellar artery (PICA) anastomosis. Posterior circulation bypass surgery has since been used to treat vertebrobasilar insufficiency, skull base tumors involving the VA and its branches, and complex or giant posterior circulation aneurysms. Current advances in endovascular techniques and the availability of intracranial stents have largely limited the need for posterior circulation bypass surgery for vertebrobasilar insufficiency. Occipital artery–PICA bypass surgery, however, remains a valuable tool in the management of fusiform aneurysms of the VA encompassing the PICA origin as well as giant and complex VA/PICA and PICA aneurysms that cannot be reconstructed with surgical clipping or endovascular coiling and require parent artery occlusion or trapping. In the context of VB insufficiency, the bypass may still have a role in the rare settings of poor endovascular access due to tortuosity or occlusion. This chapter reviews the relevant anatomy, surgical technique, perioperative care, and complications associated with OA-PICA revascularization.

ANATOMY

Occipital Artery

The OA is an ideal choice for PICA revascularization as it can be encountered during the suboccipital approach and closely approximates the size of the PICA. The course of the OA can be divided into three segments.[3]

The first segment, also known as the *digastric* segment, extends from the origin of the OA from the external carotid artery to the point of emergence from the occipital groove of the mastoid process. The OA originates from the posterior or lateral wall of the external carotid artery at the level of the angle of the mandible. The artery ascends medial to the external carotid artery and lateral to the internal jugular vein to a point posterior and medial to the styloid process. The OA then courses posteriorly and laterally superficial to the rectus capitus lateralis muscle first and then superior oblique muscle.[4] The artery is covered by the posterior belly of the digastric muscle laterally, hence known as the digastric segment. The artery then runs in the occipital groove or occasionally a true bony canal[3] medial to the mastoid notch, in which the posterior belly of the digastric muscle arises.[4]

The second segment, also known as the *suboccipital* or *horizontal* segment, extends from the emergence of the OA from the occipital groove of the mastoid process to the superior nuchal line. The OA exits the occipital groove between the superior oblique muscle and posterior belly of the digastric and is covered by the splenium capitis and sternocleidomastoid. The artery courses medially in a horizontal plane either superficial or deep to the longissimus capitus muscle, depending on whether the occipital groove is absent or present. The OA then continues superficial to the semispinalis capitis muscle just below the superior nuchal line in the upper part of the posterior triangle. The artery then changes course and runs vertically upward, piercing the fascia connecting the cranial attachment of the trapezius and sternocleidomastoid muscles to the superior nuchal line.[5] The suboccipital segment gives rise to ascending and descending muscular branches as well as transosseous branches to the dura of the posterior fossa. The diameter of the suboccipital segment ranges from 1.6 to 2.2 mm (mean 1.9 mm) and the length ranges from 75 to 85 mm (range 79.3 mm).[6]

The third segment, also known as the *occipital* or *subgaleal* segment, begins at the superior nuchal line after the OA pierces the fascial attachment of the trapezius and sternocleidomastoid muscles. In a cadaveric study, the OA was found to cross the superior nuchal line approximately 35 mm (±0.5 mm) lateral to the inion.[3] The artery continues underneath the galea and above the occipitalis muscle before dividing into its terminal branches. The diameter of the OA at the superior nuchal line is approximately 1.4 mm (±0.3 mm).[3]

PICA Artery

Segments of the PICA

It is very convenient and appropriate to subscribe to the concept advanced by Lister et al.,[7] that the PICA can be divided into five segments based on its relationship to the medulla and the cerebellum: anterior medullary, lateral medullary, tonsillomedullary, telovelotonsillar, and cortical.

The *anterior medullary* segment begins at the origin of the PICA from the VA anterior to the medulla oblongata. Congenital anomalies of the PICA include double origin, fenestration, or duplicated PICAs, a common anterior inferior cerebellar artery (AICA)–PICA configuration, a VA termination at the PICA, extradural origins at C1 and C2 levels (5% to 20%), origins at the hypoglossal, proatlantal, or posterior meningeal arteries, and at all points along the intradural VA.[8–15] From its origin, the artery runs posteriorly around the medulla past the exit of the hypoglossal nerve rootlets from the anterior border of the inferior olivary complex to the boundary between the anterior and lateral surfaces of the medulla, which is marked by a rostrocaudal line through the most prominent part of the inferior olive. The *lateral medullary* segment begins at the point where the PICA passes the most prominent part of the inferior olive and extends posteriorly around the lateral aspect of the medulla to the origin of the glossopharyngeal, vagus, and accessory rootlets from the posterior border of the inferior olivary complex. The PICA continues medially as the *tonsillomedullary* segment between the lower half of the cerebellar tonsil and the posterior aspect of the medulla oblongata. The artery makes a caudally convex curve as it passes around the lower pole of the cerebellar tonsil known as the caudal or infratonsillar loop. The caudal loop is frequently used as a recipient during OA-PICA bypasses and its diameter ranges from 0.9 to 1.4 mm (mean 1.2 mm).[6] After forming the caudal loop, the PICA ascends to the midlevel of the medial surface of the tonsil where it becomes the *telovelotonsillar* segment. The artery continues along the medial surface of the tonsil toward the roof of the fourth ventricle. The PICA then forms a rostrally convex curve referred to as the cranial or supratonsillar loop. This loop consists of proximal ascending and distal descending limbs and an apex that lies caudal to the fastigium at the center of the inferior medullary velum. The ascending limb runs posterior to the tela choroidea and inferior medullary velum toward the fastigium of the fourth ventricle. The descending limb runs posteriorly in the fissure between the vermis medially and the superomedial surface of the tonsil and cerebellar hemisphere laterally. The PICA emerges from the fissure and continues as the *cortical* segment. The artery divides into a smaller medial and a larger lateral trunk and subsequently gives rise to hemispheric, vermian, and tonsillar branches.

Branches of the PICA

The PICA gives rise to three types of branches:[7]

1. Perforating arteries
   The anterior medullary, lateral medullary, and tonsillomedullary segments of the PICA give rise to crucial brainstem

perforating arteries that must be preserved at all cost. We and others believe that sacrificing the PICA distal to the tonsillomedullary segment is generally well tolerated, unless an embryological anomaly has resulted in poor collateralization of the cortical segment vascularization zone. On the other hand, if sacrifice of the PICA within its first three segments is contemplated, a revascularization procedure must be strongly considered to avoid brainstem infarction. The anterior medullary segment gives rise to 0 to 2 (average 1.0) predominantly short circumflex perforating arteries that supply the anterior, lateral, or posterior surface of the medulla. The lateral medullary segment gives rise to 0 to 5 (average 1.8) predominantly short circumflex perforating arteries that supply the lateral or posterior surface of the medulla. The tonsillomedullary segment gives rise to 0 to 11 (average 3.3) direct or short circumflex arteries and supplies the lateral and posterior surface of the medulla.

2. Choroidal branches
   The PICA gives rise to an average of six branches that supply the tela choroidea and choroid plexus of the fourth ventricle. The choroidal arteries predominantly arise from the tonsillomedullary and telovelotonsillar segments and to a lesser extent from the lateral medullary segment. The anterior medullary segment on the other hand, does not contribute to the fourth ventricular choroidal blood supply.

3. Cortical branches
   In general, the PICA supplies the ipsilateral half of the suboccipital surface of the cerebellum hemisphere and tonsil, the ipsilateral vermis, and the anterior aspect of the tonsil. The cortical branches can be divided into hemispheric, vermian, and tonsillar groups. The hemispheric branches (range 0–9, average 2.8) usually arise from the lateral trunk and supply the medial, the intermediate, and the lateral segments of the ipsilateral suboccipital surface. The vermian branches (range 0–3, average 1.3) commonly arise from the medial trunk and supply median and paramedian segments of the vermis. The tonsillar arteries usually arise from the lateral trunk as 0 to 5 (average 1.6) branches that supply the medial, posterior, inferior, and part of the anterior surface of the tonsil.

PREOPERATIVE EVALUATION

Preoperative evaluation includes standard preoperative labs, an electrocardiogram, a chest radiograph, and assessment of the patient's general health. In contrast to dissection of the superficial temporal artery, harvesting the OA requires considerable muscle dissection and may lead to postoperative hematomas particularly if patients are on aspirin. We therefore do not give patients aspirin preoperatively and prefer to stop aspirin 1 week prior to surgery in patients on aspirin therapy for vertebrobasilar insufficiency.

Digital subtraction cerebral angiography with three-dimensional reconstruction as well as selective external carotid artery injections is essential. Aneurysm size, morphology, dome-to-neck ratio, and relation to the surrounding arteries are evaluated. The caliber and course of the OA as well as the caliber and configuration of the PICA vessel and its tributaries should be carefully studied. The course, position, and proximity of the tonsillomedullary segments of both PICAs need assessment, in order to have a side-to-side PICA-PICA bypass as an alternate plan. In cases of vertebrobasilar insufficiency, the caliber of both VAs and the presence and caliber of the posterior communicating arteries must be evaluated and if necessary an Alcock's test should be performed (carotid compression during vertebral artery injection).

Physiological imaging modalities such as positron emission tomography, xenon computed tomography, single-photon emission computed tomography, computed tomography perfusion, and magnetic resonance perfusion commonly used to detect hemodynamic compromise in anterior circulation occlusive disease are less effective in assessing the posterior circulation as a result of their limited regional resolution.[16] Furthermore, the validity of these imaging modalities in detecting posterior circulation hypoperfusion remains uncertain. Phase-contrast quantitative magnetic resonance angiography (QMRA) has become available in recent years and is capable of directly measuring volumetric blood flow (milliliters per minute) through the major vessels of the posterior (as well as anterior) circulation. The technique is now implemented and enhanced in commercially available software called the NOVA (Noninvasive Optimal Vessel Analysis) system (VasSol, Inc., Chicago, IL). Table 9–1 shows the mean blood flow values and ranges for posterior circulation vessels in 50 healthy patients.[17] In a retrospective study of 47 patients with symptomatic vertebrobasilar disease, patients with >20% reduction of blood flow in the basilar artery (<120 cc/min) and PCAs (<40 cc/min) had a higher risk of stroke as compared to patients with preserved blood flow.[17] The VERiTAS (Vertebrobasilar Flow Evaluation and Risk of Transient Ischemic Attack and Stroke) is an ongoing prospective multicenter observational study funded by the National Institutes of Health and aimed at determining the utility of QMRA in assessing patients with symptomatic

vertebrobasilar occlusive disease of ≥50%. If predictive, QMRA evaluation could help identify high-risk patients who would benefit most from either surgical revascularization or endovascular angioplasty and stenting.

SURGICAL INDICATIONS

Indications for cerebral revascularization procedures can be divided into flow augmentation and flow replacement.

Flow Augmentation

In contrast to anterior circulation occlusive disease, the role of extracranial-intracranial bypass surgery for vertebrobasilar ischemia has been less studied. This is most likely related to the higher prevalence of anterior circulation occlusive disease as well as the availability of endovascular techniques for the treatment of vertebrobasilar stenosis, which are generally less technically demanding and carry a relatively lower morbidity than posterior circulation bypass surgery. Indications for bypass surgery include patients with symptomatic occlusive vertebrobasilar disease despite maximal medical therapy who are not amenable to endovascular angioplasty and stenting as a result of access difficulties or occlusion of both VAs. Clearly the symptoms must be hemodynamic in nature and not due to embolic phenomena.

Flow Replacement

Replacement bypasses are a valuable tool in the management of appropriately located tumors, as well as fusiform, complex, and giant aneurysms of the VA/PICA and PICA. Aneurysm-related factors such as atherosclerotic changes or calcification at the neck, a dome-to-neck ratio of >1.5, the presence of major branches arising from the neck or fundus, and fusiform or blister aneurysms may preclude reconstruction with surgical clipping or endovascular coiling or pose a greater risk than trapping with revascularization.

ANESTHETIC TECHNIQUE AND NEUROPROTECTION

The surgery is performed under general anesthesia. Hypotension must be avoided during the initial part of the procedure particularly in patients with marginal cerebral perfusion. Hyperventilation and alpha-adrenergic agents are not recommended because of their vasoconstrictive effects. We routinely use modest hypothermia (33°C) throughout the procedure as well as induced blood pressure elevation to 20% to 30% of baseline during the period of temporary PICA cross-clamping to augment

Table 9–1. THE MEAN VALUE AND RANGES OF BLOOD FLOW FOR POSTERIOR CIRCULATION VESSELS IN 50 HEALTHY VOLUNTEERS.		
Vessel	Mean Flow (cc/min)	Range* (cc/min)
BA	190	150–230
LPCA	72	50–94
RPCA	68	50–86
LVA	126	94–158
RVA	110	81–139

BA, indicates basilar artery; PCA, posterior cerebral artery; VA, vertebral artery; L, left; R, right.
*Mean ± standard deviation.

collateral flow. Electrophysiologic monitoring using somato-sensory and motor-evoked potentials and brainstem auditory-evoked potentials allows early detection of ischemia or excessive retraction and manipulation. Barbiturates have been used during bypass surgery to increase tolerance to cerebral hypoperfusion. The mechanisms of barbiturate neuroprotection are multifactorial and incompletely understood. It is believed that a reversible, dose-dependent depression of cerebral blood flow occurs, with subsequent reduction in cerebral metabolic rate and intracranial pressure.[18-21] Furthermore, vasoconstriction in normal areas of the brain may result in an inverse steal phenomenon with redistribution of cerebral blood flow to ischemic tissue.[22] At a cellular level, barbiturates have been demonstrated to reduce ischemia-induced glutamate release,[23] enhance GABA-ergic transmission,[24,25] and reduce ischemia-induced intracellular calcium through inhibition of both voltage-gated calcium channels and NMDA receptors.[26] In addition to the fore mentioned neuroprotective properties, barbiturates may also act as a scavenger of membrane-damaging free radicals. Despite these potential benefits, we do not routinely use barbiturate neuroprotection during OA-PICA bypass surgery due to problems associated with circulatory and respiratory depression as well as delayed postoperative wake-up. However, if technical difficulties during the anastomosis result in excessively prolonged temporary occlusion, we may consider using barbiturates.

SURGICAL TECHNIQUE

Figures 9–1 through 9–3 show preoperative imaging of a patient diagnosed with fusiform right VA-PICA origin large aneurysm.

The patient is either placed prone (more likely for a pure ischemia case), or more commonly in a three-quarter prone position (more likely for an aneurysm or tumor case) for a far lateral approach if access to the PICA origin is necessary. For the prone position, the head is placed in moderate flexion and secured in a three-pin head holder. Proper Mayfield pin placement is crucial, as it may hinder the procedure if placed improperly. The pins are placed so that the single pin is 2 cm superior and anterior to the pinna ipsilateral to the donor OA. The paired pins are positioned so that the posterior pin is 2 cm above the contralateral ear pinna. The head is positioned above the level of the heart to reduce cerebral venous congestion. In the three-quarter prone position, the head is positioned with four movements (Figure 9–4):

1. Flexion with slight distraction, in order to uncover the suboccipital region
2. Contralateral rotation, in order to bring the ipsilateral side uppermost
3. Contralateral bending, in order to gain surgical space between the ipsilateral shoulder and the suboccipital region
4. Upward translation, in order to partially and subtly sublux the ipsilateral atlanto-occipital joint and facilitate possible condylar drilling

A portable transcutaneous Doppler probe is used to identify the course of the OA over the scalp from the mastoid to approximately 4 cm above the superior nuchal line (Figure 9–5). Scalp infiltration solutions containing vasoconstrictive agents should not be used. A hockey-stick incision is then made. The incision starts approximately at the level of the spinous process of C3 and extends superiorly in the avascular midline plane to approximately 2 cm above the superior nuchal line. The incision is then turned laterally parallel to the superior nuchal line. As this limb of the incision approaches the point at which the distal OA crosses the incision, a curved hemostat is used to dissect over and protect the OA. The

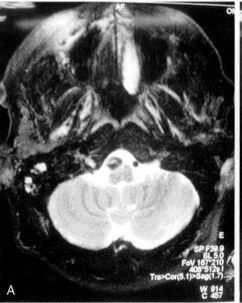
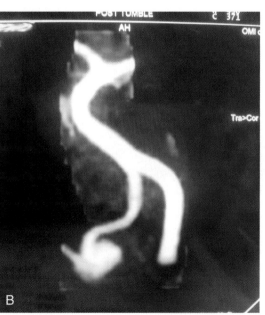

Figure 9–1. A 55-year-old man presents with headaches and right shoulder pain. A fusiform right VA-PICA origin large aneurysm is diagnosed. **A,** Magnetic resonance imaging (MRI) with T2 weighted axial sequence. **B,** Magnetic resonance angiography (MRA) with AP projection.

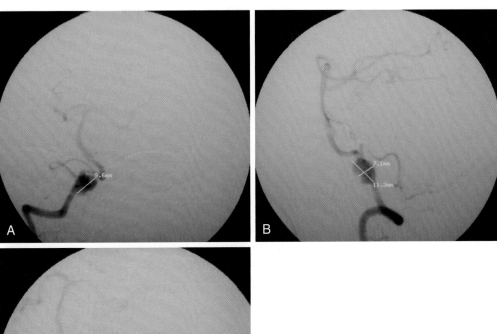

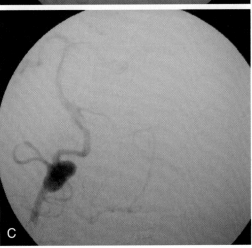

Figure 9–2. Digital subtraction angiography (DSA), right VA views. **A,** AP. **B,** Lateral. **C,** Obliques.

incision is then continued over the OA to a point immediately superior to the mastoid process. Finally, the incision is curved inferiorly to end just inferior to the mastoid tip. The distal OA is then identified and dissected proximally in its muscular plane. Although this may be performed under the operative microscope, in our opinion loupe magnification is sufficient and more efficient. Dissection of the OA is generally the most difficult part of the procedure due to the tortuosity and adherence of the artery to the surrounding tissue. The OA is typically surrounded by a venous plexus and runs with the occipital nerve in a fascial sheath. A generous cuff of periadventitial tissue is left around the artery. Small side branches are carefully coagulated using low current bipolar forceps, so as not to cause thermal injury to the parent artery. The side branches are then sectioned at a distance from their origin from the OA trunk. It is important to dissect the artery as far proximally as the occipital groove to ensure adequate length of the graft. The OA is wrapped in a papaverine-soaked cottonoid to relieve spasms related to vessel manipulation, and is left in continuity until just before it is required for the anastomosis (Figure 9–6). The suboccipital musculature is swept laterally in a subperiosteal fashion to expose the occiput as far laterally as the mastoid process as well as the arch of C1.

The skin and muscle flap are retracted inferolaterally and held in position by fish hooks. It is important to leave a muscle cuff attached to the superior nuchal line. This facilitates tight muscle closure at the end of the procedure, as a water-tight dural closure is not possible because of the necessity of creating an opening for passage of the OA.

An ipsilateral suboccipital craniotomy extending just across the midline and a C1 hemi-laminectomy are performed. The craniotomy may be extended to a far lateral transcondylar approach by exposure of the sigmoid sinus and resection of the posterior medial third of the occipital condyle if access to the PICA origin is required. Any opened mastoid air cells must be thoroughly sealed with bone wax to avoid postoperative cerebrospinal fluid leaks. The dura is opened in the midline at the level of C1 and extended in a curvilinear fashion to the superolateral extent of the exposure. An additional incision is made from the caudal end of the dural incision toward the C1/C2 joint, caudal to the vertebral artery ring. The dural flap is then sutured to the surrounding tissues with 4-0 neurolon traction sutures (Figure 9–7).

Under the operative microscope, the ipsilateral cerebellar tonsil is retracted superolaterally and the caudal loop of the PICA identified. We generally try to avoid using self-retaining

Figure 9–3. DSA, right ECA. **A,** AP. **B,** Lateral. Shows adequate right occipital artery. DSA, left VA views. **C,** AP. **D,** Lateral. Shows prominent left AICA-PICA variant.

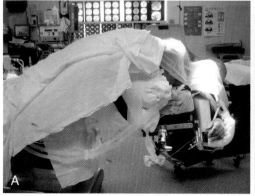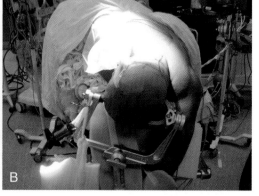

Figure 9–4. A, Surgical three-quarter prone position. Head follows four movements: flexion, contralateral rotation, contralateral bending, and subtle upward translocation. **B,** Occipital artery is traced and marked with a transcutaneous Doppler.

brain retractors, as they may actually hinder the surgical exposure. However, if retraction is necessary in spite of extensive arachnoidal lysis, then a tapered self-retaining retractor should be used on the tonsil. The caudal loop is carefully dissected by sharply dividing the arachnoidal bands anchoring the artery to the dorsal surface of the medulla. A rubber dam is then placed deep to the dissected caudal loop of the PICA. The rubber dam may be sutured to the surrounding dura or soft tissue superiorly or inferiorly to carefully elevate the caudal loop, provided that there are no perforating vessels tethering the

artery. A micromalleable self-suction device is placed in the vicinity of the anastomosis site to act as a constant drainage path for cerebrospinal fluid and blood.

The OA is then prepared for the anastomosis. A temporary clip is first applied to the proximal end of the artery, which is then cut distally at an appropriate length for the bypass. The occipital artery is notoriously tortuous and amenable to lengthening by "undoing" the various turns and loops. It is, however, critical to let the artery find its own natural contour after dissecting it, to avoid forcing an unnatural kink that

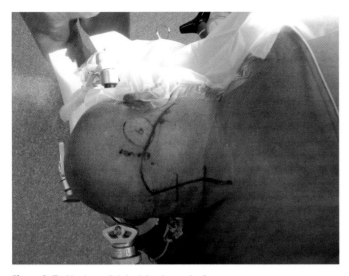

Figure 9–5. Hockey-stick incision is marked.

might result in graft occlusion. The mean length of OA required for a PICA bypass is 58 mm (range 54 to 60 mm).[6] The distal 1 cm of the artery is then stripped of its periadventitial layer. Although this step may be easier to perform while the OA is still in continuity, because of the benefit of countertraction, we prefer to first section the artery to the required length for the bypass to avoid having to repeat the periadventitial stripping if the artery proves too long. There

are several ways that the distal OA—or any donor vessel, for that matter—can be prepared, but the three most common techniques are depicted in Figure 9–8, and are as follows:

1. Straight 90-degree cut
2. Angled 45-degree cut
3. Straight 90-degree cut, with a single fishmouth on one side by a length "l" equal to half the circumference of the donor vessel (more easily thought of as the "flattened" diameter of the collapsed vessel)

The latter technique is our favored technique because it increases the cross-sectional area available for the anastomosis and provides redundancy of donor artery wall, thereby minimizing the possibility of stenosis at the site of anastomosis. We firmly believe that end-to-side anastomoses in general fare better if an "elephant foot design" is achieved, with the redundant edges of the donor allowing a flaring of the completed anastomosis and a reduced risk of stenosis or occlusion. Furthermore, the obliquity of the resulting construct allows flow to be preferentially directed toward the proximal PICA and its medullary branches. Using simple high school mathematics (Pythagorean theorem, circumference, and area formulas of circles), we can easily show in Figure 9–8 that the three different techniques result in three different anastomosis circumferences and areas at the suture line. As can be seen from the calculations, compared to the unmodified simple 90-degree, end-to-side technique (Technique 1), the 45-degree

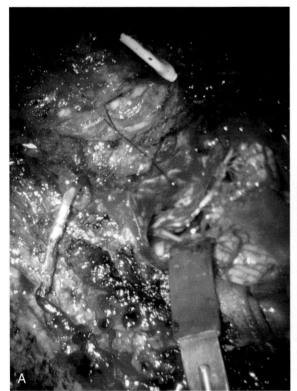

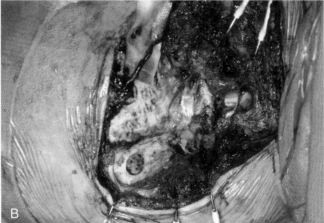

Figure 9–6. A, Myocutaneous flap is reflected inferolaterally. Occipital artery is dissected and kept in situ. **B,** In a different case, note the extradural VA visible in the sulcus arteriosus (V3).

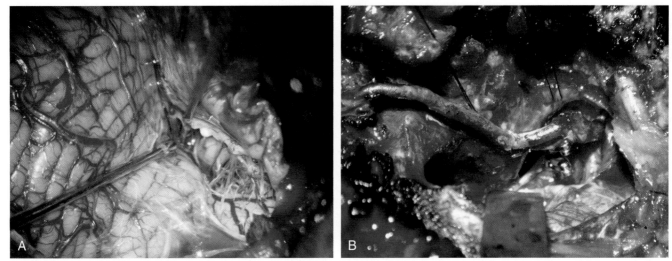

Figure 9–7. A, Intradural view of the aneurysm after dural flap reflection. Spinal accessory nerve clearly visible. **B,** View of the transposed occipital artery.

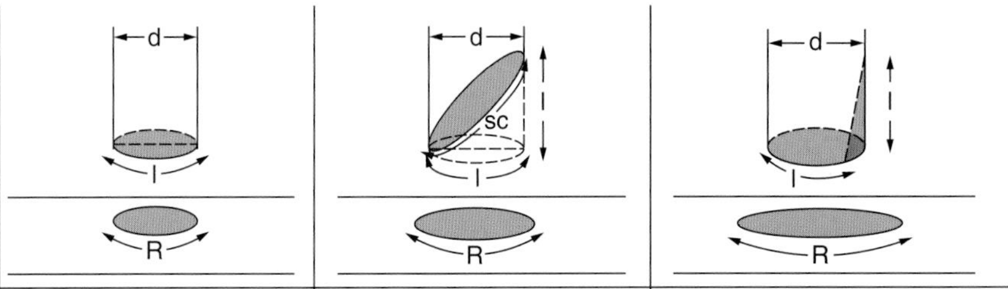

Technique	① End-to-Side, 90°	② End-to-Side, 45°	③ End-to-Side, Single fishmouth
C	$[\pi d]$	$[\pi d\sqrt{2}]$ $C = 2sc = 2(\sqrt{2l^2}) = 2l\sqrt{2}$ $= 2 \cdot \dfrac{\pi d}{2} \cdot \sqrt{2} = \pi d\sqrt{2}$	$[2\pi d]$ $C = 4l = 4\left(\dfrac{\pi d}{2}\right) = 2\pi d$
A (Shaded area)	$\left[\dfrac{\pi d^2}{4}\right]$	$[\pi d^2]$ $A = \dfrac{C^2}{4\pi} = \dfrac{(\pi d\sqrt{2})}{4\pi} = \dfrac{\pi d^2}{2}$	$\left[\dfrac{\pi d^2}{2}\right]$ $A = \dfrac{C^2}{4\pi} = \dfrac{(2\pi d)^2}{4\pi} = \pi d^2$
R	$\left[\dfrac{\pi d}{2}\right]$ $R = l = \dfrac{\pi d}{2} \approx 1.5d$	$\left[\dfrac{\pi\sqrt{2}}{2}d\right]$ $R \approx sc = l\sqrt{2} = \dfrac{\pi\sqrt{2}}{2}d \approx 2.2d$	$[\pi d]$ $R = 2l = \pi d \approx 3.1d$

Geometric effects of 3 types of End-to-Side Anastomoses on Anastomotic Circumference (C),
Cross-Sectional Area (A) and Recipient Arteriotomy Length (R)

Figure 9–8. Geometric effects of three types of end-to-side anastomoses on the following parameters: anastomotic circumference (C), anastomotic area (A), and recipient arteriotomy length (R).

cut (Technique 2) "doubles" the cross-sectional area at the suture line, but—better yet—the simple one-sided fishmouthing (Technique 3) "quadruples" it! This, of course, comes at the cost of lengthening the needed arteriotomy in the recipient vessel by a factor of 2 (Technique 3 versus Technique 1). Surgeons often wonder what the arteriotomy length in the recipient vessel needs to be, and Figure 9–8 shows clearly that, for Technique 3, it needs to be twice the "flattened" diameter of the donor, which is about three times its "true" diameter. In

summary, when focusing on the geometry of the anastomotic line, Technique 3, compared to Technique 1, results in four times the cross-sectional area and two times the circumference, at the cost of two times the recipient arteriotomy. These geometrical concepts have been clearly simplified and idealized for the purpose of approximation and illustration, and rely on the assumption that the sutured anastomosis will assume a close-to-circular configuration under flow conditions and that the vessel wall edges do not stretch significantly, both very reasonable assumptions. In addition, as a slight departure from Technique 3 as described, we often "round" (small tissue excision) very slightly the sharp corners of the 90-degree fishmouth angles to facilitate running the suture.

Regarding the arteriotomy performed on the side of the recipient artery, we prefer "incising" a straight cut, as opposed to other surgeons who actually "excise" an elliptical segment of vessel wall. Our preference is again based on the desire to maximize the circumference and orthogonal cross-sectional area of the recipient artery at the level of the anastomosis. Without getting into the mathematical details, the excision of an ellipse of tissue measuring "x" millimeters at its widest point will result in a corresponding decrease in the available recipient circumference by "x" millimeters, even though the final circumference—postanastomosis—will be augmented by the amount of the actual donor diameter "d." For a donor artery of 2 mm in diameter, a recipient artery of 2 mm in diameter, and an excision of x = 1 mm, the "excision" technique, compared to the "incision" technique, results in a relative loss of circumference and area of 25%.

We routinely make detailed intraoperative measurements of blood flow in the donor and recipient arteries during bypass surgeries, using a microvascular ultrasonic flow probe (Charbel Micro-Flow Probe, Transonic Systems, Inc.). The "cut flow," or the maximal flow carrying capacity of the donor vessel in the absence of downstream resistance, is first measured. The baseline flow in the recipient artery is also measured and gives an indication of the amount of flow that is desirable to replace or augment. Once the anastomosis has been completed, flow through the OA is measured and is known as the "bypass flow" (Figure 9–9). This measurement represents flow through the bypass and provides immediate verification of bypass patency. The ratio of the bypass flow measurement to the initial cut-flow measurement is known as the "cut-flow index" (CFI). Values greater than 0.5 have been found to be a sensitive predictor for acute and long-term postoperative bypass patency, at least in STA-MCA bypasses, primarily done for flow augmentation in ischemic cases.[27]

Going back to the technical details of the anastomosis, a temporary aneurysm clip is placed on the proximal OA, and its lumen cannulated with a blunt needle and flushed with heparinized saline to remove any blood and debris. Miniature slim-tapered temporary clips are placed on either side of the PICA segment selected for the anastomosis, generally at the telovelotonsillar segment. The patient's blood pressure is raised by 20% to 30% above baseline during the period of temporary occlusion. An arteriotomy is initially made in the PICA using a beaver blade and subsequently extended using the most delicate and sharpened microscissors. A dull instrument will destroy the delicate vessel wall. A useful alternate technique is to puncture the recipient artery first with a 27-gauge needle—with its tip bent slightly—that is attached to an arterial transducer line, with the double benefit of providing a puncture hole for the beaver blade tip to initiate the arteriotomy, as well as providing a potentially useful measurement of intraluminal recipient artery pressure (particularly in ischemia cases). Heparinized saline is used to irrigate the PICA lumen throughout the course of the suturing, and is delivered through a syringe tipped with a 27-gauge angiocatheter.

The anastomosis may be performed in several ways. We prefer to first anchor the "heel" (the apex of the fishmouth) of the distal end of the OA to one apex of the recipient arteriotomy. On the other hand, some surgeons prefer to first anchor the "toe" (the non-fishmouthed corner) of the distal end of the OA. This latter technique allows the surgeon to extend the fishmouthed corner of the donor vessel if, during suturing, it is realized that the recipient vessel arteriotomy has been made too long and that the fishmouth needs to be extended. An alternative method is to anchor both the heel and toe ends of the distal end of the OA. This latter method is useful, as it prevents errors during suturing related to unequal distances between suture throws, and is probably easier for the "novice" bypass surgeon. Despite this advantage, we prefer not to anchor both ends simultaneously, as this decreases the space available between the donor and recipient vessel walls, and therefore makes visualization of the individual vessel walls while running the suture more difficult.

The anastomosis may be carried out using interrupted stitches or a continuous suture. Although interrupted stitches have a theoretical advantage of allowing future enlargement and maturation of the bypass, we do not believe this to be a real concern unless the vessels are particularly small (<0.8 mm), and we thus generally favor the running suture for its expediency. Furthermore, we suture the back and front wall of the anastomosis separately and thereby allow some enlargement of the bypass over time, if needed. Third, since we utilize Technique 3 in most cases, we believe we are already providing a four-fold increase in cross-sectional area (see Figure 9–8),

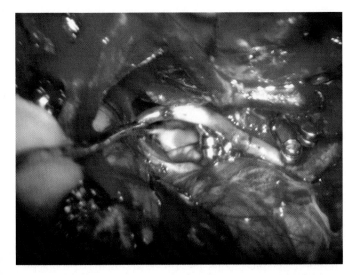

Figure 9–9. Magnified view of the end-to-end anastomosis of OA-PICA and clip trapping of the VA and aneurysm. The final measured intraoperative flow of the patent bypass was 12 cc/min, comparing favorably with a baseline flow of 16 cc/min in the native PICA and initial OA cut flow of 6 cc/min (probably an underestimate of the theoretical maximum available flow, due to dissection-related arterial spasm of the OA).

negating any concerns about stenotic complications. The initial anchoring suture is passed through the wall of the donor OA at the "heel," from outside the lumen to inside the lumen of the donor (colloquially called the "out-in" stitch), and then the needle is passed through the wall of the recipient PICA at the apex from inside the lumen to outside the lumen (colloquially called the "in-out" stitch) so that the knot ends up lying outside the lumen, naturally. The anastomosis proceeds by first suturing the more difficult (i.e., less accessible) back wall. Care must be taken to avoid grasping the luminal surface of the vessel wall with either the forceps or the needle holder, regardless of the delicacy of the instruments, as the intima may be injured. The forceps should be used to gently anchor the artery as the needle is passed through its wall. The sharp tip of the needle itself is a very useful "hook" that should be used to precisely manipulate, position, and pierce wall edges. The suture is kept loose between stitches, like the spiral binding of a book, until the entire back wall of the anastomosis has been sutured. There is a happy medium for how loose the loops should be: too loose, and they overlap on each other and interfere with each other and the passing of the next bite; too tight, and they are too close to the vessel wall and become harder to grasp later for the tightening phase. At the end of the run, the loops should ideally be equally spaced and lying parallel to each other, without interweaving. The suture is then tightened one loop at a time using two forceps starting from the initial anchoring suture. One forceps tightens the suture while the other handles the next loop, in a sequential manner, ensuring that steady tension is maintained constantly on the previously tightened suture. These forceps have to be relatively new or at least well maintained and preferably diamond-dusted, in order to provide a generous grasping surface area with less risk of slippage or of weakening the suture. The final loop is then tied to itself. Once the back wall has been sutured, the OA is rotated to expose the front wall. A new anchoring suture is placed and the front wall is then sutured in a similar manner. The lumen of the PICA is filled with heparinized saline prior to completion of the final stitch. The anastomosis is carried out using a 10-0 monofilament suture. We prefer a BV 75-3 (Ethicon, Johnson & Johnson, Somerville, NJ) tapered point needle. The needle forms three-eighths of a circle, and therefore minimizes the degree of wrist rotation required during suturing as compared to needles forming one-half of a circle. We do not use a silicon splint in the recipient, as some surgeons do.

Blood flow is restored after completion of the anastomosis by first removing the temporary clips off the recipient artery and re-measuring the recipient flow, prior to unclamping the donor OA. An intraluminal thrombus or stitch-occlusion would be detectable now. Only after this is ruled out and after adequate native recipient flow is re-established, do we then unclip the OA. Slight oozing along the suture line usually stops with a single layer of surgicel (Johnson & Johnson) and gentle pressure with a cottonoid applied over the arteriotomy. Occasionally it may be necessary to place an additional interrupted suture at a specific point if the bleeding does not abate with light pressure. A final assessment of vessel patency is made with the quantitative flow probe. Intraoperative angiography, but more likely and easily, indocyanine green (ICG) videoangiography may also be used.

Following completion of the bypass, any associated VA–PICA or PICA aneurysms should be ideally trapped in the same setting. Alternatively, if there are important perforators arising from the body of the aneurysm, or if access to one end of the aneurysm is not possible surgically or endovascularly, then proximal or distal occlusion may be considered.

The self-suction device and rubber dam are removed. The dura is then closed with or without a dural graft. As previously mentioned, a water-tight dural closure is not possible because of the necessity of creating an opening for passage of the OA. A sheet of DuraGen (Integra Life Sciences, Plainsboro, NJ) may be placed over the dural opening and reinforced with a tissue sealant. A small opening is made in the bone flap to allow an uncompromised passage of the occipital artery. The bone flap is then replaced and fixed with miniplates and screws. The wound is copiously irrigated with antibiotic solution. The muscle is reapproximated to the muscle cuff along the superior nuchal line. A multilayer meticulous closure of the muscle and fascia is crucial to avoid cerebrospinal fluid leaks and may be facilitated by taking the patient partially out of the flexed neck position. The skin is closed in two layers using 2-0 inverted vicryl stitches followed by a 3-0 running locking prolene suture. Sutures are left in place for 2 weeks. The patient is given an aspirin (300 mg) suppository in the operating room prior to extubation, and oral 325 mg daily. Aspirin is continued postoperatively indefinitely.

POSTOPERATIVE CARE

Patients are monitored in an intensive care unit for 1 to 2 days (Figure 9–10). Neurological examinations and assessment of bypass graft patency with bedside Doppler are performed every hour. Patients are kept normotensive. Postoperative hypertension should be avoided particularly in patients with vertebrobasilar ischemia, as it may predispose to parenchymal hemorrhage or cerebral edema. Computed tomography angiography (CTA) or preferably a digital subtraction angiography (DSA) is routinely performed 1 to 2 days after surgery. Patients are generally placed on daily aspirin (325 mg) for life.

Complications and Their Avoidance

In addition to general postoperative complications such as wound, urinary, and respiratory infections; deep venous thrombosis; and pulmonary embolism, there are inherent risks to OA-PICA bypass surgery.

Wound healing problems secondary to scalp ischemia from OA diversion can be prevented by performing a wide-based flap sparing the posterior auricular artery. Furthermore, meticulous wound closure and avoidance of skin strangulation

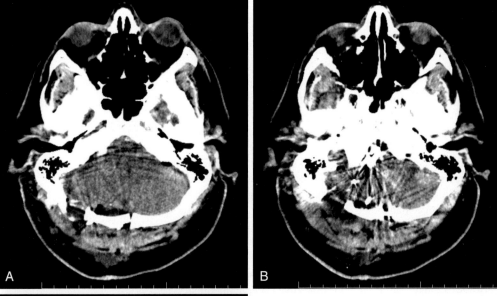

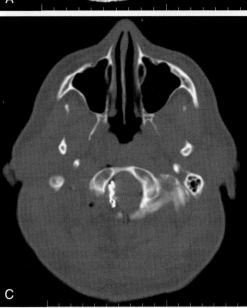

Figure 9–10. A and **B,** Computerized tomography (CT) scanning on postop day 1. **C,** The craniotomy reaches the midline, the trapping clips are visible, and there is evidence of partial condylar drilling.

by the suture can prevent such problems. Wound bed, subdural, and epidural hematomas may result from leakage at the anastomosis or from muscle ooze related to dissection of the OA. Such complications can be minimized by careful surgical technique and hemostasis at all stages of the procedure. As mentioned above, water-tight dural closure is not possible and thus patients are prone to developing cerebrospinal fluid leaks and pseudomeningoceles. This can be prevented by thoroughly waxing any open mastoid air cells and by performing a careful multilayer closure of the muscles and fascia.

Complications related to the OA include damage during dissection, thrombosis with subsequent emboli formation or occlusion, overstretching, and kinking. Injury during dissection can be prevented by careful preoperative assessment of the course and tortuosity of the OA and meticulous surgical technique, including avoidance of thermal injury during coagulation of side branches. Overstretching or kinking of the

artery can be prevented by dissecting the artery proximally to its exit from the occipital groove of the mastoid to ensure that there is adequate length to reach the anastomotic site. Damage or compromise of the OA during closure can be avoided by creating an adequate opening in the bone flap for unhindered passage of the OA as well as careful muscle closure to avoid inadvertent stitching of the artery.

The vertebral artery is at risk for injury during the exposure, and this may be prevented by careful sharp muscle dissection, stripping of the cervical musculature in a subperiosteal fashion, and avoiding the use of Bovie coagulation in the vicinity of the artery near the sulcus arteriosus at C1. In the event of inadvertent vertebral artery injury, it is much easier to repair a sharply made arteriotomy than that produced by a thermal injury. Preoperative knowledge of the anatomy and caliber of the contralateral vertebral artery is also helpful in guiding decisions regarding whether to repair or sacrifice the injured artery. The PICA is also vulnerable to injury at several stages of the procedure. Injuries may occur during the exposure, particularly if the PICA originates extradurally, as it may be mistaken for a muscular branch or for the posterior meningeal artery. The PICA and its perforators can also be injured or occluded intradurally during aneurysm dissection or clipping.

Inadvertent injury to the lower cranial nerves is a major cause of morbidity. Injuries usually result from manipulating the nerve rootlets during dissection and clipping of the aneurysm or inadvertent/deliberate inclusion of nerve rootlets in the clip. These cranial nerves are very sensitive to manipulation, necessitating very gentle retraction and sharp dissection. Lower cranial nerve injury may result in dysphagia, dysarthria, dysphonia, and inadequate airway protection; thus patients should be extubated and started on an oral diet only after a formal evaluation of lower cranial nerve function has been performed. Brainstem injury may result from either excessive retraction or vascular injury. Compromise of the PICA or its perforators may result in postoperative lateral medullary (Wallenberg) syndrome.

Failure of the bypass is usually the result of technical errors or poor patient selection. Technical mistakes may occur during vessel preparation and suturing of the anastomosis and can be minimized by meticulous surgical technique and intraoperative detection using ICG video-angiography and microvascular ultrasonic flow probe measurements. Poor patient selection in ischemic cases as a result of underestimation of collateral circulation will frequently lead to bypass failure due to an insufficient demand for the additional blood flow.

COMMON ALTERNATIVES TO OA-PICA IN POSTERIOR FOSSA REVASCULARIZATION

The following alternatives to OA-PICA bypass are performed by using a variety of donor and recipient vessels:

1. PICA-PICA (in situ bypass): This is the most likely alternative to the OA-PICA bypass and may be performed side-to-side or end-to-side. The similarity in vessel caliber, the ease of dissection, and the proximity of the telovelotonsillar segments of the two PICAs make this bypass appealing. Indications include flow augmentation in cases of hypoperfusion in the PICA or lower basilar artery territories, or flow replacement in the management of fusiform PICA aneurysms that require trapping or parent vessel occlusion. Pitfalls include the necessity to place both distal PICA territories at ischemic risk and the difficulty encountered by some in performing a side-to-side anastomosis, particularly the back wall part (see Chapter 10).

2. OA–AICA bypass: May be used in the treatment of complex AICA aneurysms or midbasilar ischemia, or in the rare instances of unavailability of posterior cerebral artery (PCA), superior cerebral artery (SCA), or PICA recipients.

3. Superficial temporal artery to posterior cerebral artery (STA-PCA) or superficial temporal artery to superior cerebellar artery (STA-SCA) bypasses: These may be used to augment flow in cases of ischemia of the top of the basilar artery territory, or in the staged treatment of complex basilar aneurysms.

4. Reimplantation of PICA origin into the VA: This is specifically applicable to fusiform aneurysms encompassing the PICA origin, when there is enough PICA redundancy to reimplant its origin in the VA.

5. PICA-PICA end-to-end anastomosis: This is applicable to nonclippable aneurysms of the PICA where there is enough redundancy in the PICA to effect aneurysm excision and reapproximation of the vessel ends.

CONCLUSION

The OA-PICA bypass is a very useful tool in the armamentarium of the bypass surgeon. It is, however, rarely the first choice for a revascularization strategy in the posterior fossa because of the tedious dissection needed for the OA, and the appeal of the more user-friendly PICA-PICA side-to-side bypass in experienced hands. When the latter is simply not doable or desirable, the OA-PICA bypass may well be the only alternative and needs to be mastered.

REFERENCES

1. Yaşargil MG: Anastomosis between Superficial Temporal Artery and a Branch of the Middle Cerebral Artery, Stuttgart, 1969, Georg Thieme Verlag.
2. Ausman JI, Lee MC, Klassen AC, et al: Stroke: what's new? Cerebral revascularization, Minn Med 59(4):223–227, 1976.
3. Alvernia JE, Fraser K, Lanzino G: The occipital artery: a microanatomical study, Neurosurgery 58(Suppl 1):ONS114–ONS122, 2006.
4. Rhoton AL Jr: The far-lateral approach and its transcondylar, supracondylar, and paracondylar extensions, Neurosurgery 47(Suppl 3):S195–S209, 2000.
5. Kawashima M, Rhoton AL Jr, Tanriover N, et al: Microsurgical anatomy of cerebral revascularization. Part II: posterior circulation, J Neurosurg 102(1):132–147, 2005.
6. Ateş O, Ahmed AS, Niemann D, et al: The occipital artery for posterior circulation bypass: microsurgical anatomy, Neurosurg Focus 24(2):E9, 2008.
7. Lister JR, Rhoton AL Jr, Matsushima T, et al: Microsurgical anatomy of the posterior inferior cerebellar artery, Neurosurgery 10(2):170–199, 1982.
8. Lesley WS, Rajab MH, Case RS: Double origin of the posterior inferior cerebellar artery: association with intracranial aneurysm on catheter angiography, AJR Am J Roentgenol 189(4):893–897, 2007.
9. Fine AD, Cardoso A, Rhoton AL Jr: Microsurgical anatomy of the extracranial-extradural origin of the posterior inferior cerebellar artery, J Neurosurg 91:645–652, 1999.
10. Ahuja A, Graves VB, Crosby DL, et al: Anomalous origin of the posterior inferior cerebellar artery from the internal carotid artery, AJNR Am J Neuroradiol 13:1625–1626, 1992.
11. Lasjaunias P, Vallee B, Person H, et al: The lateral spinal artery of the upper cervical spinal cord. Anatomy, normal variations, and angiographic aspects, J Neurosurg 63:235–241, 1985.

12. Manabe H, Oda N, Ishii M, et al: The posterior inferior cerebellar artery originating from the internal carotid artery, associated with multiple aneurysms, *Neuroradiology* 33:513–515, 1991.

13. Margolis MT, Newton TH: The posterior inferior cerebellar artery. In Newton TH, Potts DG, editors: *Radiology of the Skull and Brain*, vol. 2, bk. 2. St. Louis, 1974, Mosby, pp 1719–1775.

14. Ogawa T, Fujita H, Inugami A, et al: Anomalous origin of the posterior inferior cerebellar artery from the posterior meningeal artery, *AJNR Am J Neuroradiol* 12:186, 1991.

15. Tanaka A, Kimura M, Yoshinaga S, et al: Extracranial aneurysm of the posterior inferior cerebellar artery: case report, *Neurosurgery* 33:742–744, 1993.

16. Haase J, Magnussen IB, Ogilvy CS, et al: Evaluating patients with vertebrobasilar transient ischemic attacks, *Surg Neurol* 52(4):386–392, 1999.

17. Amin-Hanjani S, Du X, Zhao M, et al: Use of quantitative magnetic resonance angiography to stratify stroke risk in symptomatic vertebrobasilar disease, *Stroke* 36(6):1140–1145, 2005.

18. Howe JR, Kindt GW: Cerebral protection during carotid endarterectomy, *Stroke* 5:340–343, 1974.

19. Michenfelder JD, Milde JH, Sundt TM Jr: Cerebral protection by barbiturate anesthesia. Use after middle cerebral artery occlusion in Java monkeys, *Arch Neurol* 33:345–350, 1976.

20. Gross CE, Adams HP Jr, Sokoll MD, et al: Use of anticoagulants, electroencephalographic monitoring, and barbiturate cerebral protection in carotid endarterectomy, *Neurosurgery* 9:1–5, 1981.

21. Imparato AM, Ramirez A, Riles T, et al: Cerebral protection in carotid surgery, *Arch Surg* 117:1073–1078, 1982.

22. Feustel PJ, Ingvar MC, Severinghaus JW: Cerebral oxygen availability and blood flow during middle cerebral artery occlusion: effects of pentobarbital, *Stroke* 12:858–863, 1981.

23. Amakawa K, Adachi N, Liu K, et al: Effects of pre- and postischemic administration of thiopental on transmitter amino acid release and histologic outcome in gerbils, *Anesthesiology* 85:1422–1430, 1996.

24. Buggy DJ, Nicol B, Rowbotham DJ, et al: Effects of intravenous anesthetic agents on glutamate release: a role for GABAA receptor-mediated inhibition, *Anesthesiology* 92:1067–1073, 2000.

25. Bieda MC, MacIver MB: Major role for tonic GABAA conductances in anesthetic suppression of intrinsic neuronal excitability, *J Neurophysiol* 92:1658–1667, 2004.

26. Zhan RZ, Fujiwara N, Endoh H, et al: Thiopentone inhibits increases in [Ca^{2+}] induced by membrane depolarization, NMDA receptor activation and ischemia in rat hippocampal and cortical slices, *Anesthesiology* 89:456–466, 1998.

27. Ashley WW, Amin-Hanjani S, Alaraj A, et al: Flow-assisted surgical cerebral revascularization, *Neurosurg Focus* 24(2):E20, 2008.

THE STATE OF THE ART IN CEREBROVASCULAR BYPASSES: SIDE-TO-SIDE IN SITU PICA-PICA BYPASS

MIIKKA KORJA; LEENA KIVIPELTO; JUHA HERNESNIEMI; CHANDRANATH SEN; DAVID J. LANGER

INTRODUCTION

Intracranial bypasses are believed to be high-risk operations with poorly studied outcome measures, and they are often considered as the last and final option in the treatment of neurosurgically demanding vascular and oncological lesions. In situ bypasses, such as middle cerebral artery (MCA) to MCA and anterior cerebral artery (ACA) to ACA bypasses, differ from conventional graft-utilizing bypasses in many aspects. For example, in situ bypasses are always occlusive bypasses, contrary to nonocclusive bypasses like ELANA bypasses,[1-3] have only one anastomotic site between two intracranial vessels, and do not utilize extracranial or harvested vessel grafts. Poor collateral network limits the use of in situ bypasses to some extent in anterior circulation and in large proximal vessels, whereas distal segments of the posterior inferior cerebellar artery (PICA) are able to tolerate temporary occlusion for indefinite periods permitting the safe creation of bypasses proximal to their vascular territory. Therefore, a side-to-side in situ PICA-PICA bypass operation can be considered a relatively safe and elegant adjunct to the treatment repertoire of, for example, complex vertebral artery (VA)-PICA vascular lesions, when other treatment options could compromise the blood flow through the anterior medullary segment of the PICA vessel.

Only a few dozen side-to-side in situ PICA-PICA bypass cases have been reported to date.[4-12] The first report of the side-to-side in situ PICA-PICA bypass was published by Takikawa and others in 1991 describing a 42-year-old man with a ruptured right VA-PICA aneurysm treated with a combination of microsurgical aneurysm trapping and the side-to-side in situ PICA-PICA bypass.[12] Due to the lack of technical reports, we will describe this modern bypass technique in the following sections in detail.

PROCEDURE

Preoperative Evaluation

A clear understanding and visualization of the PICA anatomy is of utmost importance. The PICA is a rather complex, tortuous, and variable artery,[13] which originates from the intracranial portion of the VA in 80% to 95% of cases (on average 8.6 mm above the foramen magnum and approximately 1 cm proximal to the vertebrobasilar junction).[13,14] The gold standard for visualizing the PICAs is a vertebrobasilar angiography for both vertebral arteries; 1.5-T MRA images and CT angiographies can often provide supplementary information for in situ PICA-PICA bypass planning. It is of essence to understand PICA-related anatomical structures, as it will help to clarify the approach for the revascularization procedure.

Decision Process

Although collateral networks in posterior fossa are robust for hemispheric perfusion, sacrifice of the proximal PICA segment can result in catastrophic ischemic injury. This proximal PICA segment maintains the origin of relatively small but extremely critical perforators feeding the medulla oblongata and cerebellum.[13] To evaluate the need of the PICA revascularization, the PICA should be divided into five segments and two loops as suggested previously[13,15] (Figure 10–1):

1. Anterior medullary segment (extends posteriorly from the origin of the PICA to the inferior olivary prominence and passes near the hypoglossal rootlets)

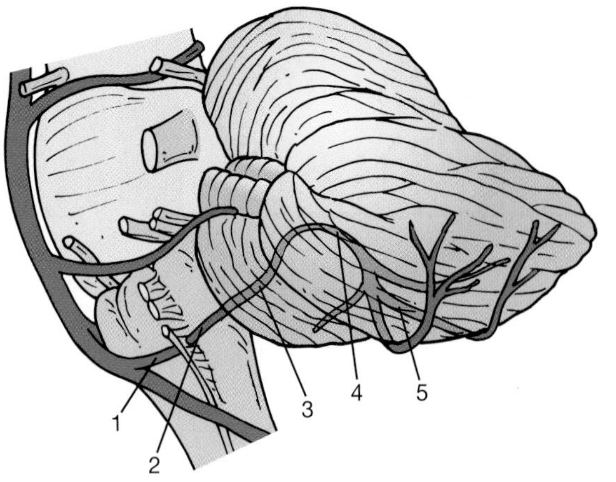

Figure 10–1. The PICA segments illustrated.
(Figure redrawn from Ramina R, et al., Distal posterior inferior cerebellar artery aneurysm: case report. Arq Neuro-psiquiatr 2005;63 (2a): 335–338, Fig. 1.)

2. Lateral medullary segment (begins at the site where the PICA passes the most prominent point of the inferior olive and ends at the origins of the 9th, 10th, and 11th cranial nerves)

3. Tonsillomedullary segment (begins at the point where the PICA passes posterior to the 9th, 10th, and 11th cranial nerves, and then extends medially across the posterior aspect of the medulla to the level of the tonsillar midportion, before which the PICA forms a so-called caudal loop at the caudal pole of the tonsils)

4. Telovelotonsillar segment (begins at the middle section of the PICA's ascent along the medial surface of the tonsils and extends to the suboccipital cortical surface of the cerebellum and includes the so-called cranial loop)

5. Cortical segment (extends to the cerebellar vermis and hemisphere)

A PICA revascularization procedure should be considered for lesions locating proximal to the telovelotonsillar segment, especially if the treatment of the lesion itself may occlude patent PICA circulation. However, the absence of perforating arteries along the very proximal portion of the anterior medullary segment permits direct clip or coil occlusion of the PICA at its very origin. Since there are no reliable PICA test occlusions, we have to rely on the anatomy-based planning of bypass surgery. In brief, the most important point in treating VA-PICA lesions is to preserve the critical perforating branches of the proximal PICA.

We next evaluate the proximity of the left and right PICAs. The distance between parallel PICAs should be less than 4 to 5 mm, if possible, which allows PICA mobilization and the side-to-side anastomosis without excessive manipulation of the vessels and their perforators. Parallel tonsillomedullary and telovelotonsillar segments may have a significant difference in diameter (ratio up to 1:2) without causing technical

problems. The suturing of the anastomosis is performed in the cistern below the cerebellar tonsils, a region that is relatively shallow and wide, making the procedure less technically challenging than those in deeper narrow corridors of the anterior or posterior circulation. We believe that neurosurgeons who are familiar with conventional cerebrovascular bypass procedures should be able to master suturing side-to-side, in situ PICA-PICA anastomoses.

Operative Technique

Patients are put on aspirin 325 g/day at 5 days before the operation, and they continue the medication indefinitely. Aspirin sensitivity is assessed with the Accumetrix system. No fractioned or unfractioned intravenous heparin is used during the operation.

Craniotomy

The neurophysiological monitoring of brainstem auditory evoked potentials (BAEPs) as well as cortical and spinal somatosensory evoked potentials (SEPs) is applied and the patient is placed in a prone position in a Sugita head frame. The midline suboccipital and upper cervical regions are scrubbed and draped, and a midline incision cranially to the nuchal line and caudally to the C1 arch is done. Self-retaining retractors are placed in the wound and a burr hole is fashioned in the midline suboccipital region. An oval-shaped or round midline suboccipital craniotomy from foramen magnum to below transverse sinuses is performed, and the dura is opened in a V- or Y-shaped fashion. It is not necessary to visualize the transverse sinuses and the craniotomy can be kept well below them. Usually, good exposure of the tonsillar region of the cerebellum is obtained.

Vessel exposure

The right and/or left cerebellar tonsil is gently retracted with the help of self-retaining retractors. Depending on the exact location of the PICA branches, less or more retraction is required. The tonsillomedullary and telovelotonsillar segments of the PICAs are well visualized at the level of the cerebellomedullary fissure. A number of brainstem perforators at the tonsillomedullary and telovelotonsillar segments may be seen, and these have to be preserved throughout the operation. Following gentle mobilization with microdissection of one or both of the vessel segments and separation of the vessels from pia/arachnoid attachments, they are brought easily to close proximity. PICA flows are then checked using the Transonic Charbel flow probe. Small temporary clips (blade length of 6 mm) are placed cranially and caudally to the anastomosis site as well as on perforating vessels originating from the same PICA segment. Blood pressure is increased during temporary clipping if changes in SEPs or in the EEG are observed, but this is a very uncommon event.

Arteriotomy and suturing

Using, for example, a back-cutting microknife, arteriotomies of approximately 4 to 6 mm (at least double the diameter of the wider PICA) of length are made on the facing surfaces of both PICAs. The lumens of the two vessels are aggressively irrigated with heparinized saline. By using a 9-0 nylon suture, a running anastomosis is made. After approximating the two arteries the first (stay) suture is placed at the apex of the arteriotomy by passing the needle from outside the vessel lumen to inside the same vessel lumen, and then from inside the other vessel lumen to outside the same vessel lumen (Figure 10–2A). The tail of the first suture is left long enough in order to use it when tightening the final suture. After making the stay suture, the needle is taken underneath the knot into the space between the two vessels (Figure 10–2B). A running suture is begun by passing the needle very close to the apical stay suture from outside to inside the vessel lumen, and then from inside to outside the other vessel lumen (Figure 10–2C). After this most crucial step of the anastomosis (Figure 10–2C), the back wall of the bypass can be sutured in a running fashion from the intravascular side (Figure 10–2D). When the other apex of the anastomosis is reached, the needle is passed from inside to outside the apex, and then from outside to inside of the adjacent apex (Figure 10–2D). Then, the anterior wall is sutured from outside the lumen using a continuous suture. (Figure 10–2E). Once the sutures are loosely placed

attaching the entire anterior wall, the bypass lumen is inspected using a small nerve hook, and flushed with heparinized saline. If the anastomosis is widely patent, the continuous suture can be tightened utilizing the long end of the very first suture or single interrupted sutures may be used for the final one to two stitches (Figure 10–2F).

Recirculation

Temporary clips are first removed distal to the bypass, then proximal to the bypass and finally from the perforators. Upon recirculation, bilateral flow volumes and directions are measured proximal and distal to the bypass and compared to the preoperative flows. Flows in the range of 8 to 12 ml/min are usually measured in both PICAs proximal and distal to the site of the anastomosis. Flow measurements can be repeated before and after an intraoperative indocyanine green (ICG) angiogram, which confirms the patency of the bypass. Flow measurements distal to the bypass can be done following a test occlusion of the proximal PICA. Minimal if any flow decrease in the occluded limb is expected if the bypass is functioning well, and the PICA origin can be sacrificed. The newly made anastomosis then allows the contralateral PICA to supply the anteromedullary segment of the proximally occluded PICA in a retrograde fashion. Should an early bypass occlusion occur, the sutures are opened, the

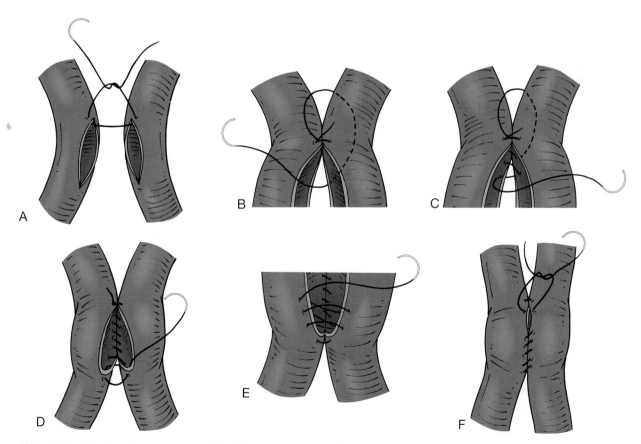

Figure 10–2. A-F, The side-to-side in situ PICA-PICA bypass procedure illustrated in detail.

lumens flushed with heparinized saline, and the anastomosis re-sutured.

Closure

A watertight dura closure is of great importance. A dural patch can be used together with tissue sealants. If any doubt of the water tightness of the dura exists, we recommend using a postoperative lumbar drain for a minimum of 2 to 3 days to avoid postoperative CSF leakage problems, which always lengthens the postoperative recovery time. The bone flap is replaced and secured with titanium microplates, a titanium mesh, or some other implant system. The wound is closed using 0-0 absorbable Vicryl sutures for the deep muscle and muscle fascia, 2-0 absorbable Vicryl sutures for the subcutaneous tissue, and an interrupted or continuous 3-0 Ethilon sutures for the skin closure.

Postoperative course

Patients undergo a CT examination and interventional angiography, if needed, on the first postoperative day. At this time, an interventional radiologist can use intravenous heparinization without a significant risk of postoperative bleeding complications. For 3 to 6 months after interventional procedures, patients usually go through first control angiographies.

DISCUSSION

We believe that PICA-PICA in situ revascularization is an essentially better option than occipital artery (OA)-PICA bypass for the following reasons:

1. It saves the neurosurgeon from tedious dissection of extracranial donor vessels.

2. Due to the midline suboccipital approach, the anastomosis procedure itself is relatively straightforward to perform.

3. The close proximity of bypass vessels eliminates problems with long bypasses and therefore diminishes the likelihood of bypass occlusion.

4. The caliber of the donor and recipient vessels matches most of the time.

5. Only one anastomotic site is necessary. Furthermore, the longitudinal (no end-to-side–like angles) bypass segment with a bypass ostium a few times larger than the vessel diameter may augment bypass patency in side-to-side in situ PICA-PICA bypasses. On a few occasions, we have used a multidisciplinary approach combining the side-to-side in situ PICA-PICA bypass and endovascular techniques in the treatment of VA-PICA lesions. Revascularization of the PICA using the multidisciplinary approach appears to be of low risk, because the risk of direct surgery of the aneurysm consists of the close proximity of the pathology to cranial nerves and to the lateral medulla. With a bypass in

place, interventional treatment of the target lesion becomes more straightforward with real-time assessment of bypass flow. This gives the interventionalist a safety margin when occluding the aneurysm. Time and invasiveness of surgery are thus reduced, and sparing the neurosurgeon from extensive surgical approaches to VA-PICA lesions eliminates a significant portion of morbidity.[16] Moreover, making a PICA-PICA bypass with the patient in a lateral position, which is often needed for direct surgical clipping of VA-PICA aneurysms, is technically more difficult. The multidisciplinary approach may allow more aggressive and safer interventional treatments and seems to be beneficial from various standpoints.

Some patients may tolerate PICA sacrifice at its very origin due to compensating retrograde collateral supply, which can reach to the anterior medullary segment of the PICA. However, since there are no definitive ways to reliably assess the collateral flow of the PICA territory, any treatment involving a probable proximal PICA occlusion should be performed only after PICA revascularization. The side-to-side in situ PICA-PICA bypass offers a relatively safe and feasible revascularization option in such cases.

Many neurosurgeons would not consider an in situ bypass as the first-line revascularization option: vessel occlusion or bypass failure during or after in situ bypass operation could compromise both donor and recipient vascular territories with a subsequent risk of bilateral or wide-ranging ischemic events. While this concern is theoretically valid, better revascularization options for the PICA are quite limited. Strong arguments can be made to select the PICA-PICA alternative even when there is an apparently adequate occipital donor vessel. First, there is no evidence that temporary bilateral PICA clamping is more hazardous than unilateral clamping, which is performed during conventional graft-utilizing PICA bypasses. Second, PICA-PICA bypass thrombosis would lead to occlusion of the PICA distal to the telovelomedullary segment, and therefore any resulting cerebellar hemispheric infarction is likely to be clinically mild due to the rich anastomoses through various cerebellar arteries. Third, if the bypass occluded after performing proximal PICA occlusion, resulting thrombosis of brainstem perforators could cause a lateral medullary syndrome, which would be the very same result of occlusion of conventional PICA bypasses. Fourth, not a single ischemic complication or bypass occlusion of side-to-side in situ PICA-PICA bypasses has been reported to date, not even in children;[4,6] however, publishing bias and the small number of conducted in situ bypass procedures certainly explains this extremely low complication rate.

If the treatment plan of ruptured or unruptured VA-PICA aneurysms as well as VA dissections includes occluding the VA and/or PICA at its origin, the side-to-side in situ PICA-PICA bypass can be readily and safely constructed prior to treating the lesion itself. Endovascular treatments may be combined with less aggressive direct surgical procedures, and this combination strategy may reduce the risks of cranial nerve or brainstem compromise.

REFERENCES

1. Tulleken CA, Verdaasdonk RM: First clinical experience with Excimer assisted high flow bypass surgery of the brain, *Acta Neurochir (Wien)* 134:66–70, 1995.
2. Tulleken CA, Verdaasdonk RM, Beck RJ, et al: The modified excimer laser-assisted high-flow bypass operation, *Surg Neurol* 46:424–429, 1996.
3. Tulleken CA, Verdaasdonk RM, Berendsen W, et al: Use of the excimer laser in high-flow bypass surgery of the brain, *J Neurosurg* 78:477–480, 1993.
4. Chandela S, Alzate J, Sen C, et al: Treatment of a complex posterior fossa aneurysm in a child using side-to-side posterior inferior cerebellar artery–posterior inferior cerebellar artery bypass, *J Neurosurg Pediatrics* 1:79–82, 2008.
5. Kakino S, Ogasawara K, Kubo Y, et al: Treatment of vertebral artery aneurysms with posterior inferior cerebellar artery–posterior inferior cerebellar artery anastomosis combined with parent artery occlusion, *Surg Neurol* 61:185–189, 2004; discussion 189.
6. Khayata MH, Spetzler RF, Mooy JJ, et al: Combined surgical and endovascular treatment of a giant vertebral artery aneurysm in a child. Case report, *J Neurosurg* 81:304–307, 1994.
7. Lemole GM Jr, Henn J, Javedan S, et al: Cerebral revascularization performed using posterior inferior cerebellar artery–posterior inferior cerebellar artery bypass. Report of four cases and literature review, *J Neurosurg* 97:219–223, 2002.
8. Nussbaum ES, Madison MT, Myers ME, et al: Dissecting aneurysms of the posterior inferior cerebellar artery: retrospective evaluation of management and extended follow-up review in 6 patients, *J Neurosurg* 109:23–27, 2008.
9. Nussbaum ES, Mendez A, Camarata P, et al: Surgical management of fusiform aneurysms of the peripheral posteroinferior cerebellar artery, *Neurosurgery* 53:831–834, 2003; discussion 834–835.
10. Quinones-Hinojosa A, Lawton MT: In situ bypass in the management of complex intracranial aneurysms: technique application in 13 patients, *Neurosurgery* 57:140–145, 2005; discussion 140–145.
11. Sanai N, Zador Z, Lawton MT: Bypass surgery for complex brain aneurysms: an assessment of intracranial-intracranial bypass, *Neurosurgery* 65:670–683, 2009; discussion 683.
12. Takikawa S, Kamiyama H, Nomura M, et al: [Vertebral dissecting aneurysm treated with trapping and bilateral posterior inferior cerebellar artery side-to side anastomosis; case report], *No Shinkei Geka* 19:571–576, 1991.
13. Lister JR, Rhoton AL Jr, Matsushima T, et al: Microsurgical anatomy of the posterior inferior cerebellar artery, *Neurosurgery* 10:170–199, 1982.
14. Fine AD, Cardoso A, Rhoton AL Jr: Microsurgical anatomy of the extracranial-extradural origin of the posterior inferior cerebellar artery, *J Neurosurg* 91:645–652, 1999.
15. Hudgins RJ, Day AL, Quisling RG, et al: Aneurysms of the posterior inferior cerebellar artery. A clinical and anatomical analysis, *J Neurosurg* 58:381–387, 1983.
16. Horowitz M, Kopitnik T, Landreneau F, et al: Posteroinferior cerebellar artery aneurysms: surgical results for 38 patients, *Neurosurgery* 43:1026–1032, 1998.

10

RADIAL ARTERY HARVEST FOR CEREBRAL REVASCULARIZATION: TECHNICAL PEARLS

11

JUSTIN M. SWEENEY; DEANNA M. SASAKI-ADAMS;
SALEEM I. ABDULRAUF

INTRODUCTION

Cerebral revascularization remains an important technique in the armamentarium of vascular neurosurgeons. Originally described by Yasargil et al.[1] for the treatment of occlusive cerebrovascular disease, the indications for bypass surgery have expanded to include the management of fusiform or giant aneurysms and complex skull-based tumors.[2-6] The choice of bypass conduits has evolved concomitantly. The selection criteria for an appropriate conduit is dependent upon a number of factors, including the extent of blood flow augmentation required, graft length, recipient vessel size, long-term occlusion rates, and the ease, availability and safety of the graft's harvest.[6-8] The radial artery is frequently an ideal candidate. Although extensively described for use in coronary circulation bypass, the evaluation of employing radial artery grafts for cerebral revascularization has not been paid a similar service. In this chapter, we focus on the preoperative evaluation and technical nuances of radial artery harvest for cerebrovascular bypass.

RADIAL ARTERY BYPASS GRAFTS

The use of the radial artery as a conduit for vascular bypass was first reported by Carpentier et al.[9] in the treatment of coronary artery disease. In 1978, Ausman et al.[10] described the use of a radial artery interposition graft for PICA distribution revascularization in the neurosurgical literature. However, its subsequent popularity as a bypass conduit diminished initially due to difficulties with vasospasm-induced graft failure and trauma during skeletonized harvesting.[11,12] Advancements in calcium channel blockade and the use of the pressure distention technique[13] led to its resurgence in the late 1990s.[14] The first large series introducing radial artery conduits as a viable alternative to saphenous vein and pedicled arterial grafts for EC-IC bypass was reported by Sekhar et al.[13] in 2001. Following that landmark study, it remains the conduit of choice for high flow bypass at many institutions.

The radial artery is a medium-sized vessel with a diameter of ~3.5 mm and a flow rate of 40 to 70 ml/min.[15] It originates at the bifurcation of the brachial artery in the antecubital fossa, supplies muscular branches to the radial forearm, and terminates in the superficial and deep palmar arcades. Here it anastamoses with the ulnar artery to supply the hand (Figure 11–1). The radial artery is comparable in caliber to common sites of cerebrovascular attachment, namely the M2 and P1 segments, which facilitates anastamosis construction and prevents flow mismatch. It is most commonly used in high flow bypasses, following temporary or permanent occlusion of medium to large vessels, when significant flow augmentation is required. With time and demand, radial artery grafts have been shown to distend appreciably and achieve larger flow rates.[3] In comparison to saphenous vein grafts, radial arteries have many advantages. They lack the valves and varices present in venous conduits, which increase the risk of graft thrombosis and induce directionality to the conduit. Arterial walls are thick and facilitate anastamosis construction, minimize kinking, and are physiologically designed to carry arterial blood flow and can adapt to changes in pressure and flow. Radial artery grafts have also been shown to better tolerate temporary occlusion and in the long-term are less susceptible to intimal hyperplasia and graft atherosclerosis than vein grafts.[16] They also have improved long-term patency rates as compared to saphenous vein counterparts in both the cardiothoracic[17,18] and neurosurgical[19,20] revascularization literature. In addition, harvest of the radial artery is relatively straightforward given its constant anatomical location within the radial forearm. Donor site morbidity is minimal and includes vascular insufficiency, forearm or hand dysesthesias and weakness, and a low but measurable harvest site infection rate.[21] The major limiting factor for the use of the radial artery is its length. Frequently, lengths of 20 to 25 cm are required to create a tension-free anastomosis from the neck to a cranial attachment. Poor preoperative screening for this limitation can lead to intraoperative abandonment of the graft. Contraindications for its use as a bypass conduit include forearm ischemia on preoperative testing, severe atherosclerosis or calcification within the graft, and dissection from prior cannulation.

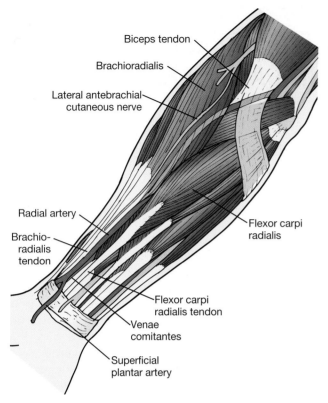

Figure 11–1. Anatomical drawing of the radial artery and surrounding structures in the forearm.

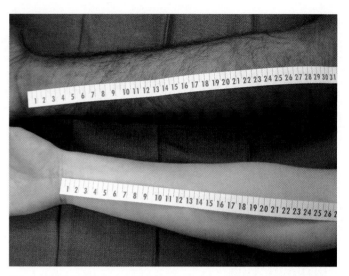

Figure 11–2. Forearm length measured from the proximal transverse furrow of the wrist to the elbow crease overlying the antecubital fossa. A difference of nearly 6 cm was noted between the two subjects, which highlights the variability of graft length.

Preoperative Diagnostic Evaluation for Radial Artery Harvest

The preoperative assessment of the intended radial harvest graft is crucial to ensure adequate length and prevent postoperative vascular insufficiency within the hand. The nondominant side is preferred; however, either forearm may be used. If appropriate, the arm contralateral to the planned craniotomy allows for multiple teams to proceed simultaneously in the operative room. Short arms may foreshadow a radial artery graft with an inadequate length, requiring more extensive evaluation (Figure 11–2).

The first step in the evaluation of a potential radial artery graft should be an Allen's test to confirm adequate ulnar collateral circulation to the palmar arcades. This test is inexpensive, easy to perform, and is highly reliable. It is conducted by occluding both the radial and ulnar arteries within the forearm until pallor is appreciated in the hand. The ulnar artery is then released and the pallor should be replaced by hyperemic rubor, which will gradually fade to normal hues. If the ulnar artery supply is insufficient, the hand pallor will remain. The modified Allen's test employs the use of pulse oximetry while conducting the assessment.[22] The probe is placed on the index finger, and a baseline amplitude is measured. Allen's test is then conducted, and, if the amplitude of the curve is low or the value does not return to baseline within 10 seconds, the harvest of that artery is abandoned. In a prospective study in 2001, Meharwal and Trehan[21] used this technique for the

preoperative evaluation of 3977 radial artery grafts and reported no postoperative ischemic hand complications. Alternatively, pulse oximetry can be measured intraoperatively following temporary clipping of the radial artery. Digital plethysmography and duplex ultrasonography have also been reported as adjunct measures to assess the relative flow within the radial and ulnar arteries and confirm the patency of the palmar arcade.[23,24]

There are many imaging modalities currently available to preoperatively evaluate the caliber and length of the intended radial artery. These include ultrasound, CT angiography, and intraluminal catheter based angiography (Figures 11–3 through 11–5).

Once the decision to harvest a radial artery graft is made, swift evaluation and site selection should be made so that arterial lines and blood gas analysis are avoided on that side.

TECHNIQUE FOR RADIAL ARTERY HARVEST AND PREPARATION

The technique for radial artery bypass harvest for cerebral revascularization is an evolving process. As detailed above, the preoperative evaluation process is imperative for graft selection and harvest safety profiles. The critical aspect of the procedure involves harvesting a graft of adequate length to enable the creation of a tension-free anastomosis. Various techniques have been reported, including open and endoscopic approaches.[25,26] We employ an open technique similar to those previously detailed;[8,13] however, over time our technique has evolved to include several new variations.

Following extensive preoperative evaluation as described above, the chosen forearm is prepared by the harvesting team.

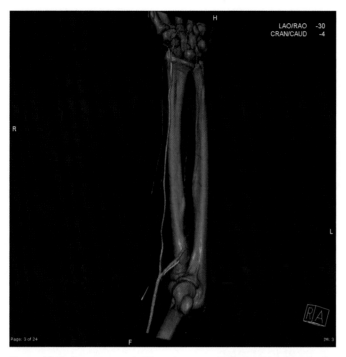

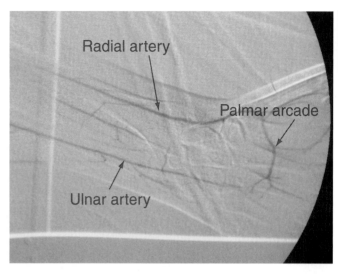

Figure 11–5. Digitally subtracted angiogram of the forearm with a brachial artery injection showing flow in the radial artery, ulnar artery, and palmar arcade. Quantitative measurements can be carried out to determine adequate graft length and luminal diameter. In addition, qualitative analysis of collateral flow can also be assessed.

Figure 11–3. Reconstructed CT angiograms of the radial artery in the forearm of the left upper extremity allowing for measurements of length.

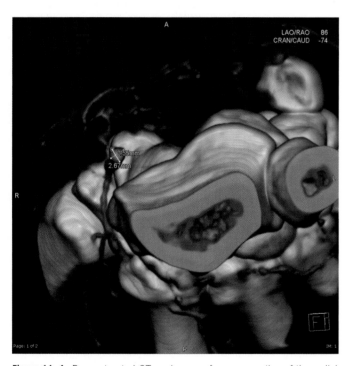

Figure 11–4. Reconstructed CT angiogram of a cross-section of the radial artery in the left distal forearm.

Assisted by palpation and a Doppler probe, an incision overlying the artery is marked from the proximal transverse furrow of the wrist to the antecubital fossa. The arm is prepped and then opened in distal to proximal fashion, depending upon the length necessary for that particular case. Care is taken to avoid injury to the lateral cutaneous nerve of the forearm,

which crosses the artery from lateral to medial near the distal end. The radial artery is identified in the deep fascia, between the brachioradialis and the flexor carpi ulnaris. Muscular branches are coagulated 1 mm from the parent vessel with the use of a harmonic scalpel (Starion CardioForceps, Sunnyvale, CA). Meticulous dissection is employed and care is taken not to injure or manipulate the radial artery. The venae comitantes is left attached to the artery, as it is thought that this may prolong the life of the graft.[27] We locate one or two large muscular branches at either end of the graft for use as outlets following anastamosis construction. These branches are divided ~0.5 to 1 cm from the parent artery and preserved with placement of a temporary aneurysm clip. They will be used later for flushing out clot and evaluation of graft patency (Figure 11–6). The artery is then measured for length and marked on its superficial surface to prevent kinking and rotation during the tunneling process (Figure 11–7). The artery remains in situ, covered in wet gauze until the cranial and cervical dissections are complete. The artery is then stitch ligated proximally and distally, preserving the patency of the ulnar and common interosseous arteries. The most common anomaly of the brachial artery bifurcation is a high division of the radial artery, occurring in up to 15% of cases.[28] This can be advantageous for conduit harvest, allowing for increased graft length. The artery is then extracted and flushed with a cocktail of heparinized saline, papaverine, and a calcium channel blocker to remove clots and help prevent vasospasm.[13] Various antispasmotic agents have been employed both directly and systemically for this purpose.[29] The pressure distention technique as described by Sekhar et al.[13] is then undertaken. This involves blunt canalization of the radial artery graft followed by meticulous sequential dilation with heparinized saline. Any remaining patent side branches are cauterized closed with

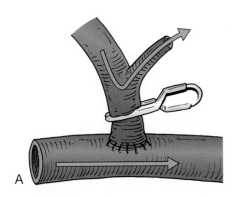

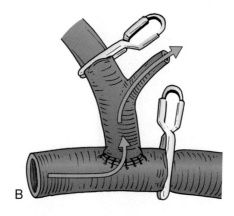

Figure 11–6. A, Diagram showing outlet branch for flushing radial artery prior to revascularization. **B,** Diagram showing the utility of an outlet branch in determining anastomosis patency.

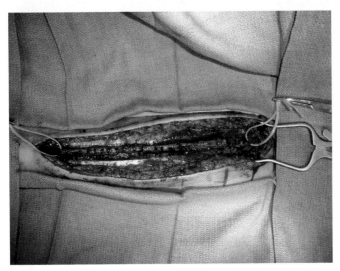

Figure 11–7. In situ radial artery graft awaiting harvest. The anterior wall is marked to avoid torsion of the artery during tunneling.

care to avoid injury to the parent vessel. The adventitia is then stripped from both ends of the graft for 1 to 1.5 cm to help facilitate a "clean" anastamosis. The graft remains in a heparinized saline bath until it is ready for implantation. Following proper hemostasis, the forearm is closed in two layers and the skin closed in subcuticular fashion with absorbable suture.

Construction of the extra and intracranial anastomosis and tunneling of the graft are then undertaken with a technique discussed extensively elsewhere.[30] Prior to releasing the vascular clamps on the cranial circulation, the preserved large muscular side branches are used to flush out any remaining clot in a manner similar to that of the external carotid artery during a carotid endarterectomy to prevent showering embolic stroke (Figure 11–6A). This technique also ensures patency of the graft and donor vessels immediately following anastomosis construction and can allow for graft evaluation without the use of an additional arteriotomy should micro-Doppler analysis reveal poor flow (Figure 11–6B). Many flow probes exist for evaluation of the graft, including micro-Doppler ultrasonography (Mizuho America, Inc., Ithaca, NY, and Transonic Systems, Inc., Beverly, MA). Pulsatility within the graft is encouraging; however, it is not definitive for patency. On-lay vasodilators

can assist in temporarily maximizing graft flow. Intraoperative angiography remains the gold standard to confirm flow. Additionally, ICG video-angiography has become an integral tool within the vascular neurosurgeon's arsenal and has been shown to be a valid measure of bypass patency.[31]

COMPLICATIONS

Complications attributable to graft occlusion are limited in the neurosurgical literature. Sekhar and Kalavakonda published their series documenting a 15-year period. A total of 24 radial arteries were harvested in 50 patients with aneurysms and 83 patients with skull base tumors requiring a revascularization procedure. The overall graft patency rate in their cohort was 95.6% with the pressure distension technique credited with overcoming the problem of arterial vasospasm previously encountered with radial artery conduits.[32] Similarly, Houkin et al. reported a 100% patency rate in 20 of 43 patients who underwent postoperative MRA and DSA following high-flow EC-IC bypass with radial artery conduits over a 10-year period.[19] In the cardiothoracic literature, excellent results have been found with the use of radial artery grafts. The short-, mid-, and long-term patency rates are 96 to 100%, 94 to 97%, and 84 o 96%, respectively;[29] however, these grafts are typically shorter in nature and may be prone to striking differences in vascular microenvironments. Saphenous vein grafts patency rates are significantly lower in the neurosurgical literature with short-, mid-, and long-term patency rates of 86%, 82%, and 73%, respectively.[33] In 2004, Desai et al.[17] enrolled 561 patients in 13 centers into a randomized controlled comparison of radial artery versus saphenous vein conduits for coronary bypass surgery. At 1 year, they found a 5.4% absolute lower occlusion rate in radial arteries as determined by follow-up angiography.

Intraoperative graft occlusions are often secondary to technical issues or hypercoagulable states and are addressed immediately. Postoperative occlusion can occur at any time point and have a number of etiologies related to anastomosis failure, donor or recipient vasculopathy, graft kinking, graft stenosis, flow mismatch, and graft spasm. In addition, intimal hyperplasia and disruption of the vaso vasorum have been implicated as possible etiologies of late occlusion.[11,27]

The majority of literature describing donor site complications of employing the radial artery as a vascular conduit stems from the thoracic literature as it has been used extensively in coronary bypass surgery. General surgical complications such as wound infection, hematoma formation, and wound dehiscence are encountered rarely. Wound infection of radial artery donor sites range between 2% and 12% with a preoperative diagnosis of diabetes mellitus and a surgical duration of greater than 5 hours identified as independent risk factors.[21,34–36] The most common organism encountered is *Staphylococcus aureus*.[36] Postoperative hematomas were observed to develop in 0.3 to 6.4% of cases.[21,34,37,38] Wound dehiscence requiring resuturing is encountered very rarely with one study documenting the incidence at 0.16%.[21] Neurologic or vascular compromise as a sequelae of radial artery harvest is a rare event and is typically self-limiting in nature. In one study of 560 patients, neurologic complications were reported in 30% with a sensory abnormality in 18% and decreased thumb strength observed in 5%. However, only 12% of patients reported sensory or motor abnormalities that did not improve within 8 months.[39] Another study employing the radial artery in 3477 patients found that initially 28% of patients complained of paresthesias and 12% complained of limitation of hand activity that decreased to 3% and 1.22%, respectively, after 6 months.[21] In the majority of cases, it appears that the sensory deficits correlate to involvement of the lateral antebrachial cutaneous nerve.[37,40] Although hand ischemia has been described in the literature, the incidence of blood flow abnormalities postoperatively was not found to be significant in those patients who had a negative Allen's test preoperatively.[21,40,41]

CONCLUSION

The selection of an appropriate bypass graft is made on a case-by-case basis. The neurovascular surgeon should be facile with the harvest, implantation, and management of complications arising from the gamut of graft choices. Radial artery grafts offer a number of advantages and should be given thoughtful consideration when planning a bypass procedure. They have been proven to be safe, durable, and relatively straightforward to use. Thorough preoperative evaluation will aid in establishing graft length and minimizing an already low complication profile. The intraoperative outlet technique described above can aid in stroke prevention and graft evaluation should a thrombus arise.

REFERENCES

1. Yasargil MG, Krayenbuhl HA, Jacobson JH 2nd: Microneurosurgical arterial reconstruction, *Surgery* 67:221–233, 1970.
2. Lawton MT, Hamilton MG, Morcos JJ, et al: Revascularization and aneurysm surgery: current techniques, indications, and outcome, *Neurosurgery* 38:83–92, 1996; discussion 92-94.
3. Sekhar LN, Bucur SD, Bank WO, et al: Venous and arterial bypass grafts for difficult tumors, aneurysms, and occlusive vascular lesions: evolution of surgical treatment and improved graft results, *Neurosurgery* 44:1207–1223, 1999; discussion 1223–1224.
4. Spetzler RF, Fukushima T, Martin N, et al: Petrous carotid-to-intradural carotid saphenous vein graft for intracavernous giant aneurysm, tumor, and occlusive cerebrovascular disease, *J Neurosurg* 73:496–501, 1990.
5. Sundt TM Jr, Piepgras DG, Marsh WR, et al: Saphenous vein bypass grafts for giant aneurysms and intracranial occlusive disease, *J Neurosurg* 65:439–450, 1986.
6. Surdell DL, Hage ZA, Eddleman CS, et al: Revascularization for complex intracranial aneurysms, *Neurosurg Focus* 24:E21, 2008.
7. Baaj AA, Agazzi S, van Loveren H: Graft selection in cerebral revascularization, *Neurosurg Focus* 26:E18, 2009.
8. Liu JK, Kan P, Karwande SV, et al: Conduits for cerebrovascular bypass and lessons learned from the cardiovascular experience, *Neurosurg Focus* 14:e3, 2003.
9. Carpentier A, Guermonprez JL, Deloche A, et al: The aorta-to-coronary radial artery bypass graft. A technique avoiding pathological changes in grafts, *Ann Thorac Surg* 16:111–121, 1973.
10. Ausman JI, Nicoloff DM, Chou SN: Posterior fossa revascularization: anastomosis of vertebral artery to PICA with interposed radial artery graft, *Surg Neurol* 9:281–286, 1978.
11. Curtis JJ, Stoney WS, Alford WC Jr, et al: Intimal hyperplasia. A cause of radial artery aortocoronary bypass graft failure, *Ann Thorac Surg* 20:628–635, 1975.
12. Fisk RL, Brooks CH, Callaghan JC, et al: Experience with the radial artery graft for coronary artery bypass, *Ann Thorac Surg* 21:513–518, 1976.
13. Sekhar LN, Duff JM, Kalavakonda C, et al: Cerebral revascularization using radial artery grafts for the treatment of complex intracranial aneurysms: techniques and outcomes for 17 patients, *Neurosurgery* 49:646–658, 2001; discussion 658–659.
14. Acar C, Jebara VA, Portoghese M, et al: Revival of the radial artery for coronary artery bypass grafting, *Ann Thorac Surg* 54:652–659, 1992; discussion 659–660.
15. Kamiyama H: [Bypass with radial artery graft], *No Shinkei Geka* 22:911–924, 1994.
16. Shi Y, Patel S, Davenpeck KL, et al: Oxidative stress and lipid retention in vascular grafts: comparison between venous and arterial conduits, *Circulation* 103:2408–2413, 2001.
17. Desai ND, Cohen EA, Naylor CD, et al: A randomized comparison of radial-artery and saphenous-vein coronary bypass grafts, *N Engl J Med* 351:2302–2309, 2004.
18. Motwani JG, Topol EJ: Aortocoronary saphenous vein graft disease: pathogenesis, predisposition, and prevention, *Circulation* 97:916–931, 1998.
19. Houkin K, Kamiyama H, Kuroda S, et al: Long-term patency of radial artery graft bypass for reconstruction of the internal carotid artery. Technical note, *J Neurosurg* 90:786–790, 1999.
20. Kocaeli H, Andaluz N, Choutka O, et al: Use of radial artery grafts in extracranial-intracranial revascularization procedures, *Neurosurg Focus* 24:E5, 2008.
21. Meharwal ZS, Trehan N: Functional status of the hand after radial artery harvesting: results in 3,977 cases, *Ann Thorac Surg* 72:1557–1561, 2001.
22. Johnson WH 3rd, Cromartie RS 3rd, Arrants JE, et al: Simplified method for candidate selection for radial artery harvesting, *Ann Thorac Surg* 65:1167, 1998.
23. Abu-Omar Y, Mussa S, Anastasiadis K, et al: Duplex ultrasonography predicts safety of radial artery harvest in the presence of an abnormal Allen test, *Ann Thorac Surg* 77:116–119, 2004.
24. Jarvis MA, Jarvis CL, Jones PR, et al: Reliability of Allen's test in selection of patients for radial artery harvest, *Ann Thorac Surg* 70:1362–1365, 2000.
25. Connolly MW, Torrillo LD, Stauder MJ, et al: Endoscopic radial artery harvesting: results of first 300 patients, *Ann Thorac Surg* 74:502–505, 2002; discussion 506.

26. Gonzalez LF, Patterson DL, Lekovic GP, et al: Endoscopic harvesting of the radial artery for neurovascular bypass, *Neurosurg Focus* 24:E10, 2008.

27. Dietl CA, Benoit CH: Radial artery graft for coronary revascularization: technical considerations, *Ann Thorac Surg* 60:102–109, 1995; discussion 109–110.

28. Doyle JR, Botte MJ: *Surgical Anatomy of the Hand and Upper Extremity*, Philadelphia, 2003, Lippincott Williams & Wilkins.

29. Kobayashi J: Radial artery as a graft for coronary artery bypass grafting, *Circ J* 73:1178–1183, 2009.

30. Abdulrauf SI: Extracranial-to-intracranial bypass using radial artery grafting for complex skull base tumors: technical note, *Skull Base* 15:207–213, 2005.

31. Woitzik J, Horn P, Vajkoczy P, et al: Intraoperative control of extracranial-intracranial bypass patency by near-infrared indocyanine green videoangiography, *J Neurosurg* 102:692–698, 2005.

32. Sekhar LN, Kalavakonda C: Cerebral revascularization for aneurysms and tumors, *Neurosurgery* 50:321–331, 2002.

33. Regli L, Piepgras DG, Hansen KK: Late patency of long saphenous vein bypass grafts to the anterior and posterior cerebral circulation, *J Neurosurg* 83:806–811, 1995.

34. Hata M, Shiono M, Sezai A, et al: Comparative study of harvest-site complications following coronary artery bypass grafting between the radial artery and the saphenous vein in identical patients, *Surg Today* 35:711–713, 2005.

35. Saeed I, Anyanwu AC, Yacoub MH, et al: Subjective patient outcomes following coronary artery bypass using the radial artery: results of a cross-sectional survey of harvest site complications and quality of life, *Eur J Cardiothorac Surg* 20:1142–1146, 2001.

36. Trick WE, Scheckler WE, Tokars JI, et al: Risk factors for radial artery harvest site infection following coronary artery bypass graft surgery, *Clin Infect Dis* 30:270–275, 2000.

37. Budillon AM, Nicolini F, Agostinelli A, et al: Complications after radial artery harvesting for coronary artery bypass grafting: our experience, *Surgery* 133:283–287, 2003.

38. Greene MA, Malias MA: Arm complications after radial artery procurement for coronary bypass operation, *Ann Thorac Surg* 72:126–128, 2001.

39. Denton TA, Trento L, Cohen M, et al: Radial artery harvesting for coronary bypass operations: neurologic complications and their potential mechanisms, *J Thorac Cardiovasc Surg* 121:951–956, 2001.

40. Chong WC, Ong PJ, Hayward CS, et al: Effects of radial artery harvesting on forearm function and blood flow, *Ann Thorac Surg* 75:1171–1174, 2003.

41. Fox AD, Whiteley MS, Phillips-Hughes J, et al: Acute upper limb ischemia: a complication of coronary artery bypass grafting, *Ann Thorac Surg* 67:535–536, 1999; discussion 536–537.

SAPHENOUS VEIN GRAFTS FOR HIGH-FLOW CEREBRAL REVASCULARIZATION

12

CHRISTOPHER S. EDDLEMAN; CHRISTOPHER C. GETCH;
BERNARD R. BENDOK; H. HUNT BATJER

INTRODUCTION

The maintenance of adequate cerebral blood flow and perfusion may require cerebral revascularization in the face of occlusive disease or as a result of treatment for complex intracranial vascular lesions. With refined criteria and improvements in patient selection, cerebral revascularization has seen resurgence over the last decade. While the most commonly used bypass graft has been the superficial temporal artery (STA), some patients require a higher demand for blood flow, and therefore need a graft that can capacitate these increased needs. Flow requirements *can be determined* by balloon test occlusion (BTO). Sacrifice of a large parent artery, such as the internal carotid or vertebral artery, may necessitate a high-flow bypass graft, especially if there is minimal collateral reserve demonstrated by BTO. Ultimately, careful patient selection is the most important predictor of successful revascularization strategies. The most commonly utilized high-flow bypass grafts are the radial artery (RA) and the saphenous vein (SV). In this chapter, we discuss the indications and uses of the SV for high-flow augmentation in cerebral revascularization.

INDICATIONS FOR HIGH-FLOW REVASCULARIZATION

Intracranial and extracranial occlusive vascular disease, can lead to progressive compromise of cerebral blood flow that may necessitate augmentation of cerebral blood flow. Trauma may result in loss or compromise of a major arterial supply to the brain and hence a need for revascularization. Further, as a greater number of complex aneurysm recurrences are seen after endovascular treatment, revascularization strategies have increased in importance. Treating these complex vascular lesions may require complex clip reconstruction techniques requiring extended temporary artery occlusion times or parent artery sacrifice. Lesions located on the M1 and P1 segments may require prophylactic bypass due to the frequent presence

of perforating vessels and low tolerance of temporary occlusion in these territories. Further, many vascular lesions involve extensive atherosclerotic changes in the neck, very broad based, or giant in size, thus potentially necessitating branch or parent artery sacrifice. Finally, previously endovascularly treated vascular lesions may require complex vascular reconstructions at retreatment, that is, removal of coil mass, potentially demanding, long parent artery occlusion times. The choice of the anastomosis site is selected based on the location of the lesion, intended territory of revascularization, and properties of the donor and recipient vessels. BTO can facilitate decision making in most cases (Table 12–1). After temporary occlusion of a parent artery, the global cerebral hemodynamics are examined, with particular attention to the vascular reserve provided by the leptomeningial and circle of Willis vessels and subsequently the flow dynamics including venous washout are carefully studied.

While angiographic study of the collateral circulation around a particular lesion is helpful, it does not provide a clinical assessment of the patient's potential cerebral blood flow requirements. In order to determine clinically significant changes regarding the need for reserve flow, the BTO includes clinical examinations, electroencephalogram (EEG), hypotensive challenges with clinical examinations, and single-photon emission computed tomography (SPECT) imaging after performance of the BTO and removal of the balloon. Clinical exams are performed at baseline and every 5 minutes after balloon inflation. If the patient fails the BTO and develops deficits at normotension (120 to 140 systolic), then we feel the patient should undergo a high-flow bypass.

SAPHENOUS VEIN CONSIDERATIONS

The saphenous vein graft has been used for decades for bypass procedures with relatively great success. Lougheed is credited for performing the first intracranial bypass using a saphenous vein graft in 1971.[1] Despite an overall decrease in the use of intracranial SV bypasses due to an increased use of

Table 12–1. BALLOON TEST OCCLUSION DETERMINATION OF AMOUNT OF REQUIRED CEREBRAL BLOOD FLOW.

Cerebral Blood Flow Needed	Balloon Trial Occlusion Results
No bypass	No clinical deficits or SPECT abnormalities
Low-flow bypass	Clinical deficits during hypotensive state with/without EEG changes; no SPECT abnormalities
High-flow bypass	Clinical deficits with SPECT abnormalities

EEG, electroencephalogram; SPECT, single-photon emission computed tomography.

endovascular techniques for complex intracranial vascular disease and an increased experience and usage of radial artery grafts, the SV graft still provides a highly flexible and adaptable bypass graft for a variety of uses, including a primary conduit from the carotid artery or superficial temporal artery or as an interposition graft. The saphenous vein has a measured flow rate between 70 and 200 ml/min and an average diameter of ~5 mm.[2,3] The advantages of the SV graft are the ease of harvest, autologous source, length of graft able to be obtained, absence of atherosclerotic changes throughout the length of the vessel, absence of vasospasm, and large caliber of graft able to be harvested. Several disadvantages of SV grafts exist and are most commonly frequent caliber mismatch between donor and recipient vessels, which can often lead to intraluminal turbulent flow and eventual thrombosis, the presence of valves that can be sites of thrombus formation, greater possibility of reperfusion hemorrhage, and the potential for kinking at the site of the recipient due to the thick surrounding tissue and vessel wall. Saphenous vein bypass grafts require two separate anastomosis sites and separate incisions for graft harvest, which increases the potential for complications. Although long-term patency rates have not been directly compared between RA and SV grafts, the average patency rate at 5 years postimplantation has been reported to be ~90% for RA grafts and ~80% for SV grafts. In the coronary literature, RAs have been consistently reported to have higher patency rates compared to SVs.[2–4]

Patients undergoing revascularization procedures are usually placed on aspirin therapy before or immediately after the revascularization procedure. In cases of hypercholesterolemia, a statin can be administered pre- and post-operatively, which has been suggested to positively affect long-term graft patency.[2,3,5] All patients receive preoperative antibiotics within 1 hour prior to incision. The utilization of a neuroanesthesia team has several advantages during all phases of the procedure. Throughout the procedure—adequate cerebral perfusion is maintained adequate pharmacological brain protection, as well as optimal brain relaxation—which reduces the necessity of brain retraction. Postoperatively, controlled emergence, that is, avoidance of hypo- and hyper-tension, and rapid emergence from anesthesia are important so that an adequate neurological exam can be completed without compromising the bypass graft. Intraoperative neurophysiological monitoring is also performed, which includes EEG and somatosensory evoked potentials (SSEPs). Other neuromonitoring, such as brainstem-evoked potentials or cranial nerve monitoring, may be employed depending on the site of surgery and necessity of cranial nerve manipulation. Intraoperative graft patency monitoring can be assessed with ICG video-angiography, micro-Doppler ultrasound, or invasive intraoperative angiography via the femoral arterial rout or via direct cervical arterial puncture.

The patient is positioned with regard to the side of the lesion and the anastomosis site. For anterior circulation lesions, the patient is placed supine with the head turned to the opposite side of the lesion. The vascular grafts are often harvested from the opposite side of the lesion. For posterior circulation lesions, the patient is often placed in the lateral position.

HARVEST AND BYPASS PROCEDURE

The most common path of the greater SV is just anteromedial to the tibia at the ankle, and, toward the knee, it gradually travels more posterior. Vein mapping can be done with a macro-Doppler or ultrasound machine. In the lower thigh, the SV runs just posterior to the adductor tubercle where it then courses proximally along the lateral surface of the femoral artery. The caliber and shape of the SV is more uniform in the lower thigh and upper leg. At our institution, the dissection of the SV is often started near the ankle, due to its easy identity with ultrasound at this location. Some institutions prefer to harvest the vein from the upper leg using endoscopic techniques. The SV is normally harvested from the side opposite to the site of revascularization. Branches of the SV are ligated and divided as the dissection proceeds more proximally. Once the adductor tubercle is reached, the dissection normally ceases as the more proximal the dissection proceeds; the drainage of the thigh becomes more dependent on the femoral vein. The orientation of the SV graft is extremely important, as the presence of valves puts the graft at risk of thrombosis if placed in the incorrect orientation. As such, the distal end of the SV graft is marked with a suture to ensure the correct orientation. The graft is then removed and placed in a basin filled with heparinized saline. The adventitia, which can be thick, should be carefully removed with tedious and meticulous care. It is particularly important for adventitia to be removed at the anastomotic end, as the suture can become embedded and leave gaps where leakage sites can occur. The orientation of the graft should be reconfirmed by flushing saline through the graft and assessing ease of flow and directionality of valves. To assess the twisting of the graft, a blue ink line is place along the long axis of the SV. The SV graft is then maintained in a basin with heparinized saline until use.

It is important for the bypass procedure to flow efficiently. As such, the intracranial and cervical dissections are performed first. After the exposure of the bypass sites is completed, a subcutaneous tunnel for the bypass graft is made. A large clamp or Betcher is used to dissect a subcutaneous tunnel that runs just superior to the zygoma toward the intracranial or lateral incision, depending on the site for the anastomoses. The subcutaneous tunnel can be made in front or behind the ear, depending on the surgeon's preference. The subcutaneous tunnel should be large enough to accommodate the graft during passage and without future risk of compression, and is often large enough if it can accommodate the fifth digit. A Penrose drain can be placed in the tunnel space until the graft is ready to be passed. To better accommodate the SV graft, a groove can be made in the zygoma so that bony compression is reduced and the cosmetic footprint on the face is improved. The graft can be passed through the tunnel with a suture attached to one end. The graft is then assessed for twisting by examining the blue ink line drawn along the graft.

The extracranial carotid anastomotic site should be able to accommodate an arteriotomy of at least 4 to 5 mm for the SV graft. Temporary clips are placed on either side of the target anastomotic site. The most common extracranial proximal anastomosis sites are the ICA, ECA, CCA, or VA. When the bypass is to the carotid circulation, the site of anastomosis is usually just distal to the superior thyroid artery on the ECA. The type of anastomosis is an end-to-side to the ECA using beveled ends sutured with a running Proline suture. Using 8- or 9-0 Proline, anchoring sutures are normally initially placed at each of the anastomotic ends, followed by a running 8- or 9-0 Proline. Running suture lines are acceptable as there is no need to compensate for bypass growth. Proline is a more suitable suture type since it is a monofilament and its strength is adequate for the thickness of the graft adventitial tissue. Braided suture is not recommended due to the likelihood of passing adventitial tissue into the suture line. Monofilament Proline suture passes through the graft tissue with less effort and with minimal damage to the graft. The contralateral side is usually sutured first. Since the SV graft is normally much larger than the recipient vessel, the amount of graft tissue will of course be greater than that of the recipient. As a result, the sutures in the graft should be placed with larger gaps than that of the recipient, which will result in an undulated graft. This ensures a more appropriate size-matched anastomotic site. Otherwise, tissue gaps may persist, which will lead to leakage along the suture line. After the contralateral wall has been completed, the suture line is examined for completeness and to ensure that no inclusion of the opposing arterial wall has taken place. The temporary clips are removed from the proximal parent vessel and a temporary clip is placed flush with the proximal anastomosis site. The graft is flushed with heparinized saline to clear the graft of residual blood or clots. The distal end of the SV graft is then positioned near the sight of the estimated distal anastomosis site and trimmed so that mild tension exists in the graft. The graft will often expand, sometimes significantly, after restoration of blood flow, and the intentional mild tension often prevents kinking at the distal anastomotic site. The patient is then systemically anticoagulated to prevent graft thrombosis and clotting during the proximal anastomosis. The arteriotomy in the proximal vessel should be slightly larger than the distal anastomosis site; approximately 6 to 8 mm. Temporary clips are placed on the target vessel around the anastomotic site. The same suture technique is used on the ipsilateral wall of the distal target vessel. Before the anastomosis is completed, the graft is again flushed with heparinized saline and redistended. A clip is then placed onto the SV graft at a site that is flush with the distal anastomosis site to prevent leakage and blood products from pooling in the graft. Subsequently, the proximal temporary clip is removed. After a final inspection of the graft and the anastomosis sites, including evaluation for suture line and kinking, the distal clip can be removed.

ASSESSMENT OF BYPASS PATENCY

Intraoperative assessment of bypass patency and functionality is paramount and can avoid complications due to premature graft stenosis or occlusion. While intraoperative catheter angiograms remain the gold standard, this technique requires additional costs and risks to the patient. Micro-Doppler assessment can provide qualitative assessments of flow and patency. Flow through the bypass graft can be nicely evaluated with indocyanine green (ICG) video angiography, which provides visual assessment of patency with little to no risk to the patient.[2] With this technique, direction of flow can be assessed, and, if the graft needs to be opened or revised, this technique can be performed multiple times to evaluate the graft.

The most common causes for acute graft failure are proximal stenosis or thrombosis at either anastomotic site. Stenosis is likely related to technical errors with the anastomoses. Thrombosis is likely a result of extended graft occlusion time while the distal anastomosis is being completed. If graft patency is not present, the bypass graft is then reopened at the proximal anastomotic site, flushed, and distended with heparinized saline. Once the bypass graft is patent, the graft is again distally clipped, filled with heparinized saline, and the proximal anastomosis is repeated. If clot or stenosis is still present, a 2F Fogerty balloon may be inserted into the graft, inflated, and then carefully pulled out of the graft, thus removing any residual clot within the graft. If adequate back-flow of blood occurs, then the proximal anastomosis is once again completed. If the graft continues to be clotted, the distal anastomosis must be examined using the same steps.

COMPLICATIONS

Cerebral revascularization with SV bypass grafts is more prone to complications than their low-flow counterparts. The most serious complication to avoid is reperfusion injury. The incidence of intracranial hemorrhage after autologous, including SV grafts, is approximately 10%.[6] These patients have likely had long-standing cerebral perfusion deficits and as such, are likely dysautoregulated and at a higher risk for reperfusion hemorrhage. In addition, patients may be at risk for reperfusion injury from poorly controlled blood pressure or blood flow mismatch changes, especially after high-flow revascularization.[4,6–8] For these reasons, patients are monitored closely in the ICU setting and blood pressure is strictly controlled. Also, most patients requiring high-flow cerebral revascularization do not have vascular reserve, as demonstrated by BTO, so prolonged temporary occlusion times can often lead to territorial infarcts with and without changes in intraoperative neurophysiological monitoring. As such, temporary occlusion times should be minimized. That is, having an efficient and well thought out operative strategy as well as a well-executed plan is paramount. Thromboembolic complications can be encountered after bypass procedures from several different sources, namely the anastomotic sites, turbulent flow and thrombosis within the graft, alterations in intracranial hemodynamics, as well as residual parent artery vascular stumps. Preoperative antiplatelet medications as well as intraoperative anticoagulation can reduce these thromboembolic events. In a delayed fashion, SV grafts can undergo proatherogenic changes after implantation, which can also eventually lead to occlusion. Furthermore, other complications may involve the site of graft harvest, such as infection, lymphadema, or hematoma, or within the graft tunnel itself, such as hematoma. While these complications are very low, close attention should be rendered to the graft harvest site, as these complications can often be overlooked due to the focus on the cerebral manifestations of the revascularization procedure.

POSTOPERATIVE CONSIDERATIONS

It is of paramount importance to proactively minimize the potential for postoperative complications. Patients are normally maintained on antiplatelet, usually aspirin, therapy indefinitely and, depending on the patient's mobility, on prophylactic doses of heparin beginning 24 to 48 hours postoperatively for deep venous thrombosis/pulmonary embolism prevention. Patients are usually monitored in the intensive care unit for at least 24 to 48 hours after revascularization. Blood pressure monitoring is strict and maintained at normopressure. Graft patency can

be assessed after the procedure with Doppler, computed tomography angiography, or magnetic resonance angiography (MRA). Perfusion imaging can be used to assess the status of brain hemodynamics. Cerebral angiography can also be performed when there is concern for graft patency or for routine assessment. The advantage of invasive angiography is the ability to intervene if a problem with the graft is encountered. Follow-up imaging can be performed with MRA/MR perfusion or Doppler ultrasonography.

CONCLUSION

Cerebral revascularization is necessary in some cases of complex vascular disease. High-flow cerebral revascularization can be successfully completed using harvested saphenous vein vascular grafts. Success is dictated by careful patient selection, meticulous surgical technique, thoughtful planning, vigilant peri-operative care, and mindful knowledge of the potential pitfalls and complications that can accompany cerebral revascularization procedures.

REFERENCES

1. Lougheed WM, Marshall BM, Hunter M, et al: Common carotid to intracranial internal carotid bypass venous graft. Technical note, *J Neurosurg* 34:114–118, 1971.
2. Surdell DL, Hage ZA, Eddleman CS, et al: Revascularization for complex intracranial aneurysms, *Neurosurg Focus* 24:E21, 2008.
3. Bisson EF, Visioni AJ, Tranmer B, et al: External carotid artery to middle cerebral artery bypass with the saphenous vein graft, *Neurosurgery* 62:134–138, 2008; discussion 138–139.
4. Jafar JJ, Russell SM, Woo HH: Treatment of giant intracranial aneurysms with saphenous vein extracranial-to-intracranial bypass grafting: Indications, operative technique, and results in 29 patients, *Neurosurgery* 51:138–144, 2002; discussion 144–146.
5. Kocaeli H, Andaluz N, Choutka O, et al: Use of radial artery grafts in extracranial-intracranial revascularization procedures, *Neurosurg Focus* 24:E5, 2008.
6. Diaz FG, Pearce J, Ausman JI: Complications of cerebral revascularization with autogenous vein grafts, *Neurosurgery* 17:271–276, 1985.
7. Quinones-Hinojosa A, Du R, Lawton MT: Revascularization with saphenous vein bypasses for complex intracranial aneurysms, *Skull Base* 15:119–132, 2005.
8. Santoro A, Guidetti G, Dazzi M, et al: Long saphenous-vein grafts for extracranial and intracranial internal carotid aneurysms amenable neither to clipping nor to endovascular treatment, *J Neurosurg Sci* 43:237–250, 1999; discussion 250–251.

IC-IC BYPASSES FOR COMPLEX BRAIN ANEURYSMS

MICHAEL LAWTON; NADER SANAI

INTRODUCTION

EC-IC bypass surgery has been essential in the management of brain aneurysms that are too complex for conventional clipping or endovascular coiling, despite its well-publicized failure to benefit patients with ischemic stroke in the EC-IC Bypass Trial.[1,3,5,11,22,27] Revascularization of a territory distal to a giant, dolichoectatic, or thrombotic aneurysm enables the aneurysm to be occluded without risk of ischemic complications, or the parent artery's blood flow to be reversed or reduced safely. The superficial temporal artery to middle cerebral artery (STA-MCA) bypass was the prototype, and subsequently an array of bypasses was developed with the same concept of redirecting extracranial blood flow from scalp arteries or cervical carotid arteries to the brain, either directly with one anastomosis or with interposition grafts and two anastomoses. In recent years, innovative bypasses have been introduced anecdotally that revascularize intracranial arteries with other intracranial arteries, without contribution from extracranial donor arteries.[7-9,15,16,20] These intracranial to intracranial (IC-IC) bypasses are simple, elegant, and more anatomical than their EC-IC counterparts. IC-IC bypasses require no harvest of extracranial donors, spare patients a neck incision, shorten any interposition grafts, are protected within the cranium, and use caliber-matched donor and recipient arteries. These advantages of IC-IC bypasses appeal to experienced bypass surgeons, and their use has increased noticeably. For example, Sekhar and colleagues performed at least 11 IC-IC bypasses in an overall experience with 119 bypasses in 115 patients.[26] Similarly, Spetzler and colleagues performed 28 IC-IC bypasses (44%) in an overall experience with 63 bypasses in 61 patients.[15]

The development of an array of IC-IC bypasses represents an important evolution of bypass surgery for brain aneurysms. We have embraced IC-IC bypasses in our aneurysm practice at the University of California, San Francisco, and categorize IC-IC bypasses into four types of intracranial arterial reconstruction: in situ bypass, reimplantation, reanastomosis, and intracranial bypass grafts.

EVOLUTION OF BYPASS SURGERY FOR BRAIN ANEURYSMS

Bypass surgery for brain aneurysms began with the introduction and popularization of the STA-MCA bypass by Yasargil.[29] This simple bypass revascularized the MCA territory and protected patients from ischemic complications after deliberate arterial occlusion during the treatment of MCA and some ICA aneurysms. Bypass surgery for aneurysms evolved with the development of an array of EC-IC bypasses that used other extracranial donor arteries and interposition grafts connected to proximal donor sites in the neck.[2,4,6,10,12-15,17-19,21,23,25,28,30] Even though these second-generation EC-IC bypasses yield excellent results, bypass surgery for aneurysms is evolving further with the development of an array of IC-IC bypasses that eliminates extracranial donor arteries and reconstructs the cerebral circulation in ways that resemble normal cerebrovascular anatomy. In this report, we analyzed this third generation of IC-IC bypasses in a large clinical series, categorized the techniques into four types, and demonstrated aneurysm and patient outcomes comparable to traditional EC-IC bypasses. Aneurysm obliteration rates, bypass patency rates, and neurological results (late GOS and change in GOS) were similar in EC-IC and IC-IC bypass patients, supporting this progression toward intracranial vascular reconstruction.

EC-IC bypasses are technically easier to perform than IC-IC bypasses. For example, an STA-MCA bypass requires one end-to-side anastomosis that is usually straightforward, particularly when the donor artery is large and mobilizes to visualize both suture lines. In contrast, an in situ bypass between two MCA branches requires a more challenging side-to-side anastomosis between arteries with limited mobility. Similarly, an ECA-MCA bypass requires a proximal anastomosis in the neck that can be performed in a superficial cervical site with no ischemia from cross-clamping an intracranial artery. In contrast, an A1 anterior cerebral artery (ACA)–MCA intracranial bypass graft requires a proximal anastomosis in a narrow surgical corridor that is even deeper than the distal anastomosis to the MCA. Although cross-clamping the A1 ACA does not produce ischemia in patients with a competent anterior communicating artery (ACoA), temporary clips on a major intracranial artery inevitably induce some time pressure. Therefore, IC-IC bypasses add a degree of difficulty.

BYPASS DEMOGRAPHICS

Patients were divided into two groups according to the type of bypass: EC-IC versus IC-IC. EC-IC bypass involved donors arteries from external carotid artery branches (STA and occipital artery (OA)), cervical carotid arteries (common carotid artery (CCA), internal carotid artery (ICA), and external carotid artery (ECA)), or other extracranial arteries (e.g., subclavian artery). IC-IC bypass involved intracranial donor arteries, and were further categorized as in situ bypass (adjacent donor artery), reimplantation (aneurysm branch artery onto parent artery), reanastomosis (primary repair of parent artery), and intracranial bypass graft (graft interposed between donor and recipient arteries).

During a 10-year period between November 1997 and November 2007, 1984 aneurysms were treated microsurgically in 1578 patients by the senior author (MTL). Of these patients, 82 (5%) underwent cerebral revascularization surgery as part of the management of an intracranial aneurysm. Overall, there were 50 women and 32 men, with a mean age of 53 years (range, 12–78 years) (Table 13–1). Twenty-one patients presented with

subarachnoid hemorrhage (26%). Hunt-Hess Grade III was the most common clinical grade (48%), and four patients presented with poor Hunt-Hess grade. Fifty-six patients (68%) presented with unruptured aneurysms and neurological symptoms, with cranial neuropathy or hemiparesis from mass effect present in 38 patients (68%). Eight patients (14%) presented with transient ischemic attacks or stroke in association with thrombotic aneurysms. Five patients presented with incidental, unruptured aneurysms (6%).

ANEURYSM CHARACTERISTICS FOR IC-IC BYPASS PATIENTS

Aneurysms were distributed throughout the intracranial circulation, with the most common locations being the cavernous ICA (19 aneurysms, 23%), MCA (16 aneurysms, 20%), and posterior inferior cerebellar artery (PICA) (10 aneurysms, 12%) (Table 13–2). The majority of aneurysms were giant in size (46 aneurysms, 56%). Only 15 aneurysms (18%) had saccular morphology, and the remaining 67 aneurysms (82%) had fusiform or dolichoectatic morphology. Thirty-one patients (38%) had thrombotic aneurysms. Eight aneurysms (10%) had been treated endovascularly with coils, of which three were incompletely treated and five were recurrent. Fifteen patients (19%) had multiple aneurysms, with 26 other aneurysms diagnosed.

Table 13–1. STUDY DEMOGRAPHICS.

		Total	%	EC-IC Bypass	%	IC-IC Bypass	%
Total patients		82		47	57	35	43
Median age (range)		53 (12–78)		57 (12–77)		45 (15–78)	
Women		50	61	35	74	15	43
Ruptured aneurysm patients	All	21	26	8	17	13	37
	Grade I	6	29	2	25	4	31
	Grade II	1	5	1	13	0	0
	Grade III	10	48	3	38	7	54
	Grade IV	4	19	2	25	2	15
	Grade V	0	0	0	0	0	0
Unruptured aneurysm patients (symptomatic)	All	56	68	37	79	19	54
	Headache	22	39	15	41	7	37
	Cranial neuropathy	29	52	22	59	7	37
	Hemiparesis	9	16	6	16	3	16
	Seizure	3	5	2	5	1	5
	TIA/stroke	8	14	4	11	4	21
	Hydrocephalus	4	7	2	5	2	11
	Incomplete coiling or recurrence	7	13	2	5	5	26

(Continued)

Table 13–1. STUDY DEMOGRAPHICS.—CONT'D

		Total	%	EC-IC Bypass	%	IC-IC Bypass	%
Unruptured aneurysm patients (incidental)	All	5	6	2	4	3	9
Aneurysm characteristics							
	Mean diameter (range)	23.8 mm (4–60)		28.5 mm (6–60)		17.2 mm (4–49)	
	Saccular	15	18	10	21	5	14
	Fusiform, dolichoectatic	67	82	37	79	30	86
	Giant	46	56	34	72	12	34
	Thrombotic	31	38	18	38	13	37
Outcome measures							
Mean preoperative GOS		4.5		4.7		4.4	

Table 13–2. ANEURYSM DEMOGRAPHICS.

Aneurysm Location INTERNAL CAROTID ARTERY	Total	%	EC-IC Bypass	%	IC-IC Bypass	%
Cavernous	19	23	17	36	2	6
Supraclinoid	9	11	9	19	0	0
Ophthalmic	3	4	3	6	0	0
Terminus	2	2	2	4	0	0
MIDDLE CEREBRAL ARTERY						
Total	16	20	7	15	9	26
ANTERIOR CEREBRAL ARTERY						
Anterior communicating artery	3	4	0	0	3	9
Pericallosal	2	2	0	0	2	6
Distal anterior cerebral artery	1	1	0	0	1	3
BASILAR ARTERY						
Basilar bifurcation	2	2	2	4	0	0
Posterior cerebral artery	2	2	2	4	0	0
Superior cerebellar artery	2	2	1	2	1	3
Basilar trunk	8	10	4	9	4	11
POSTERIOR INFERIOR CEREBELLAR ARTERY						
Posterior inferior cerebellar artery	10	12	0	0	10	29
Vertebral artery	3	4	0	0	3	9
Total	82	100	47	100	35	100

PATIENT SELECTION

Patient selection is one of the most important elements for successful aneurysm revascularization. Although balloon test occlusion is not always reliable for determining the necessity for revascularization, our reviewed experience employed balloon test occlusion (BTO) to a select 26 patients for aneurysm management with a bypass, all of them with cavernous or supraclinoid ICA aneurysms. Ten patients failed the test with balloon inflation alone, and 16 patients failed with additional hypotensive challenge (lowering mean arterial pressure with nitroprusside drip by 20 mm Hg, or 25% of mean arterial pressure, whichever was greater). Failed BTO can be used as an indication for bypass. High-flow bypass should be used in patients who fail BTO immediately, and low-flow bypass in patients who fail BTO after hypotensive challenge. The decision to perform a bypass with aneurysms in other locations should be based on patients' angiographic anatomy, specifically the presence or absence of collateral circulation from the circle of Willis.

IN SITU BYPASS TECHNIQUE

In situ bypass requires donor and recipient arteries that lie parallel and in close proximity to one another. Four sites have this anatomy: bilateral ACAs as they course through the interhemispheric fissure over the corpus callosum's genu and rostrum (A3 and A4 segments); MCA branches (M2 and M3 segments) and the anterior temporal artery (ATA) as they course through the Sylvian fissure; posterior cerebral artery (PCA, P2, and P3 segments) and superior cerebellar artery (SCA) as they course through the ambient cistern around the cerebral peduncle; and bilateral PICAs as they course through the cisterna magna to meet behind the medulla underneath the cerebellar tonsils. In situ bypasses require one side-to-side anastomosis.

REIMPLANTATION TECHNIQUE

Complex aneurysms with branches that originate from the aneurysm base or side wall can often be reconstructed with tandem clipping techniques that preserve important branch arteries (a fenestrated clip encircling the branch origin and a stacked straight clip closing the fenestration). In cases where clip reconstruction fails, the neck can be clipped to exclude the aneurysm, preserve the parent artery, and sacrifice the branch artery. The occluded branch artery can then be reconstituted with reimplantation onto the parent artery (Figure 13–1). Alternatively, the branch artery can be reimplanted to an adjacent donor artery that is not the parent artery, as long as that donor artery lies in close proximity to the branch (Figure 13–2). Like in situ bypasses, this favorable anatomy occurs with MCA, ACA, and PICA aneurysms. Reimplantation requires one end-to-side anastomosis.

REANASTOMOSIS TECHNIQUE

Reanastomosis requires trapping the aneurysm, completely detaching afferent and efferent arteries, and reconnecting cut ends with an end-to-end anastomosis (Figure 13–3). This technique works well with fusiform aneurysms that are small or medium in size. Saccular aneurysms at bifurcations with more than two or more efferent arteries are difficult to reconstruct with primary reanastomosis because the second branch must either be reimplanted or bypassed with an extracranial donor artery. Large and giant aneurysms may be difficult to reanastomose because ends of the parent artery can be widely separated after excising an aneurysm. Mobilizing the ends of afferent and efferent arteries may enable the first stitch to pull them together with minimal tension. If the gap in the parent artery is too long and the tension too great, the suture will tear through the artery wall as it is tightened and ruin the repair. Some large aneurysms in PICA and MCA territories have an unusually redundant parent artery that will allow primary reanastomosis despite their size. Reanastomosis requires one end-to-end anastomosis.

INTRACRANIAL BYPASS TECHNIQUE WITH GRAFTS

These bypasses use interposition grafts to connect donor and recipient arteries that are entirely intracranial, differentiating them from traditional EC-IC bypasses that utilize extracranial donor arteries (Figures 13–4 through 13–6). In contrast to EC-IC bypasses that use saphenous vein grafts to span from the neck to the Sylvian fissure, intracranial bypass grafts are shorter and radial artery grafts are sufficiently long. Radial artery grafts are preferred over saphenous vein grafts because they are composed of arterial tissue, have higher long-term patency rates, and match the caliber of intracranial arteries. Preoperatively, an Allen's test with Doppler ultrasound is performed to ensure adequate perfusion of the hand with the ulnar artery and a competent palmar arch.

Intraoperatively, the forearm can be accessed to harvest the radial artery more easily than the thigh, particularly when the patient is positioned laterally or prone for posterior circulation aneurysms. Vasospasm in radial artery grafts has been described, but can be avoided by using pressure distension to dilate the graft before implantation, and by bathing the graft in a mixture of nitroprusside and heparin. Unlike the other IC-IC techniques, intracranial bypass grafts require at least two anastomoses and may require end-to-side, end-to-end, or side-to-side anastomoses. The anastomoses are planned to minimize brain ischemia during the time that intracranial arteries are temporarily occluded and sutured.

Figure 13–1. Recipient reimplantation. This thrombotic ACA aneurysm, seen on axial T1-weighted magnetic resonance image (**A**), originated at the bifurcation of the pericallosal (PC) and callosomarginal (CM) arteries (**B**), right ICA angiogram, lateral view). **C** and **D,** The aneurysm (An) was exposed in the interhemispheric fissure through a bifrontal craniotomy, using gravity to retract the right hemisphere. Attempts to clip reconstruct the neck were unsuccessful; intraluminal thrombus caused the clips to occlude the pericallosal artery. The pericallosal artery was clip occluded, transected, and mobilized to the callosomarginal artery (**E**). An end-to-side PC-CM anastomosis was performed: back wall (**F**), front wall (**G**), and after completion (**H**). **I,** The CM artery supplied blood flow to the entire distal ACA territory.

(Adapted from Sanai N, Zador Z, Lawton MT: Bypass surgery for complex brain aneurysms: an assessment of intracranial-intracranial bypass, Neurosurgery 2009;65:670–683.)

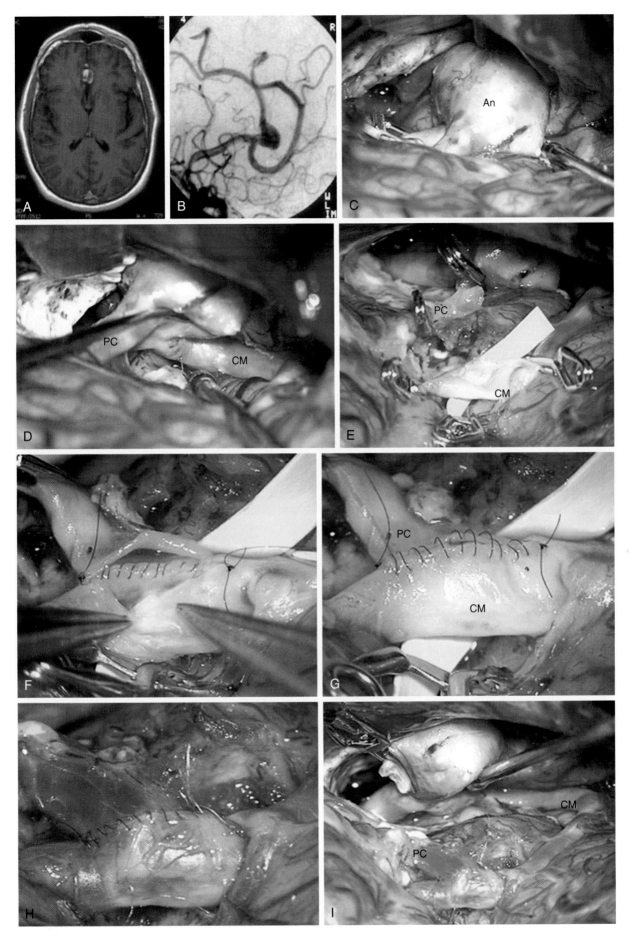

Figure 13–1. For legend, see facing page.

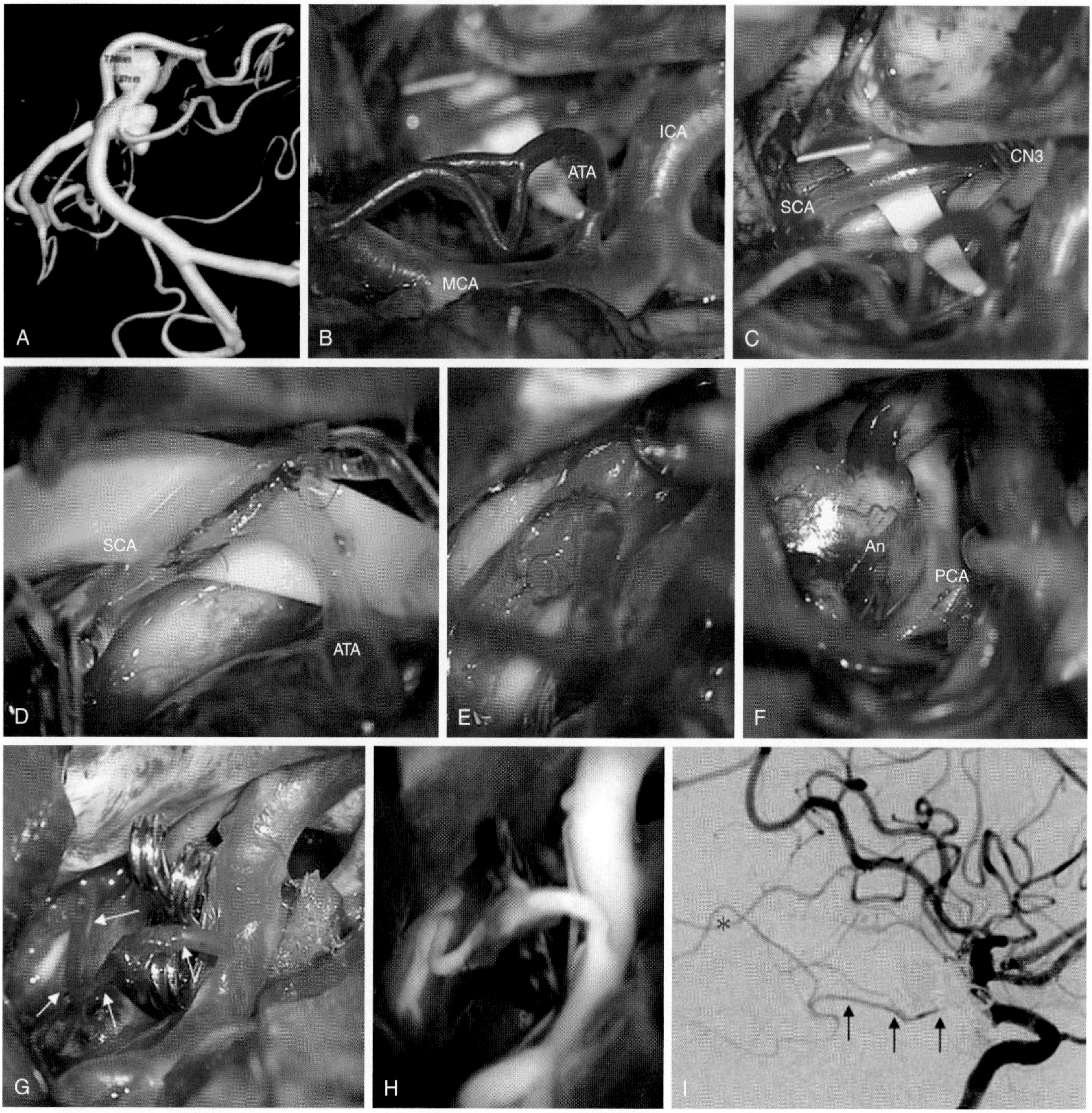

Figure 13–2. Donor reimplantation. This multilobulated left SCA aneurysm, seen on rotational angiogram with three-dimensional reconstruction (**A**), was incompletely coiled, leaving residual neck to preserve the SCA origin. After inspecting the anatomy intraoperatively, it seemed unlikely that the aneurysm could be clipped with occluding SCA and likely that a bypass would be needed to preserve it. **B,** A prominent ATA was found in the Sylvian fissure. **C,** This ATA had sufficient length to reach the SCA. **D,** The ATA was transected distally and reimplanted onto SCA with an end-to-side anastomosis. **E,** After bypass patency was confirmed, the aneurysm (An) was neck was dissected (**F**) and clipped (**G**) (*arrows*). **H,** Indocyanine green videography confirmed good flow in the ATA-SCA bypass, as did the postoperative angiogram (**I**) (left ICA injection, lateral view, with opacification of the left SCA [*arrows*]). Note the course of the SCA over the cerebellar vermis (*asterisk*). MCA, middle cerebral artery; ICA, internal carotid artery; PCA, posterior cerebral artery; CN3, oculomotor nerve.

(Adapted from Sanai N, Zador Z, Lawton MT: Bypass surgery for complex brain aneurysms: an assessment of intracranial-intracranial bypass, Neurosurgery 2009;65:670–683.)

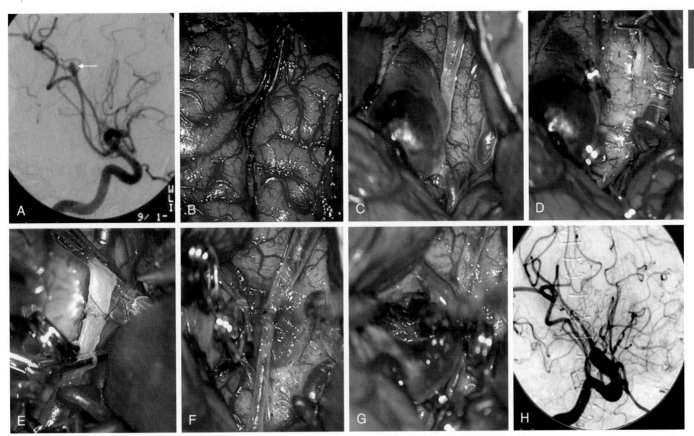

Figure 13-3. Reanastomosis. **A,** Digital subtraction angiogram (right internal carotid injection, lateral view) showed a distal middle cerebral artery aneurysm. After opening the distal Sylvian fissure (**B**), this large thrombotic aneurysm was exposed (**C**). The aneurysm was trapped between two permanent clips (**D**), and the afferent and efferent arteries were joined with an end-to-end anastomosis (**E**) to re-establish blood flow (**F**). **G,** Intraluminal thrombus prevented direct clipping. **H,** Postoperative angiography (right internal carotid injection, lateral view) confirmed exclusion of the aneurysm and preservation of angular branches.

(Adapted from Sanai N, Zador Z, Lawton MT: Bypass surgery for complex brain aneurysms: an assessment of intracranial-intracranial bypass, Neurosurgery 2009;65:670–683.)

Selection of the Microsurgical Corridor

As can be expected, surgical approach depends on aneurysm location (see Table 13–2). ICA aneurysms are approached through a pterional craniotomy in most cases, with an orbitozygomatic craniotomy used for additional exposure with giant aneurysms. Similarly, a pterional craniotomy is adequate for most MCA aneurysms, with an orbitozygomatic craniotomy used with two giant aneurysms. ACA aneurysms are exposed through bifrontal craniotomies to access the interhemispheric fissure, with the midline of the head positioned parallel to the floor and angled up 45 degrees to allow gravity to retract the dependent hemisphere. All bypasses for basilar apex aneurysms are performed through orbitozygomatic craniotomies, capitalizing on its additional trans-Sylvian exposure for these deep bypasses. The VA-SCA bypass for basilar trunk aneurysms is performed through a combined far lateral-subtemporal craniotomy. PICA bypasses are performed through far lateral craniotomies, although the PICA-PICA bypass does not require extensive resection of the occipital condyle or much lateral exposure when performed without accessing the aneurysm, as with a staged endovascular occlusion (three patients).

Selection of the Bypass

Aneurysm location influenced bypass design. In our institutional experience, 31 of 33 patients with ICA aneurysms underwent EC-IC bypass. EC-IC bypasses are preferable and easier than IC-IC bypasses for these aneurysms at the skull base with limited proximal donor sites intracranially. The petrous-to-supraclinoid ICA bypass is the only IC-IC bypass used for ICA aneurysms. Similarly, nine of 14 aneurysms involving the basilar artery apex or trunk were managed with EC-IC bypass because of their deep location and limited proximal donor sites. IC-IC bypasses for basilar artery aneurysms include MCA-PCA bypass with radial artery grafts, VA-SCA bypass, and ATA-SCA reimplantation. In contrast to ICA and basilar artery aneurysms, ACA and PICA aneurysms are revascularized exclusively with IC-IC bypasses. The distal ACA territory is far removed from extracranial donor arteries in the neck, making IC-IC bypasses more appealing. IC-IC bypass options were numerous with PICA aneurysms and eliminated the tedious dissection required to harvest the occipital artery. Bypasses for MCA aneurysms are typically split between EC-IC and IC-IC bypasses.

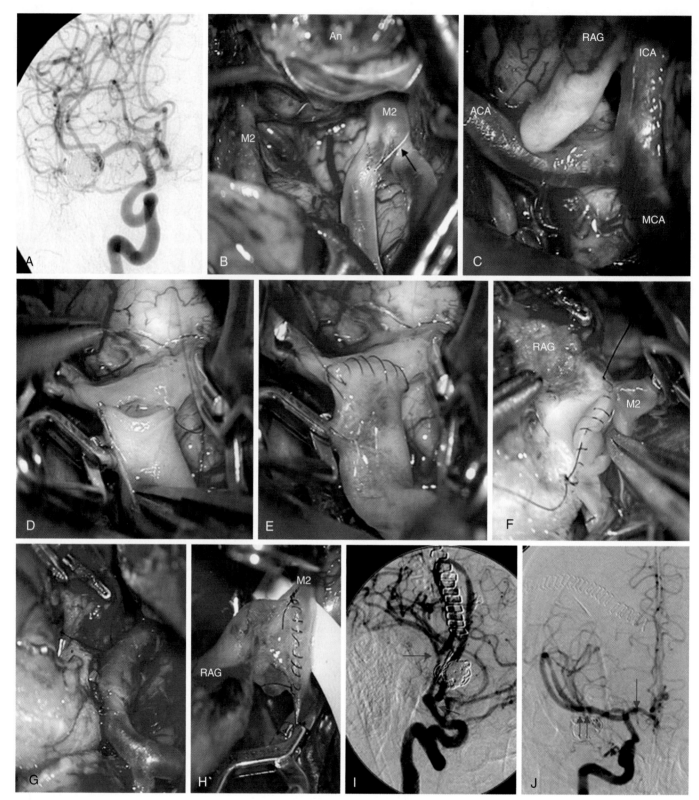

Figure 13–4. Intracranial bypass graft with double reimplantation. **A,** This ruptured right MCA aneurysm was coiled, and recurred 6 months later (right ICA angiogram, anterior oblique view). **B,** Intraoperatively, the two M2 MCA trunks originated from the aneurysm (An) base and could not be kept open with direct clipping. Note the strand of coil in the lumen of the temporal M2 trunk (*arrow*). **C,** The A1 segment of the ACA was used as the donor for a radial artery graft (RAG) that was sutured with an end-to-side anastomosis (**D** and **E**). The frontal M2 trunk was reimplanted onto the RAG with a side-to-side anastomosis: (**F**) shown after suturing the deep suture line intraluminally and (**G**) after completing the superficial suture line. **H,** The end of the RAG was looped to the temporal M2 trunk and sewn with an end-to-side anastomosis. Postoperative angiography (right ICA injection, lateral [**I**] and anterior-posterior views [**J**]) confirmed patency of the bypass and filling of both MCA trunks (*arrows* indicate anastomoses).

(Adapted from Sanai N, Zador Z, Lawton MT: Bypass surgery for complex brain aneurysms: an assessment of intracranial-intracranial bypass, Neurosurgery 2009;65:670–683.)

13

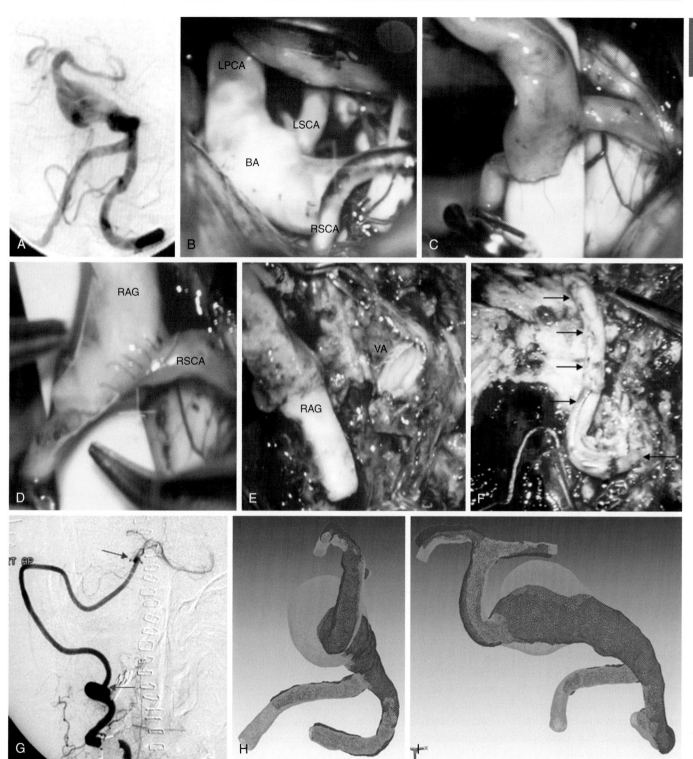

Figure 13–5. Intracranial bypass graft. **A,** This fusiform, giant basilar trunk aneurysm (left VA angiogram, anterior oblique view) was treated with a VA-SCA bypass. **B,** A combined far lateral-temporal craniotomy provided a subtemporal view of the basilar artery (BA) apex. **C** and **D,** A RAG was anastomosed to the right SCA. **E,** The proximal end of the graft was connected to the side of extradural VA at the foramen magnum. **F,** The course of the VA-SCA bypass is shown intraoperatively (*arrows*) and (**G**) angiographically (right VA injection, anterior-posterior view, with anastomoses indicated by the *arrows*). VA-SCA bypass and clip occlusion of the right VA resulted in thrombosis of the aneurysm lumen, shown preoperatively in blue and postoperatively in red on overlaid volumetric images generated from contrast-enhanced magnetic resonance angiography: lateral view (**H**) and anterior-posterior view (**I**).

(Adapted from Sanai N, Zador Z, Lawton MT: Bypass surgery for complex brain aneurysms: an assessment of intracranial-intracranial bypass, Neurosurgery 2009;65:670–683.)

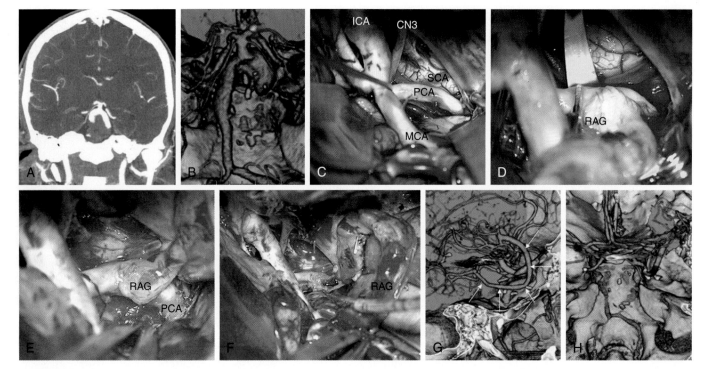

Figure 13–6. Intracranial bypass graft. An MCA-PCA bypass was used to treat this fusiform, giant basilar trunk aneurysm seen on coronal reformatted computed tomography angiogram (**A**) and three-dimensional reconstruction (**B**). Note the large amount of intraluminal thrombus and filling defect. **C,** The recipient PCA was accessed through a trans-Sylvian, pretemporal exposure. **D** and **E,** A radial artery graft (RAG) was connected with end-to-side anastomosis. **F,** The distal end of the RAG was connected to a donor M2 MCA branch, after which the basilar artery was clip occluded below the SCA, distal to the aneurysm. **G,** Postoperative CTA demonstrated patency of the bypass graft (*white arrows*). **H,** Thrombosis of the aneurysm below the clip. ICA, internal carotid artery; CN3, cranial nerve 3.

(*Adapted from Sanai N, Zador Z, Lawton MT: Bypass surgery for complex brain aneurysms: an assessment of intracranial-intracranial bypass, Neurosurgery 2009;65:670–683.*)

Intraoperative Considerations

Brain relaxation is achieved with mannitol (1 g/kg) and cerebrospinal fluid drainage through a ventriculostomy, fenestration in the lamina terminalis, or dissection into a subarachnoid cistern. During the anastomosis, when parent arteries are temporarily occluded, mild hypothermia and barbiturate-induced electroencephalographic burst suppression can be used to increase tolerance to cerebral ischemia. In our experience, the average intracranial cross-clamp time for EC-IC bypass was 46 minutes (range, 32–63 minutes), and for IC-IC bypass was also 46 minutes (range, 26–76 minutes). Blood pressure was increased with pressor agents during this time if changes in somatosensory evoked potentials or the electroencephalogram were detected, but electrophysiological changes were rarely encountered. Heparin irrigation is used liberally in the surgical field during the anastomosis, but systemic heparin is not used.

The University of California, San Francisco Bypass Experience

In our institutional experience, of the 82 patients with aneurysms requiring a bypass, 47 patients (57%) received EC-IC bypasses and 35 patients (43%) received IC-IC bypasses.[24] EC-

IC bypasses included 16 low-flow bypasses with STA donors in 15 patients and OA donor in one patient (Table 13–3). High-flow EC-IC bypasses were performed in 31 patients using saphenous vein grafts in 27 patients and radial artery grafts in four patients. IC-IC bypasses consisted of in situ bypasses in nine patients (26%), reimplantation in six patients (17%), reanastomosis in 11 patients (31%), and intracranial bypass grafts in nine patients (26%) (Table 13–4). Unlike extracranial bypass grafts, intracranial bypass grafts used radial artery more frequently than saphenous vein (six patients vs. three patients, respectively). Seven patients had complex bypass configurations like double reimplantations or additional STA-MCA bypasses (Table 13–5), of which five were categorized as IC-IC bypass patients and two as EC-IC bypass patients.

Aneurysm occlusion was performed during the surgery in 54 patients and consisted of 27 aneurysm trappings (33%), 16 proximal aneurysm occlusions (20%), six distal aneurysm occlusions (7%), and five aneurysm clippings (6%) (Tables 13–6 and 13–7). The remaining 28 patients (34%) underwent staged endovascular occlusion of their aneurysms. Twenty-two of these endovascularly treated patients were in the EC-IC bypass group, reflecting the large number of ICA aneurysms. In contrast, half of the aneurysms in the IC-IC bypass group were trapped during surgery, reflecting the accessibility of these more distally located aneurysms. The small number of aneurysms clipped

Table 13–3. DISTRIBUTION OF OPERATIVE APPROACHES.

ANEURYSM	Pterional	Orbitozygomatic	Bifrontal	Far Lateral	Torcular	Combined	Total
ICA	29	4	0	0	0	0	33
MCA	14	2	0	0	0	0	16
ACA	0	1	5	0	0	0	6
BASILAR APEX	0	11	0	0	1	2	14
PICA	0	0	0	13	0	0	13
TOTAL	43	18	5	13	1	2	82

ICA, internal carotid artery; MCA, middle cerebral artery; ACA, anterior cerebral artery; PICA, posterior inferior cerebellar artery.

Table 13–4. EC-IC BYPASSES.

Technique	Patients	Graft	Flow	Anastomosis	Technique
LOW-FLOW BYPASS					
STA-MCA	9	No	Low	1	E-S
STA-PCA	3	No	Low	1	E-S
STA-SCA	3	No	Low	1	E-S
STA-AICA	0	No	Low	1	E-S
OA-PCA	1	No	Low	1	E-S
OA-PICA	0	No	Low	1	E-S
HIGH-FLOW BYPASS					
CCA-MCA	6	Yes	High	2	E-S
ECA-MCA	16	Yes	High	2	E-S, E-E
ICA-MCA	5	Yes	High	2	E-S, E-E
Sublavian-MCA	3	Yes	High	2	E-S
CCA-PCA/SCA	0	Yes	High	2	E-S
ECA-PCA/SCA	1	Yes	High	2	E-S, E-E
ICA-PCA/SCA	0	Yes	High	2	E-S, E-E

STA, superficial temporal artery; OA, occipital artery; CCA, common carotid artery; ICA, internal carotid artery; ECA, external carotid artery; MCA, middle cerebral artery; PCA, posterior cerebral artery; SCA, superior cerebellar artery; AICA, anterior inferior cerebellar artery; PICA, posterior inferior cerebellar artery; E-S, end-to-side; E-E, end-to-end.

directly reflects the nonsaccular morphology of these aneurysms. Endovascular staging was typically performed 2 to 3 days after the bypass procedure. Patients were started on aspirin (350 mg qd) immediately after surgery.

Angiography was performed after surgery in all patients to evaluate patency of the bypass and exclusion of the aneurysm. Overall, 80 of 82 aneurysms treated with a bypass were obliterated angiographically (97.6% obliteration rate). All four clipped and 26 trapped aneurysms were completely excluded. Of the 15 aneurysms that were proximally occluded, 14 were angiographically occluded postoperatively. Of the five aneurysms that were distally occluded, four were angiographically occluded postoperatively. Two fusiform aneurysms were filling angiographically after surgery, but had new intraluminal

thrombosis, smaller angiographic size, and reduced flow. The 28 aneurysms that were treated with staged endovascular therapy were completely occluded, 16 of them with coils and 12 with proximal balloons. All six aneurysms with IC-IC bypasses were treated with direct coil occlusion, whereas only nine of 21 aneurysms with EC-IC bypasses were treated with direct coil occlusion. Aneurysm obliteration was comparable in the EC-IC and IC-IC bypass groups (97.9% and 97.1%, respectively).

Overall, 75 of 82 bypasses were patent on postoperative angiography (91%). Three EC-IC bypasses and four IC-IC bypasses occluded, with comparable patency rates in the two groups (94% and 89%, respectively). Intraoperative events predicted later occlusion in four cases. Two bypass grafts from the cervical carotid to MCA became limp at the end of the cases and both bypasses were revised (one proximally, and one proximally and distally). One patient with a gunshot-related dissecting ACA aneurysm had damaged parent arteries that were reanastomosed after aneurysm excision. The initial repair occluded, the parent artery was excised back to more normal tissue, and the anastomosis was revised, albeit under increased tension. One MCA thrombosed after clipping of a large M1 segment aneurysm. The aneurysm was excised, the M1 segment was thrombectomized, and reanastomosis restored MCA flow. Despite intraoperative recognition of bypass occlusion and immediate revision in these four cases, the bypasses occluded postoperatively. The remaining three bypass occlusions were unexpected. One of these patients had a saphenous vein with significant varicosities, and one MCA reanastomosis required an STA interposition graft to bridge the gap in the parent artery.

Three patients died in the perioperative period (surgical mortality, 3.7%), all of them with basilar trunk aneurysms. These patients underwent uncomplicated bypass procedures to revascularize the upper basilar artery (STA-SCA, STA-PCA, and ECA-SCA), but subsequent endovascular therapy resulted in aneurysm re-rupture during coiling, basilar artery thrombosis after bilateral vertebral artery occlusions, and intracerebral hemorrhage while on heparin after bilateral vertebral artery occlusions.

Permanent neurological morbidity was observed in four patients (4.9%), all related to bypass occlusions. These patients suffered MCA strokes after occlusion of high-flow EC-IC bypasses in three patients and an MCA reanastomosis

Table 13–5. IC-IC BYPASSES.

IN SITU BYPASS	Technique	Patients	Graft	Flow	Anastomosis	Technique
	ATA-MCA	1	No	Low	1	S-S
	MCA-MCA	1	No	Low	1	S-S
	ACA-ACA	2	No	Low	1	S-S
	PCA-SCA	0	No	Low	1	S-S
	PICA-PICA	5	No	Low	1	S-S
REIMPLANTATION						
	MCA-MCA	1	No	Low	1	E-S
	PC-CM	1	No	Low	1	E-S
	ATA-SCA	1	No	Low	1	E-S
	PICA-VA	3	No	Low	1	E-S
REANASTOMOSIS						
	MCA	5	No	Low	1	E-E
	ACA	1	No	Low	1	E-E
	PICA	5	No	Low	1	E-E
IC BYPASS GRAFT						
	Petrous-supraclinoid ICA	2	Yes	High	2	E-S
	ICA-MCA	0	Yes	High	2	E-S
	ACA-MCA	1	Yes	High	2	E-S
	MCA-ACA	1	Yes	High	2	E-S
	ACA-ACA	1	Yes	High	2	E-S
	MCA-PCA	2	Yes	High	2	E-S
	VA-SCA	2	Yes	High	2	E-S

ICA, internal carotid artery; ATA, anterior temporal artery; ACA, anterior cerebral artery; MCA, middle cerebral artery; PCA, posterior cerebral artery; SCA, superior cerebellar artery; AICA, anterior inferior cerebellar artery; PICA, posterior inferior cerebellar artery; VA, vertebral artery; PC, pericallosal artery; CM, callosomarginal artery; E-S, end-to-side; E-E, end-to-end.

Table 13–6. COMPLEX BYPASS TECHNIQUES.

DOUBLE REIMPLANTATION		EC-IC Bypass Group	IC-IC Bypass Group
	ECA-MCA-MCA	1	0
	ACA-MCA-MCA	0	1
	ACA-PC-CM	0	1
IC-IC PLUS EC-IC			
	MCA-MCA Reanast + STA-MCA	0	1
	ATA-MCA + STA-MCA	0	1
REANASTOMOSIS WITH INTERPOSITION STA			
	MCA-STA-MCA	0	1
DOUBLE EC-IC			
	STA-MCA, double barrel	1	0

in one patient. Two other bypass occlusions (after aneurysm excision and reanastomosis) did not cause any permanent neurological deficits, and one bypass occlusion caused only transient neurological deficits. In addition to this patient with transient neurological deficits related to bypass occlusion, three patients had postoperative epidural hematomas with deficits that resolved completely (transient neurological morbidity, 4.9%).

Excluding the three surgical mortalities and three additional patients lost to follow-up, final neurological outcomes

Table 13–7. OPERATIVE AND CLINICAL OUTCOMES FOLLOWING EC-IC AND IC-IC BYPASS.

		Total		EC-IC Bypass		IC-IC Bypass	
BYPASSED ANEURYSMS		82		47		35	
ANEURYSM OCCLUSION							
	Clipping	5	6%	2	4%	3	9%
	Trapping	27	33%	10	21%	17	49%
	Proximal occlusion	16	20%	11	23%	5	14%
	Distal occlusion	6	7%	2	4%	4	11%
	Endovascular occlusion	28	34%	22	47%	6	17%
ANEURYSM OBLITERATION		80	98%	46	98%	34	97%
BYPASS PATENCY		75	91%	44	94%	31	89%
PATIENTS		82		47		35	
SURGICAL MORTALITY		3	4%	3	6%	0	0%
TRANSIENT NEUROLOGICAL MORBIDITY		4	5%	1	2%	3	9%
LATE OUTCOME							
	GOS 5	59	78%	34	81%	25	74%
	GOS 4	9	12%	4	10%	5	15%
	GOS 3	4	5%	1	2%	3	9%
	GOS 2	0	0%	0	0%	0	0%
	Dead	4	5%	3	7%	1	3%
	Total	76		42		34	
	Lost	3		2		1	
CHANGE IN GOS AT LATE FOLLOW-UP							
	Improved	15	20%	8	19%	7	21%
	Unchanged	53	70%	28	67%	25	74%
	Worse	4	5%	3	7%	1	3%
	Dead	4	5%	3	7%	1	3%

GOS, Glasgow Outcome Scale.

were assessed in 76 patients (93%). Mean duration of follow-up was 41 months (range, 1–125 months), and did not differ significantly between EC-IC and IC-IC bypass groups (38.6 months and 42.7 months, respectively). Four patients died after hospital discharge, three from complications in rehabilitation and one from delayed growth of a basilar trunk aneurysm with resulting brainstem compression. Three of the four late deaths were in the EC-IC bypass group. Good outcomes (GOS 5 or 4) were measured in 68 patients (90%) overall, and were similar in EC-IC and IC-IC bypass groups (91% and 89%, respectively) (Table 13–7). At late follow-up, 15 patients (20%) were improved and 53 (70%) were unchanged, relative to preoperative neurological condition, excluding lost patients. Changes in outcome by GOS were slightly more favorable in the IC-IC bypass group than the EC-IC bypass group (6% vs. 14% worse or dead in IC-IC vs. EC-IC bypass groups, respectively). Mean final GOS scores reflected a similar trend, with a mean GOS of 4.3 in the EC-IC bypass group and 4.6 in the IC-IC bypass group. Relative to preoperative neurological condition, mean GOS decreased 0.30 in the EC-IC bypass group and increased 0.21 in the IC-IC bypass group.

Conversion of EC-IC to IC-IC

Easy conversion from EC-IC to IC-IC bypass is needed to embrace this progression to intracranial vascular reconstruction. Every current EC-IC bypass can be translated to an IC-IC bypass presented in this clinical experience (Table 13–8). ACA and PICA territories were particularly amenable to intracranial reconstruction, and even though MCA and basilar apex territories were divided between EC-IC and IC-IC techniques, growing experience with A1 ACA-MCA and MCA-PCA bypasses have made them preferred choices for their respective territories.

Selecting a bypass from amongst the four IC-IC techniques depends on aneurysm anatomy, suitability of the donor artery, depth of the surgical field, and type of anastomosis. Fusiform aneurysms lend themselves to reanastomosis because frequently they are distally located away from bifurcations or origins of branch arteries, with one afferent and one efferent artery. The success of an end-to-end repair hinges on the excising aneurysm back to healthy arterial tissue on both ends, and on joining those ends without tension. Mobilizing

Table 13–8. EC-IC TO IC-IC CONVERSION CHART.

	MCA	ACA	Basilar Apex	PICA
EC-IC				
Low-flow bypass	STA-MCA	STA-ACA (bonnet)	STA-PCA/SCA	OA-PICA
High-flow bypass	ECA-MCA	ECA-ACA (bonnet)	ECA-PCA/SCA	
IC-IC				
In situ bypass	MCA-MCA/ATA	ACA-ACA	PCA-SCA	PICA-PICA
Reimplantation	MCA-MCA	PC-CM	ATA-SCA	VA-PICA
Reanastomosis	MCA	ACA		PICA
Intracranial bypass graft	ACA-MCA	MCA-ACA	MCA-PCA	VA-PICA
		ACA-ACA	VA-SCA	

ECA, external carotid artery; ATA, anterior temporal artery; ACA, anterior cerebral artery; MCA, middle cerebral artery; PCA, posterior cerebral artery; SCA, superior cerebellar artery; AICA, anterior inferior cerebellar artery; PICA, posterior inferior cerebellar artery; VA, vertebral artery; PC, pericallosal artery; CM, callosomarginal artery; STA, superficial temporal artery; OA, occipital artery.

redundant artery and resecting trapped aneurysm can help bring the arteries together. If the anatomy is favorable, end-to-end anastomosis is the easiest to do. Tips of the forceps can be held in the lumen to visualize translucent arterial walls and guide the needle through its bites; the number of bites needed to complete the anastomosis is small; and the arteries rotate freely to visualize the two suture lines.

In contrast to fusiform aneurysms, saccular aneurysms occur at bifurcations with two or more efferent arteries and other reconstructive techniques are required. In situ bypass and reimplantation are effective when a saccular aneurysm is obliterated while preserving one of the efferent arteries. For example, the ACA-ACA in situ bypass works when clipping or coiling an ACoA aneurysm sacrifices one A2 ACA. The other patent A2 ACA supplies the distal bypass and restores flow to the opposite ACA. In situ bypasses require a side-to-side anastomosis, which is probably the most difficult anastomosis because the deep suture line is sewn inside the lumen. After approximating the two arteries with sutures at each end of the arteriotomies, the first bite must transition the needle from outside the lumen where the knot is tied, to inside the lumen where the running bites are taken. The neurosurgeon must work between two outer layers of arterial wall, keeping track of four translucent layers. The last bite must transition the needle again from inside to outside the lumen to tie the knot. The arteriotomy length with side-to-side anastomosis should be three times the diameter of the arteries in order to create generous communication between arteries. Therefore, side-to-side anastomoses require more bites than other anastomoses. Tracking all four walls and long suture lines make this a more difficult anastomosis that should be avoided in deep, narrow surgical fields. Side-to-side anastomosis can be performed comfortably in the Sylvian fissure, cisterna magna, and interhemispheric fissure, but it has not been attempted at the depths of the basilar apex. The superficial suture line is performed from outside the lumen and is much easier.

Reimplantation is the other basic reconstructive technique that salvages a branch artery compromised by aneurysm occlusion. An end-to-side anastomosis to the parent artery,

the other efferent artery, or an uninvolved bystander will rescue this branch. PICA-VA reimplantation was the most frequent location for this technique, but it also works well in the MCA and ACA territories (pericallosal to callosomarginal reimplantation). These recipient reimplantations connect the proximal end of a branch to the side of the donor, but donor reimplantations can also connect the distal end of a branch to a recipient artery to rededicate the branch artery to supplying a new vascular territory. For example, the ATA supplies a silent vascular territory, and when reimplanted onto the SCA, it can assume the supply of the SCA or even the basilar apex. The ATA-SCA bypass therefore demonstrates another facet of the reimplantation technique. Technically, end-to-side anastomosis is identical to that used with STA-MCA bypass. A generous arteriotomy is made in the donor (at least two times the diameter of the artery), and the end of the reimplanted recipient is spatulated to cover the arteriotomy. Simple continuous sutures are loosely placed and tightened after all bites have been taken. The site of reimplantation should be selected to make the reimplanted artery as slack as possible because a mobile artery can be shifted from one direction to another to better visualize the two suture lines.

Complex reconstructions are required when multiple efferent arteries are compromised. For example, the double reimplantation technique completely rebuilds a bifurcation with three anastomoses. A radial artery graft is first connected proximally to a donor artery to ready the bypass graft. The first efferent artery is reimplanted on the live graft and blood flow is restored immediately. The second efferent artery is reimplanted distally on the graft, allowing the graft to supply the first reimplanted artery during this second reimplantation. Placement of a temporary clip distal to the first and proximal to the second anastomosis redirects blood flow to the reimplanted trunk while keeping the other surgical site dry. This successive reimplantation of branch artery minimizes ischemia, with temporary occlusion times for each of the efferent arteries equal to the time needed to complete one anastomosis. This double reimplantation technique adapts to triple reimplantation for trifurcated anatomy. Other intracranial bypass grafts replenish cerebral blood flow with fewer anastomoses. For example, the MCA-PCA bypass revascularizes the quadrifurcated anatomy of the basilar apex with a single deep anastomosis. The superficial anastomosis site is already accessible after the exposure of the recipient P2 PCA site. Intracranial bypass grafts like the MCA-PCA bypass do not fully reconstruct the arterial anatomy and may not enable complete exclusion of the aneurysm, but may reverse flow or create more benign hemodynamics inside the aneurysm.

Bypass selection ultimately depends on an intraoperative assessment of the aneurysm and surrounding anatomy. We typically devise a primary bypass strategy, several contingency strategies (Table 13–8), and make preparations for each (like prepping a graft site). At surgery, there may be several viable options (e.g., PICA-PICA bypass and PICA reimplantation), no options (e.g., P3 segment PCA aneurysm), or serendipitous anatomy presenting unexpected options (e.g., ATA-SCA bypass). We select the bypass that facilitates aneurysm occlusion, restores normal blood flow, and is technically most feasible.

Limitations of IC-IC Bypasses

IC-IC bypasses can potentially replace EC-IC bypasses, as intracranial reconstructive techniques represent an evolution of bypass surgery for aneurysms. However, these conclusions are based on our comparative analysis between two groups of patients that are different and highly selected. While IC-IC bypasses can be applied to ACA, PICA, basilar apex aneurysms, and many MCA aneurysms, EC-IC bypasses will remain the preferred choice for petrous, cavernous, and supraclinoid ICA aneurysms because intracranial carotid reconstruction is technically difficult and associated with risks from exposing the petrous ICA (hearing loss, facial weakness, etc.). Therefore, the progression from EC-IC to IC-IC bypass does not encompass all aneurysms. The STA-MCA bypass will forever be a versatile technique and we are not suggesting that it be abandoned.

Seventeen different bypasses have been performed in the course of our clinical experience, indicating that a wide variety of reconstructions can be created. Some bypasses discussed here were not performed, like the PCA-SCA bypass and the petrous ICA-MCA bypass graft. Indications for these bypasses are few and technical demands are high. Other intracranial bypasses, like Spetzler's "figure-8 anastomosis," were not a part of our experience but should be included in menu of IC-IC bypasses. Innovative neurosurgeons will add to this menu over time and we will have a deepening armamentarium of intracranial bypasses for most aneurysms.

Bypass with aneurysm occlusion is a good strategy for managing giant, dolichoectatic, thrombotic, or previously coiled aneurysms because it avoids the unpredictable strategy of thrombectomy with clip reconstruction. It also avoids risky adjuncts like hypothermic circulatory arrest. However, deliberate hemodynamic alteration with bypass and aneurysm occlusion can also be risky and unpredictable. Poor outcomes can be encountered with flow reversal in basilar trunk aneurysms due to basilar

artery thrombosis or occlusion of perforators. Other complications come from heparinization to decelerate aneurysm thrombosis, with subsequent intracranial hemorrhage. Bypass with incomplete aneurysm occlusion relies on some degree of intraluminal aneurysm thrombosis, with unavoidable dangers. This management of basilar trunk aneurysms may not be the best strategy for this difficult disease. We are hopeful that stents or other endovascular devices will offer reconstructive options without open surgery. However, such endovascular therapies are not available presently and will need to be evaluated critically before they replace surgical bypass strategies.

CONCLUSIONS

Despite the added complexity of IC-IC bypasses, the extra effort is justified for several reasons. First, the caliber of extracranial scalp arteries is highly variable and sometimes too diminutive to revascularize an occluded efferent artery. Although scalp arteries can dilate over time to meet demand, they may not be able to restore blood flow immediately. Deep bypasses to midline or paramedian arteries can require 8 cm or more of scalp artery and are often too small at the anastomotic depth to be safe. In contrast, in situ bypass, reanastomosis, and reimplantation techniques use donor arteries that match or exceed the caliber of recipient arteries. Second, EC-IC bypasses that use the cervical carotid artery as a donor require long interposition grafts at the limit of the radial artery graft. Therefore, saphenous veins were used more frequently than radial arteries with our EC-IC bypasses, introducing significant caliber mismatches between the graft and intracranial artery. Longer grafts are also associated with lower patency rates long-term. In contrast, intracranial bypass grafts are shorter and enabled us to use radial artery grafts more frequently. Their smaller caliber closely resembles that of intracranial arteries and enhances the anastomosis. Although late patency rates were not measured in this study, shorter grafts with arterial composition are more likely to remain patent. Third, IC-IC bypasses eliminate cervical incisions, minimizing invasiveness and improving cosmesis. Intracranial bypasses are less vulnerable than EC-IC bypasses to neck torsion, injury, and inadvertent occlusion with external compression. Fourth, IC-IC bypasses eliminate the need to harvest an extracranial donor artery, saving time and tedious effort. Intracranial donor arteries reside in the surgical field that is already dissected, and typically require minimal preparation for the bypass. Finally and importantly, temporarily occluding an intracranial artery for bypass is well tolerated in the territories of most IC-IC bypasses. In situ bypasses and reimplantations require temporary occlusion of two intracranial arteries to perform the anastomosis, instead of just temporarily occluding one recipient artery with a traditional EC-IC bypass. However, neurophysiological changes are rarely encountered during these occlusion times and always resolved with a boost in arterial pressure. In our experience, we have not observed any neurological morbidity related to temporarily occluding an intracranial artery during anastomosis, or related to an intracranial donor artery that would not have been involved in an EC-IC bypass.

In our opinion, these advantages of IC-IC bypass justify their use. They are more technically challenging to perform, but well within the expertise of experienced bypass neurosurgeons. The end result is an array of elegant and more anatomical bypasses that we think represents the next generation of bypass surgery for aneurysms.

REFERENCES

1. Failure of extracranial-intracranial arterial bypass to reduce the risk of ischemic stroke. Results of an international randomized trial. The EC/IC Bypass Study Group, *N Engl J Med* 313:1191–1200, 1985.
2. Auguste KI, Quinones-Hinojosa A, Lawton MT: The tandem bypass: subclavian artery-to-middle cerebral artery bypass with dacron and saphenous vein grafts. Technical case report, *Surg Neurol* 56:164–169, 2001.
3. Ausman JI, Diaz FG: Critique of the extracranial-intracranial bypass study, *Surg Neurol* 26:218–221, 1986.
4. Barnett DW, Barrow DL, Joseph GJ: Combined extracranial-intracranial bypass and intraoperative balloon occlusion for the treatment of intracavernous and proximal carotid artery aneurysms, *Neurosurgery* 35:92–97, 1994; discussion 97–98.
5. Barnett HJ, Sackett D, Taylor DW, et al: Are the results of the extracranial-intracranial bypass trial generalizable? *N Engl J Med* 316:820–824, 1987.
6. Baskaya MK, Kiehn MW, Ahmed AS, et al: Alternative vascular graft for extracranial-intracranial bypass surgery: descending branch of the lateral circumflex femoral artery, *Neurosurg Focus* 24:E8, 2008.
7. Bederson JB, Spetzler RF: Anastomosis of the anterior temporal artery to a secondary trunk of the middle cerebral artery for treatment of a giant M1 segment aneurysm. Case report, *J Neurosurg* 76:863–866, 1992.
8. Candon E, Marty-Ane C, Pieuchot P, et al: Cervical-to-petrous internal carotid artery saphenous vein in situ bypass for the treatment of a high cervical dissecting aneurysm: technical case report, *Neurosurgery* 39:863–866, 1996.
9. Evans JJ, Sekhar LN, Rak R, et al: Bypass grafting and revascularization in the management of posterior circulation aneurysms, *Neurosurgery* 55:1036–1049, 2004.
10. Friedman JA, Piepgras DG: Current neurosurgical indications for saphenous vein graft bypass, *Neurosurg Focus* 14:e1, 2003.
11. Goldring S, Zervas N, Langfitt T: The Extracranial-Intracranial Bypass Study. A report of the committee appointed by the American Association of Neurological Surgeons to examine the study, *N Engl J Med* 316:817–820, 1987.
12. Hadeishi H, Yasui N, Okamoto Y: Extracranial-intracranial high-flow bypass using the radial artery between the vertebral and middle cerebral arteries. Technical note, *J Neurosurg* 85:976–979, 1996.
13. Kato Y, Sano H, Imizu S, et al: Surgical strategies for treatment of giant or large intracranial aneurysms: our experience with 139 cases, *Minim Invasive Neurosurg* 46:339–343, 2003.
14. Langer DJ, Van Der Zwan A, Vajkoczy P, et al: Excimer laser-assisted nonocclusive anastomosis. An emerging technology for use in the creation of intracranial-intracranial and extracranial-intracranial cerebral bypass, *Neurosurg Focus* 24:E6, 2008.
15. Lawton MT, Hamilton MG, Morcos JJ, et al: Revascularization and aneurysm surgery: current techniques, indications, and outcome, *Neurosurgery* 38:83–92, 1996; discussion 92–94.
16. Lemole GM Jr, Henn J, Javedan S, et al: Cerebral revascularization performed using posterior inferior cerebellar artery–posterior inferior cerebellar artery bypass. Report of four cases and literature review, *J Neurosurg* 97:219–223, 2002.
17. Mohit AA, Sekhar LN, Natarajan SK, et al: High-flow bypass grafts in the management of complex intracranial aneurysms, *Neurosurgery* 60:ONS105–ONS122, 2007; discussion ONS122–ONS123.
18. Morgan MK, Sekhon LH: Extracranial-intracranial saphenous vein bypass for carotid or vertebral artery dissections: a report of six cases, *J Neurosurg* 80:237–246, 1994.
19. Quinones-Hinojosa A, Du R, Lawton MT: Revascularization with saphenous vein bypasses for complex intracranial aneurysms, *Skull Base* 15:119–132, 2005.
20. Quinones-Hinojosa A, Lawton MT: In situ bypass in the management of complex intracranial aneurysms: technique application in 13 patients, *Neurosurgery* 57:140–145, 2005; discussion 140–145.
21. Regli L, Piepgras DG, Hansen KK: Late patency of long saphenous vein bypass grafts to the anterior and posterior cerebral circulation, *J Neurosurg* 83:806–811, 1995.
22. Relman AS: The extracranial-intracranial arterial bypass study: what have we learned? *N Engl J Med* 316:809–810, 1987.
23. Rivet DJ, Wanebo JE, Roberts GA, et al: Use of a side branch in a saphenous vein interposition graft for high-flow extracranial-intracranial bypass procedures. Technical note, *J Neurosurg* 103:186–187, 2005.
24. Sanai N, Zador Z, Lawton MT: Bypass surgery for complex brain aneurysms: an assessment of intracranial-intracranial bypass, *Neurosurgery* 65:670–683, 2009; discussion 683.
25. Santoro A, Guidetti G, Dazzi M, et al: Long saphenous-vein grafts for extracranial and intracranial internal carotid aneurysms amenable neither to clipping nor to endovascular treatment, *J Neurosurg Sci* 43:237–250, 1999; discussion 250–251.
26. Sekhar LN, Natarajan SK, Ellenbogen RG, et al: Cerebral revascularization for ischemia, aneurysms, and cranial base tumors, *Neurosurgery* 62:SHC1373–SHC1408, 2008; discussion SHC1408–SHC1410.
27. Sundt TM Jr: Was the international randomized trial of extracranial-intracranial arterial bypass representative of the population at risk? *N Engl J Med* 316:814–816, 1987.
28. Ustun ME, Buyukmumcu M, Ulku CH, et al: Radial artery graft for bypass of the maxillary to proximal middle cerebral artery: an anatomic and technical study, *Neurosurgery* 54:667–670, 2004; discussion 670–671.
29. Yasargil M: Anastomosis between Superficial Temporal Artery and a Branch of the Middle Cerebral Artery, Stuttgart, 1969, Georg Thieme Verlag.
30. Zhang YJ, Barrow DL, Day AL: Extracranial-intracranial vein graft bypass for giant intracranial aneurysm surgery for pediatric patients: two technical case reports, *Neurosurgery* 50:663–668, 2002.

EC-IC BYPASS USING ELANA TECHNIQUE 14

SHAMIK CHAKRABORTY; TRISTAN VAN DOORMAAL;
LEENA KIVIPELTO; DAVID J. LANGER

INTRODUCTION

High-flow EC-IC bypass using transplanted conduits in the form of radial artery and saphenous vein is a high-risk procedure performed infrequently. It is reserved for the treatment of aneurysms emanating from or in tumors in close proximity to large proximal intracranial vessels where vessel sacrifice and cranial blood flow replacement remains the safest treatment option for otherwise highly dangerous pathologies. The operations themselves, however, are also highly morbid in nature due to the risks associated with creating a novel conduit for blood flow from an extracerebral source to an intracerebral target with a transplanted vessel. The risks can be broken down into three categories: graft and attachment, occlusion time and associated maneuvers to protect the brain from ischemia and thrombus, and treatment of the aneurysm or tumor itself. The excimer laser–assisted nonocclusive anastomosis (ELANA) is a device combined with a technique designed to limit the risks associated with the second of these risk categories, or those associated with temporary vessel occlusion.

ELANA represents the results of the ideas and investigation of C. A. F. Tulleken and his group at the University Medical Centre in Utrecht, Holland, and spans a period from 1993 to the present. Their efforts arose partly in response to the EC-IC Bypass Study in the mid-1980s, which had disappointing results regarding the viability of STA-MCA bypasses in treating ischemic patients. Tulleken believed that the results of the study may have been different had the bypasses been more proximal in the circle of Willis with its resultant higher flows. However, making such high-flow bypasses would be problematic in the ischemic patient who was less likely to tolerate the temporary occlusion of the large proximal cerebral arteries while constructing the bypasses. In general, the incidence of perioperative stroke in creating high-flow bypasses is approximately 9.5%.[1–3] Therefore, a nonocclusive method of augmenting flow would be of particular benefit to these patients.

The Utrecht group began to investigate the use of laser technology to develop a nonocclusive method of creating intracranial anastomoses. In the early 1990s, they developed a laser catheter and suction system designed to create a consistent attachment to the artery wall and a more consistent arteriotomy. The addition of a separate small platinum ring that allows the laser catheter to better interface with the recipient wall has led to an efficient system of creating nonocclusive cerebral bypasses. The stages of the development of ELANA have been reviewed in the literature[4] with the first human cases performed in 1993. Minor modifications were made between 1993 and 1995 with the current technique and technology remaining quite stable over the past 15 years with minimal substantive change. This technique has similarly been reviewed previously in the literature.[4] The ELANA system is currently being utilized in primarily three centers in Europe, one in Canada, and four in the United States. This chapter aims to review the ELANA system and technique, examine the data from clinical studies in human cases, and discuss its benefits along with its disadvantages over conventional high-flow bypass techniques while updating current thinking on its future with an eye toward future modifications that may make the technique even more desirable.

TECHNIQUE

The ELANA technique is in actuality a simple modification of the steps involved in conventional conduit transplant bypass. The key difference lies in the intracranial arteriotomy step and the method of suturing the distal anastomosis. In conventional technique, temporary occlusion is performed to create an arteriotomy in the recipient vessel, which is then followed by microsurgically suturing the donor and recipient to one another prior to recirculation. The ELANA technique circumvents the temporary occlusion step by having the operator attach the vessels to one another before the arteriotomy step, thus allowing the arteriotomy to be performed after the anastomosis has already been created. In order to create this arteriotomy, a specialized ELANA catheter and a ring

145

device have been developed to not only create the hole but to remove the flap of vessel wall as well. ELANA is not truly an anastomotic device but rather a laser-assisted hole-making system.

Two unique steps are necessary to create an ELANA anastomosis. First, a platinum ring of 2.6 to 2.8 mm in diameter is attached to the distal part of the donor vessel at a side table by flipping the distal end of the donor around the ring and microsurgically suturing using 4-8 8-O nylon sutures to secure

it in place. Second, following microsurgically attaching the donor/ring construct to the recipient using 8-10 8-O prolene sutures and after the proximal anastomosis has been created, the ELANA catheter is used to create the arteriotomy using an excimer laser energy source with removal of the arterial "flap" using vacuum suction within the catheter (Figures 14–1 and 14–2). The laser catheter is composed of an outer array of laser fibers representing the "cutting" element surrounding an inner core of central suction (see Figure 14–2). The ELANA

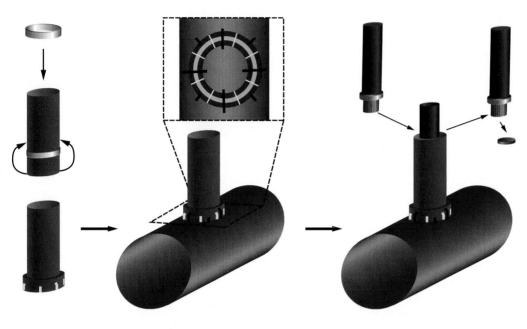

Figure 14–1. Steps of the ELANA arteriotomy system. A platinum ring is attached to the distal part of the donor vessel, which is flipped around the ring and sutured in place using 4-8 8-O nylon. The donor/ring is sutured to the recipient using 8-10 8-O prolene sutures. The ELANA catheter is used to create the arteriotomy with removal of the arterial "flap" using vacuum suction.

(Adapted from figure courtesy Tristan van Doormaal, University Medical Center, Utrecht.)

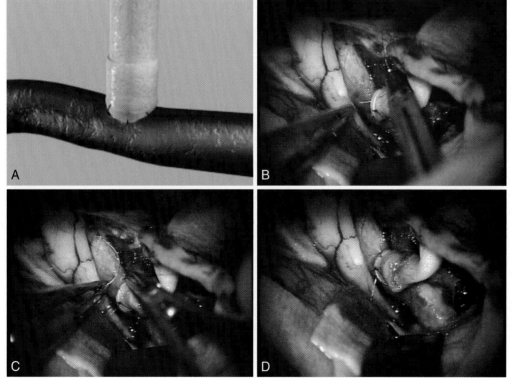

Figure 14–2. A, Computer-generated drawing of the donor/ring complex following anastomosis to recipient artery. **B** to **D,** Intraoperative photographs showing the ring/graft complex being sewn to the ICA wall with eight interrupted microsutures.

(From Langer DJ, Van Der Zwan A, Vajkoczy P, et al., Excimer laser-assisted nonocclusive anastomosis. An emerging technology for use in the creation of intracranial-intracranial and extracranial-intracranial cerebral bypass, Neurosurg Focus 2008;24 (2):E6.)

catheter is passed through the open end of the donor vessel or through a side slit of the donor to the recipient outer wall (Figure 14–3) and after 2 minutes of suction activation, the laser is activated for two to three 10-second bursts to create the arteriotomy. After the arteriotomy has been made, the catheter is withdrawn with the arterial flap attached to the central suction core (Figure 14–4).

Once the laser step has been completed, a temporary clip is placed just proximal to the anastomosis on the donor side. This prevents back bleeding through the proximal open end of the donor graft or through the side slit (Figure 14–5). Bypasses can be created in a single-piece or two-piece fashion. A one-piece graft is the same as conventional except for the creation of a temporary side slit in the donor to allow catheter access to the anastomosis. A two-piece graft can also be performed with the distal portion of the donor sewn to the proximal portion, which is attached to an extracranial carotid source (Figures 14–6 and 14–7). ELANA can also be used to create novel IC-IC bypasses where the proximal donor source is an intracranial vessel such as A1, M1, or the internal carotid, and the distal target is to nearly any target vessel of sufficient caliber. The proximal arteriotomy is made using ELANA, while the distal arteriotomy is created using ELANA or conventional technique.

The ELANA technique thus allows creation of an EC-IC or novel IC-IC bypass throughout the cerebral vasculature in a nonocclusive fashion. The nonocclusive nature of ELANA allows conventional types of bypasses to be performed without flow arrest, arguably improving safety while also offering options in cases too high risk to bypass using conventional occlusive techniques due to concerns regarding temporary occlusion time.

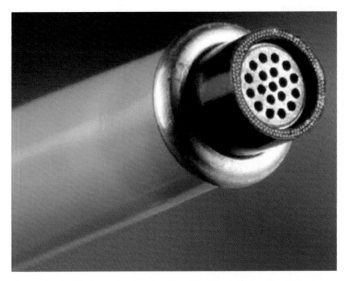

Figure 14–3. Photograph showing the ELANA catheter tip. Note inner suction surrounded by outer laser array.

(From Langer DJ, Van Der Zwan A, Vajkoczy P, et al., Excimer laser-assisted nonocclusive anastomosis. An emerging technology for use in the creation of intracranial-intracranial and extracranial-intracranial cerebral bypass, Neurosurg Focus 2008;24(2):E6.)

Figure 14–4. A, Cutting a side slit on the distal end of the graft vessel. **B,** Insertion of a catheter through the slit. **C,** View of the catheter flush against the distal end of the ring/donor graft complex. **D,** Intra-operative picture of the ELANA catheter inserted through side slit.

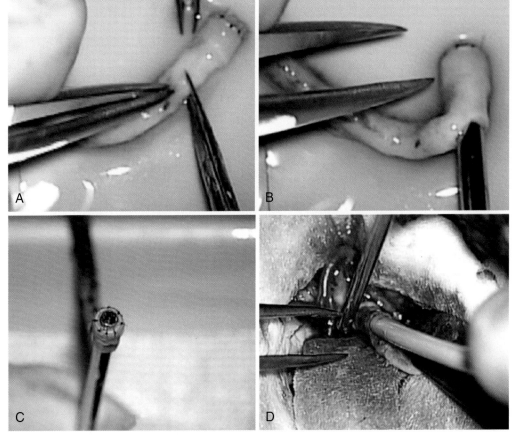

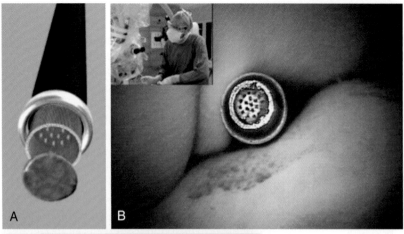

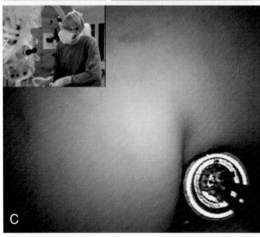

Figure 14–5. A, Computer-generated drawing of the retrieved arteriotomy flap at the tip of the laser catheter. Intraoperative photographs showing the arterial wall flap, which is seen attached to the catheter tip (**B**) and removed (**C**).

(From Langer DJ, Van Der Zwan A, Vajkoczy P, et al., Excimer laser-assisted nonocclusive anastomosis. An emerging technology for use in the creation of intracranial-intracranial and extracranial-intracranial cerebral bypass, Neurosurg Focus 2008;24(2):E6.)

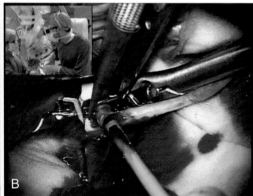

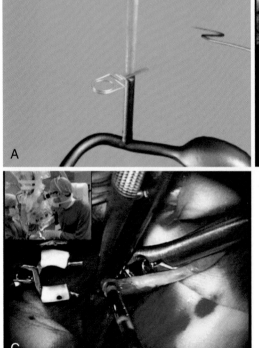

Figure 14–6. A, Computer-generated drawing showing removal of catheter following arteriotomy, with a temporary clip applied to the donor vessel to prevent back bleeding. **B,** Intraoperative photograph showing a silicone tube–covered fenestrated clip used to hold the vein graft around the catheter. The clip is removed prior to withdrawal of the catheter. **C,** The laser catheter is then withdrawn and a temporary clip is placed on the graft.

(From Langer DJ, Van Der Zwan A, Vajkoczy P, et al., Excimer laser-assisted nonocclusive anastomosis. An emerging technology for use in the creation of intracranial-intracranial and extracranial-intracranial cerebral bypass, Neurosurg Focus 2008;24(2):E6.)

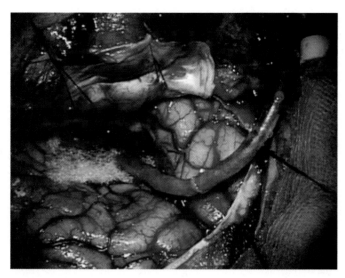

Figure 14–7. Intraoperative photograph taken after the side slit of the vein graft has been closed with a continuous suture, the temporary clips are removed, and the bypass is opened. The proximal anastomosis in the ECA has been completed before the lasering step is performed.

(From Langer DJ, Van Der Zwan A, Vajkoczy P, et al. Excimer laser-assisted nonocclusive anastomosis. An emerging technology for use in the creation of intracranial-intracranial and extracranial-intracranial cerebral bypass, Neurosurg Focus 2008;24(2):E6.)

Patient Selection and Use

Between 1993 and 2008 in Utrecht, Holland, 252 patients (116 male and 136 female) were treated using the ELANA technique. There were 318 anastomoses made creating 255 bypasses over the course of 277 surgeries. Of these patients, 170 of the patients presented with an aneurysm not suitable for coil embolization or clip ligation. EC-IC or IC-IC bypass with the ELANA technique was used as protection to treat the aneurysm by subsequent direct trapping or via endovascular means. Similarly, 71 patients were treated for prevention of stroke or TIAs due to ICA occlusion. Ten patients required ELANA bypass due to a tumor affecting a major artery, and one patient was treated for an ICA malformation unsuitable for endovascular surgery.

Although most patients with aneurysms were selected for the ELANA bypass following failure of a balloon test occlusion (BTO), early in the ELANA experience this was not the case. BTO failure indicates an increased risk for ischemia if patients undergo conventional bypass with temporary occlusion. It also indicates the extent of collateral flow in patients, an important piece of information as collateral flow may shunt blood away from a bypass, leading to subsequent bypass occlusion. Therefore, patients who have insufficient collateralization of cerebral blood flow would benefit most from having ELANA bypass.

Neuroprotective Considerations

To create most high-flow bypasses, the donor or recipient vessels must be temporarily occluded to allow for the construction of the anastomoses. Creating high-flow bypasses in the presence of inadequate collateral blood flow has a high morbidity rate due to the need for prolonged temporary clipping during the creation of the anastomosis. These patients are at high risk for ischemia and subsequent cerebral infarction due to the high occlusion times necessary for this complex procedure.[5,6] Ogilvy et al.[7] demonstrated that the risk for cerebral infarction increases when temporary occlusion exceeds 20 minutes. In high-flow bypass surgery, occlusion times can be up to 45 to 60 minutes and require neuroprotective protocols not often used for most neurosurgical procedures such as moderate to deep hypothermia, pentobarbital administration, and induction of arterial hypertension to prevent ischemia.[5,8–15] These modalities help to protect the brain during temporary occlusion by suppressing metabolic demand and improving nutrient delivery to the brain. However, these protective strategies themselves have been associated with side effects that can contribute to poor outcomes in patients who are already at high risk due to the complexities of cerebral bypass surgery.

ELANA allows for the creation of complex end-to-side, high-flow bypasses without the need for temporary clipping. It minimizes the risk of cerebral ischemia and eliminates time constraints for the construction of the bypass since the vessel stays open throughout and blood flow is uninterrupted. The complex brain-protective strategies that would otherwise be necessary can be avoided. This was confirmed by Muench et al.[5] who were able to successfully treat 29 patients who required high-flow bypasses for treatment of giant aneurysms or tumors. Rather than using brain-protective strategies as noted above, they were able to achieve good results by using standard induction protocols typical of most other intracranial cerebrovascular procedures. They also noted that ELANA allows for less retraction of the brain and less manipulation as compared to conventional bypass techniques, helping to reduce incidence of brain swelling and edema.[1,5]

Large/Giant ICA Aneurysms

The natural history for aneurysms above 1 cm in diameter is grave,[16,17] and they are typically treated aggressively. Direct coil embolization can be unsafe due to the large size and broad neck of the aneurysm. Due to their complex angiographic anatomy, giant aneurysms are not very amenable to endovascular treatment, which results in a complete occlusion rate of 64%, a mortality rate of 9%, and a major morbidity rate of 12.7%.[18] It is thought that cerebral bypass using high-flow anastomoses can assist with the direct surgical treatment of these lesions in order to achieve a higher treatment rate with fewer complications. Van Doormaal et al.[19] reported treating 34 patients with aneurysms of the ICA proximal to the bifurcation. They reported a mean age of 53 years and aneurysm sizes ranging from 10 to 30 mm. Patients presented with symptoms of cranial nerve compression, a history of SAH, or were asymptomatic. All were thought to be at risk of ICA occlusion without the bypass due to failed BTOs or poorly developed collateral vessels on angiography. In all patients, a bypass was constructed between the ECA using a conventional technique, and the intracranial ICA, M1, or A1 segment using the ELANA technique.

The results of the study were favorable: the ICA was occluded by an endovascular procedure postoperatively, or directly ligated intraoperatively, which is done for all patients now. The bypass patency rate was 97%. Two patients died early in the trial during the waiting period between their successful bypass and a subsequent endovascular procedure—one due to an air embolism from a central line, while the other patient had presented with a Hunt and Hess grade IV SAH and died due to aneurysm rupture following a successful bypass. Non-fatal complications involved intraoperative ischemia due to thrombosis of the aneurysm, cranial nerve (CN) deficits due to aneurysm thrombosis, aneurysm hemorrhage before endovascular treatment, and postoperative ischemia due to thrombosis of the bypass. Complications due to aneurysm rupture or thrombosis in the period between bypass and endovascular treatment has been eliminated by directly ligating the ICA immediately following the bypass procedure. Long-term follow-up data is positive, as 79% had a score of 2 or better on the modified Rankin Scale. Cranial nerve recovery was seen in 42% of patients. These results suggest that surgical bypass using ELANA is beneficial when compared with the natural history of large ICA aneurysms and conventional treatment modalities.

Strokes and ICA Occlusions

Ischemic strokes associated with ICA occlusions result in a compromised hemodynamic state and have a risk of recurrent stroke as high as 9% to 18% per year. In patients for whom there are no other treatment options, EC-IC bypass is a consideration. The STA-MCA bypass was not shown to be effective in preventing stroke in patients with symptomatic ICA bypass.[20] The drawback to the EC-IC Bypass Study may be due to lack of control for patients who were not hemodynamically compromised, and that STA-MCA flow may be inadequate. On average, STA-MCA bypass provides 15 to 25 ml/min. More proximal, high-flow bypasses may be able to better protect these patients from future ischemic events. In patients who have undergone cerebral revascularization for treatment of ischemic events in the setting of ICA occlusion, ELANA has been used to establish a high-flow bypass from the ECA to the intracranial ICA, proximal MCA, or ACA. In a smaller subset of patients treated for ICA occlusion with ELANA bypass, there were favorable results, with mean flow rates of 130 ml/min and no symptoms of hyperperfusion.[16] Currently studies are underway to investigate the efficacy of high-flow ELANA bypasses in patients with symptomatic carotid artery occlusive disease. Indeed, ELANA was originally designed to treat such patients and prevent further ischemia resulting from surgical treatment.

Blood Flow in ELANA Bypasses

In general, the mean flow in the ICA is approximately 250 ml/min. Distal branches of the MCA may have flows ranging from 40 to 140 ml/min.[1,3,21] Van der Zwan et al.[1] quantified ELANA bypass flow in 36 patients who underwent high-flow ELANA EC-IC bypass for treatment of giant aneurysms or symptomatic occlusive disease of the ICA. They found that mean bypass flow was 140 ml/min, ranging from 60 to 220 ml/min. This far exceeds common flows through conventional STA-MCA bypasses described in the literature, which range from 15 to 20 ml/min.[3] This is most likely because of the higher caliber of the recipient and graft vessels. The larger the recipient artery is, the larger its peripheral vascular tree; thus, the bypass graft encounters less peripheral resistance. By bringing in higher flow to the proximal circle of Willis, the bypass is able to make a greater contribution to distal cerebral circulation.

Patency of ELANA Bypasses

As the goal of bypass surgery is to provide long-term revascularization, examining the patency of ELANA bypasses as compared to conventional bypasses is necessary. Regli et al.[22] found that EC-IC bypasses using conventional saphenous vein grafts were more likely to occlude when flow was below 50 ml/min, and that the overall patency rate of such conventional bypasses was approximately 86%. Bremmer et al.[23] examined the patency rate of 159 consecutive ELANA bypasses in a prospective study. They found that intraoperative ELANA patency was 95%, and although intraoperative patency predicted long-term patency, the postoperative patency rate of ELANA bypasses was 77%. This may have been due to delayed aneurysm deconstruction, as opposed to immediate intraoperative vessel sacrifice. In addition, a number of the aneurysms bypassed required distal anastomoses at the A2 or M2 segments with somewhat lower flows obtained.[24]

In addition, Bremmer et al.[23] noted that ELANA patency rates were highest in older patients, perhaps because collateral pathways can be more effectively recruited in younger patients. There was an increased risk of occlusion of the bypass in female patients, as female patients tended to have lower bypass flows. The administration of heparin to the patients during the bypass procedure increased intraoperative patency rates, but did not have a significant impact on postoperative patency rates, even though intraoperative patency predicted long-term patency. In addition, intraoperative trapping of the aneurysm improved bypass flows and improved patency rates. ELANA bypass patency rates are best when there is careful patient selection via test occlusion, immediate intraoperative entrapment of the aneurysm, and a patent intraoperative bypass. Intraoperative angiograms and infrared indocyanine green video angiography[25] may assist in checking the patency of the bypass.

ADVANTAGES AND DISADVANTAGES

The ELANA system carries with it some clear advantages as well as disadvantages and its adoption will depend on the valuation of these factors with each individual surgeon.

The biggest single advantage of ELANA over conventional bypass is clearly the lack of temporary occlusion. This permits the operating surgeon to not only perform a high-flow bypass without ischemia time but also allows the creation of bypasses that could not be safely performed with conventional techniques such as bypasses to the ICA, P1, and the basilar artery. Grafting to larger, more proximal recipient vessels may be superior to more peripheral bypass and may provide more physiological inflow.[1] In addition grafting into more proximal vessels such as the ICA or P1 provides more direct high-pressure flow to small perforating vessels as compared to bypasses to M2/3 or P3 in which perforators are more distal from the inflow zone putting them at risk. IC-IC operations such as M1-M2 or M3 as well as ICA to P1 can be more safely performed.[26] By keeping the grafts entirely intracranial, the graft length is reduced with the elimination of a neck incision thus reducing morbidity related to neck dissection, graft compression, and thrombosis.

A second advantage related to the lack of temporary occlusion concerns the maneuvers associated with the act of occluding the recipient vessel. First, no temporary clips are required, permitting a smaller portion of the target vessel to be exposed allowing less brain manipulation and retraction to be required. Lack of temporary clips makes sewing at depth somewhat easier as the loops of suture cannot get caught on the high-profile clips. Second, medical and anesthesia management are simplified. Blood pressure can be maintained without the need to provide pressor support, heparin use is minimized if not completely eliminated, and the use of barbiturates or other forms of cerebral protection is not necessary. Each of these maneuvers incrementally increases the risk of conventional bypass and is not necessary in an ELANA procedure.

The elimination of temporary occlusion also has subjective benefits as well. With ischemia time eliminated, the morbidity related to the temporal aspect of the distal anastomosis is eliminated, improving the surgeons anxiety related to the speed with which one performs deep microsuturing.

There are, however, distinct disadvantages that may affect the adoption of the ELANA technique throughout neurosurgery. First, the ELANA technique adds time to the surgical procedure because of its extra steps. In addition, flap retrieval is not 100%, and at this point hovers around 85% to 90%. Flap retrieval remains a clear technical hurdle that needs to be overcome. The surgical technique can be modified to retrieve a residual flap by incising the donor vessel close to the anastomosis under a short period of temporary occlusion (Figure 14-8). This allows the flap retrieval rate to be close to 100% but increases the technical factors that work against its adoption.

The biggest factors that need to be overcome when considering using ELANA are cost and training versus the perceived

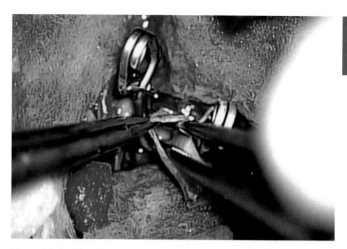

Figure 14–8. Microforceps within the graft to retrieve retained flap. Note temporary clips on the recipient vessel.

benefit to the patient. The ELANA catheter kit costs over $10,000 per use with the laser costs somewhat higher every year. The technical skill required to perform ELANA is no different than that for conventional bypass, but the technique is not straightforward[27] and requires a commitment to laboratory training and mentoring that is time-consuming. These factors would probably play less of a role if high-flow EC-IC and IC-IC were commonly done. Unfortunately, they are rare. The total number of high-flow bypasses performed nationwide probably does not exceed 1000 per year, and in all likelihood this number will continue to erode with the advent of flow-diverter technology. When these factors are balanced against the perceived benefit of a nonocclusive technique, they weigh heavily and clearly work against its adoption. Most bypass surgeons believe that the risk of stroke related to temporary occlusion time is decidedly low or simply is not high enough to warrant the cost and effort of learning a new technique that adds operative time and requires an investment in training. ELANA is clearly the only safe option for patients with aneurysms and tumors on or around vessels that cannot be occluded at all, but these remain a tiny subset of an already small patient group.

THE FUTURE OF ELANA

Currently the disadvantages of ELANA weigh heavily against its broad adoption. However, improvements in design of the ELANA ring may impact its clinical efficacy and eliminate some of these disadvantages. A newly designed ring (Figures 14–9 and 14–10) will potentially permit the creation of a nonocclusive sutureless bypass—sutureless ELANA or SELANA. This improvement will permit the surgeon to perform the distal intracranial and, with modification, the proximal extracranial anastomosis without microsuturing, vastly shortening operative time and making the operation much easier to perform. Studies evaluating the safety and efficacy of SELANA are ongoing in Holland with its clinical introduction expected in 2010.

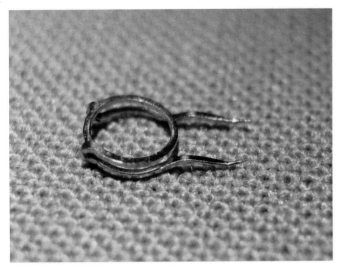

Figure 14–9. Sutureless ELANA ring. Note the prongs that allow for end-to-side grafting of the bypass onto recipient vessel without the need for sutures to anchor the bypass in place.

(Courtesy Tristan van Doormaal, University Medical Center, Utrecht.)

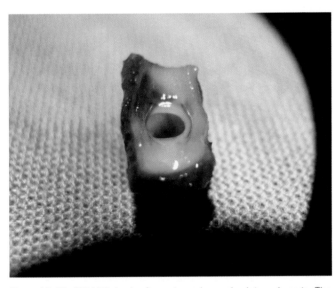

Figure 14–10. SELANA ring/graft anastomosis opening into a pig aorta. The aorta has been incised to allow for a view from within the lumen.

(Courtesy Tristan van Doormaal, University Medical Center, Utrecht.)

CONCLUSION

The ELANA system represents the results of the creativity and vision of its inventor, with clinical data currently proving its safety and efficacy. Hurdles remain to its adoption; however, with continued innovation and research it is likely that the excimer laser–based technique will impact vascular neurosurgery in a novel and significant way.

REFERENCES

1. van der Zwan A, Tulleken CA, Hillen B: Flow quantification of the non-occlusive excimer laser-assisted EC-IC bypass, *Acta Neurochir (Wien)* 143(7):647–654, 2001.
2. Iwai Y, Sekhar LN, Goel A, et al: Vein graft replacement of the distal vertebral artery, *Acta Neurochir (Wien)* 120(1–2):81–87, 1993.
3. Sekhar L, Kalavakonda C: Saphenous vein and radial artery grafts in the management of skill base tumors and aneurysms. In Spetzler RF, Schmiedeck P, eds: *Extra-Intracranial Bypass Surgery*, vol. 2, *Operative Techniques in Neurosurgery*, Philadelphia, 1999, WB Saunders, 129–141.
4. Langer DJ, Vajkoczy P: ELANA: Excimer laser assisted nonocclusive anastomosis for extracranial-to-intracranial and intracranial-to-intracranial bypass: a review, *Skull Base* 15:191–204, 2005.
5. Muench E, Meinhardt J, Schaeffer M, et al: The use of the excimer laser-assisted anastomosis technique alleviates neuroanesthesia during cerebral high-flow revascularization, *J Neurosurg Anesthesiol* 19 (4):273–279, 2007.
6. Samson D, Batjer HH, Bowman G, et al: A clinical study of the parameters and effects of temporary arterial occlusion in the management of intracranial aneurysms, *Neurosurgery* 34(1):22–28, 1994; discussion 28–29.
7. Ogilvy CS, Carter BS, Kaplan S, et al: Temporary vessel occlusion for aneurysm surgery: risk factors for stroke in patients protected by induced hypothermia and hypertension and intravenous mannitol administration, *J Neurosurg* 84(5):785–791, 1996.
8. Lavine SD, Masri LS, Levy ML, et al: Temporary occlusion of the middle cerebral artery in intracranial aneurysm surgery: time limitation and advantage of brain protection, *J Neurosurg* 87(6):817–824, 1997.
9. Spetzler RF, Hadley MN, Rigamonti D, et al: Aneurysms of the basilar artery treated with circulatory arrest, hypothermia, and barbiturate cerebral protection, *J Neurosurg* 68:868–879, 1988.
10. McDermott MW, Durity FA, Borozny M, et al: Temporary vessel occlusion and barbiturate protection in cerebral aneurysm surgery, *Neurosurgery* 25:54–61, 1989; discussion 61–62.
11. Michenfelder JD, Milde JH: Influence of anesthetics on metabolic, functional and pathological responses to regional cerebral ischemia, *Stroke* 6:405–410, 1975.
12. Michenfelder JD, Milde JH: Cerebral protection by anaesthetics during ischaemia (a review), *Resuscitation* 4:219–233, 1975.
13. Michenfelder JD, Milde JH, Sundt TM Jr: Cerebral protection by barbiturate anesthesia. Use after middle cerebral artery occlusion in Java monkeys, *Arch Neurol* 33:345–350, 1976.
14. Shapiro HM: Barbiturates in brain ischaemia, *Br J Anaesth* 57:82–95, 1985.
15. Yatsu FM, Diamond I, Graziano C, et al: Experimental brain ischemia: protection from irreversible damage with a rapid-acting barbiturate (methohexital), *Stroke* 3:726–732, 1972.
16. Langer DJ, Van Der Zwan A, Vajkoczy P, et al: Excimer laser-assisted nonocclusive anastomosis. An emerging technology for use in the creation of intracranial-intracranial and extracranial-intracranial cerebral bypass, *Neurosurg Focus* 24(2):E6, 2008.
17. Tulleken CA, van der Zwan A, van Rooij WJ, et al: High-flow bypass using nonocclusive excimer laser-assisted end-to-side anastomosis of the external carotid artery to the P1 segment of the posterior cerebral artery via the sylvian route. Technical note, *J Neurosurg* 88 (5):925–927, 1998.
18. Parkinson RJ, Eddelman CS, Batjer HH, et al: Giant aneurysms: endovascular challenges, *Neurosurgery* 59(Suppl 5):S103–S112, 2006.
19. van Doormaal TP, van der Zwan A, Verweij BD, et al: Treatment of giant and large internal carotid artery aneurysms with a high-flow replacement bypass using the excimer laser-assisted nonocclusive anastomosis technique, *Neurosurgery* 59(Suppl 4):ONS328–ONS335, 2006.

20. Failure of extracranial-intracranial arterial bypass to reduce the risk of ischemic stroke. Results of an international randomized trial. The EC/IC Bypass Study Group, *N Engl J Med* 313(19):1191–1200, 1985.

21. Charbel FT, Misra M, Clarke ME, et al: Computer simulation of cerebral blood flow in moyamoya and the results of surgical therapies, *Clin Neurol Neurosurg* 99(Suppl 2):S68–S73, 1997.

22. Regli L, Piepgras DG, Hansen KK: Late patency of long saphenous vein bypass grafts to the anterior and posterior cerebral circulation, *J Neurosurg* 83(5):806–811, 1995.

23. Bremmer JP, Verweij BH, Klijn CJ, et al: Predictors of patency of excimer laser-assisted nonocclusive extracranial-to-intracranial bypasses, *J Neurosurg* 110(5):887–895, 2009.

24. Sundt TM Jr, Piepgras DG, Marsh WR, et al: Saphenous vein bypass grafts for giant aneurysms and intracranial occlusive disease, *J Neurosurg* 65(4):439–450, 1986.

25. Woitzik J, Horn P, Vajkoczy P, et al: Intraoperative control of extracranial-intracranial bypass patency by near-infrared indocyanine green videoangiography, *J Neurosurg* 102(4):692–698, 2005.

26. Tulleken CA, Streefkerk HJ, van der Zwan A: Construction of a new posterior communicating artery in a patient with poor posterior fossa circulation: technical case report, *Neurosurgery* 50(2):415–419, 2002; discussion 419–420.

27. Heros RC: Excimer laser-assisted nonocclusive anastomosis, *Neurosurg Focus* 24(2):E6a, 2008; discussion E6a.

MINIMALLY INVASIVE EC-IC BYPASS PROCEDURES AND INTRODUCTION OF THE IMA-MCA BYPASS PROCEDURE

15

SALEEM I. ABDULRAUF; JUSTIN M. SWEENEY;
YEDATHORE S. MOHAN; JEROEN R. COPPENS; JOHN D. CANTADO;
SHERI K. PALEJWALA

EC-IC bypasses are performed for a variety of cerebrovascular and neoplastic intracranial processes. There are two major classes of EC-IC bypasses, low flow and high flow, based on the level of flow that the graft is expected to support. Both classes are extensive procedures requiring large craniotomies and, often, additional lengthy incisions. We present two evolving minimally invasive EC-IC bypass procedures.

MINIMALLY INVASIVE SUPERFICIAL TEMPORAL ARTERY TO MIDDLE CEREBRAL ARTERY BYPASS THROUGH A BUR HOLE

STA-MCA bypasses are established EC-IC bypasses for low to moderate flow cerebral revascularization. A STA-MCA, low-flow, EC-IC bypass traditionally requires a large frontotemporal craniotomy to expose the distal Sylvian fissure for the anastomotic site. We describe a less-invasive procedure using a single 2- to 2.5-cm enlarged bur hole, in place of the standard craniotomy, through which the recipient and donor vessels were identified and the anastomosis performed.[1]

This procedure was performed for multiple patients with recurrent cerebrovascular ischemic episodes. One patient was awake for the procedure, with local anesthesia and propofol sedation, due to his multivessel occlusive disease and compromised vascular reserve, in an effort to avoid general anesthesia-related hypotension. With the aid of a stereotactic neuronavigation system, we minimized the size of the skin incision and the craniotomy such that the procedure could be performed effectively via an enlarged bur hole or small craniotomy (2- to 2.5-cm diameter). A CT angiogram was used preoperatively to select the donor vessel, recipient vessel, and anastomosis site. The STA was visualized, along with its frontal and parietal branches. The diameters of the branches were measured in order to identify the optimal donor vessel (Figure 15–1A). A linear skin incision was then made overlying the donor vessel. Bur hole/craniotomy placement can be planned preoperatively using a stereotactically reconstructed model based on the CT angiogram (Figure 15–1B). The recipient vessel is chosen according to its caliber and superficial location in the Sylvian fissure. The optimal recipient vessel is identified on review of the CT angiogram (Figure 15–1C). The exact location of the bur hole/craniotomy is then planned using CT angiography–based neuronavigation, and overlies the selected recipient vessel in immediate proximity to the chosen donor vessel.

The incision is performed under the microscope where the temporalis muscle is split vertically directly below the selected donor branch of the STA. A bur hole is made and enlarged to the size of a small craniotomy (~2 to 2.5 cm) under the microscope, and then 1 cm of the recipient vessel is exposed in the Sylvian fissure (Figures 15–2 and 15–3). A rubber dam is applied and the anastomosis is performed with a 9-0 nylon suture in a running fashion. The back wall is anastomosed before the front wall. Temporary clips are applied on the recipient vessel, the M4 branch of the MCA, during the anastomosis. Postoperatively, the patients were followed up with angiography or CT angiography, and clinically, disease progression was halted (Figures 15–4 through 15–7).

We were able to successfully perform minimally invasive STA-MCA bypasses with 2- to 2.5-cm craniotomies through the use of preoperative CT angiography neuronavigation. With the use of stereotaxy we were able to limit the size of both the skin incision and the bur hole/craniotomy. We anticipate the widespread incorporation of CT angiography neuronavigation into future STA-MCA bypass procedures.

Since the publication of this minimally invasive procedure, Fischer et al.[2] have described a similar minimally invasive procedure with the use of 3D virtual planning with the Dextroscope and magnetic resonance angiography in place of intraoperative stereotaxy that could serve as an alternative to the technique described above.

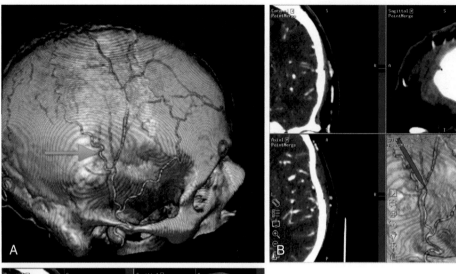

Figure 15–1. A, Image guidance workstation view of three-dimensional reconstruction of CT angiogram showing the donor vessel, parietal branch of STA (*arrow*). **B,** Image guidance workstation axial, coronal, and saggital and three-dimensional reconstruction CT angiogram views showing the preselected bur hole/craniotomy site (red dots). The overlying donor (*arrow*) and recipient vessels are seen on both sides of the bur hole location. **C,** Image guidance workstation axial, coronal, and saggital and three-dimensional reconstruction CT angiogram views showing the MCA recipient vessel in the sylvian fissure (*arrow*).

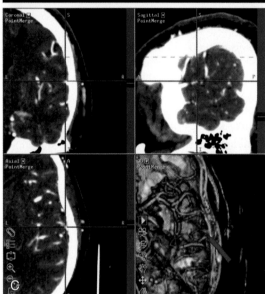

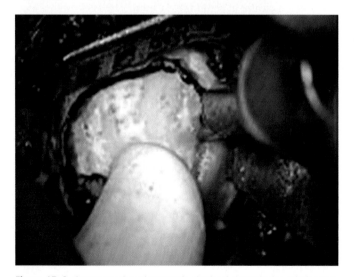

Figure 15–2. Intraoperative photograph obtained through the microscope while the bur hole/craniotomy was being performed.

(From Coppens JR, Cantando JD, Abdulrauf SI, Minimally invasive superficial temporal artery to middle cerebral artery bypass through an enlarged bur hole: the use of computed tomography angiography neuronavigation in surgical planning, J Neurosurg 2008;109(3):553–558, with permission.)

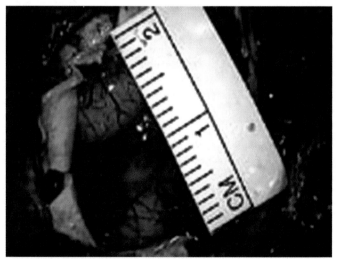

Figure 15–3. Intraoperative photograph obtained through the microscope demonstrating the maximum diameter of the bur hole/craniotomy to be ~2 cm.

(From Coppens JR, Cantando JD, Abdulrauf SI, Minimally invasive superficial temporal artery to middle cerebral artery bypass through an enlarged bur hole: the use of computed tomography angiography neuronavigation in surgical planning, J Neurosurg 2008;109(3):553-558, with permission.)

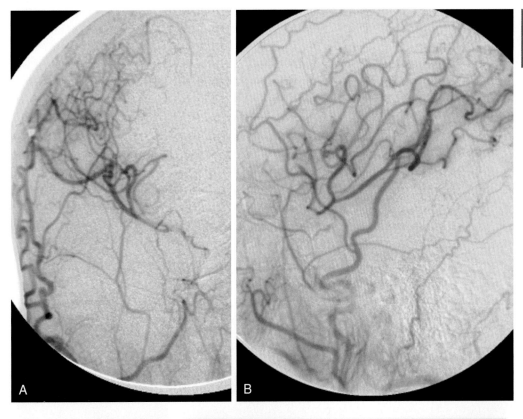

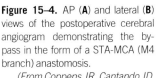

Figure 15–4. AP (**A**) and lateral (**B**) views of the postoperative cerebral angiogram demonstrating the bypass in the form of a STA-MCA (M4 branch) anastomosis.

(From Coppens JR, Cantando JD, Abdulrauf SI, Minimally invasive superficial temporal artery to middle cerebral artery bypass through an enlarged bur hole: the use of computed tomography angiography neuronavigation in surgical planning, J Neurosurg 2008;109(3):553-558, with permission.)

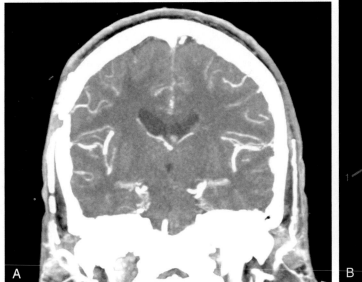

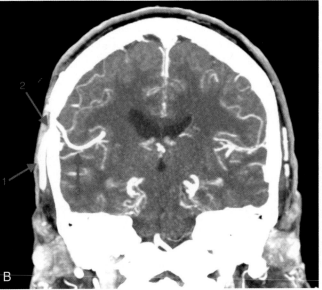

Figure 15–5 A and **B,** Sequential coronal CT angiographies showing the STA-MCA bypass entering through a bur hole (<2.5 cm in size). *Arrow 1* shows the STA, *arrow 2* points toward the bur hole opening, and *arrow 3* indicates the recipient MCA vessel.

MINIMALLY INVASIVE HIGH-FLOW BYPASS TECHNIQUE: INTERNAL MAXILLARY ARTERY TO MIDDLE CEREBRAL ARTERY EC-IC BYPASS

High-flow cerebral revascularization currently requires graft vessel harvesting, cervical incision for the proximal anastomosis, craniotomy for distal anastomosis, and parent vessel occlusion. This conventionally necessitates a large craniotomy and extensive cervical incision. Instead, we illustrate a technique that avoids a long cervical incision and allows for purely intracranial extradural access to the internal maxillary artery (IMAX) to perform a short segment high-flow anastomosis from it to the MCA, using a radial artery graft.[3]

In recent years a number of important variations have been introduced to make the high-flow EC-IC bypasses less invasive. The contributions of C. A. F. Tulleken in devising the non-occlusive, laser-assisted anastomosis have to be

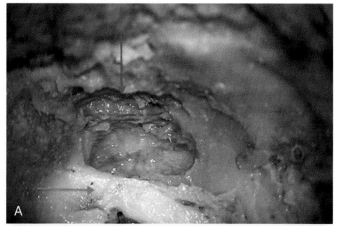

Figure 15–6. A three-dimensional reconstruction of the postoperative CT angiogram demonstrating maturation of the EC-IC bypass.

(From Coppens JR, Cantando JD, Abdulrauf SI, Minimally invasive superficial temporal artery to middle cerebral artery bypass through an enlarged bur hole: the use of computed tomography angiography neuronavigation in surgical planning, J Neurosurg 2008;109(3):553-558, with permission.)

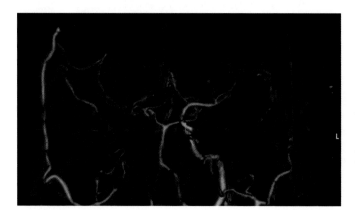

Figure 15–7. CT angiography three-dimensional reconstruction of the STA-MCA bypass using a minimally invasive technique. (Note the right carotid artery occlusion with which the patient presented.)

commended (see Chapter 14). A case report was published using the Cardica C-Port xA Distal Anastomosis System for an automated high-flow bypass. This involves an automated end-to-side anastomosis with simultaneous arteriotomy and insertion of 13 microclips into the graft and recipient vessels. This latter technique however, is very limiting because of the

size and configuration of the device and is unlikely to be used widely due to this important limitation.[4]

In this section we describe our development of the IMAX-MCA bypass technique, which we believe is much less invasive than the standard high-flow EC-IC bypass. Prior to clinical application of our bypass, we performed a series of six adult cadaveric dissections. The IMAX was dissected via a middle fossa extradural approach in the cadaveric specimens in order to confirm the middle fossa surface landmarks, location, and depth of the artery (Figure 15–8). This methodology was subsequently implemented in a clinical case as outlined below.

We drew a straight line extending anteriorly from the V2/V3 apex along the inferior edge of V2. The distance from the V2/V3 apex to the lateral rotundum was 7.8 mm $\pm$ 3.033 mm. The distance from the lateral edge of the foramen rotundum to the medial extent of the IMAX was 8.6 mm $\pm$ 2.074 mm anteriorly. We then drilled to a depth of 4.2 mm $\pm$ 1.304 mm into the greater wing of the sphenoid bone, ultimately exposing an average of 7.8 mm $\pm$ 1.643 mm of the

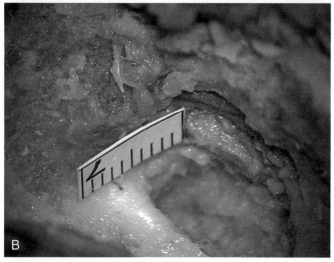

Figure 15–8. A, Cadaveric dissection showing the relationship between IMAX (*red arrow*) and V2 (*blue arrow*), via an extradural, right-sided, middle fossa approach. **B,** Cadaveric dissection showing the distal portion of the IMAX 6 mm lateral to V2.

Table 15-1. MEASUREMENTS WITH MEAN AND STANDARD DEVIATION VALUES OBTAINED FROM CADAVERIC IMAX DISSECTIONS.

Cadaver	V2/V3 Apex to Lateral Rotundum (mm)	Lateral Rotundum to Localization Point (mm)	Depth to Drill (mm)	Length of IMAX Exposed (mm)
1	—	—	4	10
2	10	10	—	—
3	5	6	3	9
4	4	7	6	6
5	10	9	5	7
6	10	11	3	7
Mean	7.8	8.6	4.2	7.8
Standard deviation	3.033	2.074	1.304	1.643

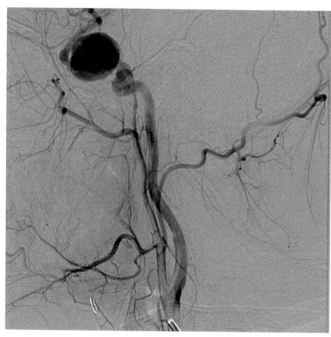

Figure 15-9. Lateral DSA of the common carotid artery of a patient with a giant aneurysm showing the proximity of the IMAX (*arrow*) to the internal carotid artery (ICA) and middle cerebral artery (MCA) for potential interposition grafting.

maxillary artery (Table 15-1). The IMAX was consistently found running just anterior and parallel to a line between the foramina rotundum and ovale.

The high-flow bypass was conducted via an extradural middle fossa approach for a patient with bilateral transitional (cavernous and clinoidal) internal carotid artery (ICA) aneurysms (Figures 15-9 and 15-10). Prior to the procedure, balloon test occlusion (BTO) was performed in order to assess the quality of the collateral vasculature (Figure 15-11). This showed that the collateral system was insufficient to support cerebral perfusion without an EC-IC bypass. Intraoperatively, the anterolateral triangle between V2 and V3 was identified. Using the aforementioned measurements taken in the laboratory, the anterior loop of the IMAX was found just anterior and parallel to a line running between the foramen rotundum

and the foramen ovale. The greater wing of the sphenoid bone was drilled at this location and the anterior loop of the internal maxillary artery was identified.

Simultaneous radial artery harvest was undertaken. Temporary clips were placed on the IMAX (Figure 15-12). An end-to-side anastomosis of the radial artery graft to the IMAX was performed (Figure 15-13), followed by an end-

Figure 15-10. DSA three-dimensional reconstruction of a complex transitional segment ICA aneurysm, AP (**A**) and lateral (**B**) views.

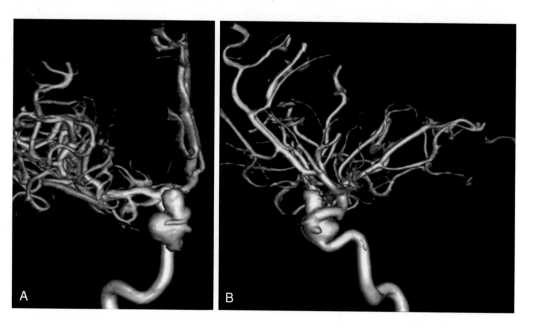

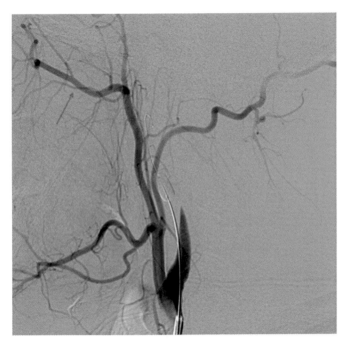

Figure 15–11. Lateral DSA of the common carotid artery during balloon test occlusion (BTO) showing the internal maxillary artery (*arrow*).

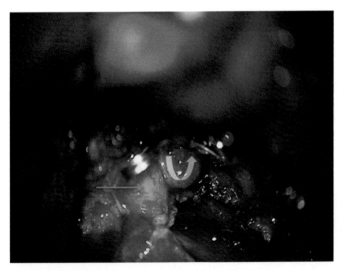

Figure 15–12. Right-sided intraoperative view of the middle fossa extradural approach showing temporary clips on anterior loop of the IMAX (*yellow arrow*), adjacent to V2 (*blue arrow*).

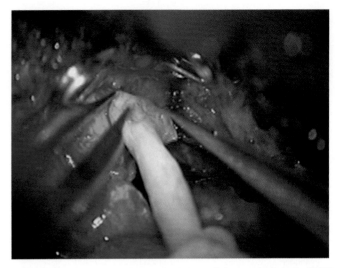

Figure 15–13. Proximal anastomosis of the radial artery graft to the IMAX in the middle fossa extradural space (intraoperative view).

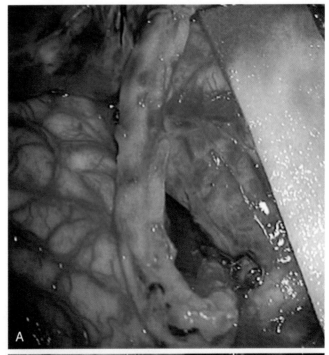

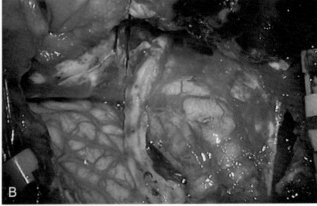

Figure 15–14. A and **B,** Radial artery interposition graft between the IMAX and the M2 segment of the MCA.

to-side anastomosis to the recipient M2 branch within the Sylvian fissure (Figure 15–14). Intraoperative ICG angiography confirmed a patent graft (Figure 15–15). The ICA was occluded both proximally and just distal to the aneurysm in the supraclinoidal segment with aneurysm clips. The proximal clipping of the ICA, in this particular case, required a very small high cervical incision (2 cm) to avoid clipping the ICA within the cavernous segment, which we hope to avoid in future cases.

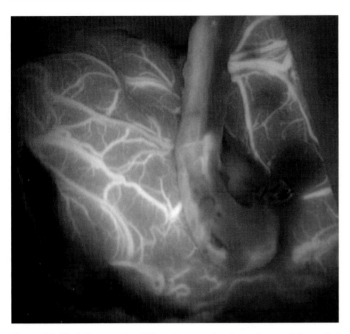

Figure 15–15. Intraoperative ICG angiogram showing patency of the radial artery graft.

Postoperatively, the patient did well, without any new neurological deficits, and underwent formal angiography ensuring graft patency (Figures 15–16 and 15–17). The patient was discharged home on postoperative day 5; at the 3-week follow-up visit she had resumed normal activity without any restrictions.

We successfully used a short segment of the radial artery to connect the IMAX with the MCA in order to circumvent the diseased internal carotid artery in a patient with bilateral giant aneurysms. With use of the IMAX as the donor vessel, we were able to minimize the transverse cervical incision traditionally used to expose the CCA, ICA, and MCA. We anticipate obviating the need for cervical incisions all together in the future.

We believe minimally invasive endeavors and technology will play key roles in the future of EC-IC bypass and cerebral revascularization, in regards to both low- and high-flow procedures.

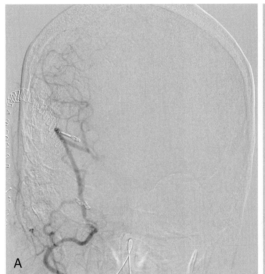

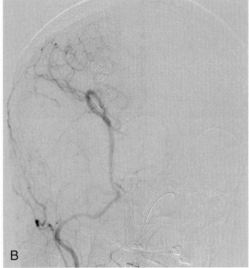

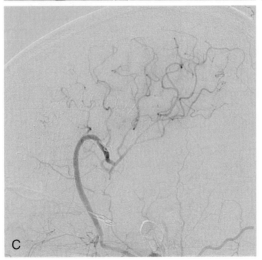

Figure 15–16. Right common carotid artery (CCA) DSA postoperative angiography showing IMAX-MCA bypass using a radial artery graft in AP (**A**), oblique (**B**), and lateral (**C**) views.

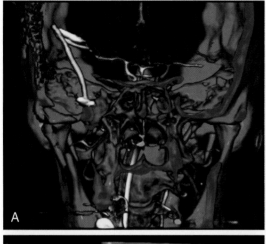
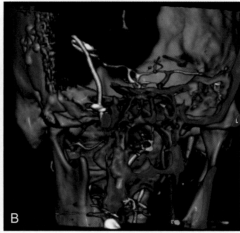
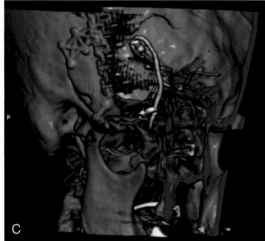

Figure 15–17. Three-dimensional DSA reconstruction of right common carotid artery (CCA) angiography showing a radial artery interposition graft coursing from the floor of the middle fossa to the MCA in AP (**A**), oblique (**B**), and lateral (**C**) views.

REFERENCES

1. Coppens JR, Cantando JD, Abdulrauf SI: Minimally invasive superficial temporal artery to middle cerebral artery bypass through an enlarged bur hole: the use of computed tomography angiography neuronavigation in surgical planning, *J Neurosurg* 109(3):553–558, 2008.
2. Fischer G, Stadie A, Schwandt E, et al: Minimally invasive superficial temporal artery to middle cerebral artery bypass through a minicraniotomy: benefit of three-dimensional virtual reality planning using magnetic resonance angiography, *Neurosurg Focus* 26(5):E20, 2009.
3. Abdulrauf SI, Sweeney JM, Mohan YS, et al: *Short Segment Internal Maxillary Artery to Middle Cerebral Artery Bypass: A Novel Technique for Extracranial-to-Intracranial Bypass,* Saint Louis, MO, 2010, Saint Louis University School of Medicine.
4. Dacey RG Jr, Zipfel GJ, Ashley WW, et al: Automated, compliant, high-flow common carotid to middle cererbal artery bypass, *J Neurosurg* 109:559–564, 2008.

SUGGESTED READING

Abdulrauf SI: Extracranial-to-intracranial bypass using radial artery grafting for complex skull base tumors: technical note, *Skull Base* 15:207–213, 2005.
Arbag H, Cicekcibasi AE, Uysal II, et al: Superficial temporal artery graft for bypass of the maxillary to proximal middle cerebral artery using a transantral approach: an anatomical and technical study, *Acta Otolaryngol* 125(9):999–1003, 2005.

Arbag H, Ustun ME, Buyukmumcu M, et al: A modified technique to bypass the maxillary artery to supraclinoid internal carotid artery by using a radial artery graft: an anatomical study, *J Laryngol Otol* 119(7): 519–523, 2005.
Baron JC, Bousser MG, Rey A, et al: Reversal of focal "misery perfusion syndrome" by extra-intracranial arterial bypass in hemodynamic cerebral ischemia. A case study with 150 positron emission tomography, *Stroke* 12:454–459, 1981.
Buyukmumcu M, Ustun ME, Seker M, et al: Maxillary-to-pertrous internal carotid artery bypass: an anatomical feasibility study, *Surg Radiol Anat* 25(5–6):368–371, 2003.
Charbel FT, Meglio G, Amin-Hanjani S: Superficial temporal artery-to-middle cerebral artery bypass, *Neurosurgery* 56(Suppl 1):186–190, 2005.
Drake CG: Giant intracranial aneurysms: experience with surgical treatment in 174 patients, *Clin Neurosurg* 26:12–95, 1979.
EC/IC Bypass Study Group: Failure of external carotid–internal carotid arterial bypass to reduce the risk of ischemic stroke. Results of an international randomized trial. The EC/IC Bypass Study Group, *N Engl J Med* 313:1191–1200, 1985.
Erickson DL: *Revascularization for the Ischemic Brain,* Armonk, NY, 1988, Futura Publishing.
Grubb RL Jr, Powers WJ, Derdeyn CP, et al: The Carotid Occlusion Surgery Study, *Neurosurg Focus* 14(3):E9, 2003.
Hanjani AS, Butler WE, Ogilvy CS, et al: Extracranial-intracranial bypass in the treatment of occlusive cerebrovascular disease and intracranial aneurysms in the United States between 1992 and 2001: a population-based study, *J Neurosurg* 103(5):794–804, 2005.

Haque R, Kellner C, Soloman RA: Spontaneous thrombosis of a giant fusiform aneurysm following extracranial-intracranial bypass surgery, J Neurosurg 110(3):469–474, 2009.

Hauck EF, Samson D: A1-A2 interposition grafting for surgical treatment of a giant "unclippable" A1 segment aneurysm, Surg Neurol 71(5): 600–603, 2009.

Karabulut AK, Ustun ME, Uysal II, et al: Saphenous vein graft for bypass of the maxillary to supraclinoid internal carotid artery: an anatomical short study, Ann Vasc Surg 15(5):548–552, 2001.

Kikuta KI, Takagi Y, Fushimi Y, et al: "Target bypass": a method for preoperative targeting of a recipient artery in superficial temporal artery-to-middle cerebral artery anastomoses, Neurosurgery 59(Suppl 4): ONS320–ONS327, 2006.

Lawton MT, Hamilton MG, Morcos JJ, et al: Revascularization and aneurysm surgery: current techniques, indications, and outcome, Neurosurgery 38(1):83–92, 1996; discussion 92-4.

Lougheed WM, Marshall BM, Hunter M, et al: Common carotid to intracranial internal carotid bypass venous graft. Technical note, J Neurosurg 56(1):205–215, 1982.

Meyer FB, Bates LM, Goerss SJ, et al: Awake craniotomy for aggressive resection of primary gliomas located in eloquent brain, Mayo Clin Proc 76:677–687, 2001.

Newell DW: Superficial temporal artery to middle cerebral artery bypass, Skull Base 15:133–141, 2005.

Nussbaum ES, Erickson DL: Extracranial-intracranial bypass for ischemic cerebrovascular disease refractory to maximal medical therapy, Neurosurgery 46:37–43, 2000.

O'Shaughnessy BA, Salehi SA, Mindea SA, et al: Selective cerebral revascularization as an adjunct in the treatment of giant anterior circulation aneurysms, Neurosurg Focus 14(3):e4, 2003.

Powers WJ, Martin WRW, Herscovitch P, et al: Extracranial-intracranial bypass surgery: hemodynamic and metabolic effects, Neurology 34:1168–1174, 1984.

Sekhar LN, Duff JM, Kalavakonda C, et al: Cerebral revascularization using radial artery grafts for the treatment of complex intracranial aneurysms: techniques and outcomes for 17 patients, Neurosurgery 49(3): 646–658, 2001; discussion 658-9.

Sundt TM Jr., Piepgras DG, Hansen KK: Saphenous vein bypass grafts for giant aneurysms and intracranial occlusive disease, J Neurosurg 65(4): 439–450, 1986.

Tulleken CA, Verdaasdonk RM, Berendsen W, et al: Use of excimer laser in high-flow bypass surgery of the brain, J Neurosurg 78(3):477–480, 1993.

Ulku CH, Ustun ME, Buyukmumcu M, et al: Radial artery graft for bypass of the maxillary artery to proximal posterior cerebral artery: an anatomical and technical study, Acta Otolaryngol 124(7):858–862, 2004.

Ustun ME, Buyukmumcu M, Ulku CH, et al: Radial artery graft for bypass of the maxillary artery to proximal middle cerebral artery: an anatomic and technical study, Neurosurgery 54(3):667–670, 2004; discussion 670-1.

Vrionis F, Cano W, Heilman CB: Microsurgical anatomy of the infratemporal fossa as viewed laterally and superiorly, Neurosurgery 39(4):777–785, 1996; discussion 785-6.

Wanebo JE, Zabramski JM, Spetzler RF: Superficial temporal artery-to-middle cerebral artery bypass grafting for cerebral revascularization, Neurosurgery 55:395–399, 2004.

Webster MW, Makaroun MS, Steed DL, et al: Compromised cerebral blood flow reactivity is a predictor of stroke in patients with symptomatic carotid artery occlusive disease, J Vasc Surg 21:338–345, 1995.

Yamauchi H, Fukuyama H, Nagahama Y, et al: Evidence of misery perfusion and risk for recurrent stroke in major cerebral arterial occlusive diseases from PET, J Neurol Neurosurg Psychiatry 61:18–25, 1996.

Yamauchi H, Fukuyama H, Nagahama Y, et al: Significance of increased oxygen extraction fraction in five-year prognosis of major cerebral arterial occlusive diseases, J Nucl Med 40:1992–1998, 1999.

Yaşargil MG, Krayenbuhl HA, Jacobson JH: Microneurosurgical arterial reconstruction, Surgery 67:221–223, 1970.

Yaşargil MG: Microsurgery Applied to Neurosurgery, Stuttgart, 1969, Georg Thieme.

Yonas H, Smith HA, Durham SR, et al: Increased stroke risk predicted by compromised blood flow reactivity, J Neurosurg 79:483–489, 1993.

Zhang YJ, Barrow DL, Cawley CM, et al: Neurosurgical management of intracranial aneurysms previously treated with endovascular therapy, Neurosurgery 52(2):283–293, 200; discussion 293-5.

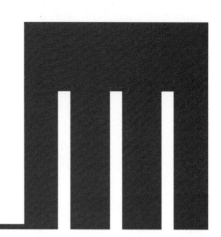

CEREBRAL ISCHEMIA

EC-IC BYPASS EVIDENCE 16

PAUL R. GIGANTE; CHRISTOPHER P. KELLNER;
E. SANDER CONNOLLY, JR

The first description of an operation intended to provide alternative cerebral blood flow (CBF) was given by German and Taffel in 1939, in which a temporalis muscle pedicle was placed over the cerebral cortex in monkeys (Figure 16–1).[1] They later subjected both treated and untreated controls to carotid and vertebral occlusion, and reported the monkeys with temporalis pedicles overlying the cortex survived, whereas untreated controls did not. In 1942, Kredel first performed the procedure in three human patients who had suffered ischemic stroke, reporting postoperative clinical improvement in all three patients.[2] However, the technique was largely abandoned over the next decade when postoperative angiograms failed to provide evidence of collateral flow through the graft.

C. Miller Fisher shed new light on the concept of re-establishing cerebral perfusion in 1951 when he postulated that extracranial to intracranial (EC-IC) arterial bypass might be performed as a treatment for occlusive vascular disease.[3] That same year, Pool and Potts created a superficial temporal artery (STA) to anterior cerebral artery (ACA) shunt during treatment of a giant ACA aneurysm. Although the shunt was successful intraoperatively, postoperative angiogram confirmed the shunt had become occluded.[4]

The first EC-IC arterial bypass was not described until 1966 when Yasargil and Donaghy successfully performed an STA to middle cerebral artery (MCA) anastomosis in a dog. Shortly thereafter, Yasargil successfully performed the same procedure in a human, providing the neurosurgical community with what was deemed a breakthrough in the treatment of intracranial atherosclerosis. Following Yasargil's description of the EC-IC arterial bypass, neurosurgeons around the world utilized the procedure with the intent of re-establishing CBF in a variety of cerebrovascular diseases. Surgeons subsequently described bypasses from the occipital and middle meningeal arteries to the MCA, from the occipital artery to the posterior inferior cerebellar artery,[5] from the occipital artery to the anterior inferior cerebellar artery (AICA), and from the STA to the superior cerebellar artery.[5,6]

Over time surgical technique improved, and the most frequently employed bypass procedure became the STA to MCA bypass for the indication of symptomatic internal carotid artery (ICA) or MCA stenosis. However, as was the case with most other surgically treated diseases at the time, there were no extant data to demonstrate that performing the procedure provided patients with any significant short- or long-term benefit. The only early report came in the form of a small retrospective series published by Sundt et al. in 1977, the utility of which was limited by multiple biases. The group reported on a retrospective series of 56 patients who underwent STA-MCA bypass for a wide variety of indications, including TIAs, "orthostatic ischemia," progressive stroke, and aneurysmal bypass. With regards to graft patency, those who had grafts prior to 1973 had low patency (25%) whereas those operated after 1974 had high patency (95%). The other outcome described was major ischemic stroke or death from the surgery, of which they reported none. The report served more to describe the acceptable safety of the procedure, rather than to examine its efficacy.[7]

As evidenced by this first series, the greatest impediments to a meaningful conglomerate of data were the lack of consistency in patient selection and evaluation, the lack of an appropriate medically treated control population, and the lack of consistent outcomes follow-up. As evidence-based medicine emerged and the Food and Drug Administration's requirements for proving pharmacologic safety and efficacy became increasingly stringent, neurologists and neurosurgeons too recognized the imperative of defining the "efficacy" of risk-containing surgical procedures. In a 1977 *Stroke* editorial introducing the initiation of the first ever EC-IC bypass study, Fletcher H. McDowell wrote,

Too often surgical treatment for a particular condition gains enthusiasm and wide use before any clear evidence of effectiveness. This problem has been particularly evident in the field of atherosclerotic vascular disease involving the treatment of its cardiac and cerebral complications. The recent suggestions for extracranial/intracranial arterial anastomosis in the prevention and treatment of stroke have without question a logical basis. This is especially true when atherosclerosis in cerebral vessels lies distal to the surgically accessible portion of the internal carotid artery. Anastomosis of the superficial temporal artery

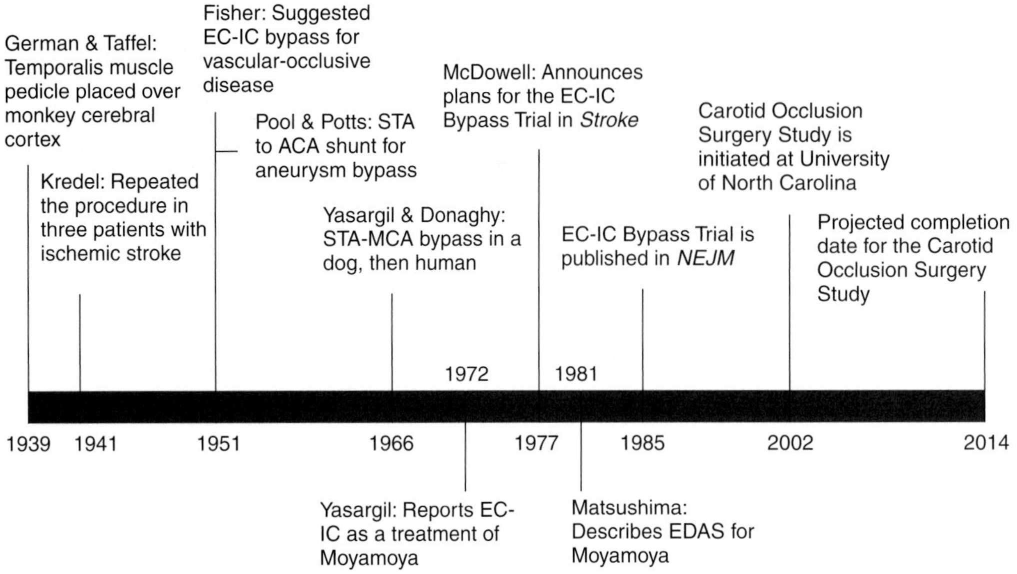

German & Taffel: Temporalis muscle pedicle placed over monkey cerebral cortex

Fisher: Suggested EC-IC bypass for vascular-occlusive disease

Kredel: Repeated the procedure in three patients with ischemic stroke

Pool & Potts: STA to ACA shunt for aneurysm bypass

McDowell: Announces plans for the EC-IC Bypass Trial in *Stroke*

Carotid Occlusion Surgery Study is initiated at University of North Carolina

Yasargil & Donaghy: STA-MCA bypass in a dog, then human

EC-IC Bypass Trial is published in *NEJM*

Projected completion date for the Carotid Occlusion Surgery Study

Figure 16–1. Outline of Advances in EC-IC Bypass Techniques.

1972   1981

1939   1941   1951   1966   1977   1985   2002   2014

Yasargil: Reports EC-IC as a treatment of Moyamoya

Matsushima: Describes EDAS for Moyamoya

to the middle cerebral artery or one of its branches to improve vertebral circulation in such situations is beginning to be carried out frequently in a number of centers across the United States. In an effort to determine the effectiveness of this therapy 20 major medical centers in the United States and three centers outside the United States have joined together in a collaborative study of this therapy.[8]

Pending the results of the EC-IC Bypass Study, neurosurgeons published a handful of case reports, series, and commentaries on the appropriate indications, safety, and utility of EC-IC bypass.[9–15] In 1983, Chater reported on 400 patients who underwent EC-IC bypass for TIAs and hemodynamic intracranial lesions, with a permanent neurological morbidity rate of approximately 2% and operative mortality of 2.5%, and an ipsilateral postoperative stroke incidence of 0.9% per year after a 55-month follow-up.[16] Chater et al. then reported on 105 patients with intracranial ICA stenosis (60% to 98%) and ischemia 1 to 3 months prior to EC-IC bypass. Of these, surgical mortality was 1%, permanent surgical morbidity was 2%, and after 54 months of follow-up, 22 patients had died, of which three were related to stroke; thus the overall late death rate was 4% per year. Although Chater's reports had begun to examine a more uniform patient population, both of his retrospective series contained no medically treated control group against which the success of surgery could be measured.[17]

INTERNATIONAL COOPERATIVE STUDY OF EC-IC ARTERIAL ANASTOMOSIS

In 1985, nearly 8 years after McDowell's introduction of the International Cooperative Study of Extracranial-Intracranial Arterial Anastomosis (termed the EC-IC Bypass Trial), the group reported the results of this randomized, prospective trial.

Of the 1377 patients enrolled in the trial, 714 (52%) were assigned to medical treatment alone (daily aspirin and aggressive hypertension control) and 663 (48%) were assigned to receive EC-IC bypass in addition to medical therapy. Inclusion and exclusion criteria are presented in Table 16–1.

Notably, patients were allowed to enroll in the trial if they had tandem stenosis (two separate stenosis lesions) of the proximal and distal ICA, the proximal lesion being amenable to carotid endarterectomy[18] and the distal lesion qualifying for EC-IC bypass. Which surgery was performed first was left to the discretion of the operating surgeons, with the caveat that CEA, if performed first, was to occur at least 30 days prior to randomization in the EC-IC Bypass Trial.

Table 16–1. INCLUSION AND EXCLUSION CRITERIA FOR THE EC-IC BYPASS TRIAL.

Inclusion Criteria

1. Must have experienced, within 3 months prior to entry, one or both of the following: (a) transient ischemic attack(s) in the carotid distribution; (b) minor completed strokes in the carotid distribution.
2. Radiologic criteria—angiogram demonstrating an appropriate atherosclerotic lesion: (a) MCA trunk, (b) ICA stenosis at or above C2, or (c) ICA occlusion.

Exclusion Criteria

1. Unable to provide self-care for most activities.
2. Does not retain some useful residual function in the affected arm or leg.
3. Unable to demonstrate intact comprehension.
4. More than mild expressive aphasia.
5. Unable to handle own oropharyngeal secretions.
6. Within 8 weeks of an acute cerebral ischemic event.
7. Within 6 months of a myocardial infarction.
8. Morbid condition causing death within 5 years.
9. Vertebrobasilar ischemia.

Patients randomized to surgery underwent end-to-side STA or occipital artery anastomosis to a cortical MCA branch. Both surgical and medical patients received aspirin 325 mg qid and optimized hypertensive control for the duration of the trial. The surgical and medical arms were matched well for age, race/ethnicity, and risk factors. Over 70% of patients had abnormal neurologic findings at entry, but preoperative functional status testing determined the majority (over 90%) had little or no functional impairment. Regarding the type of vascular disease, the majority of patients (59% in medical arm, 58% in surgical arm) had isolated ICA occlusion, and the next most common were tandem lesions followed by isolated ICA stenosis. Only 8% in each arm had MCA stenosis and 8% had MCA occlusion.

The results of the trial demonstrated that EC-IC bypass provided no significant reduction in major and fatal strokes, ipsilateral strokes, major ipsilateral strokes, or all strokes and deaths combined. Separate analyses in patients with different angiographic lesions did not identify a subgroup with any benefit from surgery. They also reported 30-day surgical mortality and major stroke morbidity rates of 0.6% and 2.5%, respectively. The graft patency rate was reported as 96%, roughly similar to previous series.[19]

The completion of such a well-run, large-scale trial was thought a major achievement in surgical literature, but its negative results served as a major blow to the perceived utility of the EC-IC bypass procedure. A sharp decline in the number of procedures performed annually followed its publication; however, neurologists and neurosurgeons remained mindful of the study's limitations.

Study Criticism

The major criticism of the EC-IC Bypass Trial was that patients were not selected for surgery based on the preoperative *physiology* of their occlusive disease, but rather were selected based on the *anatomy* of their intracranial occlusive disease. The way that intracranial occlusive disease influences flow dynamics and cerebral perfusion, and thus at-risk tissue that may benefit from bypass, was increasingly recognized as physiology far more complex than simply identifying a stenotic lesion on angiogram. Some argued that patients with a high oxygen extraction ratio (OER) and a critically under-perfused cerebral hemisphere may have been positioned to benefit in a significant way from a bypass procedure. In order to determine OER, however, advanced technology using positron emission tomography (PET) scanning was required, which was not available at the start of the trial, and upon publication of the trial was only available at a few specialized centers.

Furthermore, the bypass study contained no description of patients' collateral circulation sources into the clinically affected hemisphere. This information was considered critical with the advent of carotid endarterectomy data showing that intraoperative determination of collateral flow by radioactive xenon washout was predictive of subsequent stroke: no infarctions occurred in patients with collateral CBF greater than 40 ml/100 g/min, whereas strokes incidence was 3.4% per year when CBF was less than 25 ml/100 g/min.[20] The concept applies to EC-IC bypass in that the ideal candidate would be one with naturally available but insufficient collateral channels, for which the bypass would provide improved blood flow.

Some argued that the study was designed to select patients who were not in physiologic need of bypass—those with large numbers of low-risk or non-hemodynamic obstructions, a population that was presumed to gain little benefit from bypass surgery. The other patient population that raised concerns were those with tandem stenosis. These separate stenoses were not managed in a uniform way, or even clearly defined in the bypass trial's results.

The outcome after completion of the trial was that neurosurgeons and neurologists still believed that there was a role for EC-IC bypass in treating cerebrovascular disease, but that it would be critical to identify the small subset of patients whose preoperative flow physiology would position them best to benefit from what was now understood to be a relatively low-risk procedure with excellent postoperative patency rates.

Moyamoya Disease: EC-IC Bypass and EDAS

With the advent of angiography, Moyamoya, a disease in children and adults characterized by progressive multiple stenoses of the ICA, MCA, and ACA, was recognized as a physiologic entity distinct from the kind of adult intracranial stenosis heretofore discussed. Moyamoya occlusions result in secondary neovascularization of the lenticulostriate and leptomeningeal circulation, resulting in the characteristic "puff of smoke" appearance of collateral vessels on angiogram. As a consequence of Moyamoya, children typically present with strokes and adults typically present with intracranial hemorrhage related to friable vessels. As bypass procedures emerged, the Moyamoya population was identified as ideal for reconstituting flow for at-risk tissue. Yasargil was the first to report EC-IC bypass for Moyamoya in 1972, and a number of case reports describing STA-MCA bypass followed in the ensuing decades.[21–25] The STA-MCA bypass was generally considered the treatment of choice for Moyamoya at the time, though there were a number of patients (children, mostly) whose STA was too small to serve as an adequate pedicle.

In 1981, Matsushima et al. first described the encephaloduroarteriosynangiosis (EDAS), in which the distally intact STA and a strip of galea were mobilized, and simply placed over the cortex and sutured to the dura. The idea of the procedure was to help promote the natural tendency of the disease to develop collateral circulation.[26] The procedure was considered simple and safe because the arteries remain intact, requiring no microvascular anastomosis. Matsushima subsequently reported on 50 pediatric and four adult patients, stating that 12-month angiograms showed marked revascularization through the external carotid system.[25] Olds and Spetzler also reported early good results with unilateral or bilateral EDAS.[27]

Although no prospective studies have been performed comparing EDAS to EC-IC bypass or medical treatment, recent case series continue to support its application in the treatment of Moyamoya in both children and adults.[28–34] We recently reported long-term outcome in our series of 43 adults treated with EDAS for Moyamoya. Comparing infarct-free survival rates in surgically treated hemispheres and non-surgically treated hemispheres, we found that the 5-year, infarction-free rate was 94% versus 36% in the untreated hemispheres.[34]

Both indirect and direct revascularization procedures continue to be employed in the treatment of Moyamoya depending on patient characteristics and institutional preference. A large-scale retrospective study was published in Japan in 1997 examining 290 patients with hemorrhagic Moyamoya, including 152 patients who underwent EC-IC bypass and 138 patients who were treated conservatively with medical therapy.[35] In the surgical group, 19.1% experienced recurrent hemorrhage, while 28.3% had recurrent hemorrhage in the nonsurgical group. A large prospective trial, the Japan Adult Moyamoya Trial, is now underway in Japan to analyze the efficacy of direct EC-IC bypass for Moyamoya.[36]

At many centers in the United States, EDAS continues to be the standard of care for the neurosurgical treatment of Moyamoya. Evidence rests on large retrospective case series with a handful of prospective, long term case series now emerging. A randomized trial with appropriate patient selection is needed to quantify the clinical benefits of this procedure.

Intracranial Aneurysms, Tumors, and EC-IC Bypass

Aneurysm treatment has been historically linked to carotid occlusion since the first intracranial aneurysm was treated with Hunterian ligation of the internal carotid artery. The publication of the Cooperative Study of Intracranial Aneurysms in 1966 first presented the risk of developing neurological deficits in the event of surgical carotid occlusion: 12% in the treatment of unruptured aneurysms. In both ruptured and unruptured aneurysms, abrupt occlusion of the carotid artery led to neurologic symptoms 59% of the time if the ICA was occluded and 32% if the CCA was occluded.[37] With the development of Yasargil's STA-MCA bypass technique, aneurysm treatment became a clear indication for EC-IC bypass, but its utility quickly decreased as clipping and eventually coiling supplanted parent vessel sacrifice as the major treatment modalities for intracranial aneurysms.

In modern-day neurosurgical practice, EC-IC bypass is an important adjunct when a vessel must be sacrificed due to the presence of a complex aneurysm or skull base tumor. In these cases, practice varies among centers, but often a balloon test occlusion is performed to test for dependency on the vessel to be sacrificed and if neurological symptoms develop, a bypass is performed prior to vessel sacrifice. Given the risks of performing a balloon test occlusion and the possibility that patients might develop ischemic symptoms even if the test is

negative, some surgeons prefer to perform an EC-IC bypass in all cases.[38] The utility of EC-IC bypass in the treatment of skull base tumors and intracranial aneurysms has been well established and remains an important component of the cerebrovascular neurosurgeon's armamentarium in the treatment of complex lesions.

Re-Evaluation of EC-IC Bypass for Athero-Occlusive Disease

In the era since the *New England Journal of Medicine*'s 1985 publication of the EC-IC Bypass Trial results, clinicians have produced scores of critical articles that counter its conclusions or identify study groups in which EC-IC bypass surgery may be effective. Modern criticism elaborates on the responses that followed immediately in the wake of the trial, claiming that although the trial was carried out meticulously, the design itself biased the data against a surgical benefit.[39] Continued criticism has been accompanied by more focused clinical trials and a number of prospective clinical studies bolstering support for adapted indications. Finally, the field of neurosurgery has responded by applying new technologies to preoperative hemodynamic evaluation and to the performance of the operation itself.

The major criticism of the EC-IC Bypass Trial has been that patient selection biased results toward the null hypothesis by selecting too broad a group of patients, not all for whom bypass would be most effective. In the latter years of the trial and immediately afterward, it became possible to measure cerebral hemodynamic status using physiologic imaging, such as magnetic resonance spectroscopy,[40] static xenon inhalation dynamic CT (Xe-CT), or PET in response to acetazolamide (ACZ) or inhaled CO_2 to measure CBF and autoregulatory capacity. These major advances permitted surgeons to more precisely select patients who would be likely to benefit from EC-IC bypass and a number of studies have been performed focusing on patients suffering symptomatic hemodynamic failure (Table 16–2).

A recent systematic review of the direct EC-IC bypass literature between 1985 and 2007 identified 22 studies reporting outcomes using the procedure to treat patients with varying stages of cerebral hemodynamic failure.[41] A logistic regression model was constructed comparing medically treated and surgically treated patients with intracranial athero-occlusive disease using annual stroke rate as the outcome measure. Patients were stratified by the severity of cerebral hemodynamic compromise evaluated radiographically. Mild stage I hemodynamic failure was defined as decreased vascular reactivity in response to acetazolamide or inhaled CO_2. Severe stage I hemodynamic failure was defined as decreased dilatation after inhaled ACZ or CO_2, commonly referred to as "steal effect," which occurs when the arteries are already maximally dilated due to low flow or local ischemia and paradoxically decrease as blood flow is diverted to other dilated vessels. Stage II hemodynamic failure was defined as the phenomenon observed on a PET

Table 16–2. EC-IC BYPASS STUDIES FOR SYMPTOMATIC HEMODYNAMIC FAILURE.

Author	Year	# of Patients	Imaging Modality
Ma[44]	2007	12	SPECT and ACZ
Hirai[45]	2005	40	SPECT and ACZ
Tummala[46]	2003	44	Xe-CT
Neff[47]	2004	25	Xe-CT and ACZ
Murata[48]	2003	30	Xe-CT
Sasoh[49]	2003	25	PET
Przybylski[50]	1998	42	Xe-CT and ACZ
Kuwabara[51]	1998	7	PET and ACZ
Takagi[52]	1997	12	PET
Schick[53]	1996	40	CT/SPECT and ACZ
Schmiedek[54]	1994	28	SPECT/Xe and ACZ
Muraishi[55]	1993	6	PET
Yamashita[56]	1991	15	Xe-CT and ACZ
Holzschuh[57]	1991	18	Xe-CT and ACZ
Kuroda[58]	1990	5	SPECT/Xe and ACZ
Sunada[59]	1989	9	Xe-CT
Leinsinger[60]	1988	31	SPECT/Xe
Bishop[61]	1987	8	Xe-CT and hypercapnia
DiPiero[62]	1987	14	SPECT
Vorstrup[62]	1986	22	Xe-CT

Table 16–3. INCLUSION AND EXCLUSION CRITERIA FOR THE CAROTID OCCLUSION SURGERY STUDY.

Inclusion Criteria

1. Vascular imaging demonstrating occlusion of one or both ICAs.
2. TIA or ischemic stroke in the territory of one occluded carotid artery.
3. Most recent qualifying TIA or stroke occurring within 120 days prior to projected performance date of PET.
4. Modified Barthel Index >12/20 (60/100).
5. Language comprehension intact, motor aphasia mild or absent.
6. Age 18 to 85 inclusive.
7. Competent to give informed consent.
8. Legally an adult.
9. Geographically accessible and reliable for follow-up.

Exclusion Criteria

1. Non-atherosclerotic carotid vascular disease and blood dyscrasias.
2. Known heart disease likely to cause cerebral ischemia.
3. Other non-atherosclerotic condition likely to cause focal cerebral ischemia.
4. Any condition likely to lead to death within 2 years.
5. Other neurological disease that would confound follow-up assessment.
6. Pregnancy.
7. Subsequent cerebrovascular surgery planned that might alter cerebral hemodynamics.
8. Any condition which in the participating surgeon's judgment makes the subject an unsuitable surgical candidate.
9. Participation in any other experimental treatment trial.
10. Participation within the previous 12 months in any experimental study that included exposure to ionizing radiation.
11. Acute, progressing, or unstable neurological deficit.
12. If supplemental arteriography is required, allergy to iodine or x-ray contrast media, serum creatinine >3.0 mg/dl or other contraindication to arteriography.
13. If aspirin is to be used as antithrombotic therapy in the perioperative period, those with allergy or contraindication to aspirin are ineligible.
14. Medical indication for treatment with anticoagulant or antithrombotic medication that cannot be replaced with aspirin in the perioperative period if the patient is randomized to surgery.
15. Remediable medical conditions.

scan when vessels become maximally dilated and CBF actually declines in response to ACZ or CO_2 inhalation. The results demonstrated that surgically treated patients in the selected studies presenting with severe stage I failure significantly benefitted from surgery with an average annual stroke rate of 1.2% versus a stroke rate of 19.3% in the medically treated group. This meta-analysis provides the first evidence of a systematic attempt to compare stratified patient groups to equivalent groups of medically treated patients. These results clearly demonstrate that a modern clinical trial is needed, stratifying patients by the severity of cerebral hemodynamic failure.

A clinical trial, called the Japan EC-IC Bypass Trial (JET), was conducted in Japan to determine whether EC-IC bypass is superior to medical management for ICA and MCA athero-occlusive disease resulting in severe hemodynamic compromise.[42] An interim analysis briefly describes the inclusion criteria and results of 206 patients who met the following criteria:

1. Symptomatic ICA/MCA stenosis/occlusion ≥70% in diameter
2. Modified Rankin scale ≤2
3. Small or no brain infarct
4. Regional CBF of the ipsilateral MCA territory <80% of the control value and acetazolamide reactivity <10%

The authors concluded that the surgically treated patients showed a statistically significant decrease in the rate of major stroke, or death, although this data has never been formally presented.[43]

A second randomized clinical trial, the Carotid Occlusion Surgery Study trial (visit clinicaltrials.gov, NCT00029146), is currently underway with a projected completion date of 2014. This is a multicenter trial with a projected enrollment of 1400 patients. The inclusion and exclusion criteria are listed in Table 16–3. This randomized trial improves on the design of the original EC-IC Bypass Trial in that it precisely examines the cohort of patients for whom this procedures is practically applies, those who have perfusion deficits in the hemisphere ipsilateral to the occlusive lesion. This study also focuses on ICA occlusion following evidence from the original trial and subsequent prospective studies that this procedure may not benefit patients with MCA stenosis or occlusion and may even harm them.[19,43]

CONCLUSION

EC-IC bypass is an important component of the modern cerebrovascular neurosurgeon's armamentarium. A large number of case series has provided evidence for its application in Moyamoya disease, complex intracranial lesions that might require vascular sacrifice, and severe athero-occlusive disease resulting in cerebral hemodynamic compromise. To date, the EC-IC Bypass Trial has provided the only prospective, randomized trial to suggest a non-significant benefit from surgery, although its broad patient selection has received widespread criticism and raised concern that a more physiologic-based approach to selecting surgical candidates may indeed identify those who are poised to benefit significantly from surgery. Expanding indications, improving diagnostic ability, and advanced techniques demand further prospective clinical trials to evaluate the utility of surgical revascularization in carefully selected patient populations.

REFERENCES

1. German W, Taffel M: Surgical Production of Collateral Intracranial Circulation, Proc Soc Ex Biol Med 42:349–353, 1939.
2. Kredel F: Collateral cerebral circulation by muscle graft. Technique of operation with report of 3 cases, South Surg 10:235–244, 1942.
3. Fisher M: Occlusion of the internal carotid artery, AMA Arch Neurol Psychiatry 65:346–377, 1951.
4. Pool JL, Potts DG: Aneurysms and Arteriovenous Anomalies of the Brain, New York, 1964, Hoeber.
5. Scamoni C, Dario A, Castelli P, et al: Extracranial-intracranial bypass for giant aneurysms and complex vascular lesions: a clinical series of 10 patients, J Neurosurg Sci 52:1–9, 2008; discussion 9-10.
6. Yasargil MG, editor: Diagnosis and Indications for Operations in Cerebrovascular Occlusive Disease, New York, 1969, Academic Press.
7. Sundt TM Jr, Siekert RG, Piepgras DG, et al: Bypass surgery for vascular disease of the carotid system, Mayo Clin Proc 51:677–692, 1976.
8. McDowell FH: The extracranial/intracranial bypass study, Stroke 8:545, 1977.
9. Brambilla G, Paoletti P, Rodriguez y Baena R: Extracranial-intracranial arterial bypass in the treatment of inoperable giant aneurysms of the internal carotid artery. Report of a case, Acta Neurochir (Wien) 60:63–69, 1982.
10. Bushe KA, Bockhorn J: Extracranial-intracranial arterial bypass for giant aneurysms, Acta Neurochir (Wien) 54:107–115, 1980.
11. Ditmore QM, Watts C, Scharf P: Extracranial-intracranial bypass. a review, Mo Med 79:272–275, 1982.
12. Edwards MS, Chater NL, Stanley JA: Reversal of chronic ocular ischemia by extracranial-intracranial arterial bypass: case report, Neurosurgery 7:480–483, 1980.
13. Olteanu-Nerbe V, Marguth F: Extracranial-intracranial bypass operation in basal tumours, Neurosurg Rev 5:99–105, 1982.
14. Rhodes RS, Spetzler RF, Roski RA: Improved neurologic function after cerebrovascular accident with extracranial-intracranial arterial bypass, Surgery 90:433–438, 1981.
15. Rogers LA: Selection of patients for extracranial external carotid artery surgery and extracranial-intracranial bypass, Neurosurgery 11:467–468, 1982.
16. Chater N: Neurosurgical extracranial-intracranial bypass for stroke: with 400 cases, Neurol Res 5:1–9, 1983.
17. Weinstein PR, Rodriguez y Baena R, Chater NL: Results of extracranial-intracranial arterial bypass for intracranial internal carotid artery stenosis: review of 105 cases, Neurosurgery 15:787–794, 1984.
18. Donadio C, Tramonti G, Garcea G, et al: Azthreonam in the treatment of urinary tract infection: evaluation of efficacy, renal effects and nephrotoxicity, Drugs Exp Clin Res 13:167–170, 1987.
19. Failure of extracranial-intracranial arterial bypass to reduce the risk of ischemic stroke: Results of an international randomized trial. The EC/IC Bypass Study Group, N Engl J Med 313:1191–1200, 1985.
20. Whisnant JP, Sandok BA, Sundt TM Jr: Carotid endarterectomy for unilateral carotid system transient cerebral ischemia, Mayo Clin Proc 58:171–175, 1983.
21. Amine AR, Moody RA, Meeks W: Bilateral temporal-middle cerebral artery anastomosis for Moyamoya syndrome, Surg Neurol 8:3–6, 1977.
22. Boone SC, Sampson DS: Observations on moyamoya disease: a case treated with superficial temporal–middle cerebral artery anastomosis, Surg Neurol 9:189–193, 1978.
23. Holbach KH, Wassmann H, Wappenschmidt J: Superficial temporal-middle cerebral artery anastomosis in Moyamoya disease, Acta Neurochir (Wien) 52:27–34, 1980.
24. Karasawa J, Kikuchi H, Furuse S, et al: Treatment of moyamoya disease with STA-MCA anastomosis, J Neurosurg 49:679–688, 1978.
25. Matsushima Y, Suzuki R, Yamaguchi T, et al: [Effects of indirect EC/IC bypass operations on adult moyamoya patients], No Shinkei Geka 14:1559–1566, 1986.
26. Matsushima Y, Fukai N, Tanaka K, et al: A new surgical treatment of moyamoya disease in children: a preliminary report, Surg Neurol 15:313–320, 1981.
27. Olds MV, Griebel RW, Hoffman HJ, et al: The surgical treatment of childhood moyamoya disease, J Neurosurg 66:675–680, 1987.
28. Hankinson TC, Bohman LE, Heyer G, et al: Surgical treatment of moyamoya syndrome in patients with sickle cell anemia: outcome following encephaloduroarteriosynangiosis, J Neurosurg Pediatr 1:211–216, 2008.
29. Isono M, Ishii K, Kamida T, et al: Long-term outcomes of pediatric moyamoya disease treated by encephalo-duro-arterio-synangiosis, Pediatr Neurosurg 36:14–21, 2002.
30. Kim CY, Wang KC, Kim SK, et al: Encephaloduroarteriosynangiosis with bifrontal encephalogaleo(periosteal)synangiosis in the pediatric moyamoya disease: the surgical technique and its outcomes, Childs Nerv Syst 19:316–324, 2003.
31. Kim SK, Wang KC, Kim IO, et al: Combined encephaloduroarteriosynangiosis and bifrontal encephalogaleo (periosteal) synangiosis in pediatric moyamoya disease, Neurosurgery 62:1456–1464, 2008.
32. Kim SK, Wang KC, Kim IO, et al: Combined encephaloduroarteriosynangiosis and bifrontal encephalogaleo(periosteal)synangiosis in pediatric moyamoya disease, Neurosurgery 50:88–96, 2002.
33. Matsushima T, Inoue T, Ikezaki K, et al: Multiple combined indirect procedure for the surgical treatment of children with moyamoya disease. A comparison with single indirect anastomosis and direct anastomosis, Neurosurg Focus 5:e4, 1998.
34. Starke RM, Komotar RJ, Hickman ZL, et al: Clinical features, surgical treatment, and long-term outcome in adult patients with moyamoya disease. Clinical article, J Neurosurg 111:936–942, 2009.
35. Fujii K, Ikezaki K, Irikura K, et al: The efficacy of bypass surgery for the patients with hemorrhagic moyamoya disease, Clin Neurol Neurosurg 99(Suppl 2):S194–S195, 1997.
36. Miyamoto S: Group JAMT: Study design for a prospective randomized trial of extracranial-intracranial bypass surgery for adults with moyamoya disease and hemorrhagic onset—the Japan Adult Moyamoya Trial Group, Neurol Med Chir (Tokyo) 44:218–219, 2004.
37. Nishioka H: Report on the cooperative study of intracranial aneurysms and subarachnoid hemorrhage. Section VII. I. Evaluation of the conservative management of ruptured intracranial aneurysms, J Neurosurg 25:574–592, 1966.

38. Vilela MD, Newell DW: Superficial temporal artery to middle cerebral artery bypass: past, present, and future, *Neurosurg Focus* 24:E2, 2008.

39. Reichman OH, Origitano TC, Anderson DE, et al: Lies, damned lies, and statistics: a neurosurgical perspective on the international randomized trial of extracranial to intracranial arterial bypass surgery, *J Stroke Cerebrovasc Dis* 18:389–397, 2009.

40. Amin-Hanjani S, Shin JH, Zhao M, et al: Evaluation of extracranial-intracranial bypass using quantitative magnetic resonance angiography, *J Neurosurg* 106:291–298, 2007.

41. Garrett MC, Komotar RJ, Starke RM, et al: The efficacy of direct extracranial-intracranial bypass in the treatment of symptomatic hemodynamic failure secondary to athero-occlusive disease: a systematic review, *Clin Neurol Neurosurg* 111:319–326, 2009.

42. Jinnouchi J, Toyoda K, Inoue T, et al: Changes in brain volume 2 years after extracranial-intracranial bypass surgery: A preliminary subanalysis of the Japanese EC-IC trial, *Cerebrovasc Dis* 22:177–182, 2006.

43. Garrett MC, Komotar RJ, Merkow MB, et al: The extracranial-intracranial bypass trial: implications for future investigations, *Neurosurg Focus* 24:E4, 2008.

44. Ma J, Mehrkens JH, Holtmannspoetter M, et al: Perfusion MRI before and after acetazolamide administration for assessment of cerebrovascular reserve capacity in patients with symptomatic internal carotid artery (ICA) occlusion: comparison with 99mTc-ECD SPECT, *Neuroradiology* 49:317–326, 2007.

45. Hirai Y, Fujimoto S, Toyoda K, et al: Superficial temporal artery duplex ultrasonography for improved cerebral hemodynamics after extracranial-intracranial bypass surgery, *Cerebrovasc Dis* 20:463–469, 2005.

46. Tummala RP, Chu RM, Nussbaum ES: Extracranial-intracranial bypass for symptomatic occlusive cerebrovascular disease not amenable to carotid endarterectomy, *Neurosurg Focus* 14:e8, 2003.

47. Neff KW, Horn P, Dinter D, et al: Extracranial-intracranial arterial bypass surgery improves total brain blood supply in selected symptomatic patients with unilateral internal carotid artery occlusion and insufficient collateralization, *Neuroradiology* 46:730–737, 2004.

48. Murata Y, Katayama Y, Sakatani K, et al: Evaluation of extracranial-intracranial arterial bypass function by using near-infrared spectroscopy, *J Neurosurg* 99:304–310, 2003.

49. Sasoh M, Ogasawara K, Kuroda K, et al: Effects of EC-IC bypass surgery on cognitive impairment in patients with hemodynamic cerebral ischemia, *Surg Neurol* 59:455–460, 2003; discussion 460-3.

50. Przybylski GJ, Yonas H, Smith HA: Reduced stroke risk in patients with compromised cerebral blood flow reactivity treated with superficial temporal artery to distal middle cerebral artery bypass surgery, *J Stroke Cerebrovasc Dis* 7:302–309, 1998.

51. Kuwabara Y, Ichiya Y, Sasaki M, et al: PET evaluation of cerebral hemodynamics in occlusive cerebrovascular disease pre- and postsurgery, *J Nucl Med* 39:760–765, 1998.

52. Takagi Y, Hashimoto N, Iwama T, et al: Improvement of oxygen metabolic reserve after extracranial-intracranial bypass surgery in patients with severe haemodynamic insufficiency, *Acta Neurochir (Wien)* 139:52–56, 1997; discussion 56-7.

53. Schick U, Zimmermann M, Stolke D: Long-term evaluation of EC-IC bypass patency, *Acta Neurochir (Wien)* 138:938–942, 1996; discussion 942-3.

54. Schmiedek P, Piepgras A, Leinsinger G, et al: Improvement of cerebrovascular reserve capacity by EC-IC arterial bypass surgery in patients with ICA occlusion and hemodynamic cerebral ischemia, *J Neurosurg* 81:236–244, 1994.

55. Muraishi K, Kameyama M, Sato K, et al: Cerebral circulatory and metabolic changes following EC/IC bypass surgery in cerebral occlusive diseases, *Neurol Res* 15:97–103, 1993.

56. Yamashita T, Kashiwagi S, Nakano S, et al: The effect of EC-IC bypass surgery on resting cerebral blood flow and cerebrovascular reserve capacity studied with stable XE-CT and acetazolamide test, *Neuroradiology* 33:217–222, 1991.

57. Holzschuh M, Brawanski A, Ullrich W, et al: Cerebral blood flow and cerebrovascular reserve 5 years after EC-IC bypass, *Neurosurg Rev* 14:275–278, 1991.

58. Kuroda S, Takigawa S, Kamiyama H, et al: [Diagnosis of hemodynamic compromise in patients with chronic cerebral ischemia; measurement of cerebral blood volume (CBV) with 99mTc-RBC SPECT], *No Shinkei Geka* 18:259–266, 1990.

59. Sunada I: [Measurement of cerebral blood flow by single photon emission computed tomography in cases of internal carotid artery occlusion], *Neurol Med Chir (Tokyo)* 29:496–502, 1989.

60. Leinsinger G, Schmiedek P, Kreisig T, et al: [133Xe-DSPECT: significance of the cerebrovascular reserve capacity for the diagnosis and therapy of chronic cerebral ischemia], *Nuklearmedizin* 27:127–134, 1988.

61. Bishop CC, Burnand KG, Brown M, et al: Reduced response of cerebral blood flow to hypercapnia: restoration by extracranial-intracranial bypass, *Br J Surg* 74:802–804, 1987.

62. Vorstrup S, Brun B, Lassen NA: Evaluation of the cerebral vasodilatory capacity by the acetazolamide test before EC-IC bypass surgery in patients with occlusion of the internal carotid artery, *Stroke* 17:1291–1298, 1986.

EC-IC BYPASS FOR POSTERIOR CIRCULATION ISCHEMIA

17

SEPIDEH AMIN-HANJANI; ALI ALARAJ; FADY T. CHARBEL

INTRODUCTION

Posterior circulation strokes account for 30% to 40% of all ischemic strokes, and are particularly prone to devastating consequences due to the concentrated "eloquence" of brain tissue supplied by the posterior circulation.[1] Atherosclerotic occlusive disease of the vertebrobasilar system is a major etiology of posterior circulation ischemia,[2] and carries a high stroke risk despite medical therapy. Extracranial-intracranial (EC-IC) bypass for augmentation of flow to the posterior circulation is a treatment option for selected patients with hemodynamic compromise and recurrent ischemia.

ETIOLOGY

Posterior circulation ischemia can be attributable to a variety of etiologies. Similar to those encountered in anterior circulation stroke, these include atherosclerotic large vessel disease, small penetrating artery disease, embolism (cardiac origin or artery-to-artery), thrombosis, and dissection. In contrast with anterior circulation stroke, large- or small-vessel occlusive disease occurs more commonly in the posterior circulation than thromboembolism.[3,4] Large vessel atherosclerotic vertebrobasilar disease itself accounted for one-third of the strokes reported in the New England Medical Center Posterior Circulation Registry, consisting of 407 prospectively identified patients with posterior circulation ischemia.[2,5] Although thrombotically active plaques are a prominent feature of carotid disease, this mechanism appears less prominent as a cause of ischemia related to vertebrobasilar occlusive disease. The stroke mechanism for patients with posterior circulation atherostenosis is often related directly, or indirectly, to hemodynamic failure with regional hypoperfusion.[6] Beyond the direct mechanism of hypoperfusion, thrombus formation as a sequelae of low flow must also be considered,[2] in addition to an underlying low-flow state worsening the consequences of a given thromboembolic event. The potential synergy between thromboembolism and hemodynamic insufficiency can combine to confer higher risk.[7] Current medical therapies for cerebrovascular occlusive disease are directed primarily at decreasing the risk of in situ thrombosis and thromboembolism, but do not address the underlying low-flow state.

Although flow-limiting disease in the vertebrobasilar system may be well compensated hemodynamically by other collaterals, such as a contralateral vertebral artery, or flow through the posterior communicating arteries, the existence and flow capacity of such collaterals vary widely from individual to individual. Anatomic variants with the potential to affect collateral supply include hypoplastic vertebral arteries, absent posterior communicating arteries, and fetal origin of the posterior cerebral artery, all of which could limit compensatory flow to the vertebrobasilar territory in the setting of vertebrobasilar occlusive disease.

CLINICAL PRESENTATION

Patients with posterior circulation ischemia typically present with a range of symptoms, often referred to as vertebrobasilar insufficiency (VBI). Symptoms can potentially arise from any region of the distal territory of the vertebrobasilar system, including the occipital or temporal lobes, cerebellum, and brainstem with its cranial nerves. Dizziness, vertigo, headaches, diplopia, loss of vision, ataxia, numbness, and weakness involving structures on both sides of the body are frequent symptoms.[8] The most common neurologic signs are limb weakness, gait and limb ataxia, oculomotor palsies, and oropharyngeal dysfunction. Posterior circulation ischemia generally produces a collection of symptoms and signs dependent upon the area affected, rather than causing an isolated symptom. Neurological impairment can be devastating due to the dense collection of neurological functions harbored in the brainstem and posterior circulation structures at risk.

Patients presenting with VBI symptoms in the setting of vertebrobasilar occlusive disease may be suffering from hemodynamic compromise, thrombo-embolic phenomenon, microvascular disease or a combination of these factors.[5] As noted earlier, the predominant stroke mechanism for patients with

175

atherosclerotic occlusive disease, however, appears to involve regional hypoperfusion.

NATURAL HISTORY

Symptomatic vertebrobasilar disease, particularly if it affects intracranial vessels, carries a high stroke risk averaging 10% to 15% per year despite medical therapy.[9,10] These rates approach those seen with symptomatic high-grade extracranial carotid stenosis.[11] In a retrospective study of 44 patients with symptomatic distal vertebral or basilar artery stenosis of ≥50%, Moufarrij et al. reported a 27% overall incidence of vertebrobasilar ischemic events,[12] with an 80% stroke-free survival at 2 years. In another study of symptomatic vertebrobasilar disease (>50% stenosis), Qureshi et al. demonstrated that 14% of 102 patients experienced recurrent stroke, with a stroke-free survival of 72% at 2 years.[10] Retrospective analysis from the Warfarin Aspirin Symptomatic Intracranial Disease (WASID) study group of 68 patients with symptomatic intracranial vertebrobasilar 50% to 99% stenosis treated with antithrombotic therapy over a median follow-up of 13.8 months, showed stroke recurrence in 15 (22%) patients, of which four (27%) were fatal.[9] Territorial stroke risks were 7.8 and 10.7 per 100 patient-years for vertebral and basilar artery stenosis, respectively.

The prospective WASID trial of warfarin versus aspirin treatment for patients with >50% intracranial stenosis, demonstrated recurrent stroke within the territory of the stenotic artery in 15% of 569 patients with both anterior and posterior circulation disease over 2 years.[13] The incidence of stroke at 1 year was 12%, with similar stroke rates for posterior versus anterior circulation disease. Another prospective study of patients with intracranial stenosis ≥50%, GESICA (Groupe d'Etude des Stenoses Intra-Craniennes Atheromateuse symptomatiques), reported recurrent ischemic events in 42.8% of patients with vertebrobasilar disease during a mean follow-up of 23.4 months.[14] Additionally, several studies suggest that recurrent ischemic events occur predominantly within the early months following initial presentation. In Qureshi's study of 102 patients with symptomatic vertebrobasilar disease, stroke-free survival was 76% at 12 months, and 72% at 24 months, demonstrating that most events occur within 1 year.[10] Similarly, the probability of territory specific stroke from the WASID trial increased little from 12% at 1 year to 15% at 2 years in the aspirin group and 11% to 13% in the warfarin group.[13]

Ischemic stroke in general has been linked with a variety of epidemiological and clinical risk factors including age, hypertension, diabetes, smoking, dyslipidemia, coronary artery disease, peripheral vascular disease, oral contraceptive use, prior stroke, alcohol consumption, and hypercoagulable states. Specific risk factors for stroke in vertebrobasilar disease have not been extensively studied. However, some inferences can be made from data examining risk factors for stroke in both anterior and posterior circulation atherosclerotic intracranial stenosis. Retrospective data suggest that severe stenosis (≥70%)[15] and antithrombotic therapy failure[16] may indicate a higher stroke risk. In the prospective WASID trial, however, use of antithrombotic agents at the time of the qualifying event was not predictive of stroke,[17] despite retrospective data suggesting an elevated risk of recurrent events (45%/year) among such patients.[16] On multivariate analysis, severe stenosis (≥70%) and time from qualifying event were significant stroke predictors.

Given the likelihood that a hemodynamic mechanism plays a key role in vertebrobasilar stroke, determining the extent of flow compromise associated with vertebrobasilar disease is likely to be an important aspect of stroke risk prediction. Stenosis severity likely represents a surrogate marker for flow compromise, which may account for its association with stroke risk in previous studies.[15,17] However, when collateral pathways are considered, the mere presence of a severe stenosis or occlusion, in the absence of demonstrable distal territory flow reduction, may not be the most accurate stroke risk predictor. Without direct hemodynamic measurements, clinical indicators of flow compromise can be considered. In the prospective GESICA study of 102 patients with intracranial stenosis ≥50%, of which 48% were vertebrobasilar, hemodynamically significant stenosis was clinically defined as symptoms precipitated by a change in position or antihypertensive medication.[14] Overall, 27.4% of patients met the clinical criteria for hemodynamically significant disease, and had a 60.7% incidence of recurrent TIA or stroke compared to 31.7% over a mean 23.4 month follow-up. These data support the role of hemodynamic status as an important predictor for recurrent ischemia.

EVALUATION

Standard evaluation for patients presenting with VBI, as with other stroke syndromes, includes parenchymal brain imaging and cerebrovascular imaging, typically performed with a combination of magnetic resonance imaging (MRI) and magnetic resonance angiography (MRA). If vertebrobasilar occlusive disease is evident, imaging and clinical presentation can ascertain the etiology as atherosclerotic (vs. dissection or extrinsic compression). For athero-occlusive disease, given that a hemodynamic mechanism for stroke appears to be a significant factor, determining the extent of flow compromise within the vertebrobasilar system and distal arterial tree is an important element of patient assessment.

Unlike the anterior circulation, modalities for hemodynamic assessment in the posterior circulation are limited. Validated and precise techniques for assessing blood flow in the posterior circulation are lacking, especially at the tissue perfusion level. The modalities of imaging frequently employed in the anterior circulation to determine flow, by assessing vessel velocities (using transcranial

Doppler [TCD]), or tissue perfusion (using positron emission tomography [PET], xenon compute tomography [CT], single-photon emission computed tomography [SPECT], MR/CT perfusion), have been less effective in evaluating the posterior circulation.[18] Regional imaging resolution with these techniques is generally inadequate to reliably demonstrate perfusion deficits in the compact brain territories at risk with posterior circulation disease, and TCD is operator dependent and can be limited by anatomical variation, such as vascular tortuosity or skull density, for intracranial measurements.

Although the traditional methods of hemodynamic assessment have been difficult to apply to the vertebrobasilar system, a technique using phase contrast MR has become available in recent years, which provides the ability to quantify flow rates through individual craniocervical vessels, adding a new dimension to the conventional imaging modalities.[19,20] This technique of quantitative MR angiography (QMRA) allows flow measurement in cubic centimeters per minute in vessels of interest; this technology is now commercially available in a validated software called NOVA (Non-invasive Optimal Vessel Analysis, VasSol, Inc., Chicago, IL).[21] By direct measurement of volumetric blood flow through the major vessels of the posterior circulation (vertebral, basilar, and posterior cerebral arteries) QMRA can provide an assessment of local and distal flow compromise. In a retrospective study of 47 patients, such vessel flow measurements were highly predictive of recurrent stroke risk in symptomatic vertebrobasilar disease (vertebrobasilar stenosis [$\geq$50%] or occlusion).[22] The patients underwent QMRA using NOVA, and flow compromise was defined as >20% reduction below the normative lower limits of blood flow in the vessel measured. Given the potential for collateral to the posterior circulation, through routes such as the posterior communicating artery, the flows of interest in determining the overall hemodynamic status of the posterior circulation were flows in the distal downstream vessels, namely, the basilar artery and its largest terminal branches, the posterior cerebral arteries (PCA). Patients were designated as "low flow" if both the basilar and PCAs were reduced below the flow threshold: <120 cc/min for the basilar and <40 cc/min for the PCAs. Over an average of 28 months follow-up, a significantly higher risk of recurrent symptoms was evident in patients with low flow, 19% per person-year, compared to those with normal flow at 0% per person-year. The stroke-free survival was 100% at 24 months in the normal-flow group compared with 71% in the low-flow group. The utility of QMRA in evaluating patients with vertebrobasilar athero-occlusive disease is currently being investigated through a prospective multicenter National Institutes of Health–funded study, VERiTAS (Vertebrobasilar Flow Evaluation and Risk of Transient Ischemic Attack and Stroke, NCT 00590980). If predictive, QMRA flow evaluation could help to distinguish patients with flow compromise and at highest risk of recurrent symptoms. Such patients would be the most appropriate candidates for intervention to augment flow to the posterior circulation.

TREATMENT OPTIONS

At present, medical management consisting of antithrombotic therapy and risk factor modification aimed at factors such as blood pressure, cholesterol, and smoking cessation are the first line of treatment for patients with symptomatic vertebrobasilar disease. However, recurrent ischemic events can occur despite medical therapy.

Recent advances in angioplasty and stent technology offer a potential endovascular treatment strategy for vertebrobasilar lesions. Early reports indicated high mortality and morbidity rates, especially for intracranial disease. Gress et al. reported a 28% overall stroke and death risk, and 16% risk of disabling stroke and death from angioplasty for symptomatic intracranial vertebrobasilar stenosis in 25 patients treated between 1986 and 1999.[23] Levy et al. reported a 36% complication rate in 11 patients with intracranial vertebrobasilar disease undergoing stent assisted angioplasty, with two of four events being fatalities.[24] Fiorella et al. found a 26.1% periprocedural risk associated with stenting 44 patients with intracranial vertebrobasilar disease.[25] Other series, however, indicate that endovascular intervention has become less morbid and increasingly feasible in the posterior circulation. Such reports demonstrate reduced complication rates and fatalities with periprocedural event rates ranging from 8% to 18%.[26–29]

The efficacy and risks of stenting were prospectively evaluated in the Stenting of Symptomatic Atherosclerotic Lesions in the Vertebral or Intracranial Arteries (SSYLVIA) Study,[30] a multicenter feasibility study evaluating angioplasty/stenting of intracranial stenosis and extracranial vertebral stenosis >50%. Of the overall 61 study patients, 40 were treated for extra- or intracranial vertebrobasilar disease. In those patients, periprocedural stroke occurred in 7.5%, and 12.5% had a territorial stroke at 1 year. A recent study of a new self-expanding intracranial stent (Wingspan) revealed periprocedural complications (all resulting in death) in 10.7% of 28 patients with symptomatic intracranial vertebrobasilar disease.[31] The overall effectiveness of endovascular therapy however remains unproven at present, and not all vertebrobasilar disease is amenable to endovascular therapy.

Therefore, patients presenting with refractory VBI despite maximal medical therapy are potential candidates for posterior circulation EC-IC bypass. The use of bypass for revascularization in the setting of posterior fossa ischemia has been less studied than anterior circulation ischemia due to the relative prevalence of the conditions, the availability and evolution of endovascular techniques for treatment of vertebrobasilar stenosis, and the relatively higher morbidity and technical complexity of posterior circulation bypass. However, various EC-IC bypass options to the posterior circulation are feasible, including occipital artery to posterior inferior cerebellar artery (OA-PICA), superficial temporal artery to superior cerebellar artery (STA-SCA), and STA-PCA bypasses.

Overall, surgical revascularization of the posterior circulation does carry a higher risk and lower patency rate than that

17

seen with anterior circulation bypass. Patency rates for OA-PICA bypass range from 88% to 100%, with mortality rates averaging 4%.[32] For STA-PCA and STA-SCA bypass, a review of 86 bypasses compiled from several series, revealed patency rates in the 78% to 90% range, with mortality averaging 12%,[32,33] and serious morbidity of 20%. Although these series have shown improvement in symptoms in a subset of patients, the morbidity and mortality associated with such revascularization procedures have introduced caution when entertaining surgical bypass options, particularly for patients with poor neurological condition or medical comorbidities. Nonetheless, advances in microsurgical and neuroanesthetic technique since the publication of such series, as well as improvements in perioperative neurointensive care management, allow posterior circulation revascularization to be successfully undertaken in select patients without other options for management.

INDICATIONS FOR EC-IC BYPASS

Bypass for posterior circulation ischemia is restricted primarily to patients with vertebrobasilar atherosclerotic occlusive disease. The indications for EC-IC bypass in this setting are limited, as no prospective or randomized studies have been performed to assess the efficacy of surgical intervention, and the procedures carry the risk of morbidity. The EC-IC bypass study of STA-MCA bypass for carotid occlusion, published in 1985, failed to demonstrate the benefit of bypass for anterior circulation ischemia in hemodynamically unselected patients.[34] In light of those results, and given that bypass for posterior circulation ischemia typically carries a higher morbidity and mortality than the STA-MCA procedure, posterior circulation bypass can only be offered very selectively to patients with symptomatic vertebrobasilar disease.

The approach is to first optimize all medical therapeutic options, including judicious blood pressure control, aggressive lipid lowering with statins, and maximizing antiplatelet regimens, glycemic control, and smoking cessation. If the patient has recurrent ischemia despite these measures, and shows evidence of hemodynamic compromise on QMRA or alternative blood flow assessment modality, endovascular therapy can be entertained if feasible. If the underlying condition is not amenable to endovascular treatment, such as complete vessel occlusion, then bypass options will be considered, but only if comorbid cardiac or medical conditions are not prohibitive to undergoing general anesthesia and surgery with acceptable risk. Particular caution should be used in considering bypass distal to a high-grade vessel stenosis, for example, in the case of STA-SCA bypass for severe basilar stenosis. Distal bypass can create competing flow at the location of disease, which has the potential to precipitate thrombosis at the site of stenosis and cause local infarction with devastating consequence. A similar mechanism has been suspected for the poor results seen with STA-MCA bypass in the setting of severe MCA stenosis in the EC-IC Bypass Trial.

PREOPERATIVE ASSESSMENT

Patients who are considered for posterior circulation bypass should undergo angiography to delineate the intracranial vasculature with selective external carotid runs to evaluate the caliber and course of donor branches such as the STA or OA. If there is concern regarding the adequacy of the in situ donors, alternative bypass strategies using interposition grafts (saphenous vein or radial artery) can be entertained. Given that atherosclerosis is the primary etiology for the vertebrobasilar disease encountered in such patients, systemic atherosclerotic disease is also often present. Therefore, preoperative cardiac and medical clearance, including echocardiography and stress testing, for cardiac risk stratification is an important element of preoperative assessment.

PREOPERATIVE PREPARATIONS AND ANESTHETIC CONSIDERATIONS

Patients are generally already on aspirin. If not, they are instructed to take 325 mg beginning 1 week prior to surgery or at least the night prior to surgery. For patients on dual antiplatelets, such as Plavix, the second agent is discontinued 1 week prior to surgery and replaced with Lovenox or equivalent until the day prior to surgery. If the patient has been on Coumadin anticoagulation, they are converted to intravenous heparin, which is withheld 6 hours prior to surgery as antiplatelets are administered. Arterial line and central venous access are routinely obtained. Antibiotic prophylaxis is administered prior to skin incision and maintained for 48 hours postoperatively.

Throughout the surgery, normovolemia, normocapnia, and mild hypertension are maintained. For tenuous patients who are blood pressure dependent, even extreme hypertension is maintained throughout until the bypass has been completed. Lumbar drain for cerebrospinal fluid (CSF) drainage is used preferentially for brain relaxation to avoid the need for intravenous diuretics (Furosemide), hyperosmolar agents (Mannitol), or hyperventilation. Scalp electrodes for electroencephalographic (EEG) monitoring are placed outside the surgical field. This allows for induction of metabolic burst suppression during temporary vessel occlusion, using preferentially inhalational agents, which increase cerebral blood flow in comparison to barbiturates. Somatosensory-evoked potential (SSEP) and motor-evoked potential (MEP) can also be used for physiologic monitoring during the surgery, and can be useful in alerting the operative team to inadequate blood pressure maintenance during the case.

SURGICAL TECHNIQUES

The primary EC-IC bypass options for revascularization of posterior circulation ischemia are the STA-SCA bypass and the OA-PICA bypass.[35] Other described variants include the

OA-anterior inferior cerebellar artery (AICA), STA-PCA, and use of vein interposition graft to the SCA or PCA.[35-38] The general principles of positioning and approach for these variants are similar to the standard STA-SCA and OA-PICA bypasses that are described in the following text.

STA-SCA Bypass

Positioning

A subtemporal approach is traditionally used for the STA-SCA bypass. The patient is placed in lateral decubitus position with an axillary pad and appropriate padding, or supine with head turned and a shoulder roll to prevent excessive neck rotation. The head is fixed in lateral position with a rigid head holder (Figure 17–1A). The scalp is shaved, and a Doppler is utilized to map the trunk of the STA starting at the level of the zygoma, as well as both anterior and posterior branches of the vessel (see Figure 17–1A). Mapping is best performed after head fixation and pinning, which can pull the skin and displace prior skin markings. The bypass is typically performed on the right side if possible, given that manipulation of the temporal lobe is involved, making the nondominant side preferable.

Skin incision and STA dissection

The skin incision is generally planned to overlie the STA trunk just anterior to the tragus in the region of the zygoma and extend along the course of the posterior branch in a linear fashion. If the posterior branch is inadequate as a donor vessel, the incision can be curved forward to elevate a skin flap, and expose the anterior branch from the undersurface of the skin flap for dissection.

The initial incision through the epidermis and dermis is made along the midpoint of the projected course of the STA branch. Once the vessel is visualized, it is dissected proximally in the loose areolar plane above the vessel, until the main trunk of the STA is reached. The same procedure is performed distally, although the tissue is more adherent to the vessel distally and dissection must proceed with caution. These steps are performed either under loupe or microscopic magnification. The goal is to dissect at least 8 to 10 cm of STA in order to have enough length to reach subtemporally to the SCA. Once exposed, the STA and a cuff of surrounding tissue are skeletonized and lifted from the underlying temporalis muscle fascia, and wrapped in a papaverine-soaked cottonoid to alleviate vessel spasm induced by the mechanical manipulation of the vessel.

Craniotomy

The temporalis muscle is cut along the line of the scalp incision and retracted both anteriorly and posteriorly. Extending the linear incision to a T-shape or cruciate incision superiorly can facilitate retraction. The STA can be truncated at its most distal point and reflected inferiorly during the craniotomy to avoid injury to the vessel. It is important to flush the vessel with heparinized saline after truncation, placing a temporary clip proximally to avoid blood stagnating in the vessel. If the

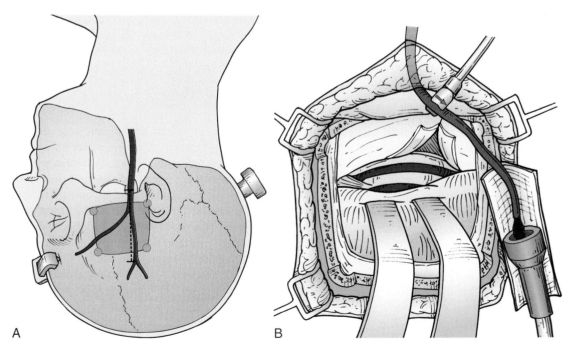

Figure 17–1. STA-SCA bypass. **A,** Incision and craniotomy. **B,** Exposure of the STA via subtemporal approach, and measurement of STA cut flow using ultrasonic flow probe.

continued

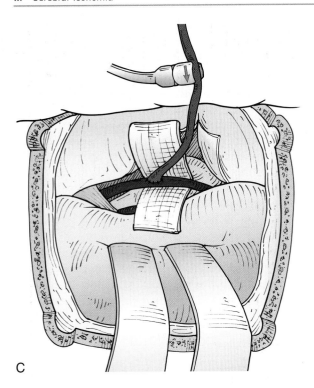

C

Figure 17-1—cont'd C, Completed STA-SCA bypass and measurement of bypass flow using ultrasonic flow probe.

anterior branch is sacrificed, leaving a stump with a temporary clip will facilitate its use as a venting branch later.

A burr hole is placed above the zygoma and along the posterior and anterior aspect of the superior temporal line, allowing a standard temporal bone flap to be elevated and centered over the insertion of the zygomatic arch (see Figure 17–1A). The zygomatic arch and prominent elevations of the middle fossa floor are drilled to create a flat plane of approach. The dura is opened as a semicircular flap that is retracted inferiorly.

Approach and preparation for anastomosis

The microscope is utilized for all intradural aspects of the procedure. Using lumbar drainage for relaxation, the temporal lobe is elevated, with coagulation of any small anterior bridging veins if needed. Once the tentorial edge is reached, the third nerve anteriorly is apparent and the arachnoid is dissected to visualize the SCA. Often it is necessary to cut the tentorium to better visualize the lateral course of the STA. The tentorium should be divided posteriorly, behind the insertion of the fourth nerve, and can be stitched laterally (Figure 17–1B). Further elevation of the temporal lobe will bring the SCA into view. Once the SCA has been identified, a perforator-free zone along its lateral course is prepared by placing a rubber dam beneath it. A papaverine soaked cotton ball can be applied to the vessel surface to alleviate spasm prior to anastomoses. Next, the required length of STA to reach the anastomotic site without tension is gauged, and marked on the vessel with a marking pen. The vessel is then

dissected free of its cuff of tissue to a point 1 inch proximal to the planned anastomosis length. Care must be taken to identify and coagulate side branches of the STA as this is performed.

Once the STA has been prepared, it is useful to check the "cut flow" of the vessel. This is performed by measuring the free flow through the cut end of the STA branch with a quantitative microvascular ultrasonic flow probe (Charbel Micro-Flowprobe; Transonics Systems Inc., Ithaca, NY).[39] The cut flow represents the flow-carrying capacity of the vessel, and indicates the maximal flow augmentation that the graft will provide to the intracranial circulation.

Performing the anastomosis

The STA-SCA anastomosis is performed in an end-to-side fashion. The STA is cut at a slight bevel and can be fishmouthed to enlarge the opening. It is important to examine the lumen of the STA carefully at this point for intimal disease or vessel dissection, which would lead to an unsuccessful bypass. Temporary mini-clips are placed proximally and then distally on the SCA. The vessel is then incised with an ophthalmic blade, and opened to the required length with microscissors. The opened vessel lumen is flushed with heparinized saline, and 10-0 nylon suture is used to place anchoring sutures at the apices of the incision. Due to the depth of the anastomoses, a continuous suture technique on each side of the anastomosis is faster and more practical than interrupted sutures. The technique for running the suture involves leaving short loops of suture along the entire length of the vessel, which are tightened sequentially just prior to tying, to achieve an even tension along the entire suture line. Placement of a small silastic stent into the SCA during suturing can help to avoid inadvertent opposite-wall suturing; this is removed prior to tightening of the suture line. Once the anastomosis is complete, the temporary clips on the SCA are released. If a venting branch is available on the STA, it is used for back-bleeding, prior to releasing the STA proximal clip. Gentle pressure is applied to the anastomosis site with cotton balls if there is any oozing. With careful attention to suture technique, additional sutures to control anastomotic leak are rarely necessary. If needed, a single 10-0 nylon suture can be placed at the bleeding site, generally without the necessity of reclipping the vessels unless there is profuse leakage.

Blood flow is again measured, now on the bypassed STA, which provides confirmation of the patency and function of the bypass (Figure 17–1C). A cut flow index (ratio of the bypass flow to the initial cut flow) is a sensitive predictor of bypass function.[39] Intraoperative conventional angiography is generally unnecessary if direct flow measurements and video indocyanine green (ICG) angiography are performed for physiologic and anatomic graft confirmation.

Closure of the craniotomy

The dura is loosely tacked or not closed with a slit created for passage of the STA, and the dural opening is covered with a piece of gelfoam. The bone is replaced, but the inferior opening is enlarged to accommodate the STA, avoiding any kinking or pressure on the vessel. The muscle is reapproximated loosely, and left open inferiorly to avoid pressure on the STA; the skin is closed with care to avoid any injury to the proximal STA trunk. The unused branch of the STA is generally ligated to optimize flow through the bypass.

OA-PICA Bypass

Positioning

A lateral suboccipital approach is traditionally used for the OA-PICA bypass. The patient is placed in prone or three-quarter prone position with the head rigidly fixed and flexed to optimize access to the posterior fossa. The scalp is shaved, and a Doppler can be utilized to map the distal OA, although the vessel is often difficult to localize prior to incision.

Skin incision and OA dissection

The skin incision is planned as a hockey-stick flap based over midline and toward the side of interest, ending over the region of the mastoid process (Figure 17–2A). The occipital artery should be identified in the midpoint of the horizontal portion of the incision, where it can be transected, flushed with heparin solution, and occluded with a temporary clip on the proximal end. The suboccipital muscles are then dissected in the

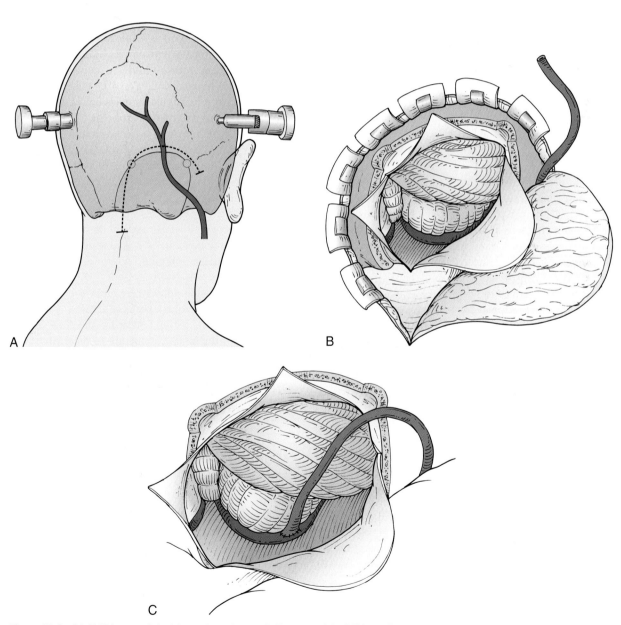

Figure 17–2. OA-PICA bypass. **A,** Incision and craniotomy. **B,** Exposure of the PICA tonsillomedullary loop and dissected OA. **C,** Completed OA-PICA bypass.

midline avascular plane. The skin and muscle flap can then be retracted laterally and inferiorly. The OA is then dissected free from the undersurface of the flap up until its exit point from the mastoid region, then wrapped in papaverine soaked cottonoids to relieve spasm. The OA is generally tortuous in its course and adherent to the surrounding tissue; therefore dissection can be tedious, but must proceed in a meticulous manner to avoid injury to the vessel.

Craniotomy

The suboccipital muscle is dissected laterally to the mastoid on the ipsilateral side, but also across midline in preparation for the craniotomy. A standard lateral suboccipital craniotomy is performed (see Figure 17–2A), extending to the edge of the sigmoid sinus laterally, and across midline including the foramen magnum. The ipsilateral bony removal helps to prevent kinking of the OA against the bony edge after muscle closure, and extension of the craniotomy across midline creates a broader and flatter working space, reducing the depth and difficulty of the subsequent anastomosis. The dura is opened in a hockey-stick fashion near midline, with an additional limb crossing midline to the contralateral side.

Approach and preparation for anastomosis

The microscope is utilized for all intradural aspects of the procedure. Using lumbar drainage and opening of the cisterna magna for relaxation, the ipsilateral cerebellar tonsil is elevated, bringing the tonsillomedullary segment of the PICA into view. This is the preferred location of anastomoses, as a lengthy perforator-free portion can be readily obtained, and the loop of vessel can be mobilized and elevated with cotton balls or gelfoam to reduce the depth of the anastomosis (Figure 17–2B). Once the recipient has been prepared, the required length of OA to reach the anastomotic site without tension is marked, and the OA is dissected free of any adherent tissue to a point 1 inch proximal to this location. Once the OA has been prepared, the cut flow of the vessel should be checked, and the vessel flushed again with heparinized saline.

Performing the anastomosis

An end-to-side anastomosis of the OA-PICA is performed. The OA is beveled and fish-mouthed. Temporary clips are placed proximally and then distally on the PICA segment. The vessel is then incised, opened to the required length, and flushed with heparinized saline. Typically due to the larger caliber of the vessels, and the greater thickness of the OA vessel wall, 9-0 nylon suture rather than 10-0 nylon suture is used for the anastomosis. The larger caliber of the vessels also allows for a running suture technique, as described previously. Temporary clips on the PICA, then the OA, are removed following completion of the anastomosis, and the flow in the

OA graft is measured to determine the cut flow index, confirming patency and function of the graft (Figure 17–2C).

Closure of the craniotomy

The dura is tacked loosely and the dural opening is covered with a piece of gelfoam. The superior portion of the bone can be replaced, but with care to avoid pressure on the graft. The lateral suboccipital musculature sometimes needs to be trimmed to prevent pressure on the exit point of the OA, and the midline muscle closure is performed with care to avoid kinking of the graft.

POSTOPERATIVE CARE

Patients are resumed on aspirin 325 mg daily starting immediately postoperatively. Patients are observed in the intensive care unit postoperatively and are kept well hydrated, with avoidance of hypotension. Pressure over the temple region (by nasal oxygen cannula, or glasses) is avoided to prevent direct mechanical occlusion of the STA trunk for STA bypasses. Blood pressure is reduced into the normal range. Hypertension is avoided given the potential risk for hyperperfusion hemorrhage, although this appears to occur less commonly in the posterior circulation, and with STA or OA grafts than larger higher-flow interposition grafts. Potential postoperative complications include epidural hematoma or wound infection. Postoperative graft occlusion is rare, given that bypass function can be well assessed intraoperatively with flow measurement, and graft revision performed at that time if necessary.

Baseline angiography, CTA, or MRA is performed postoperatively. We routinely perform QMRA instead, to confirm postoperative patency and measure the flow in the graft, as well as the intracranial vasculature to determine whether flow augmentation to the posterior circulation has been successfully achieved (Figure 17–3). Patients are discharged on daily aspirin, and can follow up with QMRA 6 weeks, 6 months, and yearly thereafter.

CONCLUSION

Surgical treatment of posterior circulation ischemia remains challenging. The bypass options themselves are more technically demanding to perform than for anterior circulation ischemia, and the patient population affected generally has significant comorbidities that increase perioperative morbidity. Success is highly dependent on attention to technique at every stage of the operation, as well as careful patient selection and perioperative medical management.

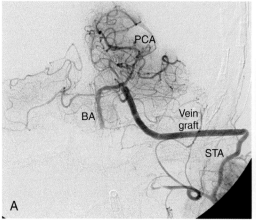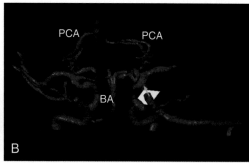

Figure 17–3. STA-PCA bypass with use of short interposition saphenous vein graft (see operative video). **A,** AP external carotid angiogram demonstrating the graft, and filling of the rostral basilar system. **B,** QMRA demonstrating anterograde flow in the bypass (*arrow*) measuring 64 cc/min.

REFERENCES

1. Caplan LR: *Posterior circulation disease: clinical findings, diagnosis, and management,* Cambridge, MA, 1996, Blackwell Science.
2. Caplan LR: Vertebrobasilar disease, *Adv Neurol* 92:131–140, 2003.
3. Caplan LR: Treatment of patients with vertebrobasilar occlusive disease, *Compr Ther* 12:23–28, 1986.
4. Bogousslavsky J, Regli F, Maeder P, et al: The etiology of posterior circulation infarcts: a prospective study using magnetic resonance imaging and magnetic resonance angiography, *Neurology* 43:1528–1533, 1993.
5. Caplan LR, Wityk RJ, Glass TA, et al: New England Medical Center Posterior Circulation registry, *Ann Neurol* 56:389–398, 2004.
6. Voetsch B, DeWitt LD, Pessin MS, et al: Basilar artery occlusive disease in the New England Medical Center Posterior Circulation Registry, *Arch Neurol* 61:496–504, 2004.
7. Caplan LR, Hennerici M: Impaired clearance of emboli (washout) is an important link between hypoperfusion, embolism, and ischemic stroke, *Arch Neurol* 55:1475–1482, 1998.
8. Savitz SI, Caplan LR: Vertebrobasilar disease, *N Engl J Med* 352: 2618–2626, 2005.
9. Anonymous: Prognosis of patients with symptomatic vertebral or basilar artery stenosis: The Warfarin-Aspirin Symptomatic Intracranial Disease (WASID) Study Group, *Stroke* 29:1389–1392, 1998.
10. Qureshi AI, Ziai WC, Yahia AM, et al: Stroke-free survival and its determinants in patients with symptomatic vertebrobasilar stenosis: a multicenter study, *Neurosurgery* 52:1033–1039, 2003; discussion 1039–40.
11. Anonymous: Beneficial effect of carotid endarterectomy in symptomatic patients with high-grade carotid stenosis: North American Symptomatic Carotid Endarterectomy Trial Collaborators [see comment], *N Engl J Med* 325:445–453, 1991.
12. Moufarrij NA, Little JR, Furlan AJ, et al: Basilar and distal vertebral artery stenosis: long-term follow-up, *Stroke* 17:938–942, 1986.
13. Chimowitz MI, Lynn MJ, Howlett-Smith H, et al: Comparison of warfarin and aspirin for symptomatic intracranial arterial stenosis, *N Engl J Med* 352:1305–1316, 2005.
14. Mazighi M, Tanasescu R, Ducrocq X, et al: Prospective study of symptomatic atherothrombotic intracranial stenoses: the GESICA study, *Neurology* 66:1187–1191, 2006.
15. Chimowitz MI, Kokkinos J, Strong J, et al: The Warfarin-Aspirin Symptomatic Intracranial Disease Study, *Neurology* 45:1488–1493, 1995.
16. Thijs VN, Albers GW: Symptomatic intracranial atherosclerosis: outcome of patients who fail antithrombotic therapy, *Neurology* 55: 490–497, 2000.
17. Kasner SE, Chimowitz MI, Lynn MJ, et al: Predictors of ischemic stroke in the territory of a symptomatic intracranial arterial stenosis, *Circulation* 113:555–563, 2006.
18. Haase J, Magnussen IB, Ogilvy CS, et al: Evaluating patients with vertebrobasilar transient ischemic attacks, *Surg Neurol* 52:386–392, 1999.
19. Guppy KH, Charbel FT, Corsten LA, et al: Hemodynamic evaluation of basilar and vertebral artery angioplasty, *Neurosurgery* 51:327–333, 2002; discussion 333–4.
20. Hendrikse J, van Raamt AF, van der Graaf Y, et al: Distribution of cerebral blood flow in the circle of Willis, *Radiology* 235:184–189, 2005.
21. Zhao M, Charbel FT, Alperin N, et al: Improved phase-contrast flow quantification by three-dimensional vessel localization, *Magn Reson Imaging* 18:697–706, 2000.
22. Amin-Hanjani S, Du X, Zhao M, et al: Use of quantitative magnetic resonance angiography to stratify stroke risk in symptomatic vertebrobasilar disease, *Stroke* 36:1140–1145, 2005.
23. Gress DR, Smith WS, Dowd CF, et al: Angioplasty for intracranial symptomatic vertebrobasilar ischemia, *Neurosurgery* 51:23–27, 2002; discussion 27–9.
24. Levy EI, Horowitz MB, Koebbe CJ, et al: Transluminal stent-assisted angioplasty of the intracranial vertebrobasilar system for medically refractory, posterior circulation ischemia: early results [see comment], *Neurosurgery* 48:1215–1221, 2001; discussion 1221–3.
25. Fiorella D, Chow MM, Anderson M, et al: A 7-year experience with balloon-mounted coronary stents for the treatment of symptomatic vertebrobasilar intracranial atheromatous disease, *Neurosurgery* 61:236–242, 2007; discussion 242–3.
26. Barakate MS, Snook KL, Harrington TJ, et al: Angioplasty and stenting in the posterior cerebral circulation, *J Endovasc Ther* 8:558–565, 2001.
27. Gomez CR, Misra VK, Liu MW, et al: Elective stenting of symptomatic basilar artery stenosis, *Stroke* 31:95–99, 2000.
28. Nahser HC, Henkes H, Weber W, et al: Intracranial vertebrobasilar stenosis: angioplasty and follow-up, *AJNR Am J Neuroradiol* 21: 1293–1301, 2000.
29. Rasmussen PA, Perl J II, Barr JD, et al: Stent-assisted angioplasty of intracranial vertebrobasilar atherosclerosis: an initial experience, *J Neurosurg* 92:771–778, 2000.
30. Stenting of Symptomatic Atherosclerotic Lesions in the Vertebral or Intracranial Arteries (SSYLVIA): study results, *Stroke* 35:1388–1392, 2004.
31. Fiorella D, Levy EI, Turk AS, et al: U.S. multicenter experience with the wingspan stent system for the treatment of intracranial atheromatous disease: periprocedural results, *Stroke* 38:881–887, 2007.
32. Hopkins LN, Budny JL: Complications of intracranial bypass for vertebrobasilar insufficiency, *J Neurosurg* 70:207–211, 1989.
33. Ausman JI, Diaz FG, Vacca DF, Sadasivan B: Superficial temporal and occipital artery bypass pedicles to superior, anterior inferior, and

posterior inferior cerebellar arteries for vertebrobasilar insufficiency, *J Neurosurg* 72:554–558, 1990.

34. Failure of extracranial-intracranial arterial bypass to reduce the risk of ischemic stroke. Results of an international randomized trial. The EC/IC Bypass Study Group, *N Engl J Med* 313:1191–1200, 1985.

35. Ausman JI, Diaz FG, Dujovny M: Posterior circulation revascularization, *Clin Neurosurg* 33:331–343, 1986.

36. Russell SM, Post N, Jafar JJ: Revascularizing the upper basilar circulation with saphenous vein grafts: operative technique and lessons learned, *Surg Neurol* 66:285–297, 2006.

37. Sundt TM Jr, Piepgras DG, Houser OW, Campbell JK: Interposition saphenous vein grafts for advanced occlusive disease and large aneurysms in the posterior circulation, *J Neurosurg* 56:205–215, 1982.

38. Hopkins LN, Budny JL, Spetzler RF: Revascularization of the rostral brain stem, *Neurosurgery* 10:364–369, 1982.

39. Amin-Hanjani S, Du X, Mlinarevich N, et al: The cut flow index: an intraoperative predictor of the success of extracranial-intracranial bypass for occlusive cerebrovascular disease, *Neurosurgery* 56:75–85, 2005.

CEREBRAL REVASCULARIZATION FOR MOYAMOYA DISEASE

18

GORDON LI; MICHAEL LIM; NADIA KHAN; GARY K. STEINBERG

MOYAMOYA DISEASE

Moyamoya disease (MMD) is a rare cerebrovascular disorder characterized by idiopathic and progressive stenosis or occlusion of the supraclinoid internal carotid arteries bilaterally with frequent involvement of the bilateral anterior and middle cerebral arteries[1] (Figure 18-1). The term *Moyamoya* meaning "a puff of smoke" in Japanese was first coined in 1969 by Suzuki and Takaku to describe the resulting characteristic abnormal vascular networks that form secondarily to the stenosis/occlusion,[2] but the disease was first described in the Japanese literature in 1957 by Takeuchi and Shimizu.[3] Although genetic links are implicated in MMD,[4] the etiology remains unknown. Moyamoya syndrome (MMS) has similar clinical and angiographic characteristics to MMD but is associated with other conditions such as Downs syndrome, neurofibromatosis type-1 (NF-1), prior irradiation, and sickle cell disease.[5] Patients with unilateral findings have MMS, although approximately 40% of these patients develop angiographic progression on the contralateral side.[6] In this chapter, we will give an overview of MMD and provide a comprehensive surgical view of cerebral revascularization for MMD, emphasizing the technical nuances and complications of the procedure.

EPIDEMIOLOGY

Although MMD was initially described in patients of Asian descent, it recently has been increasingly reported in patients of all demographic groups, although the exact incidence is not completely known.[7] Japanese studies report an annual incidence between 0.35 to 0.94/100,000 persons per year and annual prevalence between 3.16 to 10.5 per 100,000 persons.[8-10] There is a bimodal distribution of age of onset with the first peak at 5 years of age and a second peak between 45 and 49 years of age. There are twice as many female patients as compared to male patients.[8,9] The reported incidence and prevalence of MMD in the United States is significantly lower when compared to Japanese studies. A study of Moyamoya

patients from Washington and California identified 298 individuals with MMD for an incidence of 0.086/100,000 persons per year. In a subgroup of Asian Americans, however, the incidence of 0.28/100,000 was closer to those of the Japanese studies.[11] A study looking at the epidemiology of MMD in Hawaii, where the cohort was primarily of Asian descent, also revealed a higher incidence when compared to the general population in the United States.[12]

PRESENTATION

Patients with MMD generally present either with hemorrhage or with ischemia. The rate of hemorrhage is approximately seven times more common in adult patients (14.6%) when compared to pediatric patients (2.1%).[5,13] However, this was not true for the 432 patients treated at Stanford from 1991 to 2009, where ischemic symptoms were far more common than hemorrhage.[13] Some have suggested that the hemorrhage rate is higher in Asians.[14-17] Occasionally patients may also present with seizure, headaches, or behavioral changes. Some studies suggest a relation between headaches and hypoperfusion leading to cortical depression and associated migraine symptoms.[18] Others have suggested that dilation of dural and meningeal vessels irritate the pain fibers on the dura, resulting in a migraine-like headache that is refractive to medical therapies.[19] This headache initially persisted in 63% of patients even after cerebral revascularization, although it would often improve over time.

PATHOPHYSIOLOGY

On histopathologic examination, the internal carotid arteries demonstrate eccentric fibrocellular thickening of the intimal layer, proliferation of smooth muscle cells, and tortuous and often duplicated internal elastic lamina with no inflammatory or atheromatous involvement, resulting in artery stenosis/occlusion.[4] The resulting hypoxia induces collateralization through formation of dilated and tortuous perforating arteries. These

185

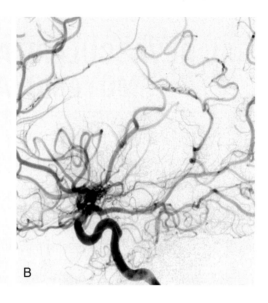

Figure 18–1. Left internal carotid artery anterior-posterior and lateral injections demonstrating supraclinoid internal carotid artery stenosis and M1 occlusion with resultant Moyamoya vessels.

A

B

"Moyamoya" vessels have thinned media with fibrin deposition in the vessel walls, fragmented elastic lamina, and microaneurysm formation that may be secondary to increased expression of numerous growth factors, including hypoxia-inducible factor 1 (HIF-1), vascular endothelial growth factor (VEGF), basic fibroblast growth factor (bFGF), transforming growth factor-beta (TGF-beta), hepatocyte growth factor (HGF), and matrix metalloproteinases (MMPs).[4]

Genetic factors play a role as up to 15% of MMD patients are familial indicating an autosomal dominant inheritance pattern with incomplete penetrance. A number of genome-wide studies from these familial carriers of MMD suggest links to chromosomal regions including 3p24.2-p26,[20] 6q25,[21] 8q23,[22] 12p12,[22] and 17q25.[23] Recently, carriers of a mutation in the vascular smooth muscle cell (SMC)–specific isoform of alpha-actin (ACTA2) were found to present with a variety of vascular diseases including premature onset of coronary artery disease, non-Marfan's thoracic artery aneurysms and dissections, non-MMD early onset stroke, and MMD.[24]

NATURAL HISTORY AND PROGNOSIS

There are limited studies on the natural history of MMD, but each of the studies has demonstrated inevitable disease progression if left untreated.[6,25,26] In one study, the 5-year cumulative risk of any recurrent ipsilateral stroke in patients treated without surgery with impaired hemodynamic reserve, as measured by increased oxygen extraction fraction on positron emission tomography (PET), was approximately 65%. In patients with bilateral disease, the stroke risk over 5 years was 82%.[14] Another North American study found a recurrent stroke rate of 18% in the first year and a 5% per year risk in subsequent years.[17] A nationwide survey in Japan of asymptomatic Moyamoya patients found a 3.2% per year stroke rate

in medically treated patients.[27] In contrast, the estimated rate of perioperative or subsequent stroke or death after surgical revascularization was between 5.5%[13] and 17%[14] over 5 years, demonstrating the need for surgical treatment of these patients.

DIAGNOSES AND TREATMENT

The diagnoses of MMD or MMS should be considered in any patient, especially in a child or young adult who presents with neurologic deficits or symptoms secondary to cerebral ischemia or hemorrhage. Radiologic evaluation can include CT, MRI, cerebral angiography, and cerebral perfusion studies, including CT perfusion, xenon-enhanced CT, or PET, MR perfusion, and SPECT or CT imaging without and with acetazolamide challenge. Cerebral angiography, CT angiography, and MR angiography imaging can reveal intracerebral vascular occlusion along with the resulting Moyamoya vessels. CT and MRI can reveal hemorrhage or ischemic changes. Cerebral perfusion studies help to characterize blood flow and elucidate the hemodynamic state preoperatively and postoperatively.[28]

Although there are no randomized studies comparing medical treatment versus surgical revascularization for patients with MMD, we believe that the stroke rate is significantly reduced in surgically treated patients. As discussed in the previous section, the natural history of these patients is to progress and the risk of recurrent stroke is extremely high with medical management only. The main medical treatment option for these patients is antiplatelet therapy. All patients are on aspirin pre- and postoperatively. Full anticoagulation drugs such as warfarin are rarely used.[5]

Patients with MMD have occlusion of the internal carotid arteries with sparing of the external carotid system. Surgical treatment uses the external carotid system to supply blood to the ischemic cerebrum by either creating a "direct" or an "indirect" revascularization bypass. A direct bypass involves dissection of a branch of the external carotid artery, specifically the superficial temporal artery (STA), which is then directly anastomosed to a distal (usually M4) cortical branch of the middle cerebral artery (MCA). An indirect bypass is performed by placement of vascularized tissue supplied by the external carotid (such as dura, the temporalis muscle, or the STA itself) onto the cortical surface of the brain leading to an ingrowth of new blood vessels to the cortex beneath it. There are no randomized studies comparing the efficacy and safety of indirect versus direct bypass, and a review of the literature failed to reveal a difference in surgical morbidity or stroke rate (perioperative or long term) between methods.[29] Many institutions will perform direct revascularization for adults and indirect revascularization for children because of the smaller and more friable caliber of the vessels in children.[30,31] However, there are many groups that perform indirect bypass for adult patients as well.[14,17,32] Our philosophy is to perform direct bypass on all patients unless the STA or MCA is too small or friable. Direct revascularization procedures have the advantage of providing immediate increase in blood flow to the ischemic cortex. In bilateral MMD, we first revascularize the symptomatic hemisphere. If there are no lateralizing signs or symptoms, we prefer to revascularize the non-dominant hemisphere because of increased incidence of transient neurologic symptoms after surgery on the dominant hemisphere. The contralateral side is generally revascularized 1 week after the first side unless there were significant complications after the first procedure.

DIRECT REVASCULARIZATION

The size of the frontal and parietal branch of the STA is determined preoperatively by cerebral angiography. The larger diameter branch is chosen as the donor vessel. The patient is positioned supine and placed in a three-point pin fixation. The head is elevated above the heart and turned to the side, bringing the frontotemporal region uppermost in the field. Stimulating and recording electrodes are placed for monitoring of bilateral somatosensory evoked potentials (SSEP) and bilateral EEG. Cooling to approximately 33°C is achieved by either a cooling blanket and bladder irrigation, or by placing an intravenous catheter (InnerCool Therapies Philips, Andover, MA) into the inferior vena cava as described previously.[33] In general, the InnerCool catheter is placed in the larger patients who are more difficult to cool and rewarm via surface techniques. The course of the superficial temporal artery is mapped out with a Doppler probe. When the parietal branch of the STA is chosen as the donor, the skin incision is planned over the artery along its course (Figure 18–2). If the frontal branch is the donor, the inferior portion of the incision follows the STA but as the artery tracks anterior to the hairline, the incision stays posterior behind the hairline for cosmetic purposes. After shaving the hair over the planned incision, the area is

prepped and draped in standard sterile fashion. The operating microscope is positioned and used for careful harvesting of the superficial temporal artery. A length of approximately 7 cm of STA with a generous cuff of soft tissue to protect it is needed for the bypass (Figure 18–3). Then the underlying temporalis fascia muscle is split and dissected from the frontotemporal bone.

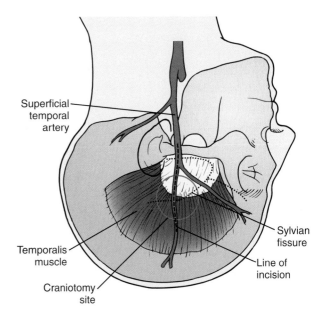

Figure 18–2. The course of the superficial temporal artery is mapped out using Doppler ultrasound and the skin incision is planned over the artery along its course.

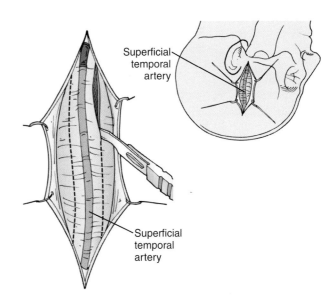

Figure 18–3. Approximately 7 cm of STA with a generous cuff of soft tissue to protect it is needed for the bypass. The artery and cuff are carefully dissected out using a combination of sharp dissection and cautery.

Burr holes are placed, the craniotomy bone flap is removed over the frontotemporal region, and the dura is opened in a cruciate manner (Figure 18–4).

Identification of a sufficiently large M4 branch of the MCA ($\geq$0.6 mm) emerging from the sylvian fissure is paramount for this procedure. The arachnoid overlying this cortical branch of the MCA is then microscopically opened. A 7-mm segment of M4 artery without branches is preferably chosen as the recipient, but any tiny branches arising from this segment can be coagulated and divided if necessary (Figure 18–5). A jeweler-type

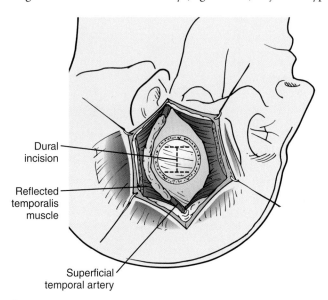

Figure 18–4. The underlying temporalis fascia muscle is split and dissected from the frontotemporal bone. Burr holes are placed, the craniotomy bone flap is removed over the frontotemporal region, and the dura is opened in a cruciate manner.

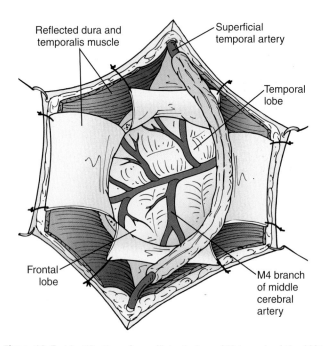

Figure 18–5. Identification of a sufficiently large M4 branch of the MCA ($\geq$0.6 mm) emerging from the sylvian fissure is paramount for this procedure.

bipolar is used. High-visibility background is placed under the M4 segment. Papaverine is intermittently instilled over the vessels to prevent spasm. Then the STA is temporarily occluded proximally and sectioned distally. The distal stump of the superficial temporal artery in the scalp is coagulated and the superficial temporal artery is truncated to the proper length for anastomosis and fish-mouthed. Temporary release of the proximal clip is performed to ensure excellent flow. The artery is temporarily occluded again proximally and flushed with heparinized saline. Intravenous thiopental is given to induce burst suppression in the EEG. The mean arterial pressure is raised and then the M4 MCA branch is temporarily occluded with Sugita aneurysm clips. An arteriotomy is made in the M4 branch, removing an elliptical portion of the superior wall, and irrigated with heparinized saline. An end-to-side anastomosis between the STA branch and the MCA branch is performed with 10-0 interrupted suture (Figure 18–6). The Sugita clips are then removed, restoring flow. Flow in all vessels is confirmed with the intraoperative Doppler. An intraoperative indocyanine green (ICG) angiogram is performed by injecting 2 ml of ICG dye intravenously and visualizing the graft with the near-infrared camera on the microscope. If the anastomosis is done correctly, the ICG demonstrates wide patency of the graft with no stenoses and good filling of the pial vasculature. It is our practice to then lay the STA with its soft tissue cuff on the cortical surface to induce an indirect bypass as well as a direct one (Figure 18–7). The dura is closed with 4-0 suture followed by synthetic dura, leaving an opening for the graft to enter without compromise. The bone is replaced using a plating system, also leaving an opening for the graft to enter unimpeded. The temporalis muscle and scalp are closed in several layers in the usual fashion. During the entire procedure care is taken to keep the mean arterial pressure high-normal for that patient and about 10 points higher during the occlusion of the cortical MCA branch for adequate perfusion. Patients are maintained normocarbic during the entire operation to prevent vasoconstriction and ischemia from hyperventilation.

INDIRECT REVASCULARIZATION

In patients in whom the STA is considered too small (<0.6 mm) or too fragile for direct revascularization, we perform an indirect revascularization (encephaloduroarteriosynangiosis or encephaloduromyosynangiosis). We have abandoned techniques such as free omental flap transplantation or pedicled omental flap transposition. In a similar fashion to the direct bypass procedure, patients are positioned and prepped, the STA and generous soft tissue cuff are harvested, and the craniotomy is performed. The arachnoid overlying the deep sulci and fissures are microscopically opened and the superficial temporal artery with the cuff of soft tissue is laid directly on the pial surface of the cortex. The closure is made in the usual fashion.

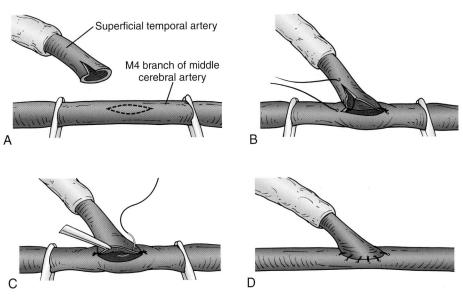

Figure 18–6. A, The superficial temporal artery is truncated to the proper length for anastomosis and fish-mouthed. **B,** An arteriotomy is made in the M4 branch, removing an elliptical portion of the superior wall. **C** and **D,** An end-to-side anastomosis between the STA branch and the MCA branch is performed with 10-0 interrupted suture.

RESULTS AND COMPLICATIONS

Patients are generally discharged after 3 to 4 hospital nights (the first night is spent in the intensive care unit). They are then evaluated clinically 1 week after the second bypass procedure (or after the first procedure in unilateral disease), and subsequently at 6 months, 3 years, and finally at 10 years. We also perform MRI, SPECT, or Xenon CT, and cerebral angiography at 6 months, 3 years, and 10 years. In addition to internal carotid and vertebral injections, external injections are included to evaluate bypass patency and extent of revascularization (Figure 18–8). In our series of 450 bypasses in 265 patients, 3% (eight patients) or 1.7% of procedures suffered postoperative ischemic stroke (four ipsilateral to the surgical hemisphere and four in the contralateral hemisphere). Fifty percent of these patients made a complete recovery by 6 months. A total of 2.6% (seven patients) suffered a postoperative hemorrhage (1.8% of procedures), all in the ipsilateral hemisphere with bleeding into prior ischemic regions. Of these seven patients, four made a full recovery by 6 months, but two died from hemorrhage within 30 days of the procedure. In nine patients (3.3% or 2.0% of procedures) transient neurologic symptoms without MRI changes occurred with full recovery by postoperative days 3 to 14. Statistical analysis for surgical risk identified several factors that trended toward increased risk; however, none were statistically significant. Patients who presented with transient ischemic attack (TIA) or stroke trended toward an increased risk of postoperative ischemic symptoms. Similarly, patients who presented with hemorrhage trended toward an increased risk of postoperative hemorrhage. Patients with MMD appeared to have a higher risk of postoperative stroke and death. Sex, ethnicity, unilateral versus bilateral, age, and type of revascularization procedure did not affect outcome.[13]

In long-term follow-up, 71.2% of our patients demonstrated improvement in quality of life. There was a significant

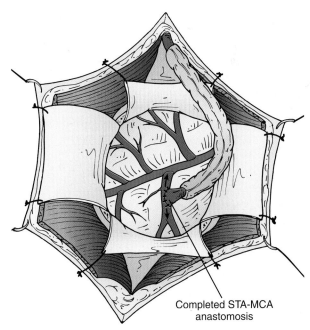

Figure 18–7. Completed bypass showing the STA with its soft tissue cuff on the cortical surface to induce both an indirect and direct bypass.

reduction in TIAs and >80% of patients who presented with headaches were headache-free at their last follow-up. The overall incidence of ischemic stroke after surgery was 3.8% (eight early and two late events) and the overall incidence of hemorrhagic stroke was 3.4% (seven early and two late events). The overall mortality rate was 2.3% (three early and three late deaths). The 5-year overall cumulative risk of postoperative stroke or death was 5.5%.[13] In another study, the 5-year risk of stroke or death was decreased from 65% in medically treated patients to 17% in surgically treated patients.[14] One study did fail to show a benefit of surgical treatment, but the authors reported an unusually high initial surgical morbidity and mortality.[17]

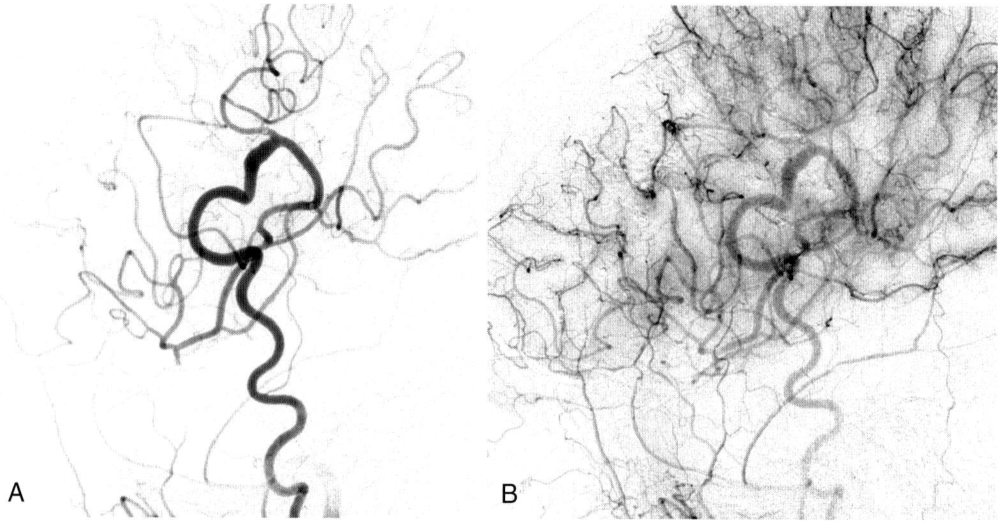

Figure 18–8. A and **B,** Left external carotid artery lateral injection demonstrating a patent superficial temporal artery to middle cerebral artery bypass supplying two thirds of the MCA territory.

A

B

CONCLUSION

In this chapter we have given an overview of MMD and provided details of surgical management of this disease, with an emphasis on the technical details and complications. Although there are risks to direct and indirect revascularization procedures for MMD, our series and the available data suggest that surgery is superior to medical management of these patients.

REFERENCES

1. Fukui M: Guidelines for the diagnosis and treatment of spontaneous occlusion of the Circle of Willis ("Moyamoya" disease). Research Committee on Spontaneous Occlusion of the Circle of Willis (Moyamoya Disease) of the Ministry of Health and Welfare, Japan, *Clin Neurol Neurosurg* 99(Suppl 2):S238–S240, 1997.
2. Suzuki J, Takaku A: Cerebrovascular "Moyamoya" disease. Disease showing abnormal net-like vessels in base of brain, *Arch Neurol* 20:288–299, 1969.
3. Takeuchi K, Shimizu K: Hypoplasia of the bilateral internal carotid arteries, *Brain Nerve* 9:37–43, 1957.
4. Achrol AS, Guzman R, Lee M, et al: Pathophysiology and genetic factors in moyamoya disease, *Neurosurg Focus* 26:E4, 2009.
5. Scott RM, Smith ER: Moyamoya disease and moyamoya syndrome, *N Engl J Med* 360:1226–1237, 2009.
6. Kelly ME, Bell-Stephens TE, Marks MP, et al: Progression of unilateral moyamoya disease: a clinical series, *Cerebrovasc Dis* 22:109–115, 2006.
7. Hoffman HJ: Moyamoya disease and syndrome, *Clin Neurol Neurosurg* 99(Suppl 2):S39–S44, 1997.
8. Baba T, Houkin K, Kuroda S: Novel epidemiological features of moyamoya disease, *J Neurol Neurosurg Psychiatry* 79:900–904, 2008.
9. Wakai K, Tamakoshi A, Ikezaki K, et al: Epidemiological features of moyamoya disease in Japan: findings from a nationwide survey, *Clin Neurol Neurosurg* 99(Suppl 2):S1–S5, 1997.
10. Kuriyama S, Kusaka Y, Fujimura M, et al: Prevalence and clinicoepidemiological features of moyamoya disease in Japan: findings from a nationwide epidemiological survey, *Stroke* 39:42–47, 2008.
11. Uchino K, Johnston SC, Becker KJ, et al: Moyamoya disease in Washington State and California, *Neurology* 65:956–958, 2005.
12. Graham JF, Matoba A: A survey of moyamoya disease in Hawaii, *Clin Neurol Neurosurg* 99(Suppl 2):S31–S35, 1997.
13. Guzman R, Lee M, Achrol A, et al: Clinical outcome after 450 revascularization procedures for moyamoya disease, *J Neurosurg* 111:927–935, 2009.
14. Hallemeier CL, Rich KM, Grubb RL Jr, et al: Clinical features and outcome in North American adults with moyamoya phenomenon, *Stroke* 37:1490–1496, 2006.
15. Yilmaz EY, Pritz MB, Bruno A, et al: Moyamoya: Indiana University Medical Center experience, *Arch Neurol* 58:1274–1278, 2001.
16. Suzuki J, Kodama N: Moyamoya disease—a review, *Stroke* 14: 104–109, 1983.
17. Chiu D, Shedden P, Bratina P, et al: Clinical features of moyamoya disease in the United States, *Stroke* 29:1347–1351, 1998.
18. Olesen J, Friberg L, Olsen TS, et al: Ischaemia-induced (symptomatic) migraine attacks may be more frequent than migraine-induced ischaemic insults, *Brain* 116(Pt 1):187–202, 1993.
19. Seol HJ, Wang KC, Kim SK, et al: Headache in pediatric moyamoya disease: review of 204 consecutive cases, *J Neurosurg* 103: 439–442, 2005.
20. Ikeda H, Sasaki T, Yoshimoto T, et al: Mapping of a familial moyamoya disease gene to chromosome 3p24.2-p26, *Am J Hum Genet* 64: 533–537, 1999.
21. Inoue TK, Ikezaki K, Sasazuki T, et al: Linkage analysis of moyamoya disease on chromosome 6, *J Child Neurol* 15:179–182, 2000.
22. Sakurai K, Horiuchi Y, Ikeda H, et al: A novel susceptibility locus for moyamoya disease on chromosome 8q23, *J HumGenet* 49:278–281, 2004.
23. Mineharu Y, Liu W, Inoue K, et al: Autosomal dominant moyamoya disease maps to chromosome 17q25.3, *Neurology* 70:2357–2363, 2008.
24. Guo DC, Papke CL, Tran-Fadulu V, et al: Mutations in smooth muscle alpha-actin (ACTA2) cause coronary artery disease, stroke, and moyamoya disease, along with thoracic aortic disease, *Am J Hum Genet* 84:617–627, 2009.
25. Imaizumi T, Hayashi K, Saito K, et al: Long-term outcomes of pediatric moyamoya disease monitored to adulthood, *Pediatr Neurol* 18:321–325, 1998.
26. Kuroda S, Ishikawa T, Houkin K, et al: Incidence and clinical features of disease progression in adult moyamoya disease, *Stroke* 36:2148–2153, 2005.
27. Kuroda S, Hashimoto N, Yoshimoto T, et al: Radiological findings, clinical course, and outcome in asymptomatic moyamoya disease: results of multicenter survey in Japan, *Stroke* 38: 1430–1435, 2007.

28. Lee M, Zaharchuk G, Guzman R, et al: Quantitative hemodynamic studies in moyamoya disease: a review, *Neurosurg Focus* 26:E5, 2009.

29. Veeravagu A, Guzman R, Patil CG, et al: Moyamoya disease in pediatric patients: outcomes of neurosurgical interventions, *Neurosurg Focus* 24:E16, 2008.

30. Mesiwala AH, Sviri G, Fatemi N, et al: Long-term outcome of superficial temporal artery–middle cerebral artery bypass for patients with moyamoya disease in the US, *Neurosurg Focus* 24:E15, 2008.

31. Scott RM, Smith JL, Robertson RL, et al: Long-term outcome in children with moyamoya syndrome after cranial revascularization by pial synangiosis, *J Neurosurg* 100:142–149, 2004.

32. Starke RM, Komotar RJ, Hickman ZL, et al: Clinical features, surgical treatment, and long-term outcome in adult patients with moyamoya disease. Clinical article, *J Neurosurg* 111:936–942, 2009.

33. Steinberg GK, Ogilvy CS, Shuer LM, et al: Comparison of endovascular and surface cooling during unruptured cerebral aneurysm repair, *Neurosurgery* 55:307–314, 2004.

18

CAROTID ENDARTERECTOMY

19

JOSHUA E. HELLER; CHRISTOPHER M. LOFTUS

INTRODUCTION

The first description of a carotid endarterectomy (CEA) for stroke was published in the *Lancet* in 1954.[5] Since that time, more clinical trials have been completed for CEA than for any other surgical procedure, first addressing the question of surgery versus best medical practice (clearly answered in favor of surgery in most cases) and, most recently, addressing the question of surgery versus endovascular carotid intervention. (These latest trials currently also favor open surgery versus endovascular intervention.)

We can review current indications for surgical intervention for carotid stenosis as follows. The first large cooperative trials randomized surgical reconstruction versus best medical therapy. The North American Symptomatic Carotid Endarterectomy Trial (NASCET) established that symptomatic patients with internal carotid artery stenoses of 50% or more benefit from surgical resection of the offending lesion.[1,3] The Asymptomatic Carotid Atherosclerosis Study (ACAS) and the European Asymptomatic Carotid Surgery Trial (ACST) trial[6,7] provided compelling evidence that asymptomatic patients with 60% or more stenosis of the cervical internal carotid artery have a more favorable outcome with endarterectomy, provided that perioperative morbidity and mortality remain low (<3%),[2] and that the patient otherwise has a 5-year life expectancy (the time needed to achieve a surgical benefit).

Surgical reconstruction (CEA) has now been randomized against carotid stenting (CAS) in several trials. To date, none has shown an advantage of CAS in either safety or efficacy. The latest trials, EVA-3S and SPACE, continue to demonstrate that open surgery is the safest and best treatment in most cases.[28,29] The SAPPHIRE trial randomized "high-risk" asymptomatic and symptomatic carotid stenosis patients to CAS or CEA.[32] Both techniques were effective, with statistically equal risk, in the treatment of symptomatic patients. For asymptomatic patients, there was a trend (p = NS) to lower risk with CAS. Questions have been raised, however, whether high-risk asymptomatic patients should be treated at all, since American Heart Association (AHA) guidelines have specified that surgical treatment is inappropriate for these patients.[4] The only true answer to this question would be a study of

CAS versus medical therapy in this group. No such study exists at present, although one large but non-randomized three-arm trial, the Japan Carotid Atherosclerosis Study (JCAS), will be forthcoming from Japan.

The National Institute of Neurological Disorders and Stroke (NINDS) and National Institute of Health (NIH)–funded Carotid Revascularization Endarterectomy versus Stenting Trial (CREST) completed enrollment of 2522 patients (53% symptomatic, 47% asymptomatic) on July 18, 2008 using the same criteria as NASCET and ACAS.[10,30] Final results of this trial have yet to be published. CREST and other similar trials in Europe (The International Carotid Stenting Study–Carotid and Vertebral Artery Transluminal Angioplasty Study [ICSS–CAVATAS 2]) and in Japan will hopefully provide level 1 evidence for therapeutic decision making. Curiously, the lead-in CREST data show that the risk of CAS, 30-day rates of stroke and death = 11.1%, is unacceptably high in elderly patients, aged >75, a group that was thought to represent excellent candidates for the procedure because of medical comorbidities.[8,10]

INDICATIONS FOR SURGERY

Patients with neurological symptoms localizing to the side of their carotid stenosis are considered symptomatic. Neurological symptoms include ipsilateral monocular blindness, contralateral motor weakness with greater involvement of the arm and face compared to the leg, contralateral sensory deficits, and aphasias (if the dominant hemisphere is involved). Symptoms may take the form of transient ischemic attacks (TIAs), reversible ischemic neurological deficits (RINDs), or cerebrovascular accidents (CVAs), the duration of the deficit being the primary difference. Non-specific neurological complaints, such as dizziness, syncope, or ill-defined visual disturbances, do not meet the criteria for symptomatic carotid stenosis.

Most patients with symptomatic carotid artery stenoses of ≥50%, as measured by the NASCET method, are offered surgery at our institution. We offer endovascular counseling to these patients particularly if they have major medical comorbidities but we educate them that there is no level 1 evidence that stenting is equivalent to surgery in any but the highest-risk cases. The patients are counseled pre-operatively about surgical risks and benefits. There is good evidence that nondiabetic men with hemispheric symptoms have the greatest benefit from surgery; diabetes certainly increases the surgical risk, and amaurosis fugax appears to be a marker for lower stroke risk carotid lesions.[26]

Asymptomatic patients with linear stenoses of 60% or more benefit from surgery, as determined by the ACAS and ACST trials. It is important to appreciate, however, that the patients should have an expected 5-year survival following surgery for the benefit to be realized; in addition, the benefit is not as great in women, and the combined surgical morbidity and mortality must remain below 3%. Asymptomatic patients with metastatic cancer, profound medical comorbidities, or other life expectancy-reducing conditions should generally not be offered treatment.

PREOPERATIVE EVALUATION AND PREPARATION

Carotid stenosis is identified in many different ways. Some patients come for surgical evaluation following workup for a TIA or stroke, where carotid duplex scanning, CTA, or MRA reveals a significant carotid lesion. Other patients present with clinically silent carotid bruits. Regardless of the referral type, we prefer catheter angiography (arch, both carotids, cervical, and cranial) for all patients being considered for surgery. This allows both accurate measurement of the stenosis using NASCET methodology and appropriate preoperative planning. The NASCET equation, where N is the linear diameter at the region of greatest narrowing and D is the greatest diameter of the normal artery distal to the carotid bulb, follows:

$$\text{Percent stenosis } (\%) = (1 - N/D) \times 100$$

Preoperative imaging should also include CT or MRI of the brain to exclude the possibility of a mass lesion mimicking cerebral ischemia. Patients should also undergo appropriate preoperative medical risk stratification and workup especially for cardiac risks factors, and their medical management of cardiac disease, hypertension, hyperlipidemia, and diabetes should be optimized.

Anticoagulation and Antiplatelet Therapies

Patients on aspirin therapy are told to continue this medication up through the day of surgery. Because of the significant operative oozing associated with clopidogrel and ticlodipine, we ask patients on these medications to switch to daily aspirin therapy for 1 week prior to their surgery. Patients on Coumadin are admitted to the hospital for institution of intravenous heparin therapy and subsequent normalization of their prothrombin time. The heparin is continued up through the arterial closure in the operating room.

SURGICAL TECHNIQUE

Principles

We have several cardinal principles of carotid reconstruction: complete knowledge of the patient's vascular anatomy, complete vascular control at all times, anatomic knowledge of the surgical field to prevent harm to surrounding structures, and finally, that a widely patent carotid repair free of technical errors must be achieved. Detailed descriptions of our carotid surgical technique with Hemashield patch graft can be found in multiple texts.[9,11,13,14,16–20,22–24,26,27,31]

CEA can easily be performed in 2 to 2.5 hours, with 30 to 40 minutes of cross-clamp time. Postoperative complications are minimized by maintaining a bloodless field and by meticulous anatomical dissection. We are not concerned about the speed of carotid repair so long as intraoperative monitoring is used (always) and collateral flow by shunt is established whenever necessary. We have not seen any complications as a result of the length of the operation in our patients.

Instruments

The Scanlan Loftus Carotid Endarterectomy Set (Scanlan International, Saint Paul, MN) contains useful high-quality instruments that facilitate the CEA procedure. The importance of a single set of instruments that includes all necessary items, eliminating the variability of different surgical teams, cannot be overstated. Our particular instrument set includes four (two large and two small) well-balanced vascular pickups, special dissecting scissors for coarse and fine work, micro ring-tip forceps (for cleaning small fragments from the artery wall prior to repair), and specialized cross-clamps, shunt clamps, and needle drivers.

Positioning

The patient is placed in the supine position with the head extended and turned away from the side of the operation (Figure 19–1). Folded sheets or pillowcases are placed beneath the shoulder blades to aid in extension of the neck; the preoperative arteriogram is reviewed to visualize the relationship between the internal and external carotid arteries (ICA and ECA) to choose the appropriate degree of head turning. Normally, the carotid vessels are superimposed in the anteroposterior plane, and rotating the head away from the operative side improves intraoperative visualization of the ICA by forcing it into a more lateral position. When the ICA is medial to the ECA (perhaps 10% of cases), no amount of head rotation will bring the ICA lateral enough, and the surgeon should recognize this and be prepared to dissect posterior and inferior to the ECA to find the "hidden" ICA and mobilize it laterally into the surgical position.

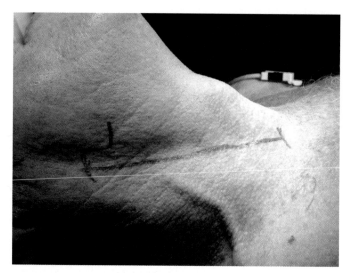

Figure 19–1. Initial positioning. The patient is in the supine position with the head extended and turned away from the operation side. The degree of rotation will be dependent on the relationship of the ICA and ECA. Generally, rotation brings the ICA into a more lateral position. Note the marking for the linear incision along the medial border of the sternocleidomastoid muscle.

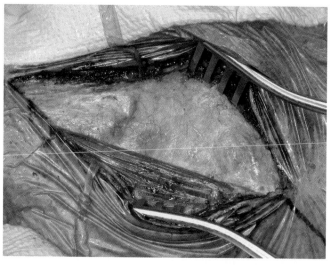

Figure 19–2. Initial dissection. After sharp and electrocautery dissection, the anterior edge of the sternocleidomastoid muscle is identified. Care is taken that the medial blunt retractor remains superficial, avoiding delicate structures below, particularly the recurrent laryngeal nerve in the tracheo-esophageal groove.

OPERATIVE TECHNIQUE

The cerebral angiogram is used to locate the height of carotid bifurcation, and the incision is planned accordingly. We prefer a linear incision along the medial border of the sternocleido-mastoid muscle (see Figure 19–1), which may extend as high as the retroaural region and as low as the suprasternal notch, as needed. Following sterile prep (never a vigorous scrub) and drape, the skin and subcutaneous tissues are dissected sharply down through the platysma, unavoidably transecting the transverse cervical nerve. (For this reason, patients should be instructed preoperatively to expect numbness anterior to the incision, which usually resolves after 6 months.) Meticulous hemostasis is obtained using monopolar and bipolar cautery superficially, and bipolar alone once the dissection is deep to the sternomastoid muscle. The medial edge of the sterno-cleidomastoid muscle is located and kept in view by placing a superficial blunt-bladed self-retaining retractor and dissecting through the overlying fat (Figure 19–2). The medial retractor blade (of this and all retractors) remains superficial to prevent injury to the recurrent laryngeal nerve in the tracheo-esophageal groove, while the lateral blade may safely be placed more deeply, on or under the sternocleidomastoid muscle.

Attention is next focused on the middle of the incision where the dissection proceeds down the sternocleidomastoid muscle until the internal jugular vein is reached. When dissection is carried under the muscle, the surgeon must be careful not to injure the laterally-placed spinal accessory nerve by inadvertent transection or over-retraction. The jugular vein is a key landmark in the dissection, and it typically lies lateral, parallel, and slightly anterior to the ICA and common carotid

artery (CCA). The medial jugular border is fully exposed, and the vein can be retracted as needed using blunt blades over a cottonoid pattie; it is crucial that the retractor blades are blunt to prevent vascular injury. In this portion of the dissection, the rather large common facial vein, and occasionally several smaller veins, are doubly ligated and divided. The common facial vein is a key landmark as it generally crosses the field at the level of the carotid bifurcation and carotid bulb (Figure 19–3).

The CCA is typically encountered first, and at first visualization we instruct the anesthesiologist to administer 5000 units of intravenous heparin, which we *do not* reverse with

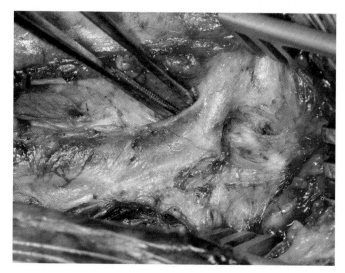

Figure 19–3. Dissection. Identification of the common facial vein is an important step in the dissection. The common facial vein often marks the level of the carotid bifurcation. We always ligate and divide the common facial vein to gain adequate carotid exposure.

protamine sulfate at the end of the procedure. The carotid is lifted and separated from surrounding structures upon opening of the carotid sheath with the aid of four sutures (4-0 silk) tied to more superficial tissue (Figure 19–4). The individual vessels (CCA, ICA, and ECA) are then dissected and encircled with 0 silk ties passed with a right-angle clamp. The carotid sinus is injected with 2 to 3 cc of 1% Xylocaine using a 25-gauge needle only if the anesthesiologist notes significant vital sign changes during vessel dissection in the region of the bifurcation. (We find this is very rarely necessary.) The CCA and ECA are not dissected free of the underlying tissue, in order to prevent postoperative kinking of these vessels; but they must, of course, be dissected circumferentially in the area where the silk ties or clamps are placed around them. The ICA is freed more extensively posteriorly, to facilitate full control of the vessel, and also where tacking sutures may later be placed.

A Rummel tourniquet is created by passing the CCA encircling silk tie through a wire loop that is then pulled through a rubber sleeve; this allows constriction of the vessel around an intraluminal shunt, should one become necessary. Mosquito clamps on the ends are used to secure the ECA and ICA ties, and to hang them over the retractor handles. The superior thyroid artery is dissected out of the surrounding connective tissue, and a double-loop 00 silk ligature is placed around the vessel; this occlusive Pott's tie is kept taut with a hanging mosquito clamp. If multiple proximal ECA branches are found, they must each be dealt with in order to prevent back-bleeding of these vessels during the procedure. Back-bleeding can also occur during the arteriotomy and repair if the ECA silk tie and subsequent cross-clamp are not placed proximal to any major external branches.

Cross-clamping of the carotid tree should not occur until the ICA is exposed and dissected well beyond the distal extent of the plaque. To obtain the critical high exposure, the plane between the lateral carotid wall and the medial jugular border is followed, allowing recognition of the hypoglossal nerve as it

travels medial to the jugular and crosses toward the midline over the ICA. The nerve is mobilized along its lateral wall adjacent to the jugular and gently retracted from the field using a vessel loop, so that its position can be easily assessed at all times. Injury to the nerve is more likely when it is blindly retracted or inadvertently coagulated because its location is not clearly known. A small ECA arterial branch to the sternocleidomastoid muscle occasionally requires ligation and transection to facilitate adequate mobilization of the hypoglossal nerve.

Avoidance of nerve injury is essential, and the carotid surgeon must understand and anticipate cervical nerve anatomy. The position of the recurrent laryngeal, hypoglossal, and spinal accessory nerves has already been discussed. Deep to the carotid, within the carotid sheath, lies the vagus nerve, which can be involuntarily cross-clamped if not properly identified. Horner's syndrome can result from injury to the sympathetic chain near the carotid, although this is extremely rare in our experience. The superior laryngeal nerve lies deep to the distal ICA and should not be inadvertently damaged with dissection, cautery, or vascular clamps.

We stress again that adequate control and exposure of the ICA distal to the plaque is imperative. A moistened finger can often feel the distal end of the hard plaque; another cue is that the vessel color returns to pinkish-blue pink distal to the hard, yellow plaque. If high exposure is necessary, the posterior belly of the digastric muscle can be divided partially with no clinical consequence.

We like to use a sterile marking pen to draw out the proposed arteriotomy (Figure 19–5), lessening the risk of a jagged or curving suture line. We then ensure that the small spring-loaded Loftus shunt clamp will fit snugly around the ICA (Figure 19–6). Next, we notify the electroencephalograph (EEG) and SSEP technicians of the impending cross-clamp.[12–21] For the past several years we have been monitoring with both modalities simultaneously and are currently acquiring data to

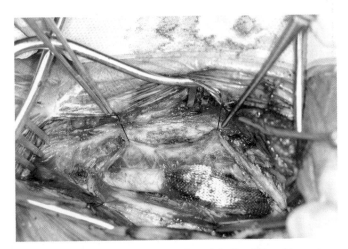

Figure 19–4. Carotid sheath stitches. Four 4-0 silk stitches (shown here pointed out by vascular pickups) between the carotid sheath and superficial soft tissue are used to lift and separate the carotid from surrounding structures. The author finds this maneuver extremely helpful.

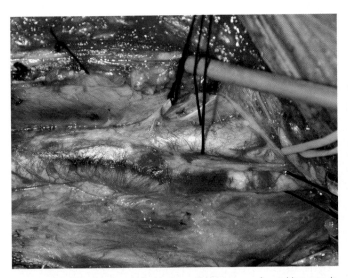

Figure 19–5. Arteriotomy. Left-sided carotid exposure. A marking pen is used to draw the proposed arteriotomy. Note in this view the double-loop ligature around the superior thyroid artery and the single loop around the ECA. A blue vessel loop is seen around the hypoglossal nerve.

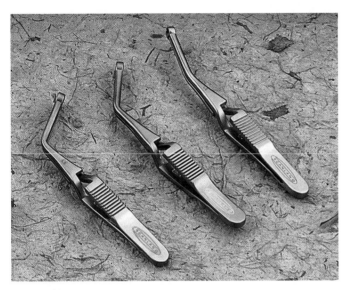

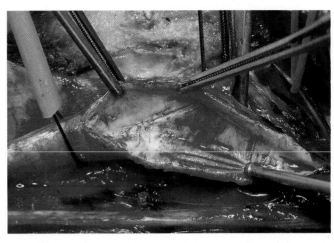

Figure 19–8. Repair of carotid back wall. The injury was repaired with a double-armed 6-0 Prolene suture with knots tied on the outside of the vessel.

Figure 19–6. Shunt clamps. A selection of Loftus shunt clamps is displayed. This unobtrusive encircling pinch clamp is used to secure the shunt in the internal carotid artery and prevent displacement or back-bleeding.

determine which modality is most sensitive in detecting ischemia. Following baseline EEG/SSEP acquisition, the ICA is occluded first with a small low closing force bulldog clamp. (Occluding the ICA first protects the brain from any debris released by clamp application elsewhere.) The CCA is then occluded with a large soft-shoe Fogarty vascular clamp and the ECA is closed with a second, larger and stronger, straight bulldog clamp. The arteriotomy is begun in the CCA with a no. 11 scalpel blade, and Potts angled scissors are used to extend the incision once the lumen is fully visualized. One needs to take care not to insert the no. 11 scalpel blade too deeply to avoid injury to the back wall of the carotid (Figures 19–7 and 19–8). The blue-marked arteriotomy line is followed from the CCA up to

the bifurcation, and then up the ICA until normal vessel is encountered. In severely stenotic vessels, identification of the lumen is not always straightforward, and great care must be taken not to cut the back wall of the carotid. The possibility of a false lumen should be excluded prior to shunt placement.

In our practice, EEG/SSEP changes in any form lead to placement of an intraluminal shunt (Figure 19–9). Our preference is the Loftus Carotid Endarterectomy Shunt (Integra LifeSciences, Plainsboro, NJ), which is a 15-cm straight silicone tube with a black marker band in the center, allowing for easy identification and correction of shunt migration; the shunt is tapered at the ends for easy insertion, and the proximal end has a bulb that facilitates anchoring by the Rummel tourniquet.[15,24,25]

The CCA is cannulated first, and the shunt is secured by pulling up on the silk ties; a mosquito clamp is used to hold the rubber sleeve in place. The shunt tubing is held shut by

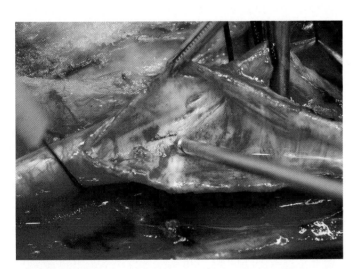

Figure 19–7. Inadvertent injury to the back wall of the carotid. This stab wound injury (indicated by the suction tip) was identified upon inspection of the back wall of the carotid for adherent plaque. The plaque in this case was very firm and this injury was likely caused by excessive downward pressure with the no. 11 scalpel blade during the first step of the arteriotomy.

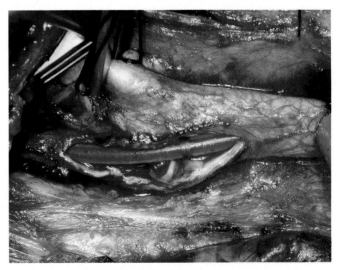

Figure 19–9. Placement of a shunt. Right-sided carotid exposure. A Loftus Carotid Endarterectomy Shunt (Integra Lifesciences, Plainsboro, NJ) is pictured in situ. The black band marks the middle of the shunt. Having the black band allows the surgeon to return the shunt to appropriate position after sliding the shunt cranially/caudally to test for proper placement.

a pair of heavy vascular forceps grasping the region of the black marker band. The tubing is cleared of air and debris by briefly releasing the vascular forceps, filling the shunt with fresh blood, and allowing confirmation of blood flow as well. The lumen of the ICA is visualized, and the distal end of the shunt is placed at the ICA orifice; the shunt is bled into the ICA to blow apart the vessel walls. The bulldog clamp on the ICA is then released and the shunt is advanced up the ICA until the black marker band lies in the center of the arteriotomy (see Figure 19–9). The shunt should slide up and down the ICA easily; no unnecessary force should be used, to avoid intimal damage and possible dissection. Our small Scanlan-Loftus custom clamp (Figure 19–6), or a Javid clamp, is then placed to secure the shunt in the distal ICA. A hand-held Doppler probe is used to confirm blood flow in the shunt.

A Scanlan plaque dissector, or a Freer elevator, is used to dissect the plaque away from the arterial wall (Figure 19–10). The wall of the vessel is held with a fine vascular pickup while the instrument is moved from side to side, first developing a plane in the lateral wall of the arteriotomy. We go approximately halfway around the wall from the lateral side when the plaque comes easily, and then repeat the dissection on the medial side of the CCA. The plaque is then transected proximally with Potts scissors, leaving a smooth transition zone, since a clean feathering away of the plaque is almost never possible in the CCA. The proximal end may create a flap despite the direction of blood flow; hence, care should be taken to ensure that the CCA endpoint is not free-floating.

Next, the plaque is dissected away from the ICA in the same manner. However, the plaque usually feathers down much more smoothly at the ICA endpoint (Figure 19–11). Occasionally, a shelf of normal tissue protrudes and must be tacked down with suture.

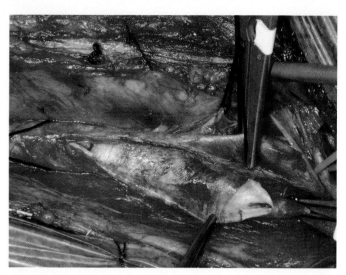

Figure 19–11. Dissection of plaque. Left-sided carotid exposure, plaque removed in toto. The plaque has been dissected along the ICA as well. Loose fragments must be avoided. The surgeon has the option of using tack-down sutures at the ICA endpoint. In this case there is a clean and smooth transition zone that will not require tacking sutures.

The ECA attachment is now the remaining point of plaque fixation. We grasp across the entire plaque at the ECA opening; traction on the plaque everts the ECA, allowing dissection a few centimeters up into the ECA. In addition, the distal ECA can be pushed (milked) proximally with the clamp or forceps. The clamp often tethers plaque to the ECA, so it is sprung while the lumen is held closed with heavy forceps to minimize bleeding, and the plaque is avulsed from the distal ECA. Quick reapplication of the clamp is tempting to stop annoying back-bleeding, but a complete plaque removal is essential. A thrombus can form and can propagate back into the carotid bulb (disastrous) if ECA plaque removal is inadequate, so if there is any question we do not hesitate to extend the arteriotomy up the ECA on an as-needed basis to ensure adequate plaque removal, and then close it with a separate suture line.

All loose fragments should be sought and removed following gross plaque removal. We use a Kittner "peanut" sponge to gently stroke areas that appear loose; the fragments should be removed in a circumferential fashion, elevating them the complete vessel width until they come free at the arteriotomy edge. (The micro-ring tip forceps in the Scanlan-Loftus set are useful for this step.) No attempt should be made to dissect firmly attached fragments that have no danger of elevating or embolizing.

Occasionally, removal of a stony hard plaque, the most difficult type, results in areas of thinning of the posterior arterial wall where only the adventitial layer remains. One or two double-armed, interrupted stitches of 6-0 prolene are used to primarily plicate the thin spot, similar to a tacking suture (from the inside out, with the knot extraluminal). Following declamping, if the arterial wall has a transparent or overly thin appearance, an encircling piece of vascular Hemashield can be used to reinforce the vessel (this is rare). The Hemashield surrounds the artery and is sewn together at the top (Figure 19–12), taking care not to pull it too snug.

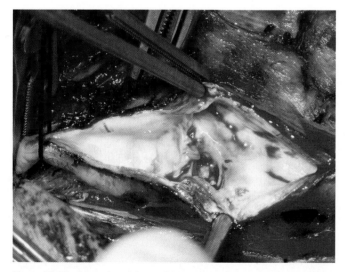

Figure 19–10. Dissection of plaque. Right-sided carotid exposure. The plaque is gently dissected from the arterial wall with a Scanlan plaque dissector or a Freer elevator. The assistant everts the borders of the arteriotomy. Note the abnormal yellow appearance of the plaque, and the deep ulceration with fresh thrombus at the carotid bulb.

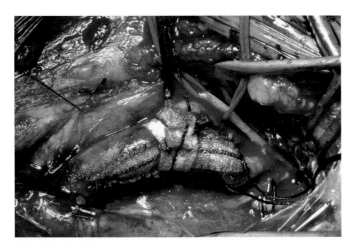

Figure 19–12. Reinforcement option. Left-sided carotid exposure. In some cases, such as heavily calcified carotid plaques, the residual arterial arterial wall appears thin, and a buttressing encircling Hemashield sling may be applied at the conclusion of the repair, taking care to ensure that no stenosis is created by pulling the sutures too tight!

While some surgeons prefer to use the microscope to perform the arteriotomy closure, we prefer to continue working under 3.5x loupe magnification. If tacking sutures in the distal ICA are required, two such sutures may be placed, at the four and eight o'clock positions. The patch material is then fashioned by placing it over the arteriotomy, cutting it to the length of the opening, and tapering the patch ends. Double-armed 6-0 prolene suture is then used to attach each of the patch ends to the arteriotomy, and rubber-shod clamps are used to secure the needles (Figure 19–13). A running, non-locking stitch is used to close the medial wall suture line from the ICA anchor to the CCA anchor; the anchors are tied together. The suture line is then inspected, and the lateral wall is closed to the level of the carotid bulb with the remaining limb of the ICA anchor stitch. The CCA anchor stitch is then

used to close the lateral CCA wall up to the ICA limb. Care must be taken to include all arterial layers and to advance the stitch in small enough intervals so that leaking will not be problematic; no stray adventitial tags or suture ends are sewn into the lumen (Figure 19–14).

If a shunt has been placed, a small opening is temporarily left on the lateral CCA wall where the shunt can be removed. After the EEG technician is notified, the shunt is double-clamped with two parallel, straight mosquito clamps and then cut between the clamps, being sure that the suture material is not entangled in the clamps. Each end of the transected shunt is then removed separately, and the vascular clamps are reapplied.

In sequential fashion, the ICA, ECA, and CCA are opened and closed to ensure that back-bleeding is present. The ICA is then opened and closed again to be certain that no debris or air has re-entered the blind sac there. A heparinized saline syringe with a blunt tip is inserted into the arterial lumen while the two stitches are held tight; the vessel is filled with heparinized saline while a surgeon's knot is thrown and laid down, and the syringe is then withdrawn, preventing air from entering the vessel. Ten more throws are placed into this final stitch. Declamping is performed in a specific, sequential manner: first the ECA, then the CCA, and after at least a 10-second pause, the ICA. This ensures that any remaining debris or small bubbles are flushed into the ECA circulation. The suture line is then inspected for leaks. Digital pressure and patience will achieve hemostasis within a few minutes; occasionally, a single throw of 6-0 prolene is needed to secure a persistent arterial bleeding point, but rarely (almost never) is reapplication of the vessel clamps necessary if the arteriotomy has been closed properly. Surgicel gauze is then used to line the repair, and all three vessels are checked for patency by a hand-held Doppler probe.

The retractors are removed and wound hemostasis is ensured by direct inspection. Carotid patency is once again confirmed with the hand-held Doppler. To protect against infection, the

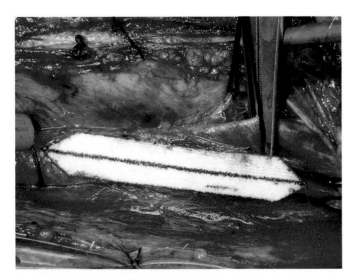

Figure 19–13. Anchoring the graft. Left-sided carotid exposure. A Hemashield patch is cut to size and sutured in position at each end with double-armed 6-0 prolene suture.

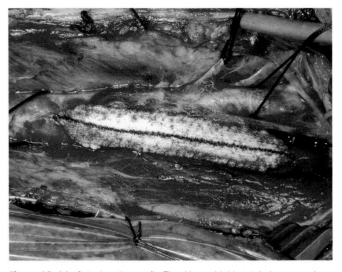

Figure 19–14. Suturing the graft. The Hemashield patch is secured on both sides with running non-locking stitches. Leaks after declamping are treated with either individual sutures or digital pressure.

carotid sheath is closed, and a Hemovac drain is left inside; the platysma is closed as a separate layer for a good cosmetic appearance. The skin edges are approximated using subcuticular stitches, interrupted or running, followed by a tissue adhesive to the skin. A dry, sterile dressing is applied. We do not give protamine.

POSTOPERATIVE CARE

Patients are continued on aspirin after surgery. The Hemovac drain is removed the first postoperative day, and patients are generally discharged on the second postoperative day. Any postoperative neurological deficit, including TIA, mandates immediate evaluation of the adequacy of the repair. High-quality, color duplex ultrasonography, CTA, or angiography should be used to check for partial or complete occlusion of the arteries (we do not find MRA to be as helpful here). If there is evidence of a postoperative occlusion the patient is returned to surgery for immediate re-exploration and repair. (This has never happened again once we began the use of routine patch grafting for CEA, which clearly reduces the frequency of this complication.)

COMPLICATIONS

As we have said, low perioperative morbidity and mortality results, commensurate with the results of the cooperative trials, are necessary to justify a recommendation of CEA over medical management. For a skilled experienced surgeon, with proper attention to patient selection and technique, these excellent results should be achievable and reproducible, and technical errors are rare. The majority of complications will be cardiac or pulmonary, and a systematic team approach to the overall care of every patent is essential to minimize this.

Complications such as wound infections or significant postoperative hematomas are rare. Wound infections should be treated with antibiotics and, as needed, exploration with washout; if the deep tissues are involved, an angiogram or CTA should be considered to exclude the possibility of an infectious false aneurysm. Small superficial hematomas usually resolve without intervention, but should be investigated with duplex, CTA, or angiography to be certain that there is no arterial disruption or leak source. In actual fact, we have never seen this happen in our practice of 25 years.

SPECIAL SITUATIONS

Concurrent Carotid Stenosis and Coronary Disease

Patients with carotid stenosis and coronary artery disease should usually undergo staged procedures, with the CEA first for neurologically symptomatic patients, unless the coronary disease prohibits safe anesthesia. In this case, a combined procedure may be acceptable, but the perioperative risks are significantly higher. For asymptomatic patients, the coronary surgery may be performed first, followed by the CEA. There is no compelling evidence that *asymptomatic* carotid stenosis increases the risk of coronary surgery, but there is significant evidence that *symptomatic* carotid disease does materially increase this risk, and such patients should have the carotid reconstructed first if at all possible.

Concurrent Carotid Stenosis and an Intracranial Aneurysm

When both a silent intracranial aneurysm and carotid stenosis are present, there is the concern that carotid repair will lead to aneurysm rupture from increased intracranial flow. There is probably a small risk of this, but incidental asymptomatic aneurysms should not prevent a surgeon from performing a CEA for symptomatic carotid disease that threatens stroke; it is generally deemed to be safe. Our policy has been that if either lesion is symptomatic, repair at that site is the first priority, followed by a later staged approach to the incidental pathology. In situations where both the carotid and aneurysm are silent, we would most often recommend primary carotid reconstruction first, followed by an endovascular approach to the aneurysm, or secondary craniotomy if an endovascular route is not feasible.

Recurrent Stenosis

Recurrent stenosis following primary CEA does occur. The only risk factor repeatedly shown to play a role is continued smoking, but other factors such as hypertension and diabetes mellitus may also contribute. The operation for recurrent stenosis is much more technically demanding and, even as performed by experienced surgeons, is clearly associated with higher risks (Figure 19–15).

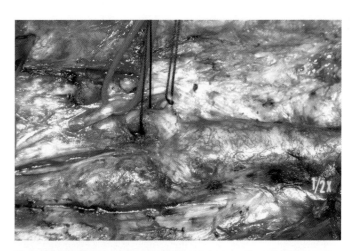

Figure 19–15. Recurrent stenosis. Right-sided reoperation carotid. Dissection and exposure of a redo carotid endarterectomy presents a challenge to any carotid surgeon. In this particular case note the presence of scar tissue, the inability to clearly identify the internal jugular vein, and loss of freely dissectible anatomic planes.

Our approach is mostly conservative for moderate-grade asymptomatic recurrent stenosis, where we offer the patient either observation for progression or a primary endovascular strategy. For symptomatic recurrent stenosis, or for rapidly progressing (to high-grade) asymptomatic recurrent disease, we are more aggressive, especially with medical therapy failure patients, and we do not hesitate to operate in such cases if the patient clearly understands the attendant risks.

CONCLUSION

Randomized clinical trial study data confirm the superiority of surgical management, by qualified surgeons, for both symptomatic (>50%) and asymptomatic (>60%) carotid artery lesions. At present, cooperative trial data shows that the best option remains surgery in most cases, despite the intrinsic appeal of less invasive endovascular procedures. Surgical correction of significant carotid artery disease by an experienced surgeon affords excellent outcomes and improves patients' quality of life.

While every patient is different, and every patient's anatomy has the potential for being more or less challenging, a standardized approach to CEA repair benefits both the surgeon and the patient. We have described the approach that works best for us and trust that this will prove helpful to surgeons at every level of expertise.

REFERENCES

1. Beneficial effect of carotid endarterectomy in symptomatic patients with high-grade carotid stenosis: North American Symptomatic Carotid Endarterectomy Trial Collaborators, *N Engl J Med* 325:445–453, 1991.
2. Endarterectomy for asymptomatic carotid artery stenosis: Executive Committee for the Asymptomatic Carotid Atherosclerosis Study, *JAMA* 273:1421–1428, 1995.
3. Barnett HJ, Taylor DW, Eliasziw M, et al: Benefit of carotid endarterectomy in patients with symptomatic moderate or severe stenosis. North American Symptomatic Carotid Endarterectomy Trial Collaborators, *N Engl J Med* 339:1415–1425, 1998.
4. Biller J, Feinberg WM, Castaldo JE, et al: Guidelines for carotid endarterectomy: a statement for healthcare professionals from a special writing group of the Stroke Council, American Heart Association, *Stroke* 29:554–562, 1998.
5. Eastcott HH, Pickering GW, Rob CG: Reconstruction of internal carotid artery in a patient with intermittent attacks of hemiplegia, *Lancet* 267:994–996, 1954.
6. Halliday A, Mansfield A, Marro J, et al: Prevention of disabling and fatal strokes by successful carotid endarterectomy in patients without recent neurological symptoms: randomised controlled trial, *Lancet* 363:1491–1502, 2004.
7. Halliday AW, Thomas D, Mansfield A: The Asymptomatic Carotid Surgery Trial (ACST). Rationale and design. Steering Committee, *Eur J Vasc Surg* 8:703–710, 1994.
8. Hobson RW II, Howard VJ, Roubin GS, et al: Carotid artery stenting is associated with increased complications in octogenarians: 30-day

stroke and death rates in the CREST lead-in phase, *J Vasc Surg* 40:1106–1111, 2004.
9. Honeycutt J, Loftus C: Carotid endarterectomy: general principles and surgical technique, *Neurosurg Clin North Am* 11:279–297, 2000.
10. Lal BK, Brott TG: The Carotid Revascularization Endarterectomy vs. Stenting Trial completes randomization: lessons learned and anticipated results, *J Vasc Surg* 50:1224–1231, 2009.
11. Loftus C: Technical aspects of carotid endarterectomy with hemashield patch graft, *Neurol Med Chir (Tokyo)* 37:805–818, 1997.
12. Loftus C: Anesthesia for carotid endarterectomy: general vs. local. In Bederson J, Tuhrim S, editors: *Treatment of Carotid Disease: A Practitioner's Manual*, Park Ridge, IL, 1998, AANS, pp 181–190.
13. Loftus C: Surgical anatomy, technique, and indications for carotid endarterectomy. In Matsuno H, editor: *Proceedings of the 12th Microsurgical Anatomy Seminar Program*, Tokyo, 1998, SciMed Publications.
14. Loftus C: Surgical management of extracranial carotid artery disease, *Surg Cerebral Stroke (Japan)* 27:7–13, 1999.
15. Loftus C: Design characteristics and clinical application of a newly designed carotid artery shunt, *Neurol Res* 22:443–448, 2000.
16. Loftus C: Surgical management of extracranial carotid stenosis. In Schmidek H, Sweet W, editors: *Operative Neurosurgical Techniques*, Philadelphia, 2000, WB Saunders, pp 1067–1079.
17. Loftus C, Biller J: Modern management of carotid atheromatosis, *Neurocirugia* 3:62–72, 1989.
18. Loftus C, Kresowik T: *Carotid Artery Surgery*, New York, 2000, Thieme.
19. Loftus C, Stanfield M: Carotid endarterectomy. In Batjer H, Loftus C, editors: *Textbook of Neurological Surgery*, Philadelphia, 2003, Lippincott, Williams and Wilkins, pp 2259–2260.
20. Loftus CM: Technique of carotid endarterectomy, *Contemp Neurosurg* 10:1–6, 1988.
21. Loftus CM: Monitoring during extracranial carotid reconstruction. In Loftus CM, Traynelis VC, editors: *Intraoperative Monitoring Techniques in Neurosurgery*, New York, 1994, McGraw-Hill, pp 3–8.
22. Loftus CM: *Carotid Endarterectomy: Principles and Technique*, St. Louis, 1995, Quality Medical Publishing.
23. Loftus CM: Carotid endarterectomy: how the operation is done, *Clin Neurosurg* 44:243–265, 1997.
24. Loftus CM: Technical fundamentals, monitoring, and shunt use during carotid endarterectomy, *Tech Neurosurg* 3:16–24, 1997.
25. Loftus CM: Overview of shunt controversy. In Loftus C, Kresowik T, editors: *Carotid Artery Surgery*, New York, 2000, Thieme Medical Publishers, pp 409–420.
26. Loftus CM: *Carotid Endarterectomy: Principles and Technique*, New York, 2007, Informa Healthcare.
27. Loftus CM, Kresowik TF: Anatomical basis and technique of carotid endarterectomy. In Loftus C, Kresowik T, editors: *Carotid Artery Surgery*, New York, 2000, Thieme Medical Publishers, pp 245–256.
28. Mas JL, Chatellier G, Beyssen B, et al: Endarterectomy versus stenting in patients with symptomatic severe carotid stenosis, *N Engl J Med* 355:1660–1671, 2006.
29. Ringleb PA, Allenberg J, Bruckmann H, et al: 30 day results from the SPACE trial of stent-protected angioplasty versus carotid endarterectomy in symptomatic patients: a randomised non-inferiority trial, *Lancet* 368:1239–1247, 2006.
30. Sheffet AJ, Roubin G, Howard G, et al: Design of the Carotid Revascularization Endarterectomy vs. Stenting Trial (CREST), *Int J Stroke* 5:40–46, 2010.
31. Snell B., Wienecke R., Loftus C.: Surgical management of extracranial vascular occlusive disease. In Lawton M, editor: *Controversies in Cerebrovascular Disease*, New York, Thieme/AANS (in press).
32. Yadav JS, Wholey MH, Kuntz RE, et al: Protected carotid-artery stenting versus endarterectomy in high-risk patients, *N Engl J Med* 351:1493–1501, 2004.

ENDOVASCULAR THERAPIES FOR CEREBRAL REVASCULARIZATION

20

C. BENJAMIN NEWMAN; YIN HU; CAMERON G. MCDOUGALL;
FELIPE C. ALBUQUERQUE

INTRODUCTION

Stroke is the third leading cause of death in the United States and the second leading cause of death worldwide. The AHA estimates that the direct and indirect costs of stroke in the United States in 2009 at $69.9 billion.[1] Stroke has been recognized as a clinical entity for millennia, dating at least to ancient Greece. Hippocrates first described and documented the syndrome of stroke, which he called "apoplexy" (from the Greek *apoplēssein*, to strike down and incapacitate). Prior to the advent and widespread accessibility of high-resolution cross-sectional imaging, neurologists and neurosurgeons could only establish the location of strokes on the basis of clinicopathological correlation. Little was known about the pathophysiology of stroke for much of the 20th century, with *in situ* thrombosis being the presumed etiology for most ischemic strokes.[2] The recognition of thromboembolic phenomena to the brain originating from the carotid artery and the description of lacunar syndromes allowed the development of strategies for stroke prevention.[3,4] However, therapies for acute stroke were not developed until the latter part of the 20th century.

Initial attempts to use systemic thrombolytic agents were complicated by the propensity of ischemic brain tissue to hemorrhage. Uncertainty about the optimal doses of thrombolytic medications, the window of time for intervention, and the identification of patients at high risk of developing complications from treatment proved challenging in developing safe and effective treatments for acute stroke.

The first three trials evaluating the use of intravenous streptokinase for the treatment of acute stroke were terminated prematurely due to an increase in mortality rate, primarily related to the hemorrhagic conversion of ischemic infarcts.[5,6] The European Cooperative Acute Stroke Study (ECASS),[7] which tested recombinant tissue plasminogen activator (r-tPA) at a dose of 1.1 mg/kg, demonstrated no overall benefit to the use of intravenous (IV) r-tPA for the treatment of acute stroke. Subgroup analysis, however, revealed significant improvement after IV t-PA administration in patients

with moderate to severe stroke without extended signs of infarction on CT. This study showed the therapeutic potential for thrombolytic agents in the treatment of acute stroke while underscoring the need to refine indications and contraindications for therapy.

The first trial to demonstrate significant clinical benefit for intravenous r-tPA with an acceptable risk of intracranial hemorrhage was the National Institute of Neurological Diseases and Stroke (NINDS) study.[8] The NINDS study used a lower dose of intravenous r-tPA (0.9 mg/kg), which was administered within 3 hours of stroke onset. The results of the NINDS study led to the approval of intravenous r-tPA by the United States Food and Drug Administration (FDA) for use in acute stroke within 3 hours of onset of stroke symptoms. The safety and efficacy of the 3-hour therapeutic window was confirmed by the Alteplase Thrombolysis for Acute Noninterventional Therapy in Ischemic Stroke (ATLANTIS) trial.[9] The ATLANTIS trial also failed to demonstrate benefit to patients who received r-tPA in a 3- to 5-hour window.

Numerous studies have subsequently demonstrated the efficacy of intravenous r-tPA when given within the 3-hour window.[10–12] Although the use of IV r-tPA was initially controversial, it has now been endorsed as class IA level of evidence by the major national guidelines development organizations.[13] Pooled results from the six major randomized, placebo-controlled IV r-tPA stroke trials[8,9,14] (ATLANTIS I & II, ECASS I & II, and NINDS I & II) included 2775 patients who were treated with IV r-tPA or a placebo. Treatment up to 3 hours after symptom onset benefitted patients, and findings suggested a benefit in treatment beyond 3 hours in certain subsets of patients. The ECASS III trial demonstrated the benefit of IV r-tPA in the 3.5- to 4-hour window in a more select group of patients.[15]

Recanalization rates, which are related to the diameter of the affected vessel, range from 20% for the ICA to 50% for occlusion of a distal branch of the MCA.[16] Ischemic stroke related to large vessel (i.e., >2 mm) occlusion carries a high risk of mortality (53% to 92%) and severe morbidity.[17,18] The presence of a hyperdense MCA sign on CT in the presence of a moderate stroke (National Institute of Health Stroke

Scale [NIHSS] stroke score of >10) portends a less favorable therapeutic outcome with IV r-tPA. This finding suggests that large proximal clots are resistant to IV r-tPA.[19] Endovascular therapies for acute stroke, particularly those related to large vessel occlusion, may overcome some limitations of systemic thrombolysis by providing superior recanalization rates in large vessel occlusions, reducing the incidence of intracranial hemorrhage, and expanding the therapeutic window.

RECANALIZATION STRATEGIES

Recanalization aims to restore antegrade blood flow by removing or dissolving occlusive thrombus, thereby allowing reperfusion of the ischemic penumbra, the functionally impaired but still viable brain tissue. Endovascular techniques for recanalization include mechanical thrombectomy, chemical thrombolysis, stenting (either temporary or permanent), or a combination thereof (Figure 20–1).

The rationale for restoring antegrade flow as rapidly as possible after stroke is intuitive. The aphorism "time is brain" accurately reflects the ephemeral nature of the ischemic penumbra and underscores the importance of rapid restoration of blood flow. The ultimate outcome of stroke is not solely dependent on the time of occlusion of the target vessel. It also depends on a number of factors and their complex degree of interactions. These factors include the site of arterial occlusion, the extent of the core of infarction, the size of the ischemic penumbra, the quality and quantity of collateral arterial supply, and the integrity of the blood-brain barrier (BBB). However, on an epidemiological level, a number of studies have documented the correlation between radiographic recanalization and improved clinical outcome as well as the critical role of rapid restoration of flow.[20]

Intracranial hemorrhage (ICH) remains the most common and dangerous complication of recanalization. Most postrecanalization ICH occurs within the core of infarcted brain tissue, suggesting that ischemia and disruption of the BBB play a major role in its pathogenesis.

Intra-Arterial Thrombolysis

Intra-arterial recanalization is occasionally used as a primary treatment modality in patients in whom IV r-tPA is contraindicated or patients who fail to demonstrate clinical improvement after administration of IV r-tPA. Primary intra-arterial thrombolysis can benefit clinical outcomes of patients who receive treatment 3 to 6 hours after symptom onset.[21,22] Compared to systemic IV thrombolysis, intra-arterial thrombolysis offers several theoretical advantages. Coaxial microcatheter techniques allow superselective access to the occluded vessel, thereby allowing infusion of thrombolytic agents directly into the thrombus. By infusing thrombolytic agents directly at the site of the thrombus, a smaller dose of fibrinolytic agent can result in more complete recanalization compared to systemic administration. Theoretically, rates of complications from systemic fibrinolysis such as ICH should be reduced.

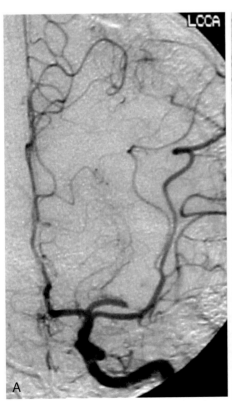 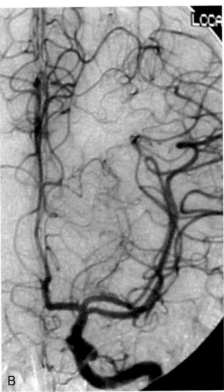

Figure 20–1. Posteroanterior projection of left internal carotid artery (ICA) injection before (**A**) and after (**B**) mechanical thrombectomy and direct intra-arterial infusion of plasminogen activator. The previously occluded M2 branch opacifies, indicating restoration of blood flow.

(Used with permission from Barrow Neurological Institute.)

The first generation of fibrinolytic agents consists of plasminogen activators. These drugs work by converting an inactive proenzyme, plasminogen, into the active form, plasmin. Plasmin degrades fibrinogen and fibrin (monomers and cross-linked) leading to clot dissolution. The plasminogen activators vary in terms of their stability and selectivity for fibrin. Urokinase and streptokinase are nonfibrin-selective agents and carry the risk of systemic hypofibrinogenemia. These drugs have a narrow therapeutic window and are no longer routinely used for intra-arterial thrombolysis since thrombolytic agents with higher selectivity for fibrin were adopted.

Alteplase (r-tPA) is a glycoprotein serine protease produced by recombinant DNA technology. It has a higher affinity and selectivity for fibrin than urokinase and streptokinase, and its use is associated with a lower rate of systemic complications than the first-generation plasminogen activators. Drawbacks to r-tPA include reduced clot penetration due to its high affinity for surface fibrin and its short half-life. Investigational trials are underway to evaluate the clinical utility of modified plasminogen activators (Reteplase, Tenecteplase, Desmoteplase) and direct fibrinolytics (Ancrod, Microplasmin, Alfimeprase) for use in intra-arterial thrombolysis.

Intra-Arterial Thrombolysis Technical Comments

Intra-arterial thrombolysis is rarely used as monotherapy for acute stroke at our institution. In general, if a patient is a candidate for an invasive stroke therapy, intra-arterial thrombosis may be employed as an adjunct to mechanical thrombolysis. The decision to use plasminogen activators is largely subjective, but the interventionalist must consider the likelihood of potentiating a hemorrhagic conversion of the infarcted brain parenchyma.

Transfemoral arterial access followed by guide catheter placement into the parent brachiocephalic artery of the target vessel is the most common approach to gain access to the lesion. Superselective microcatheter placement using standard digital subtraction roadmapping and over-the-wire navigation is then employed to position the microcatheter near the thrombus.

If used, the dose of r-tPA is low, on the order of 3 to 10 mg, and can be infused through the guide catheter or microcatheter. Abciximab is occasionally used, typically in the setting of stent placement or hyperacute thrombosis (i.e., recognition of an intraprocedural thrombotic branch occlusion or acute in-stent thrombosis).

Mechanical Thrombectomy

Ischemic stroke involving large vessel occlusions is especially morbid, and a good neurological outcome from such an event depends on rapid recanalization. The observation that clots in large intracranial vessels is relatively resistant to dissolution from intravenous plasminogen activators provides the rationale for developing endovascular techniques for revascularization. All mechanical thrombectomy devices are delivered by endovascular access and approach the lesion from the proximal/antegrade direction. The Food and Drug Administration (FDA) has approved two mechanical thrombectomy devices for the treatment of acute stroke: the Merci Retrieval System (Concentric Medical, Inc., Mountain View, CA) and the Penumbra System (PS; Penumbra, Alameda, CA). Both devices are approved for use within 8 hours of the onset of symptoms.

All patients qualified for endovascular thrombolysis are treated under general anesthesia at our institution. The use of general anesthesia in acute stroke is not universal; however, our experience suggests that the elimination of patient movement afforded by general anesthesia reduces the technical difficulty of the procedure and ultimately is safer for the patient. Transfemoral arterial access is typically employed; however, the access site selected is ultimately guided by the most favorable guide catheter stabilization needed for treatment. A baseline activating clotting time (ACT) is obtained, and the patient is heparinized to achieve an ACT between 250 to 300 seconds after arterial access is obtained.

Merci Retrieval System

The Merci Retrieval System was approved by the FDA in 2004 for the treatment of acute stroke due to thromboembolic occlusion of the intracranial vertebral artery, basilar artery, intracranial ICA, or M1 division of the MCA. The Mechanical Embolus Removal in Cerebral Ischemia (MERCI) trial was a prospective, nonrandomized, single-arm, multicenter trial that investigated the use of a novel mechanical thrombectomy device in patients with occluded large intracranial vessels within 8 hours of the onset of stroke symptoms.[23] The primary endpoint of the trial was radiographic recanalization of the target vessel with a low rate of serious adverse events. The trial enrolled 151 patients and demonstrated recanalization rates of 48% with a complication rate of 7.1%. Morbidity and mortality rates were lower in patients who demonstrated radiographic recanalization.

The Merci Retrieval System consists of the Merci Retriever, the Merci Balloon Guide Catheter (BGC), and the Merci microcatheter through which the actual retrieval device is deployed (Figure 20–2). The BGC is a 9-French catheter with a large 2.1-mm lumen and a balloon located at the distal tip. The Merci Retriever itself consists of a tapered wire with five helical loops of decreasing diameter (from 2.8 to 1.1 mm) at the distal end. The loops are constructed from memory-shaped nitinol (nickel titanium) and therefore exploit the superelastic properties of this alloy. Once the microcatheter is advanced distal to the clot, the Merci Retriever is advanced through the microcatheter in its straight configuration. Once deployed, the retriever reforms into its pre-established helical shape thereby ensnaring the thrombus. During this procedure, the balloon at the tip of the BGC (usually located in the common

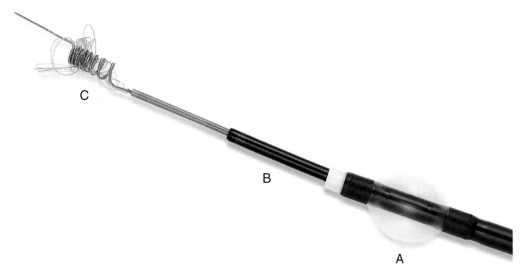

Figure 20–2. The various components of the Merci Retrieval System. **A,** Balloon Guide Catheter. **B,** Distal access catheter. **C,** Merci Retriever (V series).
(Used with permission from Concentric Medical, Inc.)

carotid artery or ICA) is inflated to minimize distal flow. A complete description of the technique can be found in the original description of the MERCI Phase I Study.[24]

On the basis of the results of the MERCI trial, the Merci Retrieval System was approved by the FDA for use in the treatment of acute stroke up to 8 hours after symptom onset. The approval of this device without a randomized trial has drawn some criticism, most notably due to the apparent increase in deaths associated with its use compared to the Prolyse in Acute Cerebral Thromboembolism (PROACT II—an earlier study evaluating the use of intra-arterial prourokinase) from 27% to 44%.[25,26] However, the MERCI investigators argued that the presence of a higher percentage of distal ICA and basilar artery occlusions may have biased their results toward worse outcomes. The discrepancies in clinical outcomes underscore the need to accurately identify which patients are most likely to benefit from aggressive intervention.

Merci System Technical Comments

After conventional catheter angiography is performed, an 8- or 9-French Merci balloon-guided (Concentric Medical, Inc., Mountain View, CA) catheter is placed in the proximal ICA (for the anterior circulation) and the subclavian or vertebral artery (for the posterior circulation). With the balloon of the guide catheter deflated, an over-the-wire microcatheter with 0.014-inch microguidewire is navigated through the thrombus. The guidewire is then exchanged for the Merci Retriever. Up to four distal loops of the retriever are deployed distal to the thrombus. With the balloon inflated to arrest proximal flow (to minimize the risk of distal embolization), the microcatheter and the retriever are retracted to engage the clot. The proximal loops of the retriever are further deployed by gentle retraction of the microcatheter. While aspirating with a syringe on the BGC, the microcatheter and retriever are

slowly withdrawn into the lumen of the guide catheter. The balloon is deflated and the thrombus is examined. Multiple passes with the retriever (as many as six passes) can be performed if the initial attempt is unsuccessful. If unsuccessful (less than thrombolysis in myocardial infarction [TIMI] grade 2 after six attempts or unable to access distal thrombus), intra-arterial tPA can be given (up to 24 mg) through the microcatheter. Postprocedural CT of the head is obtained to evaluate for intracerebral hemorrhage and the need for further management. In general, heparinization is neither reversed nor continued immediately after the procedure.

Penumbra System

The Penumbra System (PS) is a suction-based embolectomy device designed to reduce clot burden in large-vessel occlusive disease. It received FDA approval in 2008 for the treatment of acute stroke up to 8 hours after the onset of symptoms. The FDA approval was based on positive results from Phase I and II trials evaluating the safety and efficacy of the PS used for the treatment of acute stroke. The Phase II trial was a prospective, nonrandomized, single-arm, multicenter trial that enrolled patients with stroke related to an acute, large vessel occlusion that had failed to improve after treatment with IV r-tPA or patients who were not eligible to receive IV r-tPA. Like the MERCI trial, primary endpoints for the study were revascularization of the target vessel (TIMI grade 2 or 3) and the incidence of serious procedural events. Although the study lacked sufficient power to permit analysis of clinical outcomes, the authors relied on previous studies that correlated recanalization to clinical improvement. The Phase II trial investigators reported a favorable outcome (defined as 4-point improvement on the NIHSS) at discharge or on the 30-day modified Rankin Scale (mRS) of 2 or less in 41.6% of patients.

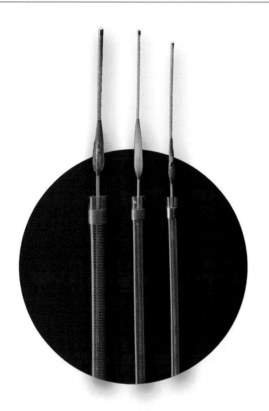

Figure 20–3. Penumbra reperfusion catheters and separators. The catheters are available with inner diameters of 0.026' (0.66 mm), 0.032' (0.81 mm), 0.041' (1.04 mm), and 0.054' (1.37 mm, not pictured). The corresponding separators are available with outer diameters of 0.022' (0.56 mm), 0.028' (0.71 mm), 0.035' (0.89 mm), and 0.045' (1.14 mm, not pictured).
(Used with permission from Penumbra, Inc.)

The PS is composed of three main components: a reperfusion catheter, a separator, and a thrombus removal ring (Figure 20–3). For aspiration, the reperfusion catheter is used coaxially with the separator while attached to an aspiration (suction) source to separate the thrombus from the vessel wall. If residual thrombus is still present after revascularization with aspiration, the thrombus removal ring can be used to directly engage and remove the residual thrombus. A complete description of the device and its use can be found in the original trial.[27]

Penumbra System Technical Comments

Again, the site of arterial access is selected on the basis of establishing stable guide catheter placement, typically through the femoral artery. A baseline ACT is obtained and the patient is given IV heparin to maintain an ACT of 250 to 300 seconds after arterial access is established.

All mechanical thrombolysis with the Penumbra System (Penumbra, Inc., Alameda, CA) is performed through a 6-French guide catheter after conventional catheter angiography is performed. Depending on the location of the thrombus, the appropriate size of the Penumbra reperfusion catheter is chosen and navigated to the proximal end of the thrombus

over a 0.014-inch guide wire. Once the target lesion is reached, the guide wire is exchanged for the same size separator. With the reperfusion catheter connected to an aspiration pump that generates a vacuum of 20 mm Hg, the separator is advanced and withdrawn into the reperfusion catheter for continuous aspiration-thrombolysis process. After multiple passes with the separator, angiography is performed to evaluate the degree of recanalization. For persistent thrombus, intra-arterial tPA can be given locally to soften the thrombus and potentially increase the efficacy of the thrombolysis. Recanalization is considered successful if TIMI grade 2 to 3 is achieved. In most cases, heparinization is neither reversed nor continued after the procedure.

Early recanalization and reperfusion have been identified as good prognostic indicators in a number of clinical trials. However, the lack of contemporaneous controls in these studies precludes the conclusion that thrombectomy definitively improves stroke outcomes. Randomized controlled trials evaluating the clinical benefit and cost-effectiveness of these invasive treatment modalities will help answer these questions and are underway.[28,29] The Phenox CRC Mechanical Thrombectomy Device (Phenox, Bochum, Germany) and the Catch Mechanical Thrombus Retriever (Balt, Montmorency, France) are approved for use in Europe.

Frequently, mechanical thrombectomy is used in conjunction with chemical thrombolysis to restore flow. Adjuvant intra-arterial thrombolysis has been evaluated in Phase I and II trials,[30] and randomized trials are ongoing.[28]

Drawbacks to intra-arterial thrombolysis include the invasiveness of the procedure, antecedent intubation, admission to an intensive care unit, and the expense of maintaining the constant availability of a dedicated interventional team. In 2007, a meta-analysis evaluating uncontrolled cohort studies of intra-arterial thrombolysis with a model predicting outcome without the use of intra-arterial thrombolysis failed to demonstrate clinical benefit. This finding indicates that more work remains to be done to identify the patients who will most benefit from aggressive intervention.

AngioJet Catheter

The AngioJet (Possis Medical, Inc., Minneapolis, MN) thrombectomy catheter uses high-pressure, pulsatile saline to fragment and aspirate clot into the lumen of the catheter. The AngioJet is used primarily in peripheral and interventional cardiac procedures, but successful intracranial use has been reported.[31,32] This device could be considered for off-label use in patients with large clot burden.

Stenting for Acute Stroke

Several case reports involving the use of self-expanding stents in the setting of recalcitrant thromboses led to interest in evaluating the use of stents for the treatment of acute stroke.

The Stent-Assisted Recanalization in Acute Ischemic Stroke (SARIS) trial was a prospective, single-arm trial to evaluate intracranial stenting as a first-line intra-arterial acute stroke treatment.[33] Primary outcome measures were safety, which is defined by the occurrence of symptomatic (>4 point worsening on the NIHSS or neurological decline in the presence of intracranial hemorrhage) or asymptomatic intracranial hemorrhage, or neurological deterioration and evidence of recanalization (evaluated by the TIMI score of the target vessel). In this small investigational study, results were encouraging and the authors recommended further analysis to evaluate the utility of intra-arterial stenting as a primary treatment modality for acute stroke.

CLINICAL TRIALS

At the time of this writing, several clinical trials are ongoing to evaluate new techniques for endovascular treatment of acute stroke. The Magnetic Resonance and Recanalization of Stroke Clots Using Embolectomy (MR RESCUE) trial randomizes patients to mechanical thrombectomy with the Merci System or to maximize medical therapy after MR or CT perfusion imaging. The MR RESCUE trial is the first trial to attempt to identify patients likely to benefit from aggressive intervention on the basis of objective, radiographic findings. The Interventional Management of Stroke Trial III (IMS-III) randomizes patients to a group receiving IV r-tPA or to a group receiving combined IV/intra-arterial r-tPA. Patients randomized to the combined IV/intra-arterial group will undergo mechanical thrombectomy (Merci Retriever, PS, or EKOS Micro-Infusion Catheter), intra-arterial r-tPA (maximum dose 22 mg), or both.

Endovascular Revascularization Techniques for Intracranial Stenosis

Large vessel atherosclerotic disease is a significant cause of intracranial ischemic events, accounting for about 10% of strokes. Important demographic disparities have been identified as well; African Americans, Asians, and Latinos are more likely to suffer from stroke related to intracranial stenosis than Caucasians, who tend to suffer from extracranial stenoses.[34]

The Warfarin versus Aspirin for Symptomatic Intracranial Disease (WASID) Trial demonstrated that certain subgroups of patients remain at a high risk of developing a stroke despite adequate medical therapy.[35] The WASID trial and the smaller Groupe d' Étude des Sténoses Intra-Crâniennes Athéromateuses symptomatiques (GESICA) both identified subgroups of patients with intracranial stenosis who are at high risk of suffering from stroke. The WASID trial studies found that the 1- and 2-year risk of stroke in patients with 50% to 69% stenosis was 6% and 10%, respectively. However, in patients with 70% to 99% stenosis, the 1- and 2-year risk rose to 18% and 20%, respectively. The GESICA trial did not quantify the degree of stenosis but identified patients with hemodynamic features (i.e., symptoms exacerbated by physical activity, change in body position, or the addition or increase in an antihypertensive medication) that increased the risk of developing recurrent vascular events.

Since its initial description by Dotter and Judkins in 1964, percutaneous transluminal angioplasty (PTA) has been used successfully to treat peripheral and coronary arterial disease.[36] Initially, coronary angioplasty balloons were used off-label to perform intracranial PTA alone. As balloon-mounted stents became the mainstay of endoluminal treatment of coronary artery disease, these devices were adopted for the treatment of intracranial atherosclerotic disease. Technological modifications were necessary to allow navigation of the more tortuous intracranial circulation with more flexible catheters and improved stent delivery systems. Initial attempts at treatment of intracranial atherosclerotic disease with stenting resulted in acceptable periprocedural rates of morbidity and mortality, but with relatively high rates of technical failure.

Initial reports of high complication rates (vessel dissection, distal embolization, vasospasm, and arterial thrombosis)[37] were probably related to inadequate technology. Angioplasty with modern over-the-wire microcatheter-guided balloons alone appears to compare favorably to medical therapy alone,[38] but is associated with higher restenosis rates than modern intracranial stenting (50% compared to 7.5%).[39]

The findings of the WASID trial that identified patients who remain at high risk of stroke despite adequate medical therapy occurred in the same year (2005) that the FDA granted a humanitarian device exemption for the Wingspan stent system (Boston Scientific, Fremont, CA). The periprocedural rates of stroke associated with the Wingspan stent were relatively low and led to widespread adoption of this technology by neurointerventionalists. At present, stenting for the treatment of intracranial atherosclerosis is reserved for patients with severe disease who have failed maximal medical therapy.

Based on the data collected from single-arm stenting trials and registries, it is probable that stenting has the potential to be an effective technique for reducing the risk of stroke in selected patients with intracranial atherosclerotic disease. The risk-benefit profile is most favorable for individuals with more than 70% stenosis of a large intracranial vessel. A number of clinical trials attempting to demonstrate this assumption are ongoing.

Stenting versus Aggressive Medical Management for Preventing Recurrent Stroke in Intracranial Stenosis (SAMMPRIS) is a randomized, controlled trial funded by the National Institutes of Health (NIH). This trial was designed to compare the Wingspan stent and Gateway balloon systems with maximal medical therapy in patients with intracranial stenosis of 70% or more with a qualifying event (stroke or transient ischemic attack) within 30 days. The Micrus Endovascular Corporation (San Jose, CA) has initiated a smaller, randomized, controlled trial comparing the Vitesse Pharos stent to medical therapy in patients with high-grade intracranial stenosis.

Complications

Major cerebrovascular complications related to angioplasty and stenting of intracranial vessels are related primarily to vessel rupture and thromboembolic phenomena. The Wingspan Intracranial Stent Registry Study Group identified possible risk factors for major complications due to angioplasty and stenting in patients with posterior circulation stenosis, low-volume centers, stenting within 10 days of a qualifying event, or stroke as a qualifying event.[40]

Restenosis represents a major source of long-term failure of endoluminal stent therapy. Restenosis occurs as a result of the elastic recoil of the vessel, neointimal hyperplasia, and vascular remodeling. In-stent stenosis occurs in approximately one third of patients who receive the Wingspan stent[41] and is most common in the anterior circulation, particularly in the supraclinoid ICA segment.[42] Revascularization by angioplasty with or without stenting in patients with restenosis is safe and effective in approximately 50% of patients with in-stent stenosis, although the durability of this therapy is unknown.[43]

At this time, the hypothesis that angioplasty and stenting for nonacute intracranial stenotic lesions is a safe and effective treatment for the reduction of stroke risk in a select group of patients is supported by class IV data. However, the degree of risk reduction for stroke that this treatment imparts is unknown.

Intracranial Stenting Technical Comments

Several standard procedural protocols are used at our institution for endovascular revascularization for cranial ischemic pathologies. All patients undergoing angioplasty and stenting as an elective procedure are given dual antiplatelet therapy for 3 days consisting of aspirin (325–350 mg/day orally) and either ticlopidine (Ticlid; Roche Pharmaceuticals, Nutley, NJ) (250 mg orally twice a day) or clopidogrel (Plavix; Bristol-Myers Squibb/Sanofi Pharmaceuticals, New York) (75 mg/day orally). In urgent situations requiring endovascular interventions, patients are given a loading dose of aspirin (650 mg) and clopidogrel (450 mg). Intraprocedural functional assays are tested to verify individual responsiveness to aspirin, clopidogrel, and abciximab, and doses of dual antiplatelet regimen may be readjusted postprocedurally. The dual antiplatelet regimen is maintained until follow-up angiography is obtained (3 to 6 months). Clopidogrel is discontinued if no in-stent restenosis is demonstrated on follow-up angiography. Aspirin is continued indefinitely unless contraindicated.

All patients are placed under general anesthesia for percutaneous transluminal angioplasty and stenting (PTAS) treatment of intracranial stenoses using the Wingspan system (Figure 20–4). Intraoperative neurophysiological monitorings (somatosensory evoked potential and electroencephalography) are used throughout the procedure. Arterial access is

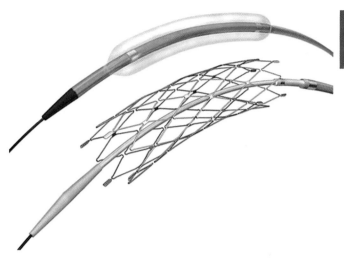

Figure 20–4. The Gateway balloon and Wingspan intracranial stent. *(Used with permission from Boston Scientific.)*

typically achieved through the common femoral artery. In rare instances, other arterial sites such as transradial, transbrachial, or direct carotid puncture are required. Heparinization is instituted with the goal of activated coagulation times between 250 and 300 seconds after arterial access is achieved. All interventions are performed through a 6-French system guide catheter.

After conventional catheter-based angiography, a microcatheter is navigated across the target lesion over a 0.014-inch guidewire. The microcatheter is then exchanged over a 0.014-inch exchange microguidewire for a Gateway angioplasty balloon and advanced across the stenotic lesion. The balloon diameter and length are sized to 80% of the normal parent vessel diameter and matched to the length of the lesion, respectively. Angioplasty is typically performed with a slow, graded inflation of the balloon to a pressure of between six and 12 atmospheres for approximately 120 seconds. After angioplasty, the balloon is removed and conventional angiography is repeated.

Next, the Wingspan delivery system is prepared and advanced over the exchange wire across the target lesion. The stent diameter is sized to exceed the diameter of the normal parent vessel by 0.5 to 1.0 mm. The stent length is selected to equal or exceed the length of the angioplasty balloon. In addition, the stent length is selected to completely cover the entire diseased segment and to allow the proximal end of the stent to be positioned so as not to preclude future endovascular access into the stented segment. The diameter of the stenotic lesion is measured using biplanar angiography and compared with a reference diameter of the normal vessel (usually proximal to the lesion), according to the technique used in the WASID study. Angiography is performed after the stent is deployed (Figure 20–5). Post-stenting angioplasty may be required if residual stenosis is present. Heparinization is typically neither reversed nor continued postoperatively.

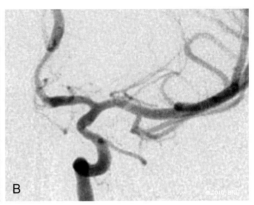

Figure 20–5. Posteroanterior angiogram of left ICA injection demonstrating high-grade, flow-limiting stenosis of the ICA terminus and M1 segment of the MCA (**A**) before and (**B**) after Wingspan stent placement and angioplasty with the Gateway balloon. *(Used with permission from Barrow Neurological Institute.)*

EXTRACRANIAL CAROTID STENOSIS

Occlusive disease of the extracranial ICA is assumed to be the cause of one-fourth of all strokes.[44] Based on numerous randomized trials, carotid artery endarterectomy (CEA) reduces the risk of stroke in patients with moderate (>50%) symptomatic or severe (>60%) asymptomatic carotid stenosis.[45,46] CEA is considered to be the best surgical treatment for carotid atherosclerotic disease, and CEA has subsequently become one of the most commonly performed surgical procedures in the United States. Certain groups of patients, however, are at high risk for complications related to CEA. Anatomic considerations (high carotid bifurcations, prior CEA, radiation-induced stenosis) can increase the technical difficulty of the operation. Patients with a history of myocardial infarction, angina, or hypertension are at increased risk of sustaining procedure-related complications. The benefits of CEA are lost if the 30-day rate of stroke or death exceeds 6% for symptomatic stenosis or 3% for asymptomatic stenosis.

Carotid artery stenting had emerged as a less invasive and effective alternative to CEA. Several randomized controlled trials comparing CEA with carotid artery stenting have yielded conflicting results. While some studies have demonstrated that carotid artery stenting was not inferior to CEA,[47,48] others have concluded that carotid artery stenting was inferior to CEA.[49] Meta-analysis and pooled risk estimates resulted in wide confidence intervals, making generalizations based on these studies very difficult.

At present, the relative benefits in reducing stroke, morbidity, and mortality between CEA and carotid artery stenting in conventional-risk patients are unknown. The Carotid Revascularization Endarterectomy versus Stenting Trial (CREST) is designed to answer these questions by randomizing conventional-risk patients with either symptomatic (≥50% by angiography or ≥70% by ultrasound) or asymptomatic (≥60% by angiography or ≥70% by ultrasound) extracranial stenosis to either carotid artery stenting or CEA. The investigational devices used are the RX Acculink stent and the RX Accunet embolic protection system (Abbott Vascular, Santa Clara, CA). The primary endpoints of CREST are stroke, myocardial infarction, all causes of mortality during a 30-day periprocedural period, and ipsilateral stroke over the 4-year follow-up period. CREST established equivalent safety profiles for endarterectomy and stenting. In terms of periprocedural complications within the first 30 days of treatment, 2.3% of endarterectomy patients suffered a stroke compared to 4.1% of stenting patients. Myocardial infarction, however, occured more frequently in patients undergoing endarterectomy (2.3%) than stenting (1.1%). The cumulative total of these adverse outcomes produced a statistically equivalent safety profile for the two procedures.

Strong evidence recommends carotid artery stenting for treating specific subsets of patients, including restenosis after CEA, radiation-induced stenosis, those with anatomically high lesions, and those at high risk for undergoing general anesthesia.[50,51]

Extracranial Carotid Stenting Technical Comments

At our institution, we prefer to perform carotid artery stenting under conscious sedation with the supervision of an anesthesiologist for hemodynamic control and comfort. Patients who undergo carotid artery stenting are typically high-risk patients for general anesthesia. Conscious sedation allows continuous neurological examination during the procedure.

The arterial access site is guided by the most favorable guide catheter stabilization needed for treatment. A baseline ACT is obtained, and the patient is heparinized to achieve an ACT between 250 and 300 prior to accessing across the stenosis. For transfemoral approach, a 5-French diagnostic catheter in coaxial fashion with a 6-French shuttle catheter is then used to selectively catheterize the targeted lesion. Opposite oblique and lateral angiograms of the carotid stenosis are obtained to minimize overlapping between the branches of the external carotid artery and the targeted stenosis in the ICA. A preprocedural angiogram of the ipsilateral anterior

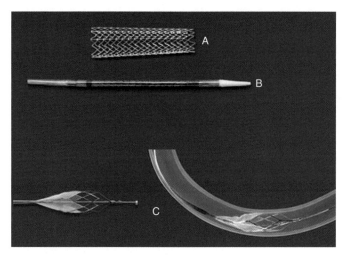

Figure 20–6. The Acculink stent (**A**), stent delivery device (**B**), and the Accunet embolic protection device (**C**).
(Used with permission from Abbott Vascular.)

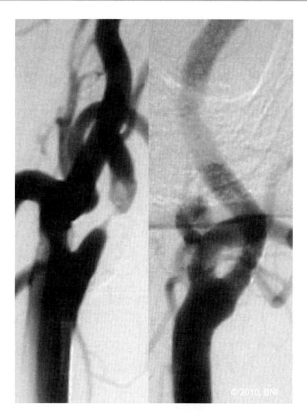

Figure 20–7. Left anterior oblique projection of a left common carotid artery injection before and after angioplasty and stenting. The high-grade stenosis seen on the left image was causing right-sided transient and ischemic attacks and aphasia. All symptoms resolved after the procedure.
(Used with permission from Barrow Neurological Institute.)

circulation is also performed as a baseline for postprocedural comparison. The following measurements are calculated on the carotid angiogram: (1) diameter and percentage of the stenosis, (2) normal proximal and distal carotid artery, and (3) length of the lesion. We also evaluate the carotid angiogram under subtracted condition to determine the stenosis in relation to the cervical bony anatomy on the lateral angiography.

All carotid artery stenting performed at our practice is executed on a monorail system with a distal protection device (DPD) (Figure 20–6). The monorail guidewire with the DPD is navigated gently across the stenosis. The DPD is deployed in the distal ICA but may require more proximal deployment if the vessel is extremely tortuous to navigate. Prestenting angioplasty with an undersize, noncompliant balloon may be required if the lesion is severely stenotic. Before angioplasty, we notify the anesthesiologist of potential vasovagal response associated with angioplasty. The vasovagal response can be dramatic, sometimes resulting in hemodynamically significant bradycardia or even asystole.[52] Occasionally, the anesthesiologist may elect to pretreat the patient with an anticholinergic agent to blunt the vasovagal reflex.

The balloon is inflated slowly with pure contrast for maximal visualization and subsequently deflated after reaching the desired inflation (6 to 10 atmospheres). A carotid angiogram is then obtained to ensure the dilation is sufficient to pass the stent. A self-expandable stent is navigated over the targeted lesion length. Using the cervical bony landmarks on a lateral angiography, the stent is deployed using a left-to-right unsheathing technique over the stent stabilizer. Poststent angioplasty may be required if residual stenosis is present. A noncompliant balloon that is approximately the diameter of the vessel is inflated slowly and under continuous fluoroscopic visualization for poststenting dilatation. An angiogram is then obtained after poststent dilatation. The DPD is recaptured with

a retrieval device. Extracranial and intracranial carotid angiography is performed to evaluate for potential thromboembolic complications (Figure 20–7). In most cases, heparinization is neither reversed nor continued postoperatively.

CONCLUSION

The array of endovascular therapies and devices available for the treatment of ischemic cerebrovascular disease has expanded substantially and at a rapid pace in the past decade. As our understanding of the pathophysiology of acute and chronic vascular occlusive disease improves and new therapies become available, rigorous clinical investigation will be required to refine the indications of these new therapies. To maximize the benefit to patients, neurointerventionalists must remain abreast of the emerging body of literature that will guide our application of these therapies.

REFERENCES

1. *Heart Disease and Stroke Statistics*, 2009, American Heart Association. Available at: www.americanheart.org/presenter.jhtml?identifier= 1200026.

2. Caplan LR: *Stroke: A Clinical Approach*, Boston, 1993, Butterworth-Heinemann.
3. Fisher M: Occlusion of the internal carotid artery, *AMA Arch Neurol Psychiatry* 65:346–377, 1951.
4. Fisher CM: Lacunes: Small, deep cerebral infarcts, *Neurology* 15:774–784, 1965.
5. Hommel M, Boissel JP, Cornu C, et al: Termination of trial of streptokinase in severe acute ischaemic stroke. MAST Study Group, *Lancet* 345:57, 1995.
6. Thrombolytic therapy with streptokinase in acute ischemic stroke: The Multicenter Acute Stroke Trial-Europe Study Group, *N Engl J Med* 335:145–150, 1996.
7. Hacke W, Kaste M, Fieschi C, et al: Intravenous thrombolysis with recombinant tissue plasminogen activator for acute hemispheric stroke. The European Cooperative Acute Stroke Study (ECASS), *JAMA* 274:1017–1025, 1995.
8. Tissue plasminogen activator for acute ischemic stroke: The National Institute of Neurological Disorders and Stroke rt-PA Stroke Study Group, *N Engl J Med* 333:1581–1587, 1995.
9. Clark WM, Wissman S, Albers GW, et al: Recombinant tissue-type plasminogen activator (Alteplase) for ischemic stroke 3 to 5 hours after symptom onset. The ATLANTIS Study: a randomized controlled trial. Alteplase Thrombolysis for Acute Noninterventional Therapy in Ischemic Stroke, *JAMA* 282:2019–2026, 1999.
10. Albers GW, Bates VE, Clark WM, et al: Intravenous tissue-type plasminogen activator for treatment of acute stroke: the Standard Treatment with Alteplase to Reverse Stroke (STARS) study, *JAMA* 283:1145–1150, 2000.
11. Asimos AW, Norton HJ, Price MF, et al: Therapeutic yield and outcomes of a community teaching hospital code stroke protocol, *Acad Emerg Med* 11:361–370, 2004.
12. Dick AP, Straka J: IV tPA for acute ischemic stroke: results of the first 101 patients in a community practice, *Neurologist* 11:305–308, 2005.
13. Adams HP Jr, Brott TG, Furlan AJ, et al: Guidelines for thrombolytic therapy for acute stroke: a supplement to the guidelines for the management of patients with acute ischemic stroke. A statement for healthcare professionals from a Special Writing Group of the Stroke Council, American Heart Association, *Circulation* 94:1167–1174, 1996.
14. Hacke W, Donnan G, Fieschi C, et al: Association of outcome with early stroke treatment: pooled analysis of ATLANTIS, ECASS, and NINDS rt-PA stroke trials, *Lancet* 363(9411):768–774, 2004.
15. Hacke W, Kaste M, Bluhmki E, et al: Thrombolysis with alteplase 3 to 4.5 hours after acute ischemic stroke, *N Engl J Med* 359:1317–1329, 2008.
16. Wolpert SM, Bruckmann H, Greenlee R, et al: Neuroradiologic evaluation of patients with acute stroke treated with recombinant tissue plasminogen activator. The rt-PA Acute Stroke Study Group, *AJNR Am J Neuroradiol* 14:3–13, 1993.
17. Brandt T, von KR, Muller-Kuppers M, et al: Thrombolytic therapy of acute basilar artery occlusion. Variables affecting recanalization and outcome, *Stroke* 27:875–881, 1996.
18. Bruckmann H, Ferbert A, del Zoppo GJ, et al: Acute vertebral-basilar thrombosis. Angiologic-clinical comparison and therapeutic implications, *Acta Radiol Suppl* 369:38–42, 1986.
19. Tomsick T, Brott T, Barsan W, et al: Prognostic value of the hyperdense middle cerebral artery sign and stroke scale score before ultraearly thrombolytic therapy, *AJNR Am J Neuroradiol* 17:79–85, 1996.
20. Gado-Mederos R, Rovira A, Varez-Sabin J, et al: Speed of tPA-induced clot lysis predicts DWI lesion evolution in acute stroke, *Stroke* 38:955–960, 2007.
21. Furlan A, Higashida R, Wechsler L, et al: Intra-arterial prourokinase for acute ischemic stroke. The PROACT II study: a randomized controlled trial. Prolyse in Acute Cerebral Thromboembolism, *JAMA* 282: 2003–2011, 1999.
22. Ogawa A, Mori E, Minematsu K, et al: Randomized trial of intraarterial infusion of urokinase within 6 hours of middle cerebral artery stroke: the middle cerebral artery embolism local fibrinolytic intervention trial (MELT) Japan, *Stroke* 38:2633–2639, 2007.
23. Smith WS, Sung G, Starkman S, et al: Safety and efficacy of mechanical embolectomy in acute ischemic stroke: results of the MERCI trial, *Stroke* 36:1432–1438, 2005.
24. Gobin YP, Starkman S, Duckwiler GR, et al: MERCI 1: a phase 1 study of Mechanical Embolus Removal in Cerebral Ischemia, *Stroke* 35:2848–2854, 2004.
25. Becker KJ, Brott TG: Approval of the MERCI clot retriever: a critical view, *Stroke* 36:400–403, 2005.
26. Wechsler LR: Does the Merci Retriever work? Against, *Stroke* 37: 1341–1342, 2006.
27. Bose A, Henkes H, Alfke K, et al: The Penumbra System: a mechanical device for the treatment of acute stroke due to thromboembolism, *AJNR Am J Neuroradiol* 29:1409–1413, 2008.
28. Broderick JP, Tomsick TA: *Interventional Management of Stroke (IMS) III Trial*, 2008, Clinical Trials.gov Available at www.clinicaltrials.gov.
29. Patil CG, Long EF, Lansberg MG: Cost-effectiveness analysis of mechanical thrombectomy in acute ischemic stroke, *J Neurosurg* 110:508–513, 2009.
30. The Interventional Management of Stroke (IMS) II Study, *Stroke* 38:2127–2135, 2007.
31. Bellon RJ, Putman CM, Budzik RF, et al: Rheolytic thrombectomy of the occluded internal carotid artery in the setting of acute ischemic stroke, *AJNR Am J Neuroradiol* 22:526–530, 2001.
32. Mayer TE, Hamann GF, Schulte-Altedorneburg G, et al: Treatment of vertebrobasilar occlusion by using a coronary waterjet thrombectomy device: a pilot study, *AJNR Am J Neuroradiol* 26:1389–1394, 2005.
33. Levy EI, Siddiqui AH, Crumlish A, et al: First Food and Drug Administration–approved prospective trial of primary intracranial stenting for acute stroke: SARIS (stent-assisted recanalization in acute ischemic stroke), *Stroke* 40:3552–3556, 2009.
34. Sacco RL, Kargman DE, Gu Q, et al: Race-ethnicity and determinants of intracranial atherosclerotic cerebral infarction. The Northern Manhattan Stroke Study, *Stroke* 26:14–20, 1995.
35. Chimowitz MI, Lynn MJ, Howlett-Smith H, et al: Comparison of warfarin and aspirin for symptomatic intracranial arterial stenosis, *N Engl J Med* 352:1305–1316, 2005.
36. Dotter CT, Judkins MT: Transluminal treatment of arteriosclerotic obstruction. Description of a new technic and a preliminary report of its application, *Circulation* 30:654–670, 1964.
37. Alazzaz A, Thornton J, Aletich VA, et al: Intracranial percutaneous transluminal angioplasty for arteriosclerotic stenosis, *Arch Neurol* 57:1625–1630, 2000.
38. Marks MP, Wojak JC, Al-Ali F, et al: Angioplasty for symptomatic intracranial stenosis: clinical outcome, *Stroke* 37:1016–1020, 2006.
39. Mazighi M, Yadav JS, Bou-Chebl A: Durability of endovascular therapy for symptomatic intracranial atherosclerosis, *Stroke* 39:1766–1769, 2008.
40. Nahab F, Lynn MJ, Kasner SE, et al: Risk factors associated with major cerebrovascular complications after intracranial stenting, *Neurology* 72:2014–2019, 2009.
41. Levy EI, Turk AS, Albuquerque FC, et al: Wingspan in-stent restenosis and thrombosis: incidence, clinical presentation, and management, *Neurosurgery* 61:644–650, 2007.
42. Turk AS, Levy EI, Albuquerque FC, et al: Influence of patient age and stenosis location on wingspan in-stent restenosis, *AJNR Am J Neuroradiol* 29:23–27, 2008.
43. Fiorella DJ, Levy EI, Turk AS, et al: Target lesion revascularization after wingspan: assessment of safety and durability, *Stroke* 40:106–110, 2009.
44. Dyken ML: *Prevention of Stroke*, New York, 1991, Springer-Verlag.
45. Barnett HJ, Taylor DW, Eliasziw M, et al: Benefit of carotid endarterectomy in patients with symptomatic moderate or severe stenosis. North American Symptomatic Carotid Endarterectomy Trial Collaborators, *N Engl J Med* 339:1415–1425, 1998.

46. Halliday A, Mansfield A, Marro J, et al: Prevention of disabling and fatal strokes by successful carotid endarterectomy in patients without recent neurological symptoms: randomised controlled trial, *Lancet* 363:1491–1502, 2004.
47. Endovascular versus surgical treatment in patients with carotid stenosis in the Carotid and Vertebral Artery Transluminal Angioplasty Study (CAVATAS): a randomised trial, *Lancet* 357:1729–1737, 2001.
48. Yadav JS, Wholey MH, Kuntz RE, et al: Protected carotid-artery stenting versus endarterectomy in high-risk patients, *N Engl J Med* 351:1493–1501, 2004.
49. Janjigian MP, Shah NR: Endarterectomy is superior to stenting in patients with symptomatic severe carotid stenosis, *J Clin Outcomes Mgt* 14:89–92, 2007.
50. Hobson RW, Mackey WC, Ascher E, et al: Management of atherosclerotic carotid artery disease: clinical practice guidelines of the Society for Vascular Surgery, *J Vasc Surg* 48:480–486, 2008.
51. Veith FJ, Amor M, Ohki T, et al: Current status of carotid bifurcation angioplasty and stenting based on a consensus of opinion leaders, *J Vasc Surg* 33(Suppl 2):S111–S116, 2001.
52. Criado E, Doblas M, Fontcuberta J, et al: Carotid angioplasty with internal carotid artery flow reversal is well tolerated in the awake patient, *J Vasc Surg* 40:92–97, 2004.

20

EXPLORING NEW FRONTIERS: ENDOVASCULAR TREATMENT OF THE OCCLUDED ICA

21

TIZIANO TALLARITA; HARRY J. CLOFT; ALEJANDRO A. RABINSTEIN; GIUSEPPE LANZINO

INTRODUCTION

Surgical revascularization of the occluded extracranial carotid artery has been established as a potential therapy in selected patients.[1] However, this procedure has not been widely applied because its intrinsic risks and the questionable benefits. Endovascular revascularization of acutely and chronically occluded femoral and coronary arteries has been performed for some time with good degree of clinical and radiological success. Application of these techniques to the extracranial carotid and vertebral arteries has lagged behind for fear of dislodging emboli. With advances in endovascular techniques, increasing experience with angioplasty and stenting of large extracranial cervical vessels, and the availability of a variety of distal protection devices, several operators have reported their results following endovascular revascularization of the acutely or even chronically occluded internal carotid artery (ICA).[2–20] In this chapter, we provide an overview of the rationale, techniques, results, and complications of endovascular revascularization of acute and chronic occlusion of the extracranial ICA.

ACUTE CAROTID OCCLUSION

Management of patients with stroke caused by acute ICA occlusion is challenging. Medical therapy alone is associated with a high rate of permanent severe neurological disability and mortality.[1] In patients with acute stroke and ICA occlusion, early restoration of flow in the occluded ICA may prevent further worsening, improve symptoms, and reduce the risk of recurrent stroke.[2] Currently, the invasive treatment of patients with acute ICA occlusion is not standardized. Acute ICA occlusion responds poorly to intravenous thrombolysis alone or in combination with intra-arterial pharmacological thrombolysis with recanalization rates ranging from 10%[21] to 50%,[22–24] and resultant mortality of 50%.[21–24] Slightly better clinical results have been reported following mechanical thrombectomy, but only a few reports are available.[25,26]

Over the past decade, several authors[2,3–11,27] have reported the feasibility of endovascular revascularization of the acutely occluded internal carotid artery with angioplasty and stenting with higher rates of recanalization and clinical improvement than reported with other methods (Table 21–1).

Technique

Symptomatic acute thrombosis of the proximal ICA often occurs in concomitance with ICA bifurcation (T-lesion) or MCA occlusion. The natural history of associated proximal ICA and central distal occlusions is poor.[2,3–10,12] Acute revascularization of the proximal ICA in such cases allows catheterization and thrombolysis of the distal segment and, by increasing distal flow, improves the chances of maintaining vessel patency after successful distal thrombolysis. In addition, stenting of the occluded ICA may "trap" thrombus against the carotid wall, potentially decreasing the risk of delayed distal emboli.

In these patients we perform a rapid diagnostic angiography with a 5F catheter and assess the status of the carotid bifurcation as well as the status of external carotid collaterals by studying the angiograms in the delayed phases. Angiography of the contralateral side is helpful to assess the presence or absence of collateral vessels. In the presence of a short ICA occlusion that does not extend to the ICA bifurcation terminus, the contralateral angiogram allows for a depiction of the anatomy of the ipsilateral MCA distribution. However, symptoms are usually related to distal MCA occlusion or the occlusion extends to the carotid bifurcation terminus and this distal occlusion also demands treatment.

After a diagnosis of the ICA occlusion and assessment of the collateral circulation, the 5F catheter is exchanged for a larger guide-catheter, which is placed in the distal common carotid artery. We prefer to perform the procedure under full heparinization. However, this is often not feasible because these patients had received variable doses of intravenous thrombolytics or intra-arterial pharmacological thrombolysis for coexistent distal occlusion. In such cases, a limited bolus of 2000 to 3000 units of heparin is administered before catheterization.

Table 21–1. RESULTS OF ENDOVASCULAR REVASCULARIZATION FOR ACUTE/SUBACUTE ICA OCCLUSION.

Author	No.	Occlusive Sites	Recanalization Rate	ICH	Mortality	Restenosis	Good Outcome	HPS	FU Length (months)
Dabitz[7]	10[a]	3 C, 1 C + P, 6 C + MCA	100%	40%	10%	0%	90%	20%	5
Imai[12]	4[b]	3 C, 1 C + MCA	100%	50%	0%	0%	50%	25%	3
Jovin, TG[2]	15[c]	10 C + CA, 5 C	100%	13%	20%	0%	47%	6.7%	1
Jovin, TG[2]	10[c]	9 C, 1 C + MCA	80%	10%	10%	0%	88%	0%	1
Komiyama[10]	1	1 C + MCA	100%	0%	0%	0%	100%	0%	5
Levy[4]	2[d]	2 C + MCA	100%	0%	0%	0%	100%	0%	10.5
Miyamoto[6]	5	1 C, 4 C + MCA	100%	0%	0%	0%	40%	0%	3
Nedeltchev[11]	25	6 C, 6 C + P, 13 C + CA	84%	8%	20%	0%	56%	0%	3
Spearman[8]	4	4 C + MCA	100%	0%	0%	25%[g]	50%	0%	6
Sugg, RM[5]	14[e]	10 C + CA, 4 C + MCA	64%	14.3%	21.4%	0%	64%	21.4%	(until discharge)
Suh, DC[3]	33[f]	13 C, 7 C + OPH, 13 C + CA	42%	27%	15%	0%	33%	15%	12
Wang[9]	6	6 C + MCA	100%	0%	0%	16.7%[h]	83%	0%	7

C, cervical carotid; CA, cavernous carotid; FU, follow-up; good outcome, rapid improvement of the mRS or is discharged home or to inpatient rehabilitation; HPS, hyperperfusion syndrome; ICH, intracranial hemorrhage; OPH, ophthalmic artery; MCA, middle cerebral artery; P, petrous carotid.
[a]*Three carotid dissections and one PTA.*
[b]*In one case alone was used.*
[c]*Ten patients with subacute occlusion (>7gg) with only one case of tandem lesion; 15 acute strokes, all associated with tandem lesions. There were one asymptomatic hemorrhage and one dissection, but it is not clear in which group.*
[d]*The second patient had a bilateral ICA occlusion due to dissection. Only one side was treated.*
[e]*Five angioplasty alone and six PTA + stenting brain protection device.*
[f]*Three cases of angioplasty alone.*
[g]*70% at 6 months.*
[h]*Reocclusion at 2 months.*

We usually try to cross the occluded segment with a filter-type distal protection. Often this is not possible and a stiffer and more steerable microguidewire is required to cross the occluded segment. The occlusion is then negotiated with a 0.014-inch or 0.018-inch steerable microguidewire. In some cases, a larger guidewire (0.035 inch) may be necessary. A microcatheter is then navigated over the microguidewire across the occluded segment and an angiogram through the microcatheter distal to the occluded segment is performed to assess the status of the carotid distal to the occlusion and the intracranial circulation.

With the microguidewire as a "buddy-wire," we try to cross the occlusion with a filter wire for distal protection. When this is possible, the protection device is landed in the distal cervical segment. A self-expandable stent is deployed in the proximal cervical carotid and poststent angiograms are obtained to confirm revascularization. Immediately after stent placement, patients are administered oral clopidrogel (300 mg) and aspirin (325 mg). Based on the findings of the post-stent angiogram further intervention is usually required. This may include thrombolysis (pharmacological or mechanical) or even further stenting of the ICA distally to the occluded segment or the proximal MCA. If a central occlusion distal to the proximal ICA occlusion exists, revascularization of the distal occlusion is critical to maximize the chance of a good functional outcome.

At the completion of the procedure, strict blood pressure control is maintained in those patients with successful recanalization (systolic pressure below 160 mm Hg in patients with acute occlusions or below 140 mm Hg when the occlusion is subacute or chronic). Clopidogrel is continued for 30 days and aspirin indefinitely. A head CT scan is routinely performed the following morning to rule out hemorrhage and to assess the extent of the infarcted area (Figure 21–1).

Results and Complications

Over the past 10 years, several authors have detailed their results with revascularization of the acutely occluded ICA. Nedeltchev and coworkers[11] studied 56 consecutive patients who suffered an MCA stroke following ICA occlusion between 1997 and 2003. Twenty-five of these patients underwent attempted endovascular revascularization (endovascular group), while 31 patients received medical treatment consisting of antiplatelet medications and, in some cases, heparin therapy (medical group). Recanalization of the ICA was achieved in 84% of patients in the endovascular group with a combination of thrombo-aspiration through an 8-French guide-catheter and stent deployment in the occluded ICA. Recanalization of the coexistent MCA occlusion (TIMI grade 2 and 3) was obtained in 52% of these patients. In the endovascular group, outcome at 3 months was favorable (modified Rankin score of 0–2) in 56% of patients and unfavorable in 24%. Twenty percent of patients died. In the medically treated group, a favorable outcome was observed in only 26% of patients. This series stresses the importance of recanalization of the coexistent distal

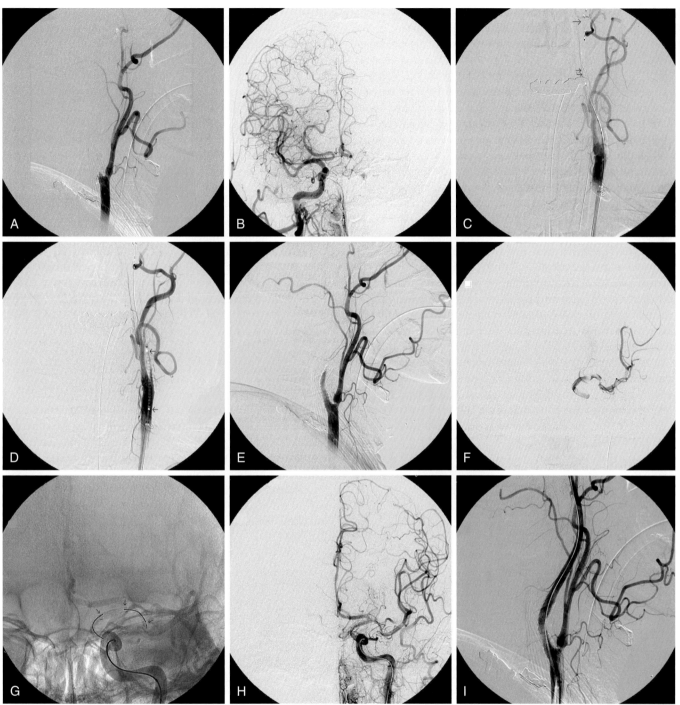

Figure 21–1. A 69-year-old man presented with acute right hemiparesis and aphasia. Cerebral angiography, left common carotid artery injection (**A**) lateral projection shows acute occlusion of the origin of the left ICA immediately distal to the bifurcation. Contralateral carotid angiography (**B**) shows hypoplastic A1 segment (*arrow*) on the right with some filling of the left distal anterior cerebral artery territory through the anterior communicating artery. A guide-catheter was placed into the distal common carotid artery. We attempted to cross the occlusion with a filter wire but this proved impossible. A 0.014 microguidewire was then advanced through the occlusion. With the microguidewire in place as a "buddy wire," we were then able to cross the occlusion with a filter wire. **C,** Shows the filter protection device deployed into the distal cervical ICA (*arrow*) and a "buddy wire" (*double arrows*) in place across the occlusion as well. A self-expandable stent was then advanced across the occlusion (**D**). Left common carotid artery injection following stent deployment, lateral projection shows flow through the stent but evidence of distal occlusion. Microcatheter injection after stent deployment shows thrombus into the cavernous ICA and occlusion of the intracranial ICA bifurcation (**E**). **F,** After mechanical and intra-arterial thrombolysis there was partial recanalization of the ipsilateral middle cerebral artery with persistent diffuse intraluminal thrombus. Telescoping enterprise (Cordis Neurovascular, Johnson and Johnson, Camden, NJ) stents placed into the M1 segment and across the intracranial ICA bifurcation: there is re-establishment of distal flow into both the anterior cerebral and middle cerebral arteries (**G** and **H**). Final lateral projection (**I**) shows re-establishment of flow through the previously occluded proximal ICA.

occlusion since MCA recanalization was the only predictor of good outcome. Symptomatic hemorrhage occurred in 8%. Although concerns exist regarding the risk of dissection and vessel perforation during blind "probing" of the occluded segment, these complications were not observed in this series.

Jovin and collaborators[2] reported a series of 23 patients who underwent successful ICA revascularization (in two additional patients crossing of the occlusion was not possible and no stent could be deployed). Of these 23 patients, 15 were revascularized within the time window for acute stroke therapy while the remaining eight had suffered subacute ICA occlusion and demonstrated ongoing symptoms related to hemodynamic compromise. A good outcome at 30 days was reported in five patients (33%) with acute ICA occlusion. Four of the five patients experiencing a good outcome did not have a coexistent intracranial occlusion and the fifth one had a coexistent MCA occlusion that was revascularized with pharmacological intra-arterial thrombolysis. No patient who had a tandem occlusion that did not revascularize achieved a good outcome. Complications related to the endovascular procedure included one asymptomatic hemorrhage and one dissection of the ICA without flow compromise. No serious complications were observed in the eight patients who had received IV tPA in conjunction with endovascular revascularization indicating the feasibility and safety of this approach. Table 21–1 provides a comprehensive summary of results and complications after revascularization of acute ICA occlusion.

CHRONIC CAROTID OCCLUSION

Endovascular revascularization of chronically occluded femoral, subclavian, and coronary arteries is an established practice in selected patients. In 2005, Terada et al.[28] reported the first patient with chronic carotid occlusion who underwent successful endovascular revascularization with flow reversal. Two years later, Kao and coworkers,[13] using a technique utilized to reopen occluded coronary arteries, reported the first series of 30 patients with chronic carotid occlusion who underwent attempted endovascular revascularization. Following these early reports, several other authors have reported successful recanalization of the chronically occluded ICA (Table 21–2).

Potential candidates for revascularization of chronic ICA occlusion must fulfill the following criteria:[13–15] (1) hemodynamic symptoms ascribed to the occluded territory, (2) hemodynamic failure demonstrated by perfusion studies, and (3) angiographic demonstration of a relatively short occluded segment.[14] This last angiographic requirement can be difficult to evaluate. Careful analysis of the angiograms with assessment of late retrograde filling of the ICA segment distal to the occlusion through collateral circulation is of critical importance to select patients who may benefit from endovascular recanalization. Assessment of the extent of occlusion can be difficult with other noninvasive angiographic techniques such as CTA and MRA, although dynamic CTA can offer valuable information.

Techniques

Technical pitfalls of chronic ICA occlusion recanalization are related primarily to crossing the occlusion while avoiding dislodgment of distal emboli.[29–31] Various techniques have been described to circumvent these problems and minimize the risk of distal emboli.

Patients are premedicated with clopidrogel 75 mg/day and aspirin 325 mg/day starting 5 days before the procedure. After obtaining femoral access, intravenous heparin is administered with the goal of maintaining the activated clotting time around

Table 21–2. RESULTS OF ENDOVASCULAR REVASCULARIZATION FOR CHRONIC ICA OCCLUSION.

Author	No.	Occlusive Sites	Recanalization Rate	ICH	Mortality	Restenosis	Good Outcome	FU Length (months)	HPS	OCs
Bhatt[19]	1	C	100%	0%	0%	0%	100%	9	0%	0%
Imai[18]	1	P/CA	100%	0%	0%	0%	100%	3	0%	0%
Lin[16]	54[a]	54 C	65%	2.9%	2.9%	5.7%	62.1%	U	0%	2.9%CCF, 2.9% PA, 2.9% CE
Kobayashi[15]	1[b]	C	100%	0%	0%	0%	100%	0	0%	0%
Komiyama[17]	1[c]	CL	100%	0%	0%	0%	100%	6	0%	BTS[f]
Terada[14]	15[d]	10 C, 4 P/CA, 1 U	93.3%	6.7%	0%	0%	93.3%	26.1	0%	27% DIS, 6.8% EMB
Thomas[20]	2[e]	2 C	100%	0%	0%	0%	100%	30 (days)	0%	0%

BTS, blue toe syndrome; C, cervical carotid; CA, cavernous carotid; CCF, carotid cavernous fistula; CE, cervical extravasation; CL, clinoid segment; DIS, dissection; EMB, embolism; FU, follow-up; good outcome, rapid improvement of the mRS or is discharged home or to inpatient rehabilitation; HPS, hyperperfusion syndrome; ICH, intracranial hemorrhage; OCs, other complications; P, petrous carotid; PA, pseudoaneurysm; U, indeterminate.

[a] In 73% cases distal protection device was used.
[b] Proximal balloon protection first and then distal protection.
[c] Angioplasty alone; proximal balloon protection device.
[d] Two cases of acute occlusion.
[e] No distal protection, but attempts were carried out.
[f] Mild BTS, first and second toes 1 month later (medical management).

300 seconds. The procedure can be done under local anesthesia and this permits careful clinical assessment during each step. However, general anesthesia is preferred in uncooperative patients or in case of difficult and tortuous proximal anatomy, which makes catheterization challenging.

The availability of "protection devices" has increased the safety of recanalization of the occluded ICA. Four types of "protection devices" are available for use in the extracranial carotid: distal occlusion balloon, distal filter, proximal occlusion catheter, and the Parodi's device.[32,33] The main disadvantage of the first two is the need to cross the lesions before device deployment with the consequent risk of cerebral microembolization before distal protection is established.[34–36]

Proximal occlusion can be achieved with one of two methods. One of these methods involves obtaining proximal occlusion with a double lumen balloon catheter positioned and inflated in the common carotid artery proximal to the occlusion. The inner lumen of the balloon allows passage of devices while the balloon is inflated though the other lumen. The goal of proximal occlusion is to prevent anterograde flow to dislodge emboli during and immediately after revascularization. Proximal common carotid occlusion alone is insufficient to prevent particles from embolizing to the brain[37] because of collateral vessels from the external carotid artery. In cases where the external carotid artery is patent, a separate small (5F) guide-catheter can be placed in the common carotid artery to allow passage of a small compliant balloon that can be separately inflated into the external carotid artery.

The other method by which proximal occlusion can be achieved is the Parodi Anti-Embolization Catheter (PAEC). This is an ingenious device originally designed to allow flow reversal during angioplasty and stenting of carotid stenosis. It consists of a triple lumen-guiding catheter with an occlusion balloon at the distal end. This balloon has a teardrop shape to prevent any dead space between the orifice of the catheter and the occlusion balloon. Occlusion of the common carotid artery is achieved by inflating this balloon while access to the lesion is possible through the main inner lumen. The main lumen has an inner diameter of 7F that allows for navigation of balloons and stents. The main lumen is connected to a three-way Y-adapter at its proximal end so that one has access to the lesion through the main lumen while suction is applied or reversal of flow is created through the other ports. In addition, the extra side port can be used for the insertion of an external carotid artery occlusion balloon, if one is needed.[33] The Parodi device also allows for activation of an arteriovenous fistula through connection with the femoral vein and this allows true flow reversal.[33]

If distal protection is used instead of proximal flow arrest, then a guide-catheter of sufficient internal diameter to allow for passage of multiple devices if needed is placed into the common carotid proximally to the occlusion (Figure 21–2).

Crossing the lesion

A microcatheter and microguidewire (0.016 inch or 0.014 inch) are typically used to cross the occluded ICA. The microcatheter is parked immediately proximal to the occlusion to provide backup support to the microguidewire as it is passed through the occluded segment. A tapered-tip stiff 0.014-inch guidewire specifically designed to cross coronary occlusions can be particularly helpful in this phase.[13] Care must be paid to avoid too much torquing or "drilling" of the microcatheter during this phase to avoid entering a false lumen with the risk of dissection or perforation. It is often difficult or even impossible to cross the occluded segment with the microguidewire. Resistance to passage of the microguidewire can be used as a criterion to judge the length and location of the occlusion.[14] Often, if the microguidewire does not cross the occluded segment, it is necessary to use a 0.035 guidewire to penetrate the occluded portion. In such cases, a 4F catheter can be passed through the occlusion over the 0.035 guidewire to gently "dilate" the channel. The guidewire is gently advanced while making sure that the microguidewire is within the true lumen of the vessel on orthogonal projections. At this point the microcatheter can be advanced distal to the occlusion and a gentle injection can be performed to confirm position into the true lumen and confirm patency of the ICA segment distal to the occlusion.

Distal Protection Technique

The microcatheter is exchanged for a small-diameter (1.5 or 2.0 mm) coronary angioplasty balloon, which is inflated to 6 to 8 atm. Percutaneous transluminal angioplasty is then performed from the distal occluded segment of the ICA to the proximal portion to predilatate the occlusion. A filter-type embolic protection device is then advanced parallel to the microguidewire and deployed distally if an adequate distal landing zone with diameter >3 mm can be identified. A self-expanding stent is then placed across the occlusion, followed by postdilation using a 4- to 6-mm–diameter balloon. A final ipsilateral intracranial angiogram is obtained to confirm re-established antegrade perfusion.

Proximal Occlusion Technique

An angioplasty balloon 20 to 40 mm in length is navigated over the microguidewire. Angioplasty of the ICA from distal to proximal is then performed. Following angioplasty, 50 to 60 ml of blood are aspirated from the double lumen balloon catheter placed in the common carotid artery to remove any debris mobilized during angioplasty. An angiogram is done by gentle injection to assess for anterograde flow. The point of occlusion can usually be identified on this angiogram as the segment (usually in proximity of the bifurcation) with the most significant residual stenosis. A self-expandable stent can then be deployed to cover this segment.

Results and complications

Recently, Lin et al.[16] updated their original experience and reported their results in 54 patients who underwent revascularization for chronic ICA occlusion. Revascularization was

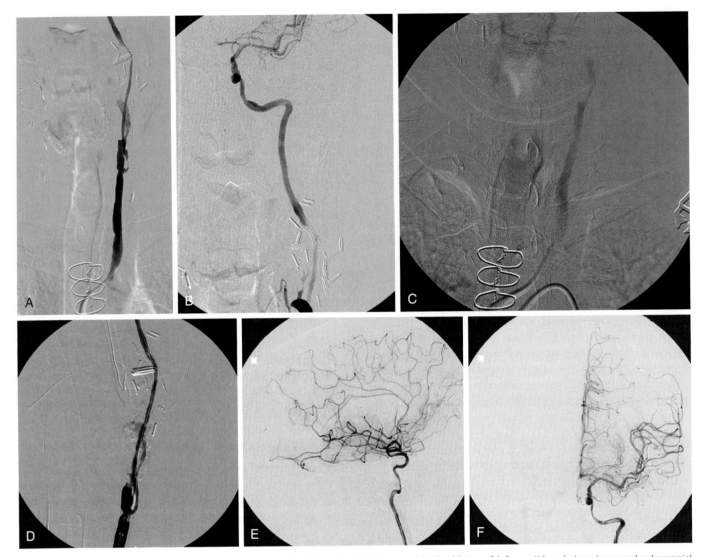

Figure 21–2. A 64-year-old female with multiple risk factors for atherosclerotic disease and prior history of left carotid endarterectomy and extracranial ICA-ICA saphenous graft elsewhere for ICA occlusion, presented with orthostatic symptoms of left hemispheric ischemia. Left common carotid artery injection shows occlusion of the ICA and external carotid artery and tandem severe stenosis of the graft (**A**) with patent ICA distal to the graft (**B**). She underwent angioplasty of the distal graft stenosis with resolution of her symptoms. She was readmitted 3 months later with recurrent symptoms of 1 month duration and catheter angiography showed occlusion of the graft (**C**). A 0.035 guidewire was negotiated through the occluded graft followed by a coronary angioplasty balloon and sequential angioplasty of the graft was performed with excellent restoration of flow through the occluded graft and the intracranial circulation (**D** to **F**).

achieved in 63% of patients. Distal protection devices were used in 73% of cases. In 10 patients, the use of distal embolic protection devices was not possible because of small distal vessel diameter. In the patients in whom technical success was achieved, the residual stenosis was 9%. The combined morbidity and mortality at 3 months was 4%. Vascular complications included an iatrogenic carotid-cavernous fistula, a delayed cervical ICA pseudoaneurysm, and extravasation of contrast in the neck during attempted crossing of ICA occlusion.

In 2009, Terada and coworkers[14] reported a series of 14 patients with a total of 15 occluded ICAs who underwent endovascular revascularization using the proximal occlusion technique and flow reversal. All of the patients were suffering from hemodynamic symptoms refractory to medical therapy.

They reported a technical success rate of 93% (14 out of 15 occlusions). Revascularized occlusions involved the cervical ICA in 10 cases and the petrous or cavernous portions of the artery in the remaining four. Complications included one case of distal MCA branch occlusion without clinical sequelae and one SAH due to microwire perforation of an MCA branch. No patient suffered recurrent symptoms at a mean follow up of 26.1 months. No cases of clinical hyperperfusion were observed.

Restenosis of the revascularized segment is a potential concern. However, experience in other vascular territories suggests that the risk of restenosis after revascularization of an occluded artery is higher in the coronary circulation[38] than in the iliac and subclavian arteries.[39,40] This observation would suggest that restenosis may be lower if the vessel diameter is greater than 3 mm. In this respect, the restenosis rate should be lower in the ICA and the largest series reported so far confirm this supposition as no restenosis >50% was observed by Terada and coworkers in their 14 cases,[14] while Kao and coworkers reported a restenosis rate of 13.6%.[13]

Cerebrovascular autoregulation in regions with chronic ischemia may be defective, and a sudden increase of perfusion after revascularization of chronic ICA occlusion raises concerns for hyperperfusion syndrome. Strict control of blood pressure after endovascular recanalization is critical to prevent or minimize the effects of this complication. Surprisingly, according to the literature, no cases of hyperperfusion syndrome were detected after revascularization of chronic ICA occlusion.[14-17,20] A summary of results and complications in published series of ICA occlusion is shown in Table 21-2.

CONCLUSION

Endovascular revascularization of ICA occlusion is feasible in cases of both acute and chronic occlusion. In patients with acute occlusion, outcome is closely dependent on revascularization of coexistent distal intracranial ICA or MCA occlusions. In patients with chronic occlusion, endovascular revascularization can be achieved in patients with short segment occlusion and retrograde partial filling of the supraclinoid ICA through collaterals. With further refinements of endovascular technique and better imaging techniques, a large proportion of patients affected by symptomatic ICA occlusion may be candidates for this procedure.

REFERENCES

1. Meyer FB, Sundt TM, Piepgras DG, et al: Emergency carotid endarterectomy for patients with acute carotid occlusion and profound neurological deficits, *Ann Surg* 203:82–89, 1986.
2. Jovin TG, Gupta R, Uchino K, et al: Emergent stenting of extracranial internal carotid artery occlusion in acute stroke has a high revascularization rate, *Stroke* 36:2426–2430, 2005.
3. Suh DC, Kim JK, Choi CG, et al: Prognostic factors for neurologic outcome after endovascular revascularization of acute symptomatic occlusion of the internal carotid artery, *Am J Neuroradiol* 28: 1167–1171, 2007.
4. Levy DI: Endovascular treatment of carotid artery occlusion in progressive stroke syndromes: technical note, *Neurosurgery* 42:186–191, 1998; discussion 91-3.
5. Sugg RM, Malkoff MD, Noser EA, et al: Endovascular recanalization of internal carotid artery occlusion in acute ischemic stroke, *Am J Neuroradiol* 26:2591–2594, 2005.
6. Miyamoto N, Naito I, Takatama S, et al: Urgent stenting for patients with acute stroke due to atherosclerotic occlusive lesions of the cervical internal carotid artery, *Neurol Med Chir (Tokyo)* 48:49–55, 2008; discussion 56.
7. Dabitz R, Triebe S, Leppmeier U, et al: Percutaneous recanalization of acute internal carotid artery occlusions in patients with severe stroke, *Cardiovasc Intervent Radiol* 30:34–41, 2007.
8. Spearman MP, Jungreis CA, Wechsler LR: Angioplasty of the occluded internal carotid artery, *Am J Neuroradiol* 16:1791–1796, 1995; discussion 1797-9.
9. Wang H, Lanzino G, Fraser K, et al: Urgent endovascular treatment of acute symptomatic occlusion of the cervical internal carotid artery, *J Neurosurg* 99:972–977, 2003.
10. Komiyama M, Nishio A, Nishijima Y: Endovascular treatment of acute thrombotic occlusion of the cervical internal carotid artery associated with embolic occlusion of the middle cerebral artery: case report, *Neurosurgery* 34:359–363, 1994; discussion 63-4.
11. Nedeltchev K, Brekenfeld C, Remonda L, et al: Internal carotid artery stent implantation in 25 patients with acute stroke: preliminary results, *Radiology* 237:1029–1037, 2005.
12. Imai K, Mori T, Izumoto H, et al: Emergency carotid artery stent placement in patients with acute ischemic stroke, *Am J Neuroradiol* 26:1249–1258, 2005.
13. Kao HL, Lin MS, Wang CS, et al: Feasibility of endovascular recanalization for symptomatic cervical internal carotid artery occlusion, *J Am Coll Cardiol* 49:765–771, 2007.
14. Terada T, Okada H, Nanto M, et al: Endovascular recanalization of the completely occluded internal carotid artery using a flow reversal system at the subacute to chronic stage, *J Neurosurg* 112(3):563–571, 2010.
15. Kobayashi N, Miyachi S, Hattori K, et al: Carotid angioplasty with stenting for chronic internal carotid artery occlusion: technical note, *Neuroradiology* 48:847–851, 2006.
16. Lin MS, Lin LC, Li HY, et al: Procedural Safety and Potential Vascular Complication of Endovascular Recanalization for Chronic Cervical Internal Carotid Artery Occlusion, *Circ Cardiovasc Interventions* 1: 119–125, 2008.
17. Komiyama M, Yoshimura M, Honnda Y, et al: Percutaneous angioplasty of a chronic total occlusion of the intracranial internal carotid artery. Case report, *Surg Neurol* 66:513–518, 2006; discussion 518.
18. Imai K, Mori T, Izumoto H, et al: Successful stenting seven days after atherothrombotic occlusion of the intracranial internal carotid artery, *J Endovasc Ther* 13:254–259, 2006.
19. Bhatt A, Majid A, Kassab M, et al: Chronic total symptomatic carotid artery occlusion treated successfully with stenting and angioplasty, *J Neuroimaging* 19:68–71, 2009.
20. Thomas AJ, Gupta R, Tayal AH, et al: Stenting and angioplasty of the symptomatic chronically occluded carotid artery, *AJNR Am J Neuroradiol* 28:168–171, 2007.
21. Christou I, Felberg RA, Demchuk AM, et al: Intravenous tissue plasminogen activator and flow improvement in acute ischemic stroke patients with internal carotid artery occlusion, *J Neuroimaging* 12: 119–123, 2002.
22. Zaidat OO, Suarez JI, Santillan C, et al: Response to intra-arterial and combined intravenous and intra-arterial thrombolytic therapy in patients with distal internal carotid artery occlusion, *Stroke* 33:1821–1826, 2002.
23. Linfante I, Llinas RH, Selim M, et al: Clinical and vascular outcome in internal carotid artery versus middle cerebral artery occlusions after intravenous tissue plasminogen activator, *Stroke* 33:2066–2071, 2002.
24. Arnold M, Nedeltchev K, Mattle HP, et al: Intra-arterial thrombolysis in 24 consecutive patients with internal carotid artery T occlusions, *J Neurol Neurosurg Psychiatry* 74:739–742, 2003.
25. Flint AC, Duckwiler GR, Budzik RF, et al: Mechanical thrombectomy of intracranial internal carotid occlusion: pooled results of the MERCI and Multi MERCI Part I trials, *Stroke* 38:1274–1280, 2007.
26. Smith WS, Sung G, Saver J, et al: Mechanical thrombectomy for acute ischemic stroke: final results of the Multi MERCI trial, *Stroke* 39: 1205–1212, 2008.
27. Meves SH, Muhs A, Federlein J, et al: Recanalization of acute symptomatic occlusions of the internal carotid artery, *J Neurol* 249:188–192, 2002.
28. Terada T, Yamaga H, Tsumoto T, et al: Use of an embolic protection system during endovascular recanalization of a totally occluded cervical internal carotid artery at the chronic stage. Case report, *J Neurosurg* 102:558–564, 2005.
29. Ackerstaff RG, Moons KG, van de Vlasakker CJ, et al: Association of intraoperative transcranial doppler monitoring variables with stroke from carotid endarterectomy, *Stroke* 31:1817–1823, 2000.

30. Jordan WD, Voellinger DC, Doblar DD, et al: Microemboli detected by transcranial Doppler monitoring in patients during carotid angioplasty versus carotid endarterectomy, *Cardiovasc Surg (London)* 7:33–38, 1999.

31. Coggia M, Goeau-Brissonniere O, Duval JL, et al: Embolic risk of the different stages of carotid bifurcation balloon angioplasty: an experimental study, *J Vasc Surg* 31:550–557, 2000.

32. Parodi JC, La Mura R, Ferreira LM, et al: Initial evaluation of carotid angioplasty and stenting with three different cerebral protection devices, *J Vasc Surg* 32:1127–1136, 2000.

33. Ohki T, Parodi J, Veith FJ, et al: Efficacy of a proximal occlusion catheter with reversal of flow in the prevention of embolic events during carotid artery stenting: an experimental analysis, *J Vasc Surg* 33: 504–509, 2001.

34. Cremonesi A, Manetti R, Setacci F, et al: Protected carotid stenting: clinical advantages and complications of embolic protection devices in 442 consecutive patients, *Stroke* 34:1936–1941, 2003.

35. Eckert B, Zeumer H: Editorial comment—carotid artery stenting with or without protection devices? Strong opinions, poor evidence!, *Stroke* 34:1941–1943, 2003.

36. Terada T, Tsuura M, Matsumoto H, et al: Results of endovascular treatment of internal carotid artery stenoses with a newly developed balloon protection catheter, *Neurosurgery* 53:617–623, 2003; discussion 623-5.

37. Theron J: Cerebral protection during carotid angioplasty, *J Endovasc Surg* 3:484–486, 1996.

38. Antoniucci D, Valenti R, Santoro GM, et al: Restenosis after coronary stenting in current clinical practice, *Am Heart J* 135:510–518, 1998.

39. Duber C, Klose KJ, Kopp H, et al: Percutaneous transluminal angioplasty for occlusion of the subclavian artery: short- and long-term results, *Cardiovasc Intervent Radiol* 15:205–210, 1992.

40. Mathias KD, Luth I, Haarmann P: Percutaneous transluminal angioplasty of proximal subclavian artery occlusions, *Cardiovasc Intervent Radiol* 16:214–218, 1993.

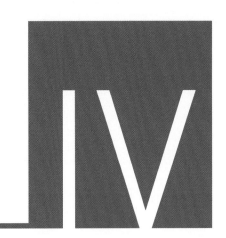

GIANT CEREBRAL ANEURYSMS

NATURAL HISTORY OF GIANT INTRACRANIAL ANEURYSMS

22

MARK J. DANNENBAUM; SCOTT Y. RAHIMI; ALBERT J. SCHUETTE; C. MICHAEL CAWLEY; DANIEL L. BARROW

INTRODUCTION

The first clinical series of giant intracranial aneurysms were reported in 1969 by Morley and Barr[1] and Bull.[2] Giant intracranial aneurysms (GIAs) are defined as those aneurysms with a greatest diameter equal to or exceeding 2.5 cm. This arbitrary designation was chosen in order to conform to the subset of the largest aneurysms in the Cooperative Study of Intracranial Aneurysms and Subarachnoid Hemorrhage.[3] Likewise smaller lesions have been shown to differ significantly with regard to their rate of rupture, the incidence of presentation with mass effect, and most importantly the difficulty with surgical treatment. GIAs are relatively infrequent compared to their smaller counterparts and therefore literature support to aid in clinical decision making is not as readily available. While once thought to represent more benign lesions with a lower incidence of hemorrhage and a more optimistic natural history, it is clear now from recent, large, multicenter studies that these lesions behave aggressively and hemorrhage more frequently than their smaller counterparts.[4,5]

PATHOLOGIC CONSIDERATIONS

Giant aneurysms are classified as either saccular or fusiform with the vast majority being the saccular type. Giant saccular aneurysms develop as a result of hemodynamic stress at arterial bifurcations and branch points similar to smaller saccular intracranial aneurysms. Once the sac has formed, both the neck and fundus will then undergo progressive enlargement. Ferguson proposed that turbulence within the aneurysm leads to endothelial injury and subsequent platelet aggregation and fibrin deposition.[6] This intraluminal cascade in giant aneurysms represents a dynamic series of events with accumulation and dissipation of platelets and fibrin-thrombus debris in an irregular fashion. Fusiform giant aneurysms most commonly result from atherosclerosis, however, may develop in patients with collagen vascular disorders such as Marfan's syndrome,

Ehlers-Danlos syndrome, and systemic lupus erythematosis. All of these diseases produce multifocal injury to the endothelial wall, resulting in weakening of an entire segment of the vessel. Fusiform lesions often present because of mass effect but not infrequently produce ischemic symptoms secondary to thromboembolic phenomena (Figure 22–1).

EPIDEMIOLOGY

Some epidemiologic differences from smaller saccular aneurysms seem to validate the separate clinical entity of giant aneurysms. In various clinical and autopsy series, the percentage of total aneurysms that are giant ranges from 3% to 13%. In one of the largest series to date, Hamburger et al. reported 1400 intracranial aneurysms and identified 58 giant aneurysms, yielding an incidence of 4.1%.[11] Based on data from three autopsy studies and six large clinical series, the aggregate incidence of giant intracranial aneurysms is 5.2%[13] (Table 22–1).

AGE AND GENDER

GIAs more commonly occur in females and most commonly come to clinical attention during the fifth to sixth decade of life. In a review of the world literature, Fox identified 693 giant aneurysms of which 60% occurred in females. This review correlates with known anatomical gender distributions with the proximal internal carotid artery location in 73% of females versus 52% for the anterior communicating complex and basilar apex.[7] Anson reviewed 14 series with 754 GIAs identified, finding 461 females and 295 males, yielding a 1.56:1 ratio.[27] In Anson's review, ages ranged from 6 months to 76 years with 67% of patients presenting between ages 40 and 70. This distribution parallels that of Fox's review of the world literature, where the median age of presentation was in the sixth decade of life.

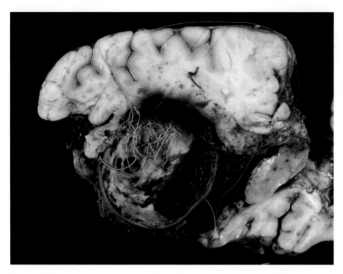

Figure 22–1. Postmortem analysis of thrombosed giant middle cerebral artery aneurysm.

Giant fusiform and dolichoectatic aneurysms probably present at a slightly younger age. Reviews from three different institutions found a mean age of presentation to be 38, 43, and 49 years with a male:female ratio of 1.5:1.[8–10]

Intracranial aneurysms are rare in children, with only 1% to 2% of all aneurysms occurring in the pediatric population. Of these, however, GIAs constitute a much higher proportion, are more common in males, and are less often present with hemorrhage. Ferrante reviewed 72 cases of pediatric aneurysms and found that 27% were giant and 50% were 1 to 2.5 cm in diameter.[11]

Table 22–1. INCIDENCE OF GIANT ANEURYSMS.

Author	Year	Total Aneurysms	Giant Aneurysms	% Giant Aneurysms
Stehbens[a]	1954	128	8[b]	6.2
Housepian and Pool[a]	1958	113	5	4.4
McCormick[a]	1970	191[c]	9	4.7
Morley and Barr	1969	658	28	4.3
Onuma and Suzuki	1979	1080	38	3.0
Sundt and Piepgras	1979	594	80	13.0
Pia	1980	522	19	3.6
Whittle et al.	1984	338	25	7.4
Hamburger et al.	1992	1400	58	4.1
Total		5024	264	5.2

[a]Autopsy series.
[b]Defined as >3 cm.
[c]Out of 136 patients.
From Day AL, Gaposchkin CG, Yu CJ, Rivet DJ, Dacey RG Jr: Spontaneous fusiform middle cerebral artery aneurysms: characteristics and a proposed mechanism of formation, J Neurosurg 99:228–240, 2003.

LOCATION

Saccular GIAs have a similar anatomic predilection as their smaller counterparts, while the distribution is different. Similarly, the internal carotid artery (ICA) is the most common site, although GIAs occur proportionately more frequently in the vertebrobasilar system and less frequently in the anterior communicating artery (ACOM) region. Drake and Peerless reported 641 GIAs treated between 1965 and 1992 in the following locations: vertebrobasilar, 390; ICA, 178; middle cerebral artery (MCA), 64; and anterior cerebral artery (ACA), 19.[12] While their data does reflect a referral bias, it supports the general trend that certain intracranial arterial segments are more vulnerable to this pathology as seen throughout the literature. Giant fusiform and dolichoectatic aneurysms have a predilection for the vertebrobasilar circulation and the MCA. These lesions, frequently referred to as "serpentine aneurysms," are often massive, partially thrombosed lesions through which runs a serpentine channel.[13]

CLINICAL PRESENTATION

GIAs may come to clinical attention in a variety of ways, including hemorrhages, as a result of their mass effect and distortion of surrounding anatomy, thromboembolic events, or by producing seizures. The duration of symptoms in patients presenting with GIAs is variable. A disproportionately high number of GIAs have been discovered in patients with symptoms for >5 years.

NATURAL HISTORY

The natural history of GIAs is dependent upon several factors, including the location of the aneurysm with respect to the subarachnoid space, the pathological form of the aneurysm (saccular vs. fusiform), the specific anatomic location, and the presence or absence of laminated thrombus and or atherosclerotic plaque within the fundus and neck of the aneurysm.[14] In Morley and Barr's original series of 28 patients, 17 had intradural aneurysms, and only four of those underwent a direct operation on their aneurysm. Of the five patients who received no definitive therapy, four died. Of the five patients with intradural aneurysms who had common carotid ligation, three died and one was disabled. They concluded that "direct surgical attack on extracavernous giant aneurysms is seldom possible or successful except in the case of MCA aneurysms."

Peerless et al. observed 31 patients with giant intracranial aneurysms (25 saccular and six fusiform). Sixty-eight percent of patients with saccular aneurysms were dead at 2 years and 85% were dead at 5 years. If patients presenting with subarachnoid hemorrhage were excluded, the 2-year mortality rate was 62%. Only four patients who were all disabled were alive at 5 years. Of the six patients with fusiform aneurysms, four were dead at 2 years, one died at 3.5 years after diagnosis, and one remained disabled.[15] Ljunggren et al. demonstrated a mortality or severe morbidity rate of 80% within 5 years in patients with untreated symptomatic GIAs.[16] Hamburger et al. reported on 58 patients with GIA and showed that 7% of patients presenting without SAH died, compared with 29% of patients presenting with SAH. Only 18% of the later group were discharged home as independent compared with 50% of the former group.[17] The Italian Cooperative Study on Giant Intracranial Aneurysms found that extensive or thick cisternal deposition of blood was associated with a significantly higher mortality rate than with thin or absent depositions.[18] Although GIAs present more commonly with mass effect or thromboembolic events, there is no evidence that they are associated with a lower rate of rupture. It is evident that the presence of thrombus in the sac does not protect against SAH and that when extensive or complete may actually have a deleterious effect on the natural history.[19–21]

The most recent and comprehensive data on the natural history of GIAs comes from the International Study of Unruptured Intracranial Aneurysms Investigators (ISUIA I & II).[4,5] In the retrospective arm, ISUIA I, 1449 patients with 1937 intracranial aneurysms were reviewed. The patients were divided into two groups. Group 1 patients (N = 727) had no history of SAH from a different aneurysm, while Group 2 (N = 722) had a history of a SAH from a previously repaired aneurysm. The rupture rate for aneurysms greater than 25 mm in diameter was 6% in the first year. In the prospective arm, ISUIA II, 4060 patients were assessed of which 1692 did not have aneurysmal repair. The 5-year cumulative rupture rates for patients who did not have a history of SAH was 40% for giant aneurysms located in the anterior circulation, and 50% for aneurysms located in the posterior circulation as well as the posterior communicating artery (PCOM).

The natural history of patients presenting with symptoms related to mass effect or ischemia from giant aneurysms is less clear. In giant paraclinoid aneurysms presenting with visual loss, the deterioration usually progresses without treatment.[22,23] Patients with symptoms of brainstem compression due to giant dolichoectatic verterbobasilar artery aneurysms also appear to have a poor prognosis without treatment. In a report by Michael, all seven patients with giant posterior circulation aneurysms treated with observation died between 2 months and 2 years after diagnosis.[24] The Italian Cooperative Study analyzed 25 patients with untreated giant aneurysms and reported mortality in seven cases (28%), which was double the mortality rate in the 86 treated cases. Morbidity was seen in 12 of the observed cases due to progressive expansion of the aneurysm mass.

The natural history of giant aneurysms presenting with mass effect is usually one of progressive enlargement. Sonntag and Stein demonstrated progressive enlargement on successive angiograms in two of 13 cases being non-surgically managed.[25]

Growth can be extremely rapid with one case in the literature documenting formation in less than 3 months.[26] There is no evidence that the presence of extensive thrombus improves the natural history of giant aneurysms. Despite the lack of luminal filling, it has been demonstrated that even extensive intra-aneursmal thrombosis does not protect against SAH. Furthermore, the presence of extensive or even complete thrombosis within a giant aneurysm may increase the risk of compressive symptoms.[27]

The risk of distal ischemic symptoms may actually increase in partially or extensively thrombosed giant aneurysms, contributing to a more ominous natural history. Sutherland and Peerless noted distal thromboembolism in 59% of cases in their series of giant aneurysms containing thrombus.[28] In addition, it is also possible for thrombus to propagate into the parent artery and cause occlusion. The risk of thromboembolic stroke from thrombosed giant aneurysms seems to be greatest in cases of fusiform or dolichoectatic vertebrobasilar artery aneurysms.[29]

INTRACAVERNOUS ANEURYSMS

Intracavernous aneurysms generally contain sacs located extradurally, and therefore, for the purposes of discussing natural history and clinical manifestations, are considered as a separate and unique clinical entity. They most commonly occur in middle aged women with a history of hypertension. Approximately 21% of intracavernous aneurysms are bilateral and 15% are giant, with intracavernous aneurysms accounting for 3% to 39% of all giant aneurysms.[30] Unlike their intradural counterparts these lesions are associated with a more benign natural history.[31] Intracavernous aneurysms may be discovered as incidental findings or as a result of compressive symptoms of the cranial nerves traversing the cavernous sinus (Figure 22–2).

The vast majority of symptomatic intracavernous aneurysms cause symptoms by compressing the intracavernous cranial nerves. The abducens nerve is the most commonly affected cranial nerve, followed by the occulomotor and later the first two divisions of the trigeminal nerve. Lateral enlargement of intracavernous aneurysms will usually result in a cavernous sinus syndrome manifesting as multiple extraocular palsies with associated facial pain or numbness. In Drake's series all nine patients with giant intracavernous aneurysms presented with compressive symptoms. Similarly 10 of 11 patients with giant intracavernous aneurysms in Morley and Barr's series presented with compressive symptoms as well.

They may also produce vascular symptoms such as subarachnoid hemorrhage, carotid-cavernous fistulae, epsitaxis, subdural hematoma, or ischemic symptoms secondary to thromboembolic processes distal to the aneurysm.

For a subarachnoid hemorrhage to occur, a portion of the sac must extend through the distal dural ring into the sella turcica and rupture through the diaphragma sella. Rupture rates

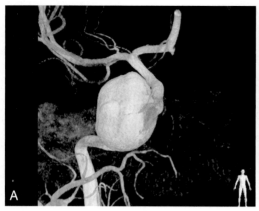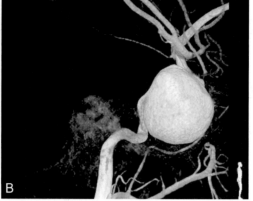

Figure 22–2. A and **B**, Giant intra-cavernous internal carotid artery aneurysm.

for intracavernous aneurysms vary widely throughout the literature; however, the overwhelming majority of these lesions do not present with subarachnoid hemorrhage.

When an intracavernous aneurysm ruptures, it most commonly produces a carotid cavernous fistula, which is the cause of most high-flow, spontaneous carotid cavernous fistulas.[32] This presentation, however, is more common with smaller intracavernous aneurysms than in those with giant sacs. The wall of the intracavernous internal carotid artery bulges into the sphenoid sinus in 71% of specimens and bone is absent between the ICA and sphenoid mucosa in 4%.[33] Because of this anatomic relationship, an intracavernous aneurysm may rupture into the sphenoid sinus and produce epistaxis, which may be life-threatening.

Spontaneous thrombosis of intracavernous aneurysms may result in occlusion of the parent ICA or in distal embolization, causing stroke. Distal vascular symptoms may be more common with giant aneurysms because of thrombus within the aneurysms. In Linskey's series, two of 37 patients had hemispheric ischemic symptoms from aneurysms between 1 and 2.5 cm in size.

NONSACCULAR VERTEBROBASILAR ANEURYSMS

This class of aneurysms warrants a separate discussion because of the unique natural history associated with these lesions. Frequently referred to as fusiform or dolichoectatic aneurysms, they are relatively uncommon compared to their saccular counterparts. In addition, they are different with respect to their clinical presentation and treatment options. These aneurysms usually cause symptoms by compressing adjacent brainstem or cranial nerves or by launching emboli from mural thrombus within the aneurysm leading to ischemia in vascular territories distal to the aneurysm. Subarachnoid hemorrhage occurs with less frequency compared to saccular aneurysms. The hemorrhage rate for dolichoectatic and fusiform aneurysms is not well understood and no clear consensus exists in

the world literature regarding the predicted behavior of these aneurysms. Drake and others have reported that the number of patients with fusiform and dolichoectatic aneurysms that present with subarachnoid hemorrhage is lower than for patients harboring saccular aneurysms.[12,34–36] Other series have demonstrated a rupture rate quite similar to that of saccular aneurysms.[37] However, because fusiform aneurysms are more likely to be diagnosed from symptoms related to compression or ischemia, there is a lower incidence of SAH at presentation.

This discrepancy in the natural history is accounted for predominantly by small case series and retrospective reviews. Flemming et al. were the first group to prospectively review the natural history of fusiform and dolichoectatic vertebrobasilar aneurysms in their analysis of 159 patients from the Mayo Clinic.[38] Patients most commonly presented initially because of symptoms associated with mass effect (22%), related ischemic stroke (28%), or hemorrhage (3%). After a mean follow-up interval of 4.4 years, they calculated the annual prospective risk of rupture to be 0.9% overall and up to 2.3% per year for certain morphological subtypes based upon their own classification system. Sixty-five patients died during follow-up. These deaths were found to be aneurysm related in 45% of patients, with the most common mechanism being ischemic cerebral infarction or thrombosis.

O'Shaughnessy and colleagues reported the progressive growth of a giant dolichoectatic vertebrobasilar artery aneurysm after complete Hunterian ligation of the posterior circulation. This report is the first such case in the English literature in which progressive lesion expansion occurred after complete Hunterian proximal arterial occlusion of the posterior circulation.[39] They demonstrated lesional expansion despite eliminating the principal orthograde inflow and proposed an alternative theory to conventional thinking of aneurysm growth and subsequent expansion as a consequence of hemodynamic stress and proposed that in vertebrobasilar dolichoectasia a more likely explanation arises from a progressive, expansile arteriopathy throughout the arterial wall that occurs independent of hemodynamic stress (Figure 22–3).

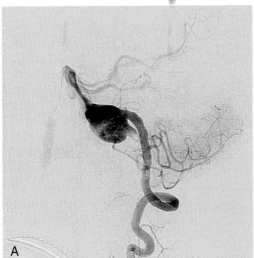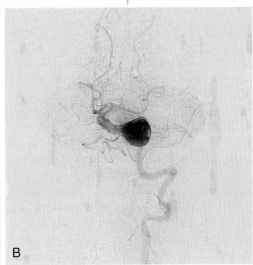

Figure 22-3. Giant dolichoectatic vertebrobasilar junction aneurysm. **A**, Lateral view. **B**, AP view.

CONCLUSION

Giant intracranial aneurysms are a heterogeneous group of lesions with numerous clinical presentations and a distinctive natural history. Because of the inherent difficulty in their definitive treatment, patients and practitioners alike in the past have chosen to observe the lesions, anticipating a more benign natural history. Clearly it has been demonstrated in large and recent series that these lesions have an aggressive behavior when left untreated and often produce catastrophic and fatal neurological outcomes. As endovascular and microneurosurgical technologies continue to evolve, it is likely that outcomes will continue to improve and these lesions may be treated more routinely with lower morbidity.

REFERENCES

1. Morley TP, Barr HWK: Giant intracranial aneurysms: diagnosis, course and management, *Clin Neurosurg* 16:73–94, 1969.
2. Bull J: Massive aneurysms at the base of the brain, *Brain* 92:535–570, 1969.
3. Locksley HB: Report on the Cooperative Study of Intracranial Aneurysms and Subarachnoid Hemorrhage. Section V, Part II. Natural history of subarachnoid hemorrhage, intracranial aneurysms and arteriovenous malformations, *J Neurosurg* 25:321–368, 1966.
4. Wiebers DO, Whisnant JP, Huston J 3rd, et al: International Study of Unruptured Intracranial Aneurysms Investigators, *Lancet* 362:103–110, 2003.
5. International Study of Unruptured Intracranial Aneurysms Investigators: Unruptured intracranial aneurysms—risk of rupture and risks of surgical intervention, *N Engl J Med* 339:1725–1733, 1998.
6. Ferguson GG: Physical factors in the initiation, growth and rupture of human intracranial saccular aneurysms, *J Neurosurg* 37:666–667, 1972.
7. Fox JL: *Intracranial Aneurysms*, New York, 1983, Springer-Verlag.
8. Little JR, Louis P, Weistein M, et al: Giant fusiform aneurysms of the cerebral arteries, *Stroke* 12:183–188, 1981.
9. Suzuki S, Takahashi T, Ohkuma H, et al: Management of giant serpentine aneurysms of the middle cerebral artery. Review of the literature and report of a case successfully treated by STA-MCA anastomosis only, *Acta Neurochir (Wien)* 117:23–39, 1992.
10. Anson JA, Lawton MT, Spetzler RF: Characteristics and surgical treatment of dolichoectatic and fusiform aneurysms, *J Neurosurg* 84:185–193, 1996.
11. Ferrante L, Fortuna A, Celli P, et al: Intracranial arterial aneurysms in early childhood, *Surg Neurol* 29:39–56, 1988.
12. Drake CG, Peerless SJ: Giant fusiform intracranial aneurysms: review of 120 patients treated surgically from 1965 to 1992, *J Neurosurg* 87:141–162, 1997.
13. Day AL, Gaposchkin CG, Yu CJ, Rivet DJ, Dacey RG Jr: Spontaneous fusiform middle cerebral artery aneurysms: characteristics and a proposed mechanism of formation, *J Neurosurg* 99:228–240, 2003.
14. Barrow DL, Alleyne C: Natural History of Giant Intracranial Aneurysms and Indications for Intervention, *Clin Neurosurg* 42:214–244, 1995.
15. Peerless SJ, Wallace MD, Drake CG: Giant intracranial aneurysms. In Youmans JR, editors: *Neurological Surgery*, ed 3, Philidelphia, 1990, WB Saunders, pp 1742–1763.
16. Ljunggren B, Brandt L, Sundbarg G, et al: Early management of aneurysmal subarachnoid hemorrhage, *Neurosurgery* 11:412–418, 1982.
17. Hamburger C, Schoenberger J, Lange M: Management and prognosis of intracranial giant aneurysms. A report of 58 cases, *Neurosurg Rev* 15:97–103, 1992.
18. Rosta L, Battaglia R, Pasqualin A, et al: Italian Cooperative Study on Giant Intracranial Aneurysms. 2: Radiological Data, *Acta Neurochir Suppl (Wien)* 42:53–59, 1988.
19. Drake CG: Giant intracranial aneurysms: experience with surgical treatment in 174 patients, *Clin Neurosurg* 26:12–95, 1979.
20. Khurana VG, Wijdicks EFM, Parisi JE, et al: Acute deterioration from thrombosis and rerupture of a giant intracranial aneurysm, *Neurology* 52:1697–1699, 1999.
21. Khurana VG, Piepgras DG, Whisnant JP: Ruptured giant intracranial aneurysms. Part I. A study of rebleeding, *J Neurosurg* 88:425–429, 1998.
22. Ferguson CG, Drake Cg: Carotid-ophthalmic aneurysms: visual abnormalities in 32 patients and the results of treatment, *Surg Neurol* 16:1–8, 1981.
23. Heros RC, Nelson PB, Ojemann RG, et al: Large and giant paraclinoid aneurysms: surgical techniques, complications and results, *Neurosurgery* 12:153–163, 1983.
24. Michael WF: Posterior fossa aneurysms simulating tumors, *J Neurol Neurosurg Psychiatry* 37:218–223, 1974.
25. Sonntag VKH, Yuan RH, Stein BM: Giant intracranial aneurysms: a review of 13 cases, *Surg Neurol* 8:81–84, 1977.
26. Fried LC, Yballe A: Rapid formation of a giant aneurysm: case report, *J Neurol Neurosurg Psychiatry* 35:527–530, 1972.
27. Anson JA. Epidemiology and natural history. In Awad IA, Barrow DL, editors: *Giant Intracranial Aneurysms*, Park Ridge, IL, 1995, American Association of Neurological Surgeons, pp. 225.

28. Sutherland GR, King ME, Peerless SJ, et al: Platelet interaction with giant intracranial aneurysms, *J Neurosurg* 56:53–61, 1982.

29. Nishizaki T, Tamaki N, Takeda N, et al: dolichoectatic basilar artery: a review of 23 cases, *Stroke* 17:1277–1281, 1986.

30. Berenstein A, Ransohof J, Kupersmith M, et al: Transvascular treatment of giant aneurysms of the cavernous carotid and vertebral arteries, *Surg Neurol* 21:3–12, 1984.

31. Linskkey ME, Sekhar LN, Hirsch WL, et al: Aneurysms of the intracavernous carotid artery: natural history and indications for treatment, *Neurosurgery* 6:933–938, 1990.

32. Barrow DL, Spector RH, Braun IF, et al: Classification and treatment of spontaneous carotid cavernous fistulas, *J Neurosurg* 56:248–256, 1985.

33. Harris FS, Rhoton AL: Anatomy of the cavernous sinus. A microsurgical study, *J Neurosurg* 45:169–180, 1976.

34. Anson JA, Lawton MT, Spetzler RF: Chararacteristics and surgical treatment of dolichoectatic and fusiform aneurysms, *J Neurosurg* 84:185–193, 1996.

35. Nishizaki T, Tamaki N, Takeda N, et al: Dolichoectatic basilar artery: a review of 23 cases, *Stroke* 17:1277–1281, 1986.

36. Anson JA: Treatment strategies for intracranial fusiform aneurysms, *Neurosurg Clin North Am* 9:743–753, 1998.

37. Vates GE, Auguste KI, Lawton MT: Fusiform, dolichoectatic and dissecting aneurysms: diagnosis and management. In LeRoux P, Winn HR, Newell D, editors: *Management of Cerebral Aneurysms*, Philadelphia, 2003, Saunders, pp 689–709.

38. Flemming KD, Wiebers DO, Brown RD, et al: Prospective risk of hemorrhage in patients with vertebrobasilar nonsaccular intracranial aneurysm, *J Neurosurg* 101:82–87, 2004.

39. O'Shaughnessy BA, Getch CC, Bendok BR, et al: Progressive growth of a giant dolichoectatic vertebrobasilar artery aneurysm after complete Hunterian occlusion of the posterior circulation: case report, *Neurosurgery* 55:1223, 2004.

EC-IC BYPASS FOR GIANT ICA ANEURYSMS

SALEEM I. ABDULRAUF; JOHN D. CANTANDO; YEDATHORE S. MOHAN; RAUL OLIVERA; JONATHON J. LEBOVITZ

INTRODUCTION

Transitional internal carotid artery (ICA) aneurysms incorporate the cavernous, clinoidal, and supraclinoidal segments of the ICA as portions of the neck of the aneurysm. In this chapter, we review the natural history, clinical course, our series, and surgical techniques/nuances for the treatment of these aneurysms.

Pure cavernous ICA aneurysms are a separate category of aneurysms, which do not extend beyond the dural ring of the ICA. In general, in the neurosurgical literature these aneurysms are considered benign, even in larger sizes.[1] However, in our experience it is possible that when these aneurysms get significantly large in size, they can cause rupture through the middle fossa dura, causing hemorrhage and potential mortality (Figure 23–1).

NATURAL HISTORY OF TRANSITIONAL SEGMENT OF ICA ANEURYSMS

Unruptured intracranial aneurysms are being diagnosed more often than in the past and these lesions pose management problems. The first series of giant aneurysms was presented in 1969 by Morley and Barr, who described giant aneurysms as >2.5 cm.[2] Giant aneurysms are relatively rare, comprising between 5% and 7% of aneurysms[3] in most series. Giant aneurysms have a female predominance with ratios as high as 3:1 in some series[4] and most commonly present in the middle decades. Giant aneurysms are most frequently located on the ICA, specifically, involving the paraclinoid segment 21% of the time.[5]

The natural history of giant aneurysms is one of a poor prognosis. Some have compared the fate of unruptured giant aneurysms to that of subarachnoid hemorrhage (SAH).[6] Patients often present with symptoms consistent with SAH or mass effect. The Italian cooperative study has shown a 28% mortality rate for untreated giant aneurysms compared to a 14% mortality rate for patients who received treatment.[7] In the same series, morbidity was seen in 48% of cases

due to expansion. Giant aneurysms, not unlike other aneurysms, continue to enlarge over time. Expansion is thought to be from growth of the lumen or thrombus formation within the sac. This progressive enlargement often causes symptoms of mass effect.[8]

Historically, it was thought that giant aneurysms were less prone to rupture; however, contemporary evidence suggests that this is inaccurate. Drake found that 62 of 174 cases did rupture.[9] Aneurysms sized ≥25 mm had a relative risk of rupture of 59% compared to aneurysms <10 mm.[10] Giant aneurysms had a 6% rupture rate in the first year compared to <1% for aneurysms <10 mm.[10] Patients with a giant aneurysm, but without previous SAH, were at a significantly increased risk for rupture based on size. The rupture rate was not dependent on the location of the aneurysm; all anterior circulation giant aneurysms were at increased risk of rupture.[3] Risk factors for aneurysm rupture include hypertension, current or former tobacco use, alcohol use greater than five drinks per day, and use of oral contraceptives.[10] It was thought that partially or completely thrombosed aneurysms would be less likely to rupture, thus not requiring treatment; however, in Drake's large series, this was not the case.[9]

The ISUIA (International Study of Unruptured Intracranial Aneurysms Investigators) trial has shown that unruptured aneurysms overall do not pose the risk they once were thought to; and that treating aneurysms, specifically small ones, puts the patient at more risk than surveillance. However, this advice should not be applied to the special case of giant aneurysms, where "the natural history is ominous."[6] Morley and Barr's original series demonstrated similar findings, with an 80% mortality rate for untreated aneurysms. Other studies have shown high 1-year mortality rates.[11] Peerless et al. found that 85% of patients with giant intracranial aneurysms were dead at 5 years.[12] Additionally, the ISUIA II found that the cumulative rupture rates for anterior circulation giant aneurysms with no previous history of SAH were 40%. Patients who present with SAH are at increased risk of mortality compared to patients without SAH.[13] We present a case of a ruptured giant aneurysm without previous history of SAH 6 months after initial diagnosis (Figure 23–2).

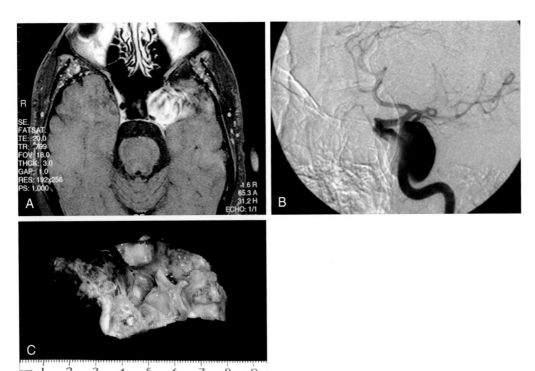

Figure 23–1. A, A 55-year-old presented with new onset diplopia. T1 axial MRI shows cavernous sinus aneurysm. **B,** Digital subtraction angiogram (DSA) showing a giant cavernous ICA aneurysm (does not extend into the supraclinoidal segment). Following balloon test occlusion in hospital, the patient had an acute headache, and became fixed and dilated. The patient subsequently died within 2 hours. **C,** Autopsy revealed a rupture through the middle fossa dura into the temporal lobe.

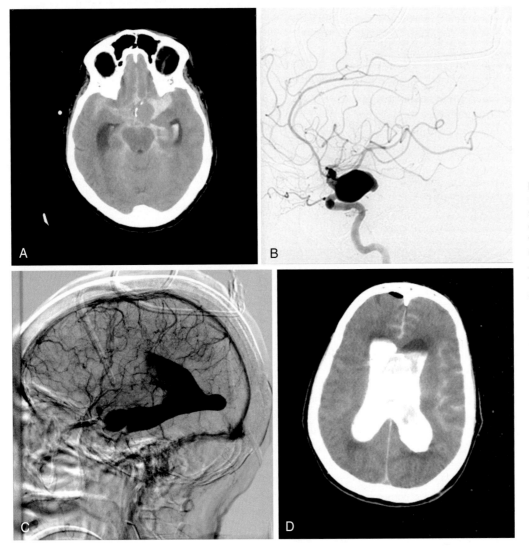

Figure 23–2. A, A patient was diagnosed with this aneurysm at an outside institution and was recommend conservative treatment. **B,** Patient was transferred to our institution 6 months after initial diagnosis with acute SAH and IVH, and underwent an angiogram. **C,** During angiography, the aneurysm reruptured (see extravagation of blood). **D,** Postangiography CT scan showing blood completely filling the lateral ventricles. The patient subsequently expired.

The Dilemma of Deliberate ICA Occlusion

Traditional neurosurgical literature and practice have held a liberal view of ICA occlusion for the treatment of giant ICA aneurysms. Historically, this has been accompanied by a relatively high risk of stroke following the ICA occlusion (Table 23–1). With recent improvements in the balloon test occlusion (BTO) paradigms, the risk is smaller but clearly not absent.

For the treatment of carotid occlusive disease, traditional neurosurgical literature and practice have strongly recommended preservation of the ICA. High-grade stenosis (i.e., 99% stenosis) is considered a relative neurosurgical emergency, requiring an endarterectomy or stenting. It is interesting that most patients who present with cervical carotid occlusive disease are usually older and generally have multiple medical comorbidities; yet performing a procedure to open the carotid artery has remained standard practice. Most cervical carotid occlusive disease symptomatology is due to embolic disease rather than hemodynamic compromise. Therefore, in the majority of cervical carotid occlusive disease, a deliberate occlusion of the ICA, in the opinion of the senior author, could be performed with a relatively low risk of morbidity, and most likely less risk of morbidity and mortality, when compared to carotid endarterectomy or stenting. However, this would be considered a complete departure from our current standards of care (Figure 23–3).

On the other hand, patients with giant ICA aneurysms are usually younger and have relatively less medical comorbidities when compared to patients with cervical carotid occlusive disease. Yet, in these cases, it is considered acceptable in neurosurgical practice to sacrifice the ICA. Long-term effects of deliberate carotid occlusion are not well studied. The risks of forming additional aneurysms, developing hemodynamic ischemic disease, and developing potential cognitive disorders have to be taken into account when this decision is made.

Therefore, it has been the practice of the senior author (SIA) to preserve flow to the hemisphere in the treatment of giant aneurysms, especially in younger patients.

Experience at St. Louis University Hospital in Treatment of Giant ICA Aneurysms

We performed a retrospective review of 55 consecutive patients treated at St. Louis University Hospital from June 1999 to June 2007. All 55 patients had transitional ICA aneurysms. The mean aneurysm size was 34.7 mm (range 25 to 70 mm). The mean age was 46 years (range 30 to 64 years). The mean follow-up period was 34.7 months (range 1 to 76 months). The objectives of this study were to assess the use of high-flow EC-IC bypass for the treatment of giant transitional ICA aneurysms, delineate surgical mortality and morbidity, and determine the long-term efficacy of the treatment and functional outcomes of these patients. The presenting symptoms were cranial neuropathy (42%), headache or incidental finding (40%), and SAH (18%) (Figure 23–4). The World Federation of Neurological Surgeons (WFNS) grade was 0 in 81%, 1 in 15%, 2 in 2%, and 3 in 2% (Figure 23–5). All 55 patients underwent a high-flow EC-IC bypass procedure.

SURGICAL TECHNIQUE

Craniotomy: A skull base approach, usually a cranio-orbital or a cranio-orbital-zygomatic access, is usually needed. We prefer a single-piece craniotomy, which entails an osteotomy of the orbital

Table 23–1. ICA SACRIFICE.

Source	Surgery	Outcomes
Sahs and Locksley, 1969[14]	ICA ligation	Stroke 30% Mortality 20.7%
Roski et al., 1981[15]	ICA ligation	TIA 16.6% Stroke 16.6% SAH 5.5% Mortality 5.5%
Linskey et al., 1994[16]	Intravascular ICA occlusion	Stroke 12.9% Mortality 3.2%
Larson et al., 1995[17]	Intravascular ICA occlusion	TIA 10.9% Stroke 3.6% SAH 3.6% Mortality 5.4%

ICA, internal carotid artery; SAH, subarachnoid hemorrhage; TIA, transient ischemic attack.

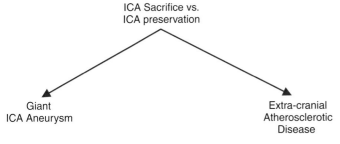

Figure 23–3. ICA sacrifice versus ICA preservation.

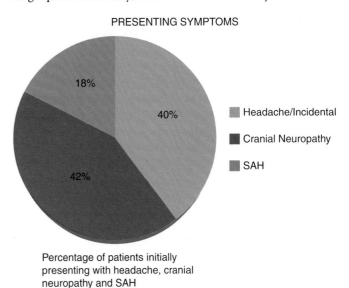

Figure 23–4. Percentage of patients initially presenting with headache, cranial neuropathy, and SAH.

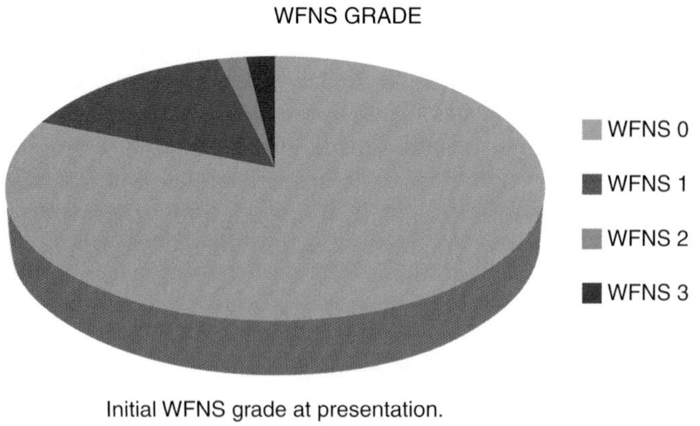

WFNS GRADE

- WFNS 0
- WFNS 1
- WFNS 2
- WFNS 3

Initial WFNS grade at presentation.

Figure 23–5. Initial WFNS grade at presentation.

roof and lateral margins. A high-speed drill is used to thin the zygomatic arch posteriorly, which allows the radial artery to lie without kinking at the zygomatic area (Figure 23–6A).

Exposure of the carotid artery in the neck: A standard incision anterior to the sternocleidomastoid muscle to expose the common, external, and internal carotid arteries (CCA, ECA, and ICA) is used. Vessel loops are applied around the CCA, ECA, and ICA. We recommend the use of the ECA as the site for the proximal anastomosis.

Radial artery harvest: The critical aspect of radial artery harvest is the length of the graft, which can be limiting. Obtaining maximal length is critical during this harvest. The senior author prefers to personally mark the superficial wall of the radial artery with a marking pen prior to removal of the graft. This step is crucial to avoid rotation during the tunneling (Figure 23–6B). Once the graft is harvested, it is placed in a heparinized saline solution.

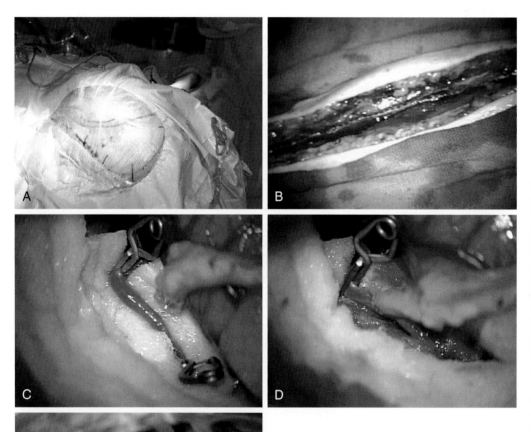

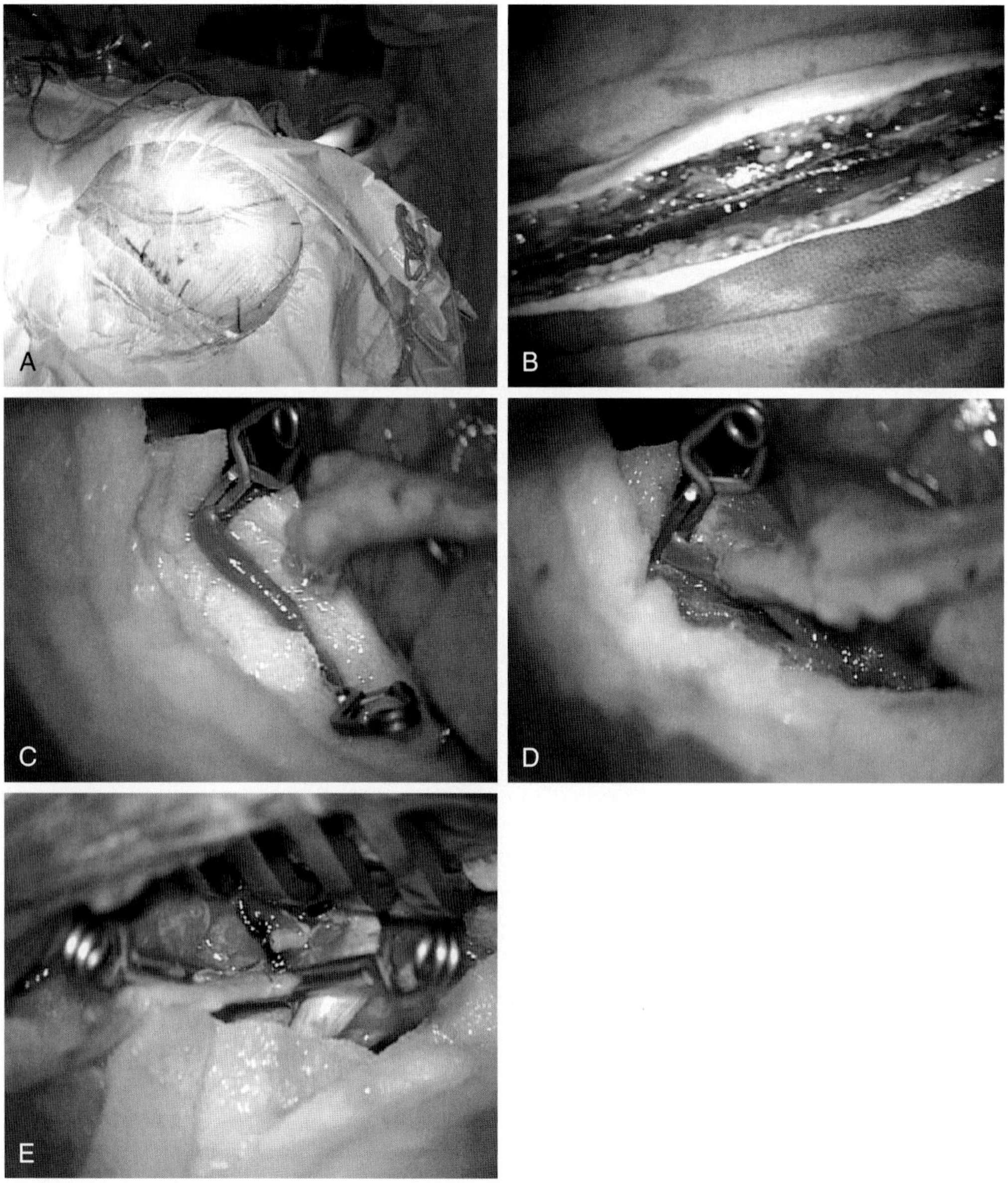

Figure 23–6. A, Operative photograph shows simultaneous planning for the craniotomy, cervical incision, and radial artery harvest. **B,** Operative photograph shows exposure of the radial artery with superficial marking. **C,** Trans-sylvian preparation for anastomosis. M3 recipient branch with temporary clips. Radial artery donor graft is shown. **D,** Completed anastomosis is shown. **E,** Anastomosis of the radial graft to the ECA in the neck and temporary clips on ECA are shown. ECA, external carotid artery.

(From Abdulrauf SI: Extracranial-to-intracranial bypass using radial artery grafting for complex skull base tumors: technical note, Skull Base 2005;15:207-213, with permission.)

Tunneling the graft: The graft is tunneled using a pediatric chest tube. The marked surface of the graft is kept most superficial.

Intracranial anastomosis: We also start the patient on aspirin (81 mg) daily for 3 days prior to surgery. Intraoperative continuous electroencephalography (EEG), somatosensory-evoked potential (SSEP), and motor-evoked potentials are monitored. The site of the anastomosis is determined based on several factors: intended revascularization territory, size of donor and recipient vessels, length of the graft, and location of the aneurysm. Mild hypothermia is used. EEG burst suppression using pentobarbital is maintained during the temporary clipping period. A color background is placed behind the recipient vessel. Temporary clips are applied (Figure 23–6C). An arteriotomy is made using an arachnoid knife. The arteriotomy is extended using a microscissors to the width of the donor vessel lumen. The lumen of the donor vessel is expanded by "fish-mouthing" the opening. We used 9-0 nylon for M2 and M3 vessels and 8-0 nylon for the supraclinoidal ICA. We prefer a running suture technique and performing the "back" wall (i.e., the more difficult anastomosis) first, followed by the front wall (Figure 23–6D). When the anastomosis is completed, retrograde flow is confirmed in the graft followed by positioning of a temporary clip on the graft just distal to the anastomosis.

Cervical carotid anastomosis: The graft length is cut to expose an area of the ECA where the proximal anastomosis is planned. Yasargil long temporary clips can be used for the ECA anastomosis. Similar technique of "back" wall and "front" wall can be utilized as described previously for the intracranial anastomosis. For this part, 7-0 prolene can be used (Figure 23–6E).

Graft inspection: Pulsatility of the graft is not enough to confirm graft potency. Micro-Doppler (Mizuho America, Inc., Beverly, MA) can be used. We now use ICG microscope-based angiography routinely for these cases. If the latter technology is not available, intraoperative angiography, in our opinion, is critical before parent vessel occlusion is performed. Flow probe technology (Transonic Systems, Inc., Ithaca, NY) has allowed us to estimate the amount of flow (cubic centimeter per minute) within the graft.

Parent vessel occlusion: Once the preceding steps, including intraoperative angiography, have documented flow in the graft, we then advocate parent vessel occlusion during the same surgical procedure, rather than delayed (staged) occlusion. In our opinion, the risk of graft occlusion would be high if competitive flow in the parent vessel were allowed to continue. We occlude the ICA at the level of the bifurcation in the cervical area and just distal to the giant aneurysm in the supra-clinoidal portion of the ICA. The distal occlusion must be performed proximal to the anterior choroidal and dominant posterior communicating arteries.[18]

Results of Giant Aneurysm Series

The outcome of this series shows that 50 patients (91%) had a Modified Rankin Scale (mRS) of 0 to 1, two patients (3.5%) had a mRS of 2 to 3, and three patients (5.5%) had a mRS of 4 to 5. Fifty-one patients (93%) had a Glasgow Outcome Scale (GOS)

of 5, two patients (3.5%) had a GOS of 3 to 4, and two (3.5%), a GOS of 1 to 2. At discharge from the hospital, 49 (89%) of the patients went home, four (7%) went to rehabilitation facilities, and two patients (4%) went to nursing homes (Figure 23–7).

Acute graft occlusion occurred in four patients (7.3%), and late graft occlusion in four (7.3%). The main complication/morbidity was reflected in our cerebrovascular accident (CVA) rate, which occurred in four patients (7.3%). Two patients

RESULTS: OUTCOME

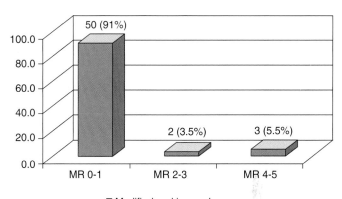

A

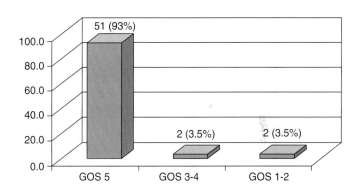

B

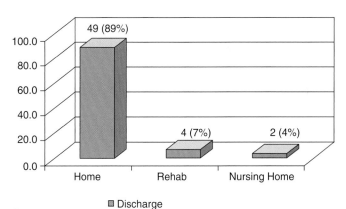

C

Figure 23–7. A total of 92.7% of patients had good GOS, 90.9% had none to no significant disability, and 89.1% went home. Only one patient died, which accounts for the 1.8% mortality.

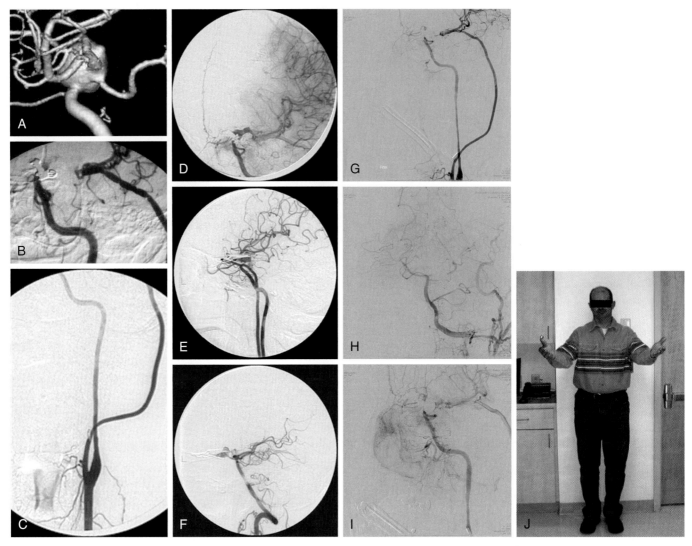

Figure 23–8. A, Fusiform aneurysm (involves the entire wall) of the lateral ICA segment. Patient failed BTO within 60 seconds. **B,** Immediate postoperative angiogram showing graft with nonsymptomatic vasospasm. **C,** Six-month follow-up showing end-to-end bypass (patient is asymptomatic.) **D,** One-year follow-up showing progression of disease into the distal ICA. **E,** Lateral view ICA injection showing the progression. **F,** Lateral view vertebral artery injection showing new formation of aneurysm in distal ICA. **G,** ICA injection following endovascular coiling of the aneurysm through the posterior communicating artery (PCA). **H,** Vertebral artery injection following endovascular coiling through the PCA. **I,** CCA injection following coiling showing the bypass as well as complete resolution of the aneurysm. **J,** At 1-year follow-up, patient is asymptomatic and aneurysm is completely treated.

had CVA secondary to acute graft occlusion, and two had CVA secondary to microsurgical manipulation of calcified aneurysms. Aneurysm recurrence was seen in only one patient (Figure 23–8). Mortality occurred in one patient from a pulmonary embolus at home 5 weeks postoperatively.

OPTIONS FOR TREATMENT OF GIANT ICA ANEURYSMS

Traditional treatment of giant aneurysms was direct microsurgical clipping. This continues to be a feasible option in certain cases. However, the risk of direct clipping of giant aneurysms is not low. Our review of major series of direct clipping of giant ICA aneurysms revealed a fair to poor outcome in

approximately 18% of the patients. In these same series, the mortality rate was 11% (Table 23–2). Endovascular treatment of giant aneurysms also poses certain challenges. In our review of major series of coiling, stent plus coiling of giant aneurysms reveals that approximately 42% of the aneurysms are completely occluded by the treatment. Thirty-seven percent of the aneurysms recanalize. Major morbidity occurred in approximately 21% of the patients. Mortality occurred in 15% of the patients (Table 23–3).

EC-IC bypass for giant aneurysms in the major published series shows relatively better outcomes than direct microsurgical clipping or endovascular treatment. Based on our review of these major series, excellent to good outcome was achieved on average in 84% of the patients. Significant morbidity was seen on average in 11% of the patients. Mortality was seen on average in 5% of the patients (Table 23–4).

Table 23–2. DIRECT CLIPPING OF GIANT ICA ANEURYSMS.

Series	# ICA Cases	Excellent/ Good Outcome	Fair/Poor Outcome	Death
Drake et al., 1979[9]	23	16 (70%)	4 (17%)	3 (13%)
Sundt and Piepgras, 1979[19]	47	40 (85%)	6 (13%)	1 (2%)
Heros et al., 1983[11]	25	20 (80%)	2 (8%)	3 (12%)
Symon et al., 1984[20]	9	5 (56%)	2 (22%)	2 (22%)
Yasargil et al., 1984	10	8 (80%)	2 (20%)	0 (0%)
Batjer and Samson, 1994[21]	10	5 (50%)	4 (40%)	1 (10%)
Lawton and Spetzler, 1994	34	25 (73%)	2 (6%)	7 (21%)
Total	158	71%	18%	11%

ICA, internal carotid artery.

TECHNICAL NUANCES IN HIGH-FLOW EC-IC BYPASS SURGERY

Importance of Atypical Appearance of Giant Aneurysms

Irregular appearance of the wall, or the pattern of more than one sac, indicates partial calcification or thrombosis. The appearance of the aneurysm on cerebral angiography is a critical factor in decision making regarding treatment. In the experience of the senior author, complex aneurysms, including those with irregular appearance of the wall, out-pouching within the dome, or the presence of calcification, may carry a higher risk with direct clipping. Partial thrombosis of the aneurysm may show a smaller aneurysm on angiography when compared to the MRI. Partially thrombosed aneurysms also carry a risk of embolic complications during microsurgical clipping or endovascular coiling (Figure 23–9).

Table 23–3. ENDOVASCULAR TREATMENT OF GIANT ICA ANEURYSMS.

	# Cases	Treatment	% Complete	% Recanalized	% Morbidity	% Mortality	F/U Angio
Gruber et al., 1999[22]	12	Coil	42	37.5	33	33	24.3 mo
Hayakawa et al., 2000[23]	10	Coil	10	90	NS	NS	NS
Mawad et al., 2002[24]	11	Stent+onyx	81	0	9	18	5 mo
Murayama et al., 2003[25]	19	Coil	25	58	NS	NS	NS
Sluzewski et al., 2003[26]	17	Coil	29	53	29	18	12.7 mo
Gonzalez et al., 2004[27]	29	Coil	24	NS	NS	NS	NS
Molyneux et al., 2004[28]	73	Balloon+Onyx	47	0	16	0	5 mo
Cekirge et al., 2006[29]	21	Stent+Onyx	76	20	19	5	12 mo
Jahromi et al., 2008[30]	16	Stent+coil	25	62.5	12.5	12.5	19.1 mo
Total	208		40%	38%	20%	14%	13 mo

Angio, angiography; F/U, follow-up; ICA, internal carotid artery; mo, months; NS, not significant; Onyx, liquid embolic system.

Table 23–4. EC-IC BYPASS FOR GIANT ICA ANEURYSMS.

Series	# ICA (total)	Graft	Excellent/Good	Poor	Death	Acute Occlusion	Late Occlusion	Late Patency
Sundt and Piepgras, 1986	NS (20)	SV	80%	15%	5%	13%	3%	84%
Lawton and Spetzler, 1996[31]	12	SV/STA-MCA	93%	5%	2%	5%	3%	92%
Sekhar et al., 2001[32]	4	SV/RA	76%	12%	12%	25% SV 6% RA	NS	94% SV 100% RA
Jafar et al., 2002[33]	12	SV	90%	7%	3%	7%	0%	93%
Tulleken et al., 2006[34]	34	SV	73.5%	20.5%	6%	NS	3%	97%
Abdulrauf, current study, 2007	55	RA	91%	7%	2%	7%	7%	86%
Total	117		84%	11%	5%	8%	3%	90%

Angio, angiography; F/U, follow-up; ICA, internal carotid artery; MCA, middle cerebral artery; mo, months; NS, not significant; Onyx, liquid embolic system; RA, right atrium; STA, superficial temporal artery; SV, saphenous vein.

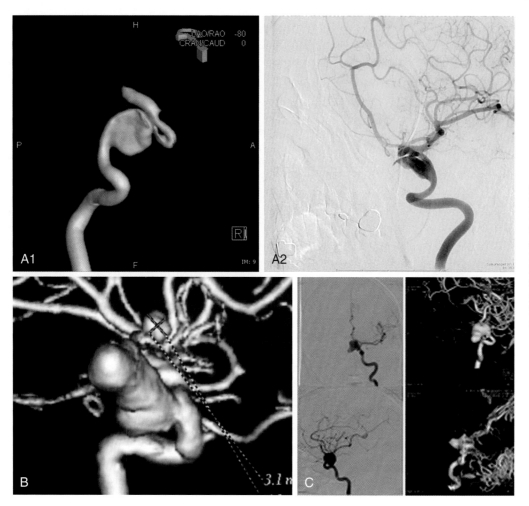

Figure 23–9. Importance of the atypical appearance of giant aneurysms: Irregular appearance of the wall, or the pattern of more than one sac should indicate partial calcification or thrombosis. **A,** DSA of partially thrombosed giant ICA aneurysm. **B,** DSA angiogram of partially calcified and partially thrombosed giant ICA aneurysm. **C,** DSA of a partially thrombosed and partially calcified ICA aneurysm.

Aneurysm size: The size of the aneurysm, although a critical factor when considering direct microsurgical clipping or endovascular coiling, is not an equally important factor when considering EC-IC bypass. In our opinion, for significantly large aneurysms, EC-IC bypass would be the least risky procedure (Figure 23–10).

EC-IC bypass for giant cavernous segment ICA aneurysm: The location of the aneurysm is an important factor when making decisions regarding treatment. Endovascular stenting plus coiling or EC-IC bypass are potential treatments of a giant cavernous segment aneurysm. Direct surgical clipping should not be considered in these cases, as it would almost certainly lead to ophthalmoplegia (Figure 23–11).

End-to-side versus end-to-end proximal anastomosis: For the proximal anastomosis, both end-to-end or end-to-side are options. The senior author prefers the use of the ECA as the donor vessel. This avoids temporary occlusion of the ICA during the procedure. The advantage of end-to-end anastomosis is, presumably, more vigorous flow into the graft. The disadvantage of end-to-end anastomosis is potential occlusion of

ophthalmic-based collaterals into the surpraclinoidal carotid artery. End-to-side anastomosis, therefore, is a reasonable option, and it is an easier anastomosis to make in comparison to end-to-end (end-to-end may create a size mismatch that may in certain occasions be difficult to compensate for) (Figure 23–12).

Competitive flow: It is important to recognize that during intraoperative angiography, the graft may only supply a single division of the recipient territory (i.e., a single M2 division). This should not be a concerning sign. In general, this is due to the fact that there is significant competitive flow coming through the ACA from the contralateral side, which is protective, and the surgeon should not change the strategy during the case (Figure 23–13).

Radial artery graft enlargement over time as graft adapts to blood flow demands: The diameter size of the graft as seen during intraoperative catheter or ICG is not concerning as long as there is no occlusion or specific area of stenosis. In our experience, the graft will expand in diameter over time to accommodate for blood flow demand (Figure 23–14).

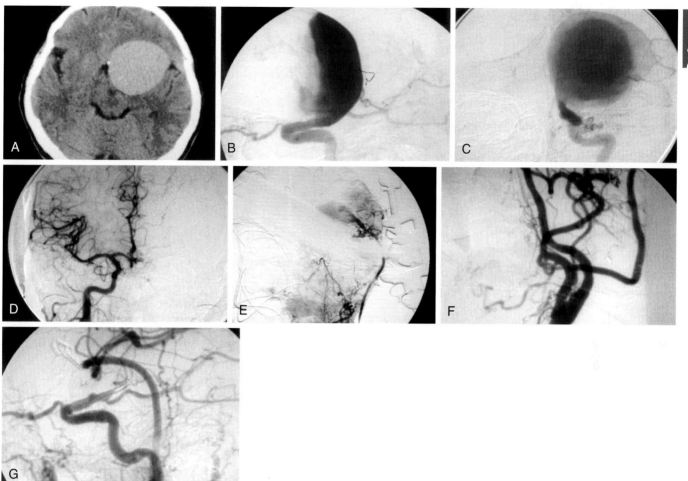

Figure 23–10. Treatment of a 9-cm "mega-giant" aneurysm using EC-IC bypass. **A,** CT of a 51-year-old female presenting with speech difficulties and hemiparesis. **B,** Lateral view of DSA showing aneurysm. **C,** Anteroposterior view showing aneurysm. **D,** Contralateral DSA shows no flow through anterior communicating artery (ACA). **E,** Intraoperative angiogram showing radial artery to MCA bypass. **F,** Postoperative angiogram. **G,** Postoperative DSA showing bypass and clip reconstruction of the aneurysm and the preservation of the PCA.

Intraoperative failure of graft: In most situations where the graft is not visible during intraoperative angiography, technical failure is assumed, and the anastomosis, as well as the tunneling, should be reinvestigated. In patients who have passed the BTO, it is possible to have such significant competitive flow that the resistance in the graft cannot match the higher contralateral flow and the graft is not necessary. It is important to look at every step of the procedure to ensure that there is no technical failure before making any other decisions. If no technical failures are found and no changes in the patient's motor and sensory evoked potentials are detected, it is reasonable to leave the graft in place. In certain circumstances, the graft may enlarge over time if demand is placed on it. While in other situations, the graft would be occluded without any neurological symptoms based on the fact that competitive flow was significantly strong and the graft was not needed to start with (Figure 23–15).

Creation of a new posterior communicating artery: EC-IC bypass surgery is an intellectual exercise given the complexity of the aneurysm. In certain situations, an intraposition graft may be needed. In some cases, an IC-IC bypass may be more appropriate than an EC-IC bypass. In other cases, the creation of a new ACA or PCA (using an interposition graft) may aid in the treatment of the specific aneurysm, whether it is microsurgical or endovascular (Figure 23–16).

Length of the graft and risk of occlusion: The length of the graft is also an important aspect. Unneeded length may lead to kinking in the cervical or cranial areas and could be a risk factor for graft occlusion. This aspect has to be well studied during the operation, as this is an important variable in achieving success in EC-IC bypass surgery (Figure 23–17).

Distal anastomosis size mismatch: From a technical standpoint of the distal anastomosis, it is important to match

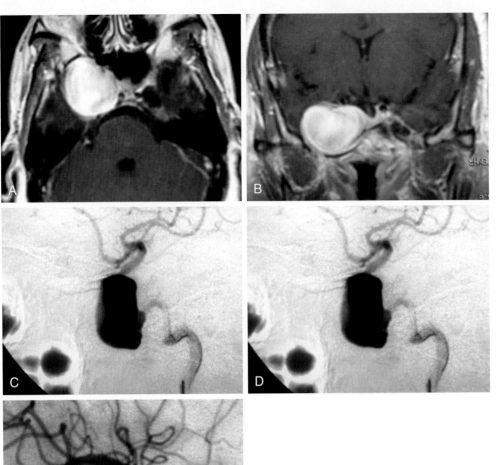

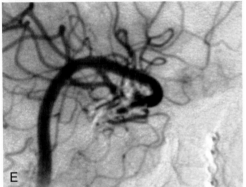

Figure 23–11. EC-IC bypass for giant cavernous segment ICA aneurysm. **A,** Axial T1+gad showing cavernous aneurysm in 45-year-old female presenting with ophthalmoplegia. **B,** Sagittal T1+gad. **C,** DCA of giant aneurysm. **D,** Intraoperative angiogram of ICA radial artery graft. **E,** Postoperative angiogram showing radial graft and occlusion of the cavernous aneurysm.

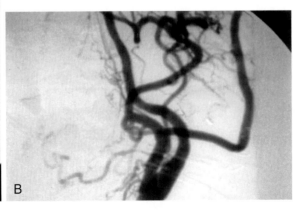

Figure 23–12. A, End-to-side radial artery graft to the ECA. **B,** End-to-end radial artery graft to the ECA.

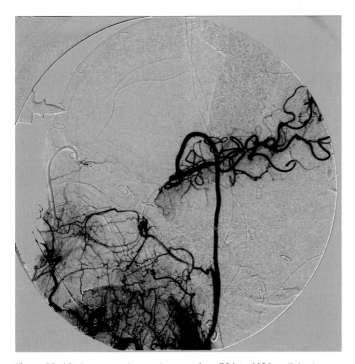

Figure 23–13. Intraoperative angiogram of an ECA to MCA radial artery bypass showing flow into a single MCA division.

the size of the donor and recipient arteries. In our opinion a significant size mismatch could have a higher risk of turbulent flow and subsequent thrombosis at the anastomosis site (Figure 23–18).

CONCLUSION

Giant intracranial aneurysms carry a high risk of morbidity and mortality. They are among the highest-risk disease processes within the field of neurosurgery. These aneurysms are potentially curable. Advances in microsurgical clipping, endovascular treatments, and EC-IC bypass have all contributed to decreasing the morbidity of these treatment modalities.

Evolving techniques in EC-IC bypass have documented a measurable decrease in the morbidity of treating these complex lesions. Minimally invasive EC-IC bypass techniques currently being developed will add to the armamentarium that will lead to less morbidity while achieving a cure.

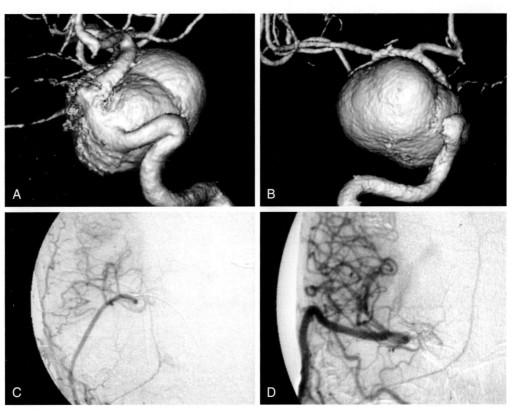

Figure 23–14. A, Lateral three-dimensional DSA reconstruction of a giant ICA transitional segment aneurysm. **B,** Anteroposterior three-dimensional DSA reconstruction of a giant ICA transitional segment aneurysm. **C,** Intraoperative angiogram showing the bypass and deliberate occlusion of the ICA. **D,** At 1-year follow-up, DSA showing increased diameter of the graft.

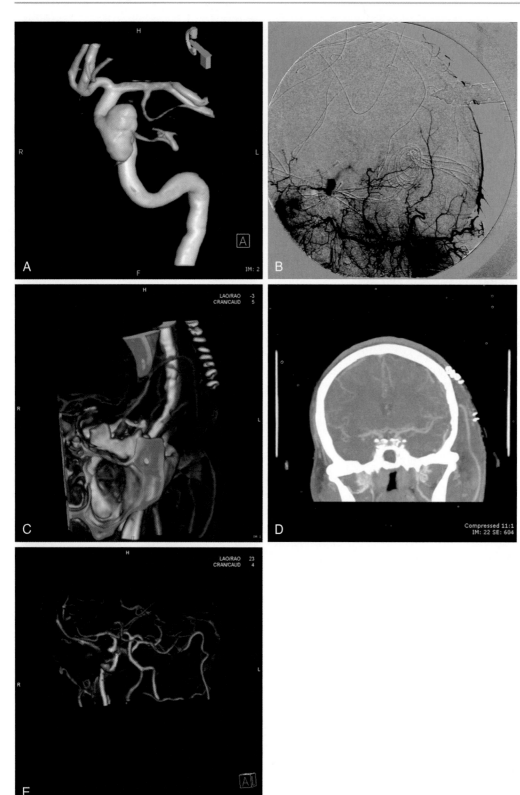

Figure 23–15. A, Three-dimensional DSA reconstruction of complex ICA partial thrombosed aneurysm. **B,** Intraoperative failure to establish flow with no change in SSEPs and motor-evoked potentials **C,** Immediate postoperative reconstruction showing graft is patent but small diameter. **D,** Immediate postoperative CTA showing small diameter graft. **E,** At 3-month follow-up, CTA reconstruction showing the expanded graft diameter.

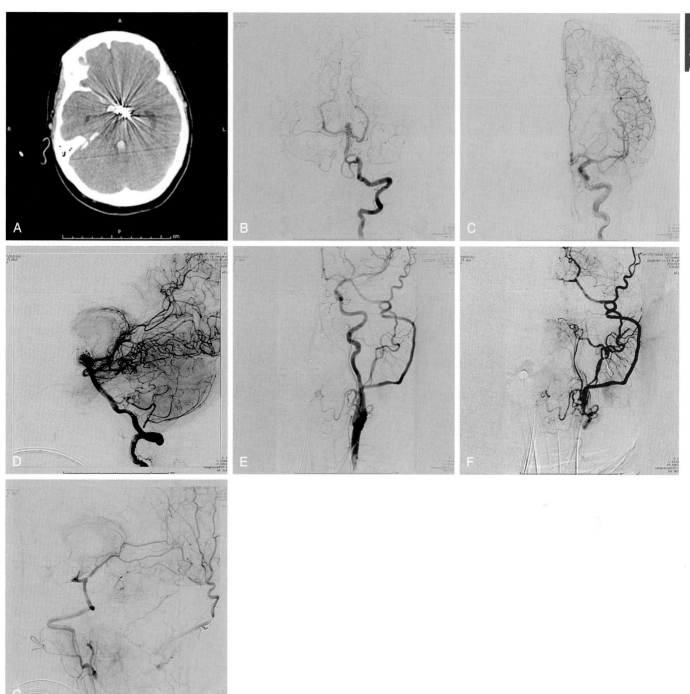

Figure 23–16. A, Patient with a third SAH following previous endovascular coiling. **B,** Anteroposterior DSA showing the coil embedded in the L P1 segment **C,** A/P DSA L ICA showing new P-Com artery. **D,** Vertebral artery DSA showing PCA flow completely dependant on the P1. **E,** ECA to PCA bypass postoperative DSA showing graft. **F,** Postoperative DSA showing flow to the PCA. **G,** Postoperative lateral view showing a PCA to radial artery graft showing PCA flow completely coming through the graft.

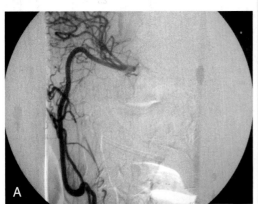

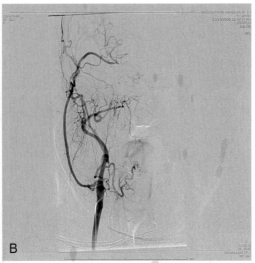

Figure 23–17. A. DSA of the R CCA showing a radial artery bypass for a giant aneurysm. The graft redundancy in the cervical area may be risky from a kinking standpoint as shown in this case. **B.** DSA of the R CCA showing a radial artery bypass for a giant aneurysm with ideal length of the graft that would minimize the risk of kinking.

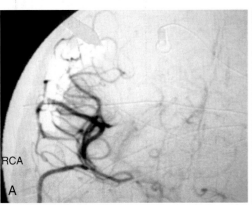

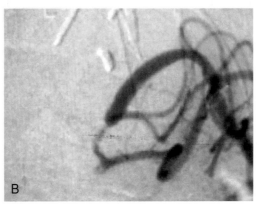

Figure 23–18. A. DSA angiogram of a radial artery bypass to the MCA showing ideal size match. **B.** DSA angiogram of a radial artery bypass to the MCA showing significant size mismatch.

REFERENCES

1. Linskey ME, et al: Aneurysms of the intracavernous carotid artery: natural history and indications for treatment, *Neurosurgery* 26 (6):933–937, 1990; discussion, 937–938.
2. Morley TP, Barr HW: Giant intracranial aneurysms: diagnosis, course, and management, *Clin Neurosurg* 16:73–94, 1969.
3. Wiebers DO, et al: Unruptured intracranial aneurysms: natural history, clinical outcome, and risks of surgical and endovascular treatment, *Lancet* 362:103–110, 2003.
4. Whittle IR, Dorsch NW, Besser M: Giant intracranial aneurysms: diagnosis, management, and outcome, *Surg Neurol* 21:218–230, 1984.
5. Nukui H, et al: [Bilaterally symmetrical giant aneurysms of the internal carotid artery within the cavernous sinus, associated with an aneurysm of the basilar artery [author's transl.], *No Shinkei Geka* 5:479–484, 1977.
6. Awad IA, Barrow DL, editors: *Giant Intracranial Aneurysms*, Park Ridge, IL, 1995, American Association of Neurological Surgeons.
7. Pasqualin A, et al: Italian cooperative study on giant intracranial aneurysms: 4. Results of treatment, *Acta Neurochir Suppl (Wien)* 42:65–70, 1988.
8. Sonntag VK, Yuan RH, Stein BM: Giant intracranial aneurysms: a review of 13 cases, *Surg Neurol* 8(2):81–84, 1977.
9. Drake CG: Giant intracranial aneurysms: experience with surgical treatment in 174 patients, *Clin Neurosurg* 26:12–95, 1979.
10. International Study of Unruptured Intracranial Aneurysms Investigators: Unruptured intracranial aneurysms—risk of rupture and risks of surgical intervention, *N Engl J Med* 339:1725–1733, 1998.
11. Heros RC, Kistler JP: Intracranial arterial aneurysm—an update, *Stroke* 14:628–631, 1983.
12. Peerless SJ, Wallace MD, Drake CG: Giant intracranial aneurysms. In Youmans JR, editor: *Neurological Surgery*, ed 3, Philadelphia, 1990, WB Saunders, pp 1742–1763.
13. Hamburger C, Schonberger J, Lange M: Management and prognosis of intracranial giant aneurysms. A report on 58 cases, *Neurosurg Rev* 15(2):97–103, 1992.
14. Locksley SA: *Intracranial aneurysms and subarachnoid hemorrhage: a cooperative study*, Philadelphia, 1969, JB Lippincott.
15. Roski RA, Spetzler RF, Nulsen FE: Late complications of carotid ligation in the treatment of intracranial aneurysms, *J Neurosurg* 54(5):583–587, 1981.
16. Linskey ME, et al: Stroke risk after abrupt internal carotid artery sacrifice: accuracy of preoperative assessment with balloon test occlusion and stable xenon-enhanced CT, *Am J Neuroradiol* 15(5):829–843, 1994.
17. Larson JJ, et al: Treatment of aneurysms of the internal carotid artery by intravascular balloon occlusion: long-term follow-up of 58 patients, *Neurosurgery* 36(1):26–30, 1995; discussion 30.
18. Abdulrauf SI: Extracranial-to-intracranial bypass using radial artery grafting for complex skull base tumors: technical note, *Skull Base* 15:207–213, 2005.
19. Sundt TM Jr, Piepgras DG: Surgical approach to giant intracranial aneurysms: operative experience with 80 cases, *J Neurosurg* 51 (6):731–742, 1979.

20. Symon L, Vajda J: Surgical experiences with giant intracranial aneurysms, *J Neurosurg* 61(6):1009–1028, 1984.
21. Batjer HH, Kopitnik TA, Giller CA, et al: Surgery for paraclinoidal carotid artery aneurysms, *J Neurosurg* 80(4):650–658, 1994.
22. Gruber A, et al: Clinical and angiographic results of endosaccular coiling treatment of giant and very large intracranial aneurysms: a 7-year, single-center experience, *Neurosurgery* 45(4):793–803, 1999; discussion 803–804.
23. Hayakawa M, et al: Natural history of the neck remnant of a cerebral aneurysm treated with the Guglielmi detachable coil system, *J Neurosurg* 93(4):561–568, 2000.
24. Mawad ME, et al: Endovascular treatment of giant and large intracranial aneurysms by using a combination of stent placement and liquid polymer injection, *J Neurosurg* 96(3):474–482, 2002.
25. Murayama Y, et al: Guglielmi detachable coil embolization of cerebral aneurysms: 11 years' experience, *J Neurosurg* 98(5):959–966, 2003.
26. Sluzewski M, et al: Coiling of very large or giant cerebral aneurysms: long-term clinical and serial angiographic results, *Am J Neuroradiol* 24(2):257–262, 2003.
27. Gonzalez LF, Zabramski JM: Anatomic and clinical study of the orbitopterional approach to anterior communicating artery aneurysms, *Neurosurgery* 54(4):1031–1032, 2004.
28. Molyneux AJ, et al: Cerebral Aneurysm Multicenter European Onyx (CAMEO) trial: results of a prospective observational study in 20 European centers, *Am J Neuroradiol* 25(1):39–51, 2004.
29. Cekirge HS, et al: Intrasaccular combination of metallic coils and onyx liquid embolic agent for the endovascular treatment of cerebral aneurysms, *J Neurosurg* 105(5):706–712, 2006.
30. Jahromi BS, et al: Clinical and angiographic outcome after endovascular management of giant intracranial aneurysms, *Neurosurgery* 63(4):662–674, 2008; discussion 674–675.
31. Lawton MT, Hamilton MG, Morcos JJ, et al: Revascularization and aneurysm surgery: current techniques, indications, and outcome, *Neurosurgery* 38(1):83–92, 1996; discussion 92–94.
32. Sekhar L, Duff JM, Kalavakonda C, et al: Cerebral revascularization using radial artery grafts for the treatment of complex intracranial aneurysms: techniques and outcomes for 17 patients, *Neurosurgery* 49(3):646–658, 2001.
33. Jafar JJ, Russell SM, Woo HH: Treatment of giant intracranial aneurysms with saphenous vein extracranial-to-intracranial bypass grafting: indications, operative technique, and results in 29 patients, *Neurosurgery* 51(1):138–144, 2002; discussion 144–146.
34. Tulleken CA, et al: Treatment of giant and large internal carotid artery aneurysms with a high-flow replacement bypass using the excimer laser-assisted nonocclusive anastomosis technique, *Neurosurgery* 59(4 Suppl 2):ONS328–ONS334, 2006; discussion ONS334–ONS335.

23

CEREBRAL BYPASS IN THE TREATMENT OF ACA ANEURYSMS

24

ADITYA S. PANDEY; B. GREGORY THOMPSON

INTRODUCTION

Cerebral revascularization has had a tumultuous history with the nadir being just after the publication of the Extracranial/Intracranial Bypass Study Group (1985)[1] Currently, cerebral revascularization has gained momentum for specific disease processes: basal occlusive disease (MMD), giant or fusiform aneurysms unamenable to clip ligation or endovascular technology, and symptomatic intracranial and/or extracranial atherosclerotic occlusive disease. In 1963, Woringer and Kunlin performed the first external to intracranial internal carotid artery bypass utilizing a saphenous vein graft.[2] Yasargil is credited with advancement of cerebral revascularization techniques with the incorporation of microinstruments, bipolar technology, as well as the microscope.[3] At present, conduits available for bypass include scalp branches such as the superficial temporal artery (STA) and occipital artery (OA), and interposition grafts such as reverse saphenous vein (SV) and radial artery (RA). More recently, intracranial vessels such as the anterior temporal artery, the posterior inferior cerebellar artery (PICA) or vessels in close proximity to each other such as the pericallosal (A2–4) segments of the anterior cerebral artery (ACA) have been used to allow for in situ bypass.

While controversy still exists regarding cerebral revascularization for occlusive disease—and indeed at the time of this writing the Carotid Occlusion Surgery Study (COSS) is still ongoing—its role in the treatment of giant/fusiform aneurysms is well documented.[4,5] In some instances, it is simply impossible to exclude an aneurismal segment of vessel without sacrificing the parent vessel. In addition, dissection of a large aneurysm may require a prolonged period of temporary flow arrest, which would require a cerebral bypass for flow augmentation and prevention of ischemic complications. In such cases, cerebral bypass provides temporary or permanent flow arrest of the parent vessel harboring the aneurysm. Current bypass techniques utilize temporary occlusion of the recipient and donor vessels; however, the ELANA (excimer-laser assisted nonocclusive anastomosis) technique popularized in Europe will allow for cerebral bypass without temporary occlusion.[6]

Aneurysms in the anterior circulation unamenable for simple clip ligation or coiling procedures include giant aneurysms, fusiform aneurysms, and dissecting aneurysms. While clip reconstruction could be performed in some, the possibility of parent or branch vessel occlusion or injury and the time required for surgical dissection lend way to utilization of a cerebral bypass so that the aneurismal segment may be safely sacrificed. Coiling of giant aneurysms is generally not practical because (1) it is rarely a durable form of treatment, and (2) endovascular treatment of distal ACA segment aneurysms is not feasible at present if a stent is required, as stents in use today are not approved for vessels <2.5 mm. However, cerebral bypass may be utilized with coil embolization to deconstruct a vessel in order to minimize cerebral retraction.[7]

METHODS

There are multiple options for bypasses within the anterior circulation, and these include both IC-IC and EC-IC bypasses. The workhorse bypasses include in situ pericallosal side-to-side grafts and interposition grafts using arterial or venous donor vessels as follows: graft to distal A1, A1 to contralateral A1, A1 to ipsilateral or contralateral A2, A2 to A2, or A3 to A3.[8]

An anastomosis performed on any portion of the ACA is difficult as there is great depth in addition to a small working area. Yokoh et al. performed autopsy based studies to better define bypass techniques within the anterior circulation.[9] A1 mobility is approximately 3 mm unless the perforators are sacrificed purposefully to increase mobility. In comparison to the A1 segment, the A2 and A3 segments have greater mobility and their surgical exposure affords a wider access to these pericallosal vessels, thus rendering them somewhat less difficult for cerebral bypass. When bypassing in the region of the A2 and A3, the recurrent artery of Heubner (RAH), orbitofrontal artery (OfA), and frontopolar (FpA) arteries may need to be reimplanted utilizing an end-to-side technique. In their study, Yokoh et al. showed that each of the perforating vessels mentioned above measured 1 mm in diameter except the RAH, which averaged at 0.7 mm.

End-to-end anastomosis is possible between the A1, A2, or A3 segments if the cut surfaces are <5 mm apart.[9] Distal ACA side-to-side anastomosis protects the pericallosal distribution from ischemic injury and can be performed with approximately 1 cm of width space.[9,10] Grafts utilizing RA, STA, and or vein can be used to bypass to the distal ACA in order to prevent ischemia with parent vessel occlusion.

ANTERIOR CIRCULATION BYPASS SCENARIOS

Scenario I: Diseased A1 Segment

A giant fusiform aneurysm involving the A1 segment could be treated with exclusion of the diseased segment and bypass of the diseased A1. If angiography reveals that the contralateral A1 is dominant and supplies bilateral A2s, then clip ligation of the aneurismal A1 should be performed without any revascularization unless the RAH emanates from the distal A1.[11] In this case, the RAH can be reimplanted onto proximal A2 in an end-to-side anastomosis. When the contralateral A1 is hypoplastic, further flow augmentation is needed within the A2 or A3. This can be achieved with an A3-A3 side-to-side anastomosis or a STA-RA graft to the ipsilateral A2.

Scenario II: Diseased A1-A2 Junction

When the segment to be bypassed is the A1-A2 junction then the ipsilateral A1 could be anastomosed to the distal A2 or contralateral A1. If this is not possible then flow augmentation needs to occur at the ipsilateral A2 level either with a STA-RA graft or with an A3-A3 side-to-side anastomosis. We have also successfully used an RA interposition graft from the ipsilateral MCA to the A3 segment for this purpose.

The RAH, FpA, and OfA may need to be reimplanted, depending on their location relative to the diseased segment. However, it is also critical to preoperatively assess for angiographic evidence of hemodynamic collateral supply around the diseased segment, particularly in the setting of giant aneurysms. By virtue of their gradually progressive mass effect on adjacent *en passage* branches they promote the development of significant collateral flow, which may obviate the need for distal branch reimplantation. For example, in the setting of a giant anterior communicating artery aneurysm, angiographic demonstration of retrograde flow in the A3 and A4 pericallosal arteries via collateral supply from the posterior pericallosal branches off the posterior cerebral artery (PCA) may obviate the need for bypass to the side(s) with significant collateral flow.

Scenario III: Diseased A3 Segment

If the A3 segment is involved then the A3-A3 or A4-A4 side-to-side anastomosis is the best flow diversion. The A3 and A4 segments are ideal for side-to-side anastomosis as they lie parallel and within millimeters of each other.[5]

PREOPERATIVE IMAGING AND SURGICAL PLANNING

Preoperative imaging is a crucial part of surgical planning. The patient's cerebral vasculature is studied utilizing both two- (2D) and three-dimensional (3D) cerebral angiography. Evaluation of the arterial, capillary, and venous phases with 2D angiography provides hemodynamic information, which is unavailable in static 3D renderings. Hemodynamic assessment of 2D angiography, for example, may demonstrate that a giant and/or partially thrombosed aneurysms may produce sufficient mass effect to slow flow in surrounding branches, and even displace supply to smaller perforating vessels.

Three-dimensional rotational angiography is superior to 2D angiography for assessment of anatomic relationships and is critical as a "virtual" surgical planning tool. Three-dimensional angiography allows for simulation of the vasculature as it would appear within the in vivo scenario.

Magnetic resonance imaging (MRI) is obtained preoperatively not only to comprehensively assess the anatomical abnormality for the purposes of surgical planning, but also to assess the adjacent brain that is at risk for ischemia. MRI evidence of recent ischemia (by diffusion weighted imaging) in brain adjacent to a partially thrombosed aneurysm is a crucial finding. It should alert the surgeon as to a risk of hemorrhagic conversion, and the necessity for careful consideration of operative timing relative to the likely age of the ischemia.

CEREBRAL BYPASS TECHNIQUE

Following administration of general anesthesia, patients are placed in the supine position with a shoulder roll, and are secured in three-point fixation utilizing radiolucent pins and a Mayfield head-holder (Integra, Plainsboro, NJ). The radiolucent head holder allows us to perform intraoperative angiography without substantial streak artifact. Both the left and right groins are prepped routinely in case cerebral angiography is required. For interhemispheric fissure (IHF) approaches we prefer that the patient's head be turned 90 degrees so that the IHF is parallel to the floor, with the vertex tipped up 30 to 45 degrees with the operative side down. This both obviates the need for brain retractors (by using gravity) and allows the surgeon to work with instruments ergonomically in a more natural working plane.

For a bypass involving the A1 segment, a pterional craniotomy with orbital osteotomy is performed in order to allow for better visualization within the chiasmatic region. If an A2 or A3 anastomosis is to be performed, then a bifrontal craniotomy is performed for access to the anterior interhemispheric region. This approach may also be combined with the pterional approach. After a segment relatively free of perforating vessels is selected, the vessel to be bypassed is dissected clear of arachnoid adhesions, which allows further freedom to manipulate the recipient vessel. The case is performed with electrophysiological monitoring and the patient is placed under burst suppression with a short-acting barbiturate such as pentothal (Hospira Inc., Lake Forest, IL). The mean arterial pressure is maintained greater than 90 mm Hg to maximize collateral flow during temporary clip ligation.

Patients are treated preoperatively with antiplatelet therapy, using aspirin 325 mg daily for a week. After a wide cranial exposure, burst suppression by EEG, normocarbia, and mild hypothermia have been obtained, a piece of durapair (TEI Biosciences, Boston, MA) is placed under the recipient vessel to provide better visualization. A self-retaining suction (size 4, French) is placed within the field as to prevent cerebrospinal fluid/blood accumulation. After exposure of the recipient vessel and harvest of the donor, but before temporary clipping, heparin (Baxter International, Deerfield, IL) boluses are given (1000 units at a time) to maintain an activated clotting time (ACT) near 200.

Both the recipient and donor vessels are highlighted with a marking pen in the region to be anastomosed to enhance visualization. End-to-end or end-to-side anastomoses are performed with 8-0 to 10-0 nylon suture (Deme Tech, Miami, FL) in an interrupted fashion, while side-to-side anastomosis are performed in a running fashion. When the anastomosis is nearly complete, we use the technique described by Dacey, which employs unclipping of a temporarily clipped side branch on the donor vessel to back-bleed and rid the anastomosis of any air or debris.[12] Indocyanine green (ICG) angiography is then performed to evaluate the patency of the bypass. Tamponade with fibrillary collagen (avitene) rather than bipolar cautery should be used to obtain hemostasis of any slow oozing at the anastomosis. Rarely since the advent of ICG angiography do we perform intraoperative catheter cerebral angiography.

Before final wound closure, the ACT is checked, and the anticoagulation is *partially* reversed with protamine 1 mg for every 10 seconds above 200 seconds. The protamine dose rarely exceeds 5 mg, should never exceed 50 mg, and should be given over at least 10 minutes, as otherwise patients can develop an enhanced anticoagulation effect as well as extreme hypotension. In the immediate postoperative period, patients are maintained on aspirin therapy with systolic blood pressure normally maintained >120 mm Hg. Follow-up cerebral angiography is performed postoperatively and at 12 months to evaluate for patency and maturation.

ILLUSTRATIVE CASE

A 32-year-old male presented to our institution with a prior history of a left ICA terminus aneurysm that had been treated by Drake 22 years ago. At the age of 10 years, the patient had

undergone craniotomy for clip ligation of the left ICA terminus aneurysm along with a cerebral bypass. Further evaluation had revealed the bypass to be thrombosed as the left cervical ICA was occluded.

After a motor vehicle accident in 2004, the patient underwent evaluation with a computer tomographic angiography (CTA) of the head that revealed continued filling of the left ICA terminus aneurysm as well as development of a large anterior communicating (ACOM) aneurysm. These findings were corroborated by a diagnostic cerebral angiogram (Figure 24–1). A 10-month follow-up angiogram revealed enlargement of the ACOM aneurysm as well as persistence of the left ICA terminus aneurysm. The patient underwent coil embolization of the left ICA terminus aneurysm without any complications. Eight months later the ICA terminus aneurysm had significant recurrence as well as further enlargement of the ACOM aneurysm.

With the presence of an enlarging ACOM aneurysm and recurrent ICA terminus aneurysm, the decision was made to proceed with clip ligation and cerebral bypass. Since the left cerebral circulation was dependent on the ACOM complex, an ECA to M3 segment bypass was performed utilizing a radial artery graft (Figure 24–2). Twenty-four hours after the procedure, cerebral angiography revealed a thrombosed left ICA terminus aneurysm.

Since the ACOM aneurysm was a fusiform aneurysm, clip ligation of the neck was not possible; instead, the patient

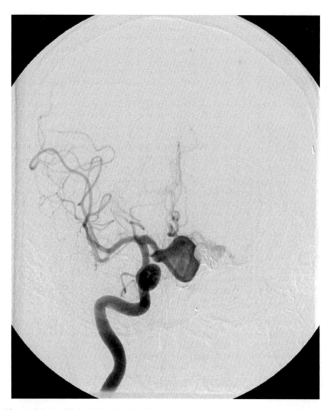

Figure 24–1. Right ICA injection in the anteroposterior projection showing a fusiform aneurysm of the ACOM as well as a recurrence of the left ICA terminus aneurysm.

required cerebral bypass and trapping of the aneurysm. First an A3-A3 side-to-side anastomosis was performed and then a radial graft was utilized to perform a right-M1 to left-A3 bypass (Figure 24–3). The right A1 was clipped distally and the A2s were not clipped to allow backfilling of perforating vessels arising from the A2. Subsequent angiography revealed thrombosis of the left ICA terminus and ACOM aneurysms. The patient tolerated these three separate procedures and made a remarkable recovery, returning to his daily life.

REFERENCES

1. The International Cooperative Study of Extracranial/Intracranial Arterial Anastomosis (EC/IC Bypass Study): methodology and entry characteristics. The EC/IC Bypass Study group, *Stroke* 16:397–406, 1985.
2. Woringer E, Kunlin J: [Anastomosis between the Common Carotid and the Intracranial Carotid or the Sylvian Artery by a Graft, Using the Suspended Suture Technique], *Neurochirurgie* 200:181–188, 1963.
3. Hayden MG, et al: The evolution of cerebral revascularization surgery, *Neurosurg Focus* 26:E17, 2009.
4. Cote R: [International cooperative study of extracranial artery bypass: development report], *Union Med Can* 113:242–244, 1984.
5. Sanai N, Zador A, Lawton MT: Bypass surgery for complex brain aneurysms: an assessment of intracranial-intracranial bypass, *Neurosurgery* 65:670–683, 2009; discussion 683.
6. Streefkerk HJ, et al: The ELANA technique: constructing a high flow bypass using a non-occlusive anastomosis on the ICA and a conventional anastomosis on the SCA in the treatment of a fusiform giant basilar trunk aneurysm, *Acta Neurochir (Wien)* 146:1009–1019, 2004; discussion 1019.
7. Kim LJ, et al: Combined surgical and endovascular treatment of a recurrent A3-A3 junction aneurysm unsuitable for stand-alone clip ligation or coil occlusion. Technical note, *Neurosurg Focus* 18:E6, 2005.
8. Kashimura H, et al: Trapping and vascular reconstruction for ruptured fusiform aneurysm in the proximal A1 segment of the anterior cerebral artery, *Neurol Med Chir (Tokyo)* 46:340–343, 2006.
9. Yokoh A, et al: Anterior cerebral artery reconstruction, *Neurosurgery* 19:26–35, 1986.
10. Kim K, et al: Giant intracranial aneurysm of the anterior communicating artery treated by direct surgery using A3-A3 side-to-side anastomosis and A3-RA graft-STA anastomosis, *Acta Neurochir (Wien)* 148:353–357, 2006; discussion 357.
11. Lownie SP, et al: Clinical presentation and management of giant anterior communicating artery region aneurysms, *J Neurosurg* 92:267–277, 2000.
12. Dacey RG, et al: Use of a side branch in a saphenous vein interposition graft for high-flow extracranial-intracranial bypass procedure, *J Neurosurg* 103:186–187, 2005.

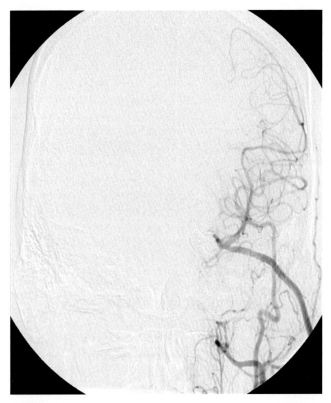

Figure 24–2. Left CCA injection in the anteroposterior projection revealing a patent ECA-M3 bypass

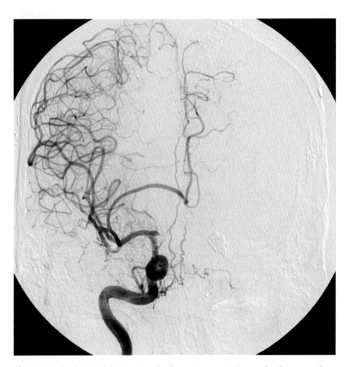

Figure 24–3. Right ICA injection in the anteroposterior projection revealing a patent M1 to left A3 bypass.

BYPASS SURGERY FOR COMPLEX MCA ANEURYSMS

DAVID H. JHO; GAVIN P. DUNN; CHRISTOPHER S. OGILVY

INTRODUCTION

Complex MCA aneurysms may be categorized into three major groups based on etiology and anatomic location along the vessel: (1) M1 segment fusiform aneurysms, (2) giant MCA bifurcation aneurysms, and (3) distal MCA infectious aneurysms. Although fusiform aneurysms are relatively uncommon, the M1 segment tends to be the region of the MCA affected, perhaps due to its relationship to atherosclerotic disease.[1] Among MCA aneurysms overall, the most common anatomic location is at the MCA bifurcation (or trifurcation) at the origin of the M2 branches, with saccular morphology and etiology likely related to hemodynamic forces. Distal MCA branches such as M2-M4 segments are a common site for infectious or mycotic aneurysms, often associated with favored flow routes of septic emboli from infective endocarditis.

Most MCA aneurysms involve simple or modestly complex saccular aneurysms at the MCA bifurcation, which can frequently be managed with surgical clipping or endovascular embolization alone. However, when obliteration of an MCA aneurysm would potentially involve compromise of the parent vessel or important distal branches, the conjunctive use of vascular bypass can be a crucial component of management to avoid significant morbidity or mortality. The designation of an MCA aneurysm as "complex" may be due to fusiform configuration, large size, intricate neck, calcifications, or incorporation of important branch vessels. It must be noted that although "giant" aneurysms are designated with a diameter size criteria of >25 mm, large aneurysms (10- to 25-mm diameter) can still present with similar treatment challenges such as mass effect to surrounding anatomy, high rupture risk, and strokes from thromboemboli or compromise of perforators.

Although this chapter will focus specifically on the bypass surgery component, the repertoire of treatment options for complex MCA aneurysms may include surgical trapping of the M1 segment with EC-IC or IC-IC bypass, surgical ligation of the internal carotid artery with EC-IC bypass, endovascular MCA takedown with EC-IC bypass, endovascular takedown of the internal carotid artery with EC-IC bypass, or bypass with possible endovascular flow remodeling if the aneurysm cannot

be safely excluded from the circulation. Among the various permutations of therapeutic combinations, IC-IC bypass is unlikely to be used with endovascular takedown of the MCA, since if the IC-IC bypass is technically feasible from a surgical standpoint then surgical trapping during the same procedure tends to be amenable. Alternative options for M1 fusiform aneurysms may include endovascular construct placements for vessel reconstruction and flow remodeling. Alternative treatment for giant MCA bifurcation aneurysms may include surgical excision with microsurgical reconstruction of the bifurcation or endovascular coil embolization (possibly with stent or balloon assistance) plus bypass if needed. Alternative therapy for distal MCA mycotic aneurysms may include Onyx embolization, coil embolization, or surgical trapping without bypass. Advantages of surgical treatments for giant MCA aneurysms are that some of the mass effect may be able to be reduced if portions of the aneurysm undergo controlled resection, and, although rupture risk may be higher with surgical manipulation compared to endovascular treatments, there may be more immediate options for managing intraprocedural aneurysm rupture surgically.

The role of bypass surgery for complex MCA aneurysms has been somewhat tempered by the infrequency of this technically demanding procedure usually done by specialized vascular neurosurgeons at institutions with an ample referral base[2] and by the rapid evolution of potential alternative endovascular therapies. Yet bypass is an essential tool in the repertoire of a vascular neurosurgeon given its sometimes crucial role in the management of complex intracranial aneurysms. In this chapter, we focus on surgical bypass treatment options for complex MCA aneurysms, including the decision-making process and details of surgical technique.

TREATMENT DECISIONS

Although many of the following steps occur in parallel, generally the sequence progresses from the history/exam to imaging, then determination is made as to optimal management options that may include observation, surgical treatments, endovascular treatments, or combined surgical-endovascular treatments. For initial imaging assessment, we use CTA with maximal intensity projections and 3D image reconstruction since it is quick, non-invasive, surveys other related neuroanatomic issues (such as mass effect for giant aneurysms or any associated hydrocephalus), identifies other coexisting aneurysms, assesses the full extent of giant or complex aneurysms (such as thrombosed components) that may not be seen on conventional angiography, and outlines relationships of the target with other anatomic structures such as the skull base or proximity to potential extracranial bypass vessels.[3–5] In complex scenarios, the CTA can easily be extended to the neck and aortic arch to help facilitate assessment for endovascular access or an array of surgical options. Bilateral cervical carotid and vertebral systems may also be assessed for outlining the individual's overall intracranial hemodynamic configuration, and ECA branches such as the superficial temporal artery (STA) can be delineated in detail including 3D reconstruction. Linkage may also be done with image-guidance systems (IGS) to facilitate STA harvest or distal MCA bypass if needed. Our second choice study for those patients who cannot undergo CTA is conventional digital subtraction angiography (DSA) that can be done with contrast-minimizing strategies if needed, or least commonly MRA.

There are multiple considerations that factor into the decision-making process in determining the optimal choices for aneurysm management:

1. Etiology
2. Size/location
3. Configuration
   a. Orientation/shape (saccular or fusiform)
   b. Aneurysm neck (wide, atheromatous, or calcified base)
   c. Thrombosis
   d. Calcifications
4. Available donor vessels for bypass
5. Overall medical condition

Fundamentally, the suspected etiology of the aneurysm is based on history, exam, and imaging. Needless to say, the presentation and management of a ruptured intracranial saccular MCA aneurysm seen in the emergency ward is distinctly different from that of an elective giant MCA aneurysm presenting with chronic progressive symptoms in the outpatient setting. Etiology can have a major impact on management, with an example being infectious (mycotic) MCA aneurysms with associated infective endocarditis and septic emboli requiring intravenous antibiotics as a major component of therapy along with cardiac valvular disease management. Based on imaging, the size and location of the aneurysm must be considered along with any other potential neuroanatomic considerations. Laterality can occasionally be a consideration in treatment decisions since left MCA involvement may have more potential functional implications than a similar lesion in the right MCA, especially in relation to aphasias, and the handedness of the patient may be considered in weighing potential stakes in motor function. Once the aneurysm is

established as MCA in location with a complex pattern, further assessment and potential treatment approach may be based on the specific aneurysm configuration.

Complex MCA aneurysms that cannot be appropriately treated by surgical or endovascular trapping with possible bypass may alternatively be treated by altering blood flow to the inflow zone using various surgical and endovascular strategies.[6] Endovascular options for complex MCA aneurysms may include coil or Onyx embolization (with possible stent or balloon assistance) versus flow alteration strategies or combined surgical-endovascular therapies with bypass followed by endovascular trapping or embolization.[7,8] Recurrences are another category that may need special consideration and may be treated with additional surgical clipping, endovascular embolization, proximal parent vessel occlusion, or bypass with surgical or endovascular trapping.[9] At our institution, complex elective cases are usually discussed in a weekly multi-disciplinary neurovascular conference involving neurosurgeons, neurologists, and interventional radiologists before final therapies are pursued. As previously mentioned, we will focus on three types of complex MCA aneurysms, which include fusiform M1 segment aneurysms, large or giant MCA bifurcation aneurysms, and distal MCA infectious aneurysms.

M1 FUSIFORM ANEURYSMS

Patients with M1 fusiform aneurysms may present with ischemic symptoms, stroke, mass effect, rupture with subarachnoid hemorrhage, or as an incidental finding. For a focal M1 segment fusiform aneurysm, treatment options include observation with expectant management, endovascular reconstruction, surgical trapping with EC-IC bypass, or combined endovascular-surgical therapies.[10] The etiology may involve acute dissection associated with trauma versus chronic fusiform aneurysm, with the natural history of the latter being poorly understood.[11] Acute dissecting aneurysms can have significant risk of associated hemorrhage.[12] For chronic fusiform aneurysms, cerebral infarction related to thrombus involving compromise of perforators or thromboembolic phenomena may occur more frequently than hemorrhagic rupture based on the natural history of the more frequently encountered vertebrobasilar dolichoectasia or fusiform aneurysms.[13] Treatment of choice may depend on whether the aneurysm is ruptured, unruptured but symptomatic, flow-limiting, or incidental upon presentation.

In addition, an important factor for determining appropriate treatment to minimize morbidity is the identification of significant perforators, which may emanate from the aneurysm itself and may not be fully recognized until intraoperatively. If perforators are not involved with the aneurysm, then the treatment goal is exclusion of the aneurysm from the circulation while preserving distal MCA flow using techniques such as EC-IC bypass with clip trapping or coil embolization (Figures 25–1A and 25–1B), with less favored alternatives being excision of aneurysm with interposition graft or aneurysmal

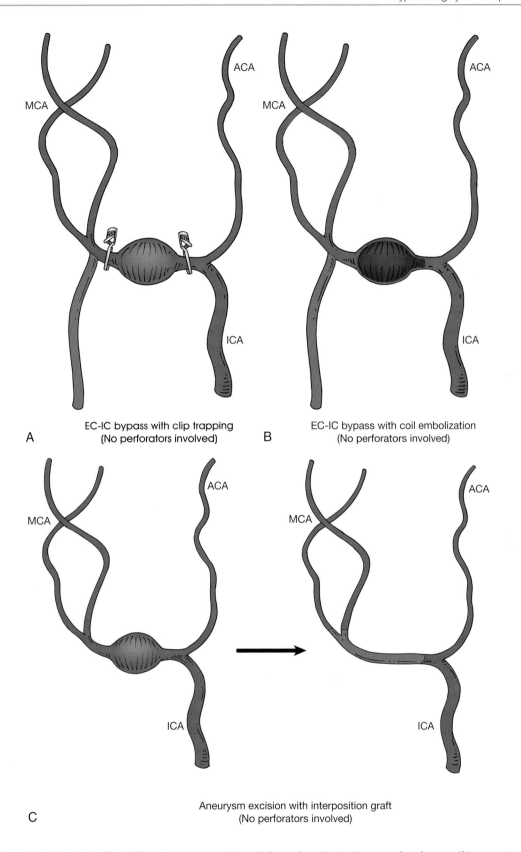

A — EC-IC bypass with clip trapping
(No perforators involved)

B — EC-IC bypass with coil embolization
(No perforators involved)

C — Aneurysm excision with interposition graft
(No perforators involved)

Figure 25–1. Treatment strategies for fusiform M1 aneurysms may be based (in part) on the involvement of perforators. If important perforators are not involved with the aneurysm, then EC-IC bypass with clip trapping **(A)** or coil embolization **(B)** is the preferred intervention. Extension of the fusiform M1 aneurysm to involve the MCA bifurcation may alternatively require excision with interposition graft **(C)** or vessel reconstruction techniques **(D)**.

Continued

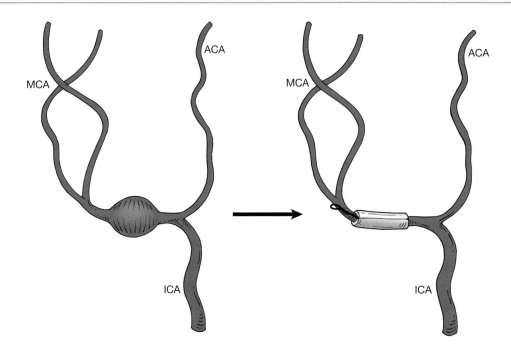

D

Hemashield and clip reconstruction
(No perforators involved)

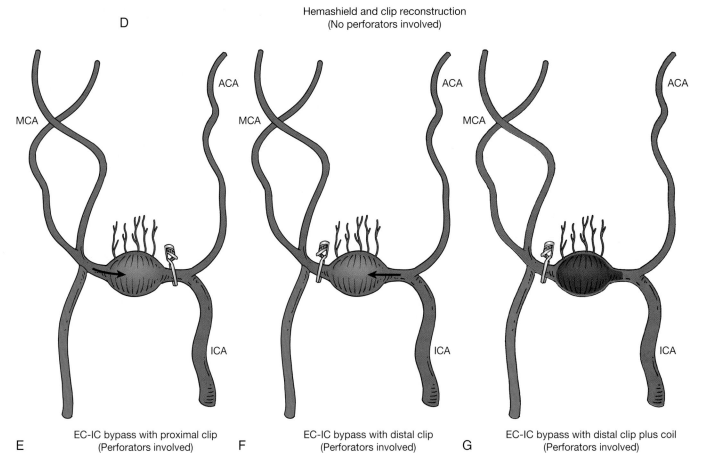

E   EC-IC bypass with proximal clip
(Perforators involved)

F   EC-IC bypass with distal clip
(Perforators involved)

G   EC-IC bypass with distal clip plus coil
(Perforators involved)

Figure 25–1.—cont'd If crucial perforators originate from the aneurysm itself, then EC-IC bypass with proximal clip **(E)** is preferred. Alternatively, EC-IC bypass with distal clip may be done **(F)**, with future supplementation by endovascular embolization as needed **(G)**.

vessel reconstruction depending on the aneurysm configuration (Figures 25–1C and 25–1D). If perforators are involved, then flow remodeling strategies to reduce hemodynamic pressures at the inflow zone may be pursued such as EC-IC bypass with proximal clip (retrograde flow supplying perforators), and less favorably EC-IC bypass with distal clip, which may be supplemented with additional endovascular embolization as needed (Figures 25–1E through 25–1G). Intraoperative angiography can be helpful in determining the optimal configuration of flow remodeling. Various techniques for IC-IC bypass with aneurysm trapping have also been described.[14,15] At least the following additional factors are also considered for therapeutic selection: overall medical condition and age of the patient along with anatomic extent of the fusiform segment. Diffuse extent of fusiform aneurysms may preclude a focused surgical therapy and warrant conservative management with observation and possibly antiplatelet or anticoagulation agents to reduce risk of thromboembolic phenomena related to turbulent flow (Figures 25–2A through 25–2C).

Acute traumatic arterial dissection involving a focal M1 segment is rare, but if the resulting fusiform aneurysm with dissected flap demonstrates significant flow limitation, associated pseudoaneurysm, or rupture in a patient whose overall medical condition would tolerate invasive therapies, options include surgical trapping with bypass, endovascular takedown with bypass, or endovascular reconstruction. EC-IC bypass followed by proximal surgical occlusion alone without distal trapping may result in reversal of blood flow in the M1 segment with preserved flow to the M1 perforators while helping the dissection subside due to the direction of orientation of the dissected flap.[16] Surgical trapping may alternatively be accomplished in conjunction with a purely intracranial IC-IC bypass.[14,15] Endovascular takedown with EC-IC bypass may be a more attractive option if the fusiform segment involves the distal internal carotid artery near the skull base in addition to the M1 segment (with ipsilateral anterior cerebral artery having potential contralateral collateral supply via the anterior communicating artery), but surgical therapy may still be achieved in this scenario.[17] Reconstructive endovascular options may include flow diverting stent placement, self-expandable stent-within-stent placement, and stent with balloon-assisted coiling.[18]

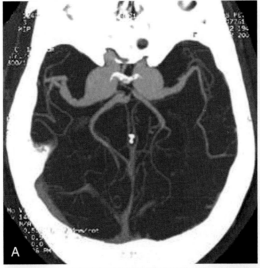

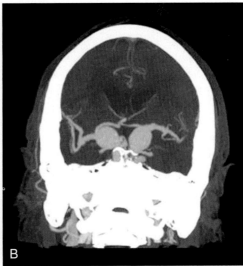

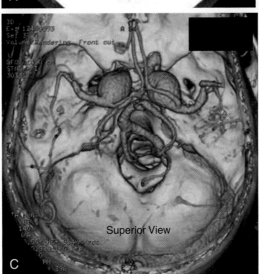

Figure 25–2. Axial (A) and coronal view CTA (B) maximal intensity projections, along with 3D reconstructions (C) show extensive fusiform dilatations of bilateral MCAs and the posterior circulation along with bilateral fusiform aneurysms of the intracranial internal carotid arteries. The patient was a highly functional 67-year-old male with work-up for near-syncopal episode, treated conservatively with anti-platelet agents.

GIANT MCA BIFURCATION ANEURYSMS

Patients with giant MCA bifurcation aneurysms may present with mass effect, seizures, ischemic symptoms, stroke, rupture with subarachnoid hemorrhage, or as an incidental finding. For giant MCA bifurcation aneurysms of saccular or fusiform morphology, the configuration of the bifurcation or trifurcation on imaging should help determine how to best preserve the M2 branches. The surgical option of simply clipping the neck of the aneurysm and preserving the direct flow from the M1 trunk to the M2 branches may be precluded by calcified atheromatous base, thick walls with giant wide neck, extensive thrombosis, or anatomic configuration of the M2 origins. Booster clips or a complex combination of clips may be required to achieve clipping of giant aneurysms, and the use of a vascular clamp for assistance has also been described.[19] Alternatively, surgical or endovascular obliteration may be performed with or without bypass.[20,21]

If the anatomic configuration is amenable, EC-IC bypass may be performed to one nonsalvageable M2 branch and clipping can then be performed across the aneurysm neck along with this revascularized M2 origin, while flow may be preserved from the M1 segment to the other salvageable M2 trunk.[22] If the giant MCA bifurcation aneurysm is to be excised instead of clipped, the bifurcation can still be microsurgically reconstructed with similar methods.[23,24] An analogous reconstruction option can include excision of the giant MCA bifurcation aneurysm with end-to-end anastomosis of the remaining M1 segment to one M2 trunk and performing STA-MCA bypass to the other M2 trunk.[25] Sometimes EC-IC or IC-IC bypass may be done to a dominant inferior (or superior) segment if the other bifurcation branch provides minimal supply or has already suffered significant previous infarct with minimal preservable cerebral tissue to salvage in that region. For large or giant MCA aneurysms distal to the bifurcation, surgical trapping may similarly be performed with possible EC-IC bypass or end-to-end anastomosis.[26]

Challenges in surgical treatment may include rupture risk with dissection around a large aneurysm dome required to reach the aneurysm neck, adhesion of the giant aneurysm to adjacent frontal and temporal lobes, adhesion of MCA branch vessels to the aneurysm dome, and thrombus within the aneurysm, which may put the patient at risk of emboli during aneurysm manipulation. Post-operative complications may include graft thrombosis, anastomotic leak, pseudoaneurysm, and ischemic or thromboembolic stroke.

DISTAL MCA INFECTIOUS ANEURYSMS

Patients with distal MCA infectious aneurysms may present with inflammatory symptoms and signs including bacteremia with possible sepsis, congestive heart failure, septic emboli with infarcts of the brain or other organs, rupture with subarachnoid hemorrhage, or as an incidental finding. As previously mentioned, distal infectious aneurysms are often associated with infective endocarditis and cardiac valvular disease, which should optimally be co-managed with infectious disease and cardiac specialists. The natural history of infectious intracranial aneurysms is not fully understood, although there appears to be a relatively high risk of rupture confounded by the fact that cerebrovascular imaging tends to be done for patients who are symptomatic and have high pre-test probability of mycotic aneurysms and septic emboli. It may be prudent to perform screening cerebral CTA on patients with new diagnosis of infective endocarditis or prior to cardiac valve repair with plans for possible anticoagulation for the procedure that could potentially worsen the consequences of an aneurysm rupture. When infectious cerebral aneurysms are noted in coexistence with severe cardiac valvular disease, it may be challenging to determine the optimum timing of whether treatment of the aneurysm versus cardiac valve repair should be undertaken first.[27,28] Cardiac valve repair has been reported without anticoagulation in the context of a ruptured infectious aneurysm and conservative management of the aneurysm with antimicrobials, having improvement in the aneurysm over several months.[29]

Patients who have <5-mm, unruptured distal MCA infectious aneurysms may be considered for expectant conservative management with antimicrobials but should have serial follow-up imaging (such as CTA) every few weeks or months, with consideration for invasive treatment within the first several months if the aneurysm demonstrates lack of improvement or worsening (such as growth or rupture). Patients in moribund condition may also be considered for conservative treatment regardless of aneurysmal configuration. Patients in poor overall medical condition but ruptured or larger distal MCA infectious aneurysms may be considered for endovascular Onyx or coil embolization, depending on the aneurysmal configuration. If the patient is in reasonable overall medical condition, surgical or endovascular trapping may be considered regardless of the size or rupture status of the infectious aneurysm. This may be performed without bypass if the distal MCA branches supply minor or noneloquent cerebral regions, or EC-IC versus IC-IC bypass may be performed if the angular branch on the dominant side or other important distal branches are involved. If the aneurysmal configuration is amenable, direct surgical clipping may even be feasible as a preferred option, but more commonly the configuration requires proximal and distal trapping with possible excision of the infectious aneurysm.[30] If it is unclear whether the involved distal MCA branches supply functionally important cerebral tissues, awake craniotomy may be undertaken for temporary clipping to determine if surgical trapping may be tolerated without EC-IC or IC-IC bypass, which can be performed in a minimally invasive fashion when used in conjunction with image-guidance systems.[31]

Challenging issues include the presence of multiple mycotic aneurysms, which may be more amenable to a single or staged endovascular interventional combination, especially if the locations are bilateral or involve the posterior circulation, although staged surgical treatment may still be feasible in select cases.[32] Involved branching or various bifurcation points can be microsurgically reconstructed in theory, but there is a potential risk of delayed pseudoaneurysm formation at the bifurcation site, such that end-to-end anastomosis of the proximal MCA to one of the distal MCA branches (with graft if needed) used in conjunction with EC-IC bypass to the other distal MCA branch is the preferred reconstruction option.

SURGICAL TECHNIQUE

I. Donor Evaluation

Donor vessel options include the STA, radial artery, greater saphenous vein graft, and cadaveric vein graft.[33,34] The sites of the ipsilateral STA, bilateral radial arteries, and bilateral greater saphenous veins should be assessed on physical exam with noting of any past surgical history involving those vessels, and portions of the STA can also be assessed on cranial vascular imaging studies. Alternatively, in situ IC-IC bypass may be an option depending on the individual anatomic configuration, which can also be assessed on imaging. IC-IC bypasses such as an in situ MCA-MCA bypass may have the advantages of having caliber-matched donor and recipient arteries along with being a relatively short graft that remains protected inside the cranium postoperatively.[15,22]

Donor vessels require a diameter of at least >1 mm with matching of donor-recipient size facilitating an optimal anastomosis. Although there can be great variability in the same donor vessels between individuals, there is debate that a STA-MCA graft provides a low-flow bypass, long arterial graft provides an intermediate-flow bypass, and a long venous graft bypass provides a high-flow bypass.[35,36] As previously mentioned, anastomotic options involve STA to MCA end-to-side or end-to-end bypass, radial artery ECA-MCA bypass, in situ MCA-MCA bypass, reversed saphenous vein graft ECA-MCA bypass, or reversed cadaveric vein graft ECA-MCA bypass. A standard STA-MCA bypass consists of end-to-side or end-to-end anastomosis of a branch of the STA to a selected MCA branch in the region of the Sylvian fissure. Radial artery ECA-MCA bypass involves harvesting the radial artery (usually from the side of the nondominant hand) using open or endoscopic techniques[33]; Allen's test has poor predictive value for evaluating collateral flow and the ulnar artery of the donor arm should not have any history of previous injury or surgery. In situ IC-IC bypass may involve MCA-MCA bypass from the anterior temporal artery to another M2 branch, reimplantation of an M2 trunk onto another M2 trunk, or other methods of direct MCA to MCA bypass depending on individual anatomy.[14,15] Saphenous vein graft ECA-MCA bypass may be done using autologous saphenous interposition vein graft taken from either leg (if sites have not previously been used for coronary artery or peripheral vascular disease).

If neither saphenous vein nor other autologous site is desirable, then cadaveric vein graft may be used for ECA-MCA bypass.

II. Positioning

The patient is usually positioned in the conventional position for a pterional craniotomy with the head turned toward the contralateral side fixed in a three-point Mayfield holder with the temporal bone parallel to the floor; ipsilateral shoulder rolls may be placed if necessary.

III. Preparation of the Donor Graft

Portable Doppler ultrasound is used to map the location and course of donor vessels. Vasoconstrictive agents such as epinephrine should not be used in local infiltration. A #15 scalpel blade is used to incise the scalp, and the STA is harvested working proximal to distal using blunt dissection along with needle-tip monopolar cautery with a cuff of surrounding soft tissue; usually either the frontal or parietal branch is used depending on dominant size, proximity to the recipient vessel, or surgeon preference. Smaller branches of the STA are ligated or carefully cauterized.

IV. STA-MCA Anastomosis

Usually a standard pterional craniotomy is performed for fusiform M1 segment aneurysms or MCA bifurcation aneurysms, which may be modified for distal MCA aneurysms (including use of image-guidance system if desired). The temporalis muscle is divided and retracted, then a standard pterional bone flap is removed, the dural is opened in a U-shaped fashion with the dura remaining attached toward the base of the Sylvian fissure, and dissection of the arachnoid layer is performed to expose an approximately 1-cm segment of recipient vessel. A rubber dam is placed as background to facilitate anastomosis, and flowprobe monitoring is performed to obtain baseline flow measurements on the donor and recipient vessels. A temporary clip is placed on the proximal STA, and then the distal STA is ligated and divided at the desired length with an oblique cut at the desired diameter. The temporary clip on proximal STA is briefly released to verify good flow, the STA is flushed with heparinized saline, and the distal tip is cleaned in preparation for anastomosis. Temporary clips are placed proximally and distally on the recipient vessel, then an arteriotomy is performed in the side wall of the MCA to prepare for an end-to-side anastomosis, the recipient vessel is irrigated with heparinized saline, and indigo carmine blue dye may be used to mark the vessel edges to facilitate suturing of the anastomosis. Interrupted stitches are placed using 8-0 or 9-0 nylon either at two ends or four corners, then the back wall may be sutured using interrupted or running stitch, followed by the front wall, making sure to include the intimal layer. Surgicel is used to line the anastomosis, temporary clips are released, and flow probe is used to check flow in the components of the anastomosis. The dura is closed with the local region of dural opening preserved around the STA-MCA bypass graft, bone flap is replaced with generous focal opening at the bypass graft with contouring as needed to avoid any vessel kinking, and the remaining layers (temporalis muscle, galeal, and skin) are closed in standard fashion being careful to avoid graft compromise.

Intraoperative monitoring with electroencephalography and evoked potentials may optionally be used. An operating microscope should be used for optimal anastomosis. Papaverine local application may be used to minimize vasospasm. Flow-probe monitoring may be used after bypass to assess flow,[37] and intraoperative cerebral angiography may be used to assess bypass patency and hemodynamic configuration. The use of laser contrast analysis has also been reported.[38]

Case Example

The surgical technique for standard right STA-MCA bypass with surgical trapping for a right distal M3/M4 infectious aneurysm is described, with similar general principles applicable for EC-IC bypass approaches for M1 fusiform aneurysms and giant MCA bifurcation aneurysms. A 36-year-old male with a history of *Staphylococcus aureus* endocarditis status post-antibiotic treatment and post-mitral valve replacement (29-mm Bjork-Shiley prosthetic valve) 19 years prior on chronic Coumadin (INR goal maintained at 2 to 3) presented with gradual onset headaches for 3 months. He reportedly had distant history of *Staphylococcus aureus* bacteremia with seeding of the mitral valve at age 17 with source unclear and denied any history of intravenous drug use. His past medical history was otherwise only notable for L4-L5 discectomy and laminectomy with posterior spinal fusion (L4-L5 pedicle screws and rods) and transforaminal lumbar interbody fusion 3 years prior followed by removal of segmental spinal instrumentation 2 years prior after bony fusion (for low back pain and left hip pain since resolved) for which he had been off construction work for the past 4 years. CTA showed a 16-mm AP x 7-mm TV x 6-mm SI bilobed aneurysm arising from a Sylvian branch of the superior division of the right MCA (Figure 25–3A), which was suspicious for a mycotic aneurysm, but radiology read suggested differential diagnosis of arteriovenous malformation (AVM) not being completely excluded. Therefore, a follow-up DSA was done that also included selective right ECA and ICA injections that confirmed the 16-mm AP x 7-mm TV x 6-mm irregular multilobulated aneurysm with partially fusiform and partially saccular configuration involving an M3/M4 junction of a distal branch of the right MCA superior division with two M4 branches projecting superior-posteriorly and inferior-posteriorly from the body of the aneurysm (Figures 25–3B and 25–3C). A prominent right ECA with right STA for

potential EC-IC bypass was noted, and there was no evidence for associated AVM.

The patient was taken for right temporal craniotomy for microsurgical right STA-MCA bypass with proximal occlusion of the complex distal right MCA aneurysm using the operative microscope, stereotactic image-guidance system, and intraoperative cerebral angiography (Figures 25–3D through 25–3I). The patient underwent general anesthesia, right common femoral artery sheath was placed for intraoperative angiography access with integration into the craniotomy sterile draping, the patient's head was turned to the left, and the right superficial temporal artery was mapped using a microvascular Doppler probe. The right parietal-temporal region was prepped and draped in a sterile fashion. After the skin incision, an operating microscope was used to dissect and isolate the right STA using pencil-tip monopolar cautery, scissors and ligation. The artery was dissected along its length from the superior border of the zygoma to its distal end at the right parietal region. Red vascular loops were used to wrap around and isolate the right STA with circumferential dissection (Figure 25–4A). The right STA was retracted anteriorly and posteriorly to open the temporalis muscle layer deep to this region with Gelpi retractor.

The stereotactic image-guidance system was then used to confirm the location of the complex right MCA aneurysm, which was located just superior to the level of the ear and within the planned craniotomy. Four burr holes were placed around the planned craniotomy with curettes used to remove the inner table, and a #3 Penfield dissector was used to separate the dura from the inner surface of the skull. The craniotome was used to connect the burr holes into a rectangular-shaped bone flap, which was then removed. The dura was opened and reflected anteriorly, revealing the partially thrombosed distal right MCA aneurysm on the surface of the brain (Figure 25–4B).

Using the operating microscope, dissection was performed circumferentially around the MCA aneurysm with dissection around the efferent vessels leaving the lesion and afferent vessel entering the lesion, consistent in appearance with the CTA and DSA. A patty was placed on the proximal end to prepare for proximal control in case rupture should occur (Figure 25–4C), and then attention was turned to the distal vessels with bipolar coagulation of two small perforators associated with the branch vessel. The aneurysm target was isolated on a rubber dam stage with placement of a microsuction device below the stage to provide constant suction for the bypass procedure and intermittent irrigation with heparinized saline (Figure 25–4D). The STA was cleaned at the site for the planned anastomosis using two 5-O jeweler's forceps and then straight microscissors. A temporary clip was placed proximal and distal to the planned anastomotic site along the STA, and then the STA was transected at a slight angle and brought to the prepared donor site on the rubber dam stage. The MCA branch was occluded proximally and distally with temporary clips (Figure 25–4E), and the donor site was incised linearly with an arachnoid knife to form an end-to-side, STA-to-MCA anastomosis with the STA angled slightly towards the angle of desired flow of the anastomosis (Figure 25–4F). A 9-O nylon suture was used to tack two sides of the graft into

25

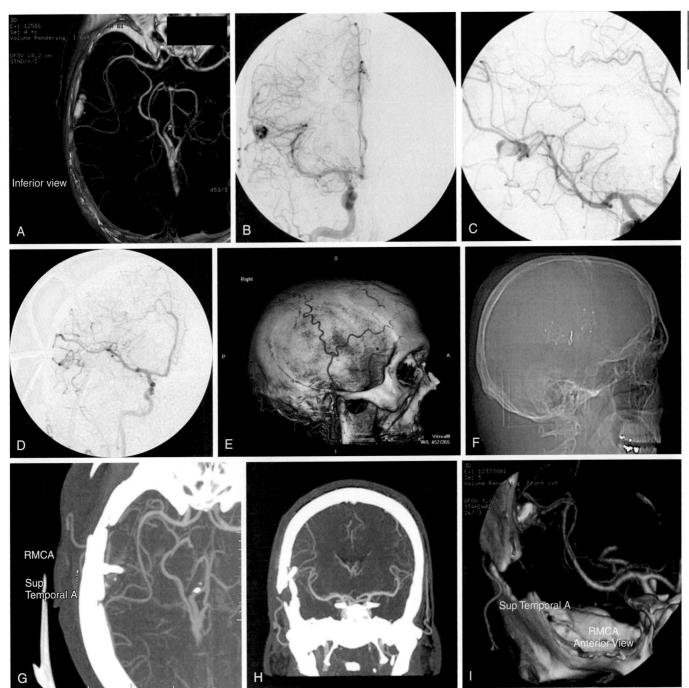

Figure 25–3. CTA 3D reconstruction **(A)** and conventional digital subtraction angiography (DSA) with AP **(B)** and right anterior oblique **(C)** views show fusiform right M3/M4 infectious aneurysm involving the distal right MCA superior division in a 36-year-old male with distant history of treated endocarditis and new headaches for 3 months. Intraoperative angiography following proximal clipping and distal STA-MCA bypass demonstrated filling of the right MCA (and ACA) but lack of aneurysmal filling **(D)**. Preoperative CTA 3D reconstruction of the right STA demonstrates serendipitous location **(E)** in relation to the recipient vessel for STA-MCA bypass as reflected in the postoperative scout X-ray **(F)** done as a component of postoperative CTA. Maximal intensity projections of the postoperative CTA with axial **(G)** and coronal **(H)** views along with 3D reconstruction **(I)** illustrate the radiographic configuration of the right M3/M4 infectious aneurysm proximal clipping and distal STA-MCA bypass.

position (Figures 25–4G and 25–4H), the graft was flipped and six interrupted sutures were placed to connect the back side, and then the graft was rotated back and six interrupted sutures were placed to connect the front side (Figures 25–4I and 25–4J). Clamps were released with one leak site at the anastomosis

noted for which the clamps were reapplied with one additional suture placed at the leak site. The clamps were again removed, and excellent flow was observed through the STA graft into the distal MCA vessels as confirmed using microvascular Doppler probe.

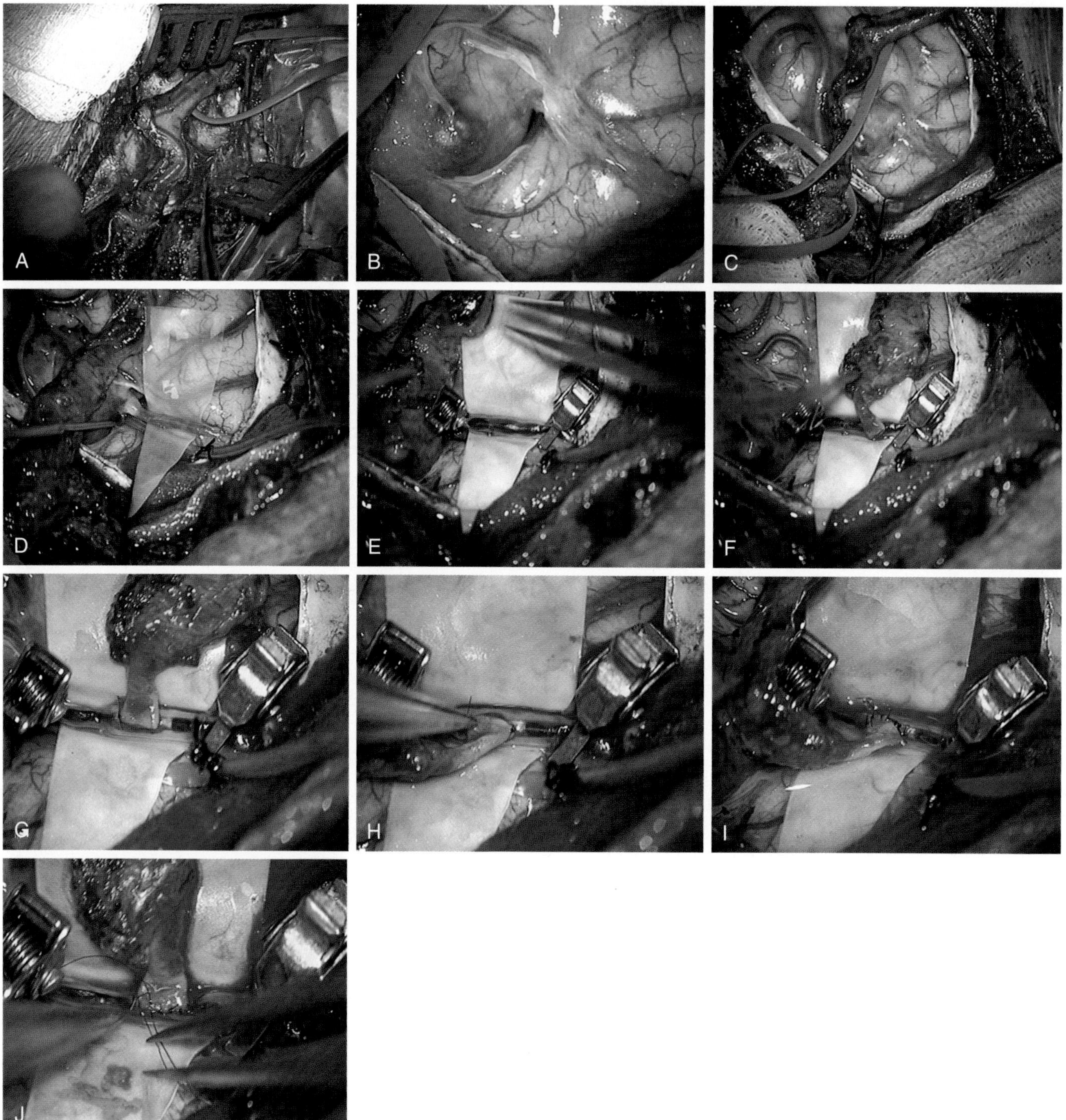

Figure 25–4. Intraoperative photographs show preparation of the right STA bypass donor with vascular loop **(A)** and intracranial exposure of the fusiform right M3/M4 infectious aneurysm **(B)** in this 36-year-old male patient. Preparation for the bypass with placement of the donor right STA into the intracranial field **(C)** and isolation of the recipient segment with rubber dam stage and microsuction placement beneath the anastomotic site **(D)** is shown. Proximal and distal temporary clips isolate the anastomotic site **(E)**, and the donor STA with perivascular cuff is brought to the site **(F)** with anchoring interrupted 9-0 nylon sutures placed at each end of the anastomosis **(G–H)**. The back wall of the anastomosis is sutured first **(I)** followed by the front wall of the graft **(J)**.

A J-shaped aneurysm clip was then placed on the afferent vessel entering the aneurysm for proximal occlusion, and then intraoperative focused cerebral angiography was performed. Intraoperative focused cerebral angiography with right common carotid artery injection showed patent right STA (posterior branch) with end-to-side anastomotic bypass to a right distal MCA (M4) branch that continued to fill further distal MCA branches, with no filling of the complex right MCA aneurysm following surgical trapping (see Figure 25–3D). At the Y-shaped junction, it was known that there was a second efferent vessel adjacent to the vessel that received bypass, which were both in close proximity to the aneurysm. Attempts for distal occlusion of the aneurysm would force the clip onto the branch vessels, and the alternative of opening the aneurysm and cleaning out the edge to place the clip without compromising the branch vessels was felt to be a higher potential risk than benefit given that the intraoperative angiography showed that the aneurysm was no longer filling with the current operative configuration. If the intraoperative angiography had shown continued filling of the aneurysm, then distal occlusion would have been pursued by placing temporary distal clips and opening the aneurysm to clean out the edge to allow the aneurysm clip to sit securely on the distal site. The patient remained neurologically intact immediately after surgery and at his 5-month follow-up visit.

Additional case examples are illustrated: EC-IC bypass with distal clip and coil embolization for a giant right fusiform M1 aneurysm (Figures 25–5A through 25–5D), vessel reconstruction with partial clip obliteration of giant fusiform M1 aneurysm involving the right MCA bifurcation having regrowth at 2 years postoperatively for which EC-IC bypass for flow remodeling using saphenous vein graft was done (Figures 25–6A through 25–6G), and distal infectious aneurysm along the right MCA inferior division treated with aneurysm excision and saphenous vein interposition graft (Figures 25–7A through 25–7G).

POTENTIAL COMPLICATIONS

Potential risks and complications include graft thrombosis, anastomotic leak, hemorrhage, stroke, vasospasm, seizures, cerebral spinal fluid (CSF) leak, pseudoaneurysms involving the bypass, aneurysm recurrence, and wound infections. Series of EC-IC bypass grafts in complex aneurysms generally quote patency rates over 84% with mortality less than 10%.[36,39,40] Care must also be taken that the patient avoids wearing compressive glasses, tight hats, or other headwear that would potentially compress and compromise EC-IC graft patency. Early compromise of the bypass graft may be surgically re-explored with thrombectomy or re-anastomosis, intraoperative prophylactic mechanical or topical medication techniques may be used for minimizing vasospasm, endovascular therapies may be attempted for delayed vasospasm, and consideration of new therapeutic approaches need to be devised if pseudoaneurysms involving the bypass graft or recurrence of aneurysm occurs at follow-up.

CONCLUSION

Bypass surgery can be an important technique in the repertoire of the vascular neurosurgeon for the treatment for complex MCA aneurysms in association with surgical or endovascular aneurysm obliteration.

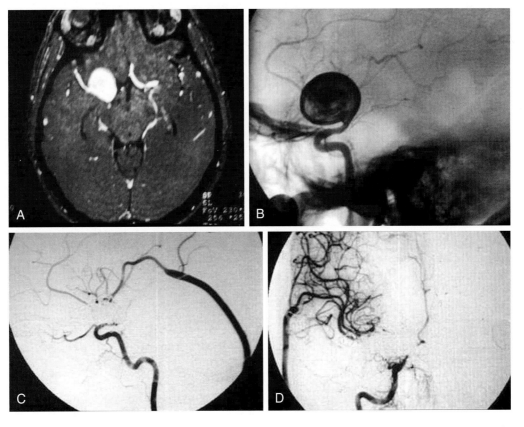

Figure 25–5. MR angiography (MRA) axial view **(A)** and digital subtraction angiography (DSA) lateral view **(B)** demonstrate a giant ~3-cm, right MCA aneurysm extending from the right M1 segment to the right MCA bifurcation in a 38-year-old female nurse having chronic headaches. Following EC-IC bypass with saphenous vein graft and distal clip placement plus endovascular coil embolization of the aneurysm, postprocedural DSA lateral **(C)** and AP **(D)** views show patent EC-IC bypass with coil obliteration of the aneurysm.

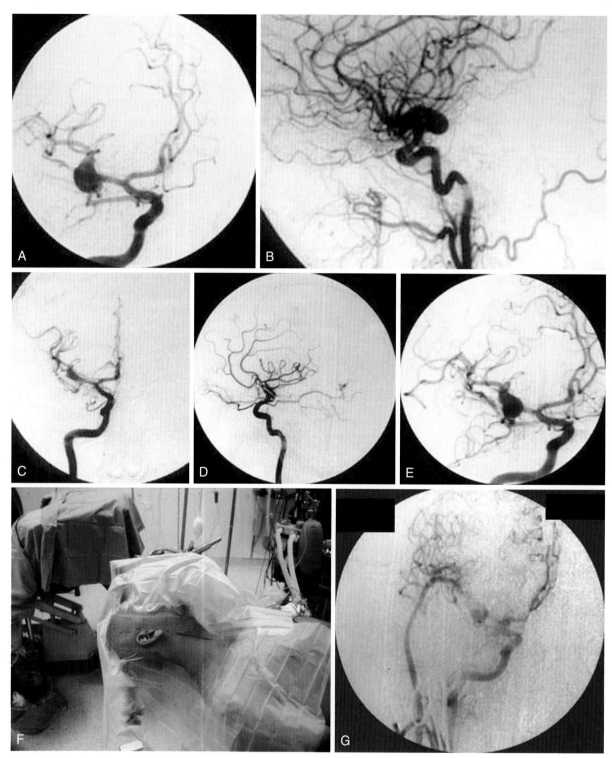

Figure 25–6. Digital subtraction angiography (DSA) with AP **(A)** and lateral **(B)** views reveal a giant fusiform right MCA aneurysm with saccular component involving the distal right M1 segment and MCA bifurcation in a 25-year-old male security guard with chronic headaches and sinus problems. Lenticulostriate perforators emerging from the proximal and distal back walls of the aneurysm were identified intraoperatively. The aneurysm was treated initially with partial clip obliteration using two giant aneurysm clips across the base of the saccular component of the aneurysm with reconstruction of the right MCA in a tubular fashion with preservation of the perforators shown in postoperative DSA in AP **(C)** and lateral **(D)** views. However, recurrence of the aneurysm was noted at 2-year follow-up as demonstrated in DSA right anterior oblique view **(E)**. Patient positioning for a right-sided EC-IC bypass is shown **(F)** with long saphenous vein graft used for end-to-side anastomosis to the donor right ECA and end-to-side anastomosis to the recipient right MCA superior division at a site 1.5 cm distal to the MCA bifurcation with clip placement on the distal M1 segment. Intraoperative DSA AP view **(G)** demonstrates patent EC-IC bypass graft with distal right MCA flow and reduced filling of the aneurysm but continued flow from the right ICA into the proximal right MCA supplying the region of the aneurysm associated with the intraoperatively visualized lenticulostriate perforators.

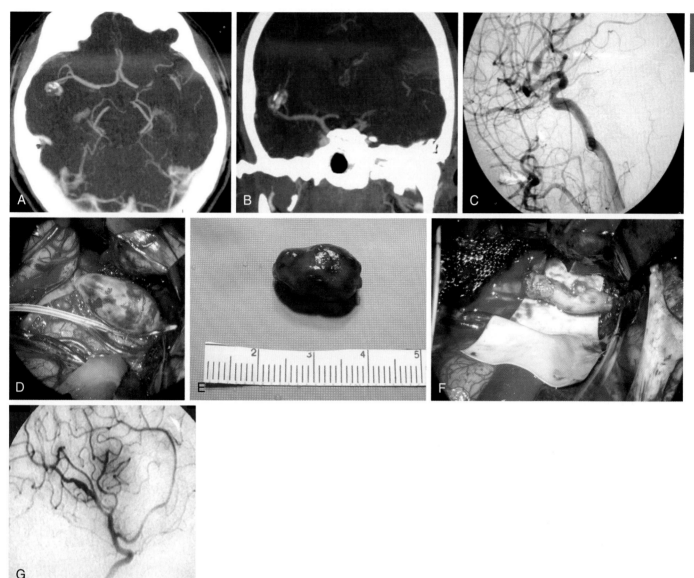

Figure 25–7. CT angiography (CTA) axial **(A)** and coronal **(B)** views along with digital subtraction angiography (DSA) oblique view **(C)** show right distal MCA mycotic aneurysm of fusiform configuration along the right MCA inferior division M2 segment. Intraoperative photograph demonstrates the fusiform right M2 infectious aneurysm with retractors and microsuction in the field **(D)**, and gross pathology specimen photograph of the excised aneurysm is shown **(E)**. Intraoperative photograph illustrates the saphenous vein interposition graft with underlying rubber dam stage **(F)**, and intraoperative DSA oblique view shows good flow through the graft into the distal right MCA **(G)**.

REFERENCES

1. Park SH, Yim MB, Lee CY, et al: Intracranial fusiform aneurysms: its pathogenesis, clinical characteristics and managements, *J Korean Neurosurg Soc* 44:116–123, 2008.

2. Amin-Hanjani S, Butler WE, Ogilvy CS, et al: Extracranial-intracranial bypass in the treatment of occlusive cerebrovascular disease and intracranial aneurysms in the United States between 1992 and 2001: a population-based study, *J Neurosurg* 103:794–804, 2005.

3. Aoki S, Sasaki Y, Machida T, et al: Cerebral aneurysms: detection and delineation using 3-D-CT angiography, *AJNR Am J Neuroradiol* 13:1115–2110, 1992.

4. Hoh BL, Cheung AC, Rabinov JD, et al: Results of a prospective protocol of computed tomographic angiography in place of catheter angiography as the only diagnostic and pretreatment planning study for cerebral aneurysms by a combined neurovascular team, *Neurosurgery* 54:1329–1340, 2004.

5. Napel S, Marks MP, Rubin GD, et al: CT angiography with spiral CT and maximum intensity projection, *Radiology* 185:607–610, 1992.

6. Hoh BL, Putman CM, Budzik RF, et al: Combined surgical and endovascular techniques of flow alteration to treat fusiform and complex wide-necked intracranial aneurysms that are unsuitable for clipping or coil embolization, *J Neurosurg* 95:24–35, 2001.

7. Chen L, Kato Y, Sano H, et al: Management of complex, surgically intractable intracranial aneurysms: the option for intentional reconstruction of aneurysm neck followed by endovascular coiling, *Cerebrovasc Dis* 23:381–387, 2007.

8. Song DL, Leng B, Zhou LF, et al: Onyx in treatment of large and giant cerebral aneurysms and arteriovenous malformations, *Chin Med Journal* 117(12):1869–1872, 2004.

9. Hoh BL, Carter BS, Putman CM, et al: Important factors for a combined neurovascular team to consider in selecting a treatment modality for patients with previously clipped residual and recurrent intracranial aneurysms, *Neurosurgery* 52:732–738, 2003.

10. Karnchanapandh K, Imizu M, Kato Y, et al: Successful obliteration of a ruptured partially thrombosed giant m1 fusiform aneurysm with coil embolization at distal m1 after extracranial-intracranial bypass, *Minim Invasive Neurosurg* 45:245–250, 2002.

11. Nakatomi H, Segawa H, Kurata A, et al: Clinicopathological study of intracranial fusiform and dolichoectatic aneurysms, *Stroke* 31:896, 2000.

12. Yonekawa Y, Zumofen D, Imhof HG, et al: Hemorrhagic cerebral dissecting aneurysms: surgical treatments and results, *Acta Neurochir Suppl* 103:61–69, 2008.

13. Flemming KD, Wiebers DO, Brown RD Jr, et al: The natural history of radiographically defined vertebrobasilar nonsaccular intracranial aneurysms, *Cerebrovasc Dis* 20:270–279, 2005.

14. Lawton MT, Zador ZE, Lu D: Current strategies for complex aneurysms using intracranial bypass and reconstructive techniques, *Jpn J Neurosurg (Tokyo)* 17:601–611, 2008.

15. Sanai N, Zador Z, Lawton MT: Bypass surgery for complex brain aneurysms: as assessment of intracranial-intracranial bypass, *Neurosurgery* 65:670–683, 2009.

16. Takeo G, Kenji O, Akimasa N, et al: Treatment of a fusiform middle cerebral artery aneurysm at M1 part which cause cerebral infarction at its perforating area: a case report, *Surg Cerebral Stroke* 34:59–63, 2006.

17. Ferroli P, Ciceri E, Parati E, et al: Obliteration of a giant fusiform carotid terminus-M1 aneurysm after distal clip application and extracranial-intracranial bypass. Case report, *J Neurosurg Sci* 51:71–76, 2007.

18. Lubicz B, Collignon L, Lefranc F, et al: Circumferential and fusiform intracranial aneurysms: reconstructive endovascular treatment with self-expandable stents, *Neuroradiology* 50:499–507, 2008.

19. Navratil O, Lehecka M, Lehto H, et al: Vascular clamp-assisted clipping of thick-walled giant aneurysms, *Neurosurgery* 64:113–120, 2009.

20. Carter BS, Ogilvy CS, Putman C, et al: Selective use of extracranial-intracranial bypass as an adjunct to therapeutic internal carotid artery occlusion, *Clin Neurosurg* 46:351–362, 2000.

21. Shi ZS, Ziegler J, Duckwiler GR, et al: Management of giant middle cerebral artery aneurysms with incorporated branches: partial endovascular coiling or combined extracranial-intracranial bypass–a team approach, *Neurosurgery* 65:121–129, 2009.

22. Seo BR, Kim TS, Joo SP, et al: Surgical strategies using cerebral revascularization in complex middle cerebral artery aneurysms, *Clin Neurol Neurosurg* 111(8):670–675, 2009.

23. Bojanowski WM, Spetzler RF, Carter LP: Reconstruction of the MCA bifurcation after excision of a giant aneurysm. Technical note, *J Neurosurg* 68:974–977, 1988.

24. Ceylan S, Karakus A, Duru S, et al: Reconstruction of the middle cerebral artery after excision of a giant fusiform aneurysm, *Neurosurg Rev* 21:189–193, 1998.

25. Zhou LF, Jiang DJ: Cerebral artery reconstruction in the treatment of large and giant intracranial aneurysms, *Chin Med J (Engl)* 107:41–46, 1994.

26. El Beltagy M, Muroi C, Imhof HG, et al: Peripheral large or giant fusiform middle cerebral artery aneurysms: report of our experience and review of literature, *Acta Neurochir Suppl* 103:37–44, 2008.

27. Tsutsumida H, Nakamura K, Matsuzaki Y, et al: A case of heart operation in infective endocarditis after brain surgery for mycotic cerebral aneurysm, *Kyobu Geka* 53:229–232, 2000.

28. Uchino T, Hirayama T, Ishikawa M, et al: A case report of early valve replacement surgery in infective endocarditis with mycotic cerebral aneurysm, *Nippon Kyobu Geka Gakkai Zasshi* 37:2025–2028, 1989.

29. Shiraishi Y, Awazu A, Harada T, et al: Valve replacement in a patient with infective endocarditis and ruptured mycotic cerebral aneurysm, *Nippon Kyobu Geka Gakkai Zasshi* 40:118–123, 1992.

30. Nakahara I, Taha MM, Higashi T, et al: Different modalities of treatment of intracranial mycotic aneurysms: report of 4 cases, *Surg Neurol* 66:405–409, 2006.

31. Luders JC, Steinmetz MP, Mayberg MR: Awake craniotomy for microsurgical obliteration of mycotic aneurysms: technical report of three cases, *Neurosurgery* 56:E201, 2005.

32. Kuki S, Yoshida K, Suzuki K, et al: Successful surgical management for multiple cerebral mycotic aneurysms involving both carotid and vertebrobasilar systems in active infective endocarditis, *Eur J Cardiothorac Surg* 8:508–510, 1994.

33. Ferroli P, Bisleri G, Miserocchi A, et al: Endoscopic radial artery harvesting for U-clip high-flow EC-IC bypass: technical report, *Acta Neurochir (Wien)* 151:529–535, 2009.

34. Mery FJ, Amin-Hanjani S, Charbel FT: Cerebral revascularization using cadaveric vein grafts, *Surg Neurol* 72:362–368, 2009.

35. Kocaeli H, Andaluz N, Choutka O, et al: Use of radial artery grafts in extracranial-intracranial revascularization procedures, *Neurosurg Focus* 24:E5, 2008.

36. Scamoni C, Dario A, Castelli P, et al: Extracranial-intracranial bypass for giant aneurysms and complex vascular lesions: a clinical series of 10 patients, *J Neurosurg Sci* 52:1–9, 2008.

37. Charbel FT, Hoffman WE, Misra M, et al: Role of a perivascular ultrasonic micro-flow probe in aneurysm surgery, *Neurol Med Chir (Tokyo)* 38:35–38, 1998.

38. Hecht N, Woitzik J, Dreier JP, et al: Intraoperative monitoring of cerebral blood flow by laser speckle contrast analysis, *Neurosurg Focus* 27:E11, 2009.

39. Cantore G, Santoro A, Guidetti G, et al: Surgical treatment of giant intracranial aneurysms: current viewpoint, *Neurosurgery* 63:279–289, 2008.

40. Sekhar LN, Duff JM, Kalavakonda C, et al: Cerebral revascularization using radial artery grafts for the treatment of complex intracranial aneurysms: techniques and outcomes for 17 patients, *Neurosurgery* 49:646–658, 2001.

BYPASS SURGERY FOR COMPLEX BASILAR TRUNK ANEURYSMS

26

NADER SANAI; ROBERT F. SPETZLER

INTRODUCTION

Mid- and lower-basilar artery aneurysms represent challenging surgical entities. Midbasilar aneurysms can be defined as those affecting the basilar trunk below the level of the superior cerebellar arteries (SCAs) and extending to the anterior inferior cerebellar artery (AICA). Lower basilar aneurysms affect the inferior basilar trunk and the vertebrobasilar junction. Anatomic variability of the vertebrobasilar tree and its branches in relationship to the surrounding anatomy and the configuration, size, and orientation of the aneurysms in this region preclude the universal application of a single operative approach. Each case requires consideration of the particular features of the lesion and selection of an approach that provides the necessary surgical corridor. Endovascular treatments have become increasingly important in the management of these difficult aneurysms, but this chapter focuses on surgical management.

MICROSURGICAL ANATOMY

The basilar artery originates at the junction of the vertebral arteries at the level of the pontomedullary sulcus and ascends anterior to the pons toward its apex in the interpeduncular fossa. The vertebrobasilar junction is typically located near the midline of the clivus at the level of the pontomedullary junction. Numerous perforating branches, in addition to the larger main branches, exit along its course.

The AICA originates near the pontomedullary sulcus and courses around the pons, typically below or between the fascicles of the abducens nerve, to the cerebellopontine angle (CPA). There, it passes between or around cranial nerves (CNs) VII and VIII, which head toward the acoustic meatus. The AICA sends branches to these nerves and to the choroid plexus before it courses posterolaterally to supply the petrosal surface of the cerebellum. The SCA, which originates at the pontomesencephalic sulcus, encircles the midbrain to supply the cerebral peduncles before it courses superiorly and medially to supply the tentorial surface of the cerebellum.

Numerous perforators arise along the entire course of the posterior and lateral surfaces of the basilar artery, but not along its anterior surface. The perforators supply cranial nerve nuclei, reticular centers, and input-output pathways for the cerebrum and cerebellum. Along the midbasilar portion, the long lateral pontine arteries exit and course laterally to supply the paramedian and lateral pons. The medial branches enter the pons near the midline.

CLINICAL PRESENTATION

Mid- and lower-basilar aneurysms are uncommon lesions, accounting for fewer than 1% of all aneurysms in most neurosurgical series.[1,2] Yamaura et al. reported a frequency of 5% (10/202) for posterior circulation aneurysms.[3] In contrast, Drake and Peerless and Peerless et al. reported that mid- and lower-basilar aneurysms accounted for 15.2% (193/1266) of all posterior circulation aneurysms.[4,5] Undoubtedly, however, this higher incidence reflected the referral bias of their institution.

The clinical features of ruptured aneurysms in the mid- and lower-basilar artery location tend to be indistinguishable from subarachnoid hemorrhage (SAH) from other cerebral aneurysms. As with any SAH, sudden headache, nuchal pain, altered mental status, nausea, and vomiting are the typical manifestations. Intraparenchymal bleeding, which can be associated with anterior circulation aneurysms, is rarely a feature of these aneurysms. As with other posterior circulation aneurysms, the natural history of these aneurysms appears to be that of high rupture rates.[5] Unruptured giant aneurysms can produce neurological symptoms specific to their anatomic location, ranging from isolated cranial neuropathies to brainstem compression syndromes.

Fusiform and dissecting aneurysms are more common in the posterior circulation than in the anterior circulation and are associated with a poor prognosis.[6] Large dolichoectatic aneurysms involving the basilar trunk and vertebral arteries may be the result of dissection with subsequent fusiform degeneration of the artery, progressive enlargement, and luminal thrombosis or may be a consequence of intracranial atherosclerosis. These lesions are particularly challenging and often require indirect approaches for their obliteration compared to the standard direct clipping techniques most often used for saccular aneurysms.

MANAGEMENT PRINCIPLES

Patients presenting with SAH from mid- or lower-basilar artery aneurysms are managed according to the same general principles as patients with aneurysmal SAH in general: cardiorespiratory and basic neurological supportive care, early ventriculostomy in patients with a poor Hunt and Hess grade, early surgery in suitable patients, and aggressive management of increased intracranial pressure and vasospasm. Patients with neurological symptoms related to the mass effect of an aneurysm are managed semi-urgently. These patients typically exhibit signs of brainstem compression or cranial nerve deficits, which must be considered when planning both the surgical approach and timing of surgery.

Standard intraoperative management is utilized. Intraoperative hypotension is avoided. In fact, intraoperative blood pressure is allowed to run mildly hypertensive, especially during temporary vessel clipping. For brain protection, all patients receive intravenous doses of barbiturates (pentobarbital) to achieve electroencephalographic burst suppression. As required, brain relaxation is achieved with hyperventilation, mannitol, barbiturates, or spinal drainage of cerebrospinal fluid (CSF). Comprehensive electrophysiological monitoring is used routinely:[7] somatosensory-evoked potentials, brainstem auditory responses (in both ears or the contralateral ear alone if ipsilateral hearing is to be sacrificed), and monitoring of the facial nerve and other appropriate CNs.

SURGICAL OVERVIEW

The general principles for surgical treatment of aneurysms located in this part of the basilar artery are the same as those for any aneurysm.[6,8–17] The main surgical difference relates to the anatomical considerations specific to the constrained aneurysm locations and the surrounding vital neuroanatomy. Regardless, the primary endpoint for the surgeon should be complete obliteration of the aneurysm from the circulation, with preservation of the parent vessels, particularly the perforators supplying the brainstem.

To achieve optimal aneurysm obliteration, maximal exposure of the basilar artery and the aneurysm itself is required. This exposure must be achieved without exposing the brain or critical structures to undue retraction while simultaneously obtaining adequate control of the parent vessel and aneurysm. Given the challenges of exposure in this region, specialized operative approaches are often necessary. In some cases, such

approaches must be combined with the technique of hypothermic cardiac standstill.[18–22] Alternatively, additional methods may be used for revascularization to allow proximal artery occlusion or trapping of the aneurysm.

SURGICAL DECISION MAKING

Depending on the specific anatomy and configuration of the aneurysm, the following approaches can be appropriate. Moving from superior to inferior, the following approaches provide overlapping access to the mid- and lower-basilar artery: subtemporal, extended orbitozygomatic approach, transpetrosal approach, lateral suboccipital-retrosigmoid, and far-lateral. Combinations of these approaches (combined supra- and infratentorial approach and combined-combined) can extend exposure as sometimes needed for large aneurysms.

The various approaches that provide overlapping amounts of exposure can be seen in Figure 26–1. Typically, the subtemporal and orbitozygomatic approaches are used for basilar tip lesions, but the extended orbitozygomatic approach can provide access to the upper two-fifths of the basilar artery. Some aneurysms of the basilar trunk below the SCAs can be approached in this manner. The transpetrosal provides exposure further inferiorly, allowing the middle three-fifths of the basilar trunk to be accessed. With the combined supra- and infratentorial approach, access can be extended down to the vertebrobasilar junction. The far-lateral approach gives access primarily to the lower two-fifths of the basilar artery and is suitable for vertebrobasilar junction aneurysms. Both the far-lateral and extended orbitozygomatic approaches

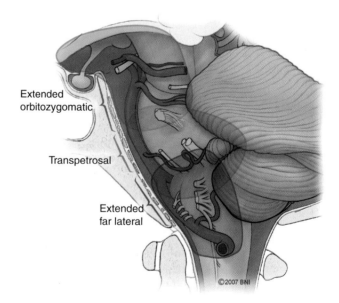

Extended orbitozygomatic

Transpetrosal

Extended far lateral

©2007 BNI

Figure 26–1 Approaches to the basilar artery, divided in thirds. The upper third can be accessed through an orbitozygomatic approach. The middle third can be approached via the transpetrosal route. The lower third is accessible through a far-lateral craniotomy.

(With permission from the Barrow Neurological Institute.)

provide a view along the aneurysm neck, allowing a clip to be applied along this line of sight. In contrast, however, the transpetrosal approach exposes the aneurysm sac between the surgeon and the neck. A right-angled clip is required, increasing the technical difficulty of clip application (Figure 26–2).

There is still a role for the standard subtemporal craniotomy and lateral suboccipital/retrosigmoid craniotomy in approaching the upper-mid and mid-lower basilar artery, respectively, especially given that the more extensive approaches such as radical petrosectomy are associated with inherent morbidity. These standard craniotomies can be used for small, favorably located, unruptured aneurysms. Adequate brain relaxation is required. A combination of diuretics and CSF drainage can be used to allow clipping without the application of undue retraction.

At our institution, a standard retrosigmoid craniotomy has been found to be adequate for small-to-medium aneurysms associated with the AICA along the lower two-thirds of the clivus. For larger aneurysms, however, the routine lateral suboccipital or retrosigmoid approach may not adequately expose the mid- or lower-basilar trunk without an unacceptable amount of cerebellar or brainstem retraction. For aneurysms involving the basilar trunk above the vertebral bifurcation, the transpetrosal approaches increase rostral exposure for distal

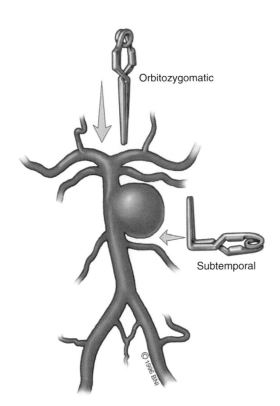

Orbitozygomatic

Subtemporal

©1996 BNI

Figure 26–2 Variations in the operative approach to the basilar artery translate to variations in surgical clip strategy. Far-lateral and extended orbitozygomatic approaches provide a view along the neck of the aneurysm, allowing a clip to be applied along this line of sight. The transpetrosal approach exposes the aneurysmal sac between the surgeon and the neck, necessitating a right-angle clip.
(With permission from the Barrow Neurological Institute.)

control and decrease the operative distance to the lesion. Even the extent of this exposure, especially for larger aneurysms, can be limited, leading to the utility of the combined approaches. The combined supra- and infratentorial approach with its appropriate variations permits exquisite surgical exposure for dealing with most aneurysms involving the mid- and lower-basilar artery. The far-lateral approach, alone or in combination with other approaches, provides excellent access to the lower basilar and vertebrobasilar junction.

OPERATIVE APPROACHES

Aneurysms of the mid- and lower-basilar artery pose a difficult challenge because they are located in a small, restricted area encased with bone and situated within a limited subarachnoid space filled with a dense collection of vital neurovascular structures. All these elements must be considered when an approach is planned. The basic principles of aneurysm surgery still apply: (1) proximal and distal vascular control, (2) preservation of parent vessels and all perforators, and (3) complete obliteration of the aneurysm.

Next, the anatomical concerns specific to this region must be accommodated. In the past, these aneurysms were treated through a subtemporal-transtentorial approach or through the suboccipital approach. A transoral or transmaxillary-transclival approach has also been used,[23] but exposure is limited and the risks of postoperative CSF leakage and meningitis are significant. Although these approaches can provide access to aneurysms of the mid- and lower-basilar artery, they seldom provide maximal exposure with minimal retraction. Consequently, the subtemporal and lateral suboccipital/retrosigmoid approaches are often superseded by more extensive skull base approaches that maximize lateral bone removal to provide a shorter and flatter route of access to the anterior brainstem and basilar artery (Figure 26–3). The basic tenets of these approaches and their application to mid- and lower-basilar artery aneurysms are reviewed.

Extended Orbitozygomatic Approach

The standard orbitozygomatic craniotomy, which has been well described for the management of tumors and aneurysms of the upper basilar artery,[14,24–27] can be modified to allow access to the upper aspect of the midbasilar trunk.

Transpetrosal

The transpetrosal approach encompasses a range of approaches with various extents of bony dissection that provide differential degrees of exposure to the anterior brainstem and clival region (Figure 26–4).[28–30] Overall, this approach provides a lateral trajectory to the basilar trunk through a presigmoid corridor by

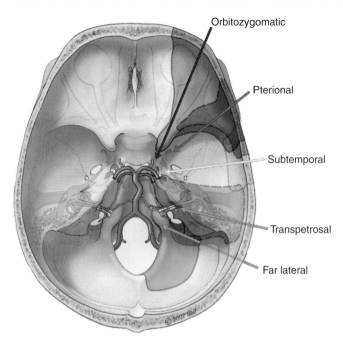

Figure 26–3 Microsurgical corridors to the skull base and basilar artery. *(With permission from the Barrow Neurological Institute.)*

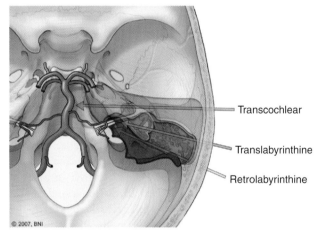

Figure 26–4 Transpetrosal approaches to the basilar trunk. *(With permission from the Barrow Neurological Institute.)*

drilling through the petrous aspect of the temporal bone. This approach can afford good proximal and distal control and is usually undertaken ipsilateral to the side of the aneurysm. The lateral angle of approach can place the aneurysm dome between the surgeon and the site of clip application at the neck of the aneurysm. However, a contralateral approach often mandates more complex clip strategies, including the use of fenestrated clips and a subsequent increase in the potential for perforator injury. The trajectory places the CNs in the foreground of the operative field, although this is true of all exposures to this region other than the direct anterior transoral or transclival.

The transpetrosal approach can be divided into three variations (see Figure 26–4): the retrolabyrinthine approach (which involves petrous bone resection between the semicircular canals anteriorly and the posterior fossa dura on the posterior aspect of the temporal bone). Hearing is preserved. The translabyrinthine approach removes more of the petrous bone (including the semicircular canals, thereby increasing exposure anteriorly to the internal auditory canal), and sacrifices hearing. The transcochlear approach involves maximal petrous bony resection by transposing the facial nerve posteriorly and allowing access for removal of the cochlea. Hearing is sacrificed and injury to the facial nerve is a risk. In each variation the amount of petrous bone resection increases with a resultant increase in exposure of the anterior brainstem and basilar trunk.

Far-Lateral Approach

The far-lateral approach extends to the unilateral suboccipital-retrosigmoid approach, which has been standard in neurosurgery for many years. This modification greatly enhances the anterior exposure of the inferior aspect of the clivus, thereby providing excellent access to the lower-basilar artery and vertebrobasilar junction. The primary principle is to achieve a flat exposure to the anterior aspect of the inferior brainstem and to the associated neurovascular structures and CNs. To do so, the inferior rim of the foramen magnum, part of the occipital condyle, and the posterolateral arch of C1 to the level of the sulcus arteriosus of the vertebral artery are removed. The dural opening afforded by this bony removal provides maximal exposure with minimal retraction of neurovascular structures.

Combined Supratentorial/Infratentorial Approach

The exposure of the basilar artery provided by the transpetrosal approach can be enhanced dramatically when combined with a supratentorial approach. Using this combined supra- and infratentorial surgical approach can provide exposure extending from the sphenoid ridge and cavernous sinus to the foramen magnum. The skills of both the neurosurgeon and neuro-otologist are combined. There are three key elements to the approach: (1) variable degrees of temporal bone dissection in conjunction with (2) a supra- and infratentorial craniotomy, and (3) division of the tentorium to connect the supra- and infratentorial compartments. These maneuvers allow extensive exposure of the clivus, medial petrous region, and associated neurovascular structures with a minimum amount of brain retraction.

Variations of this combined approach with various degrees of petrosal resection and various ways of handling the sigmoid sinus (mobilization vs. transection) have been described. Some authors have presented their experience using variations of the combined infratemporal and posterior fossa approach for the removal of large lesions involving the clivus and medial petrous region. Some have advocated preservation of the major dural sinus. Others, with appropriate consideration for the patency of the opposite transverse sinus, sacrifice the sigmoid or transverse sinus. At our institution, the initial

26

experience with the approach was associated with no operative mortality. The rates of postoperative morbidity compared favorably to previous reports: facial nerve palsy, 30%; CSF leakage, 13%; CN VI palsy, 7%; and other neurologic (aphasia, hemiparesis) and non-neurologic complications (pneumonia, hematoma), 2% to 4%.

REVASCULARIZATION

Although the primary surgical goal in the management of aneurysms is direct clip obliteration with preservation of the parent vessel, not all aneurysms are amenable to this approach.[31-33] Large aneurysms especially can incorporate the parent vessel to such an extent that clip reconstruction is infeasible. The extreme example of this situation is fusiform vertebrobasilar dolichoectatic aneurysms or dissecting aneurysms, but even large saccular aneurysms can behave in this fashion. Under these circumstances, the remaining options are trapping of the aneurysmal segment or proximal occlusion to alter the flow dynamics in the region of the aneurysm to induce regression and spontaneous thrombosis.[34,35]

For mid- and lower-basilar lesions, direct trapping may be less desirable because of the potential risk to adjacent perforators.[36] However, proximal or even distal basilar occlusion can serve to abolish the aneurysm effectively.[37] For large fusiform dolichoectatic aneurysms, proximal occlusion of one or both vertebral arteries can reverse blood flow in a similar fashion by removing the hemodynamic wall stress thought to play a role in the growth of these degenerative lesions. If the caliber of the posterior communicating arteries is insufficient to provide adequate blood flow, this strategy must be combined with a bypass to the upper basilar territory. In such cases, the donor and recipient vessels depend on blood flow requirements and the availability of suitable vessels. For basilar trunk lesions, the distal basilar territory typically needs to be revascularized.[38,39] Doing so can be accomplished with a STA donor or interposition graft from the external carotid artery anastomosed to the posterior cerebral artery or SCA. Posterior circulation bypasses tend to be technically demanding due to the depth at which the anastomosis must be performed. These procedures are associated with the general risks of any vascular surgery within the posterior circulation in addition to the more specific risks of graft failure and ischemia. In certain cases, however, revascularization and proximal occlusion strategy are the best feasible options.

Surgical approaches to the revascularization of the posterior circulation include revascularization of mid-basilar artery lesions with an STA-PCA or STA-SCA bypass. A vertebral artery aneurysm can be trapped and revascularized with a PICA-PICA in situ bypass or with an OA-PICA bypass. In either scenario, endovascular coils placed within the vertebral artery can be used to occlude the vertebral artery once the bypass has been achieved. Using the vast armamentarium of available surgical and

endovascular techniques, most giant aneurysms can be treated successfully.

FLOW REDIRECTION

Flow-redirection techniques can be used for aneurysms involving the basilar artery.[40] When an aneurysm cannot be removed from the circulation, the goal is to alter the hemodynamics at the lesion by changing the direction of blood flow. One approach involves a two-stage treatment paradigm. The first procedure consists of revascularization through an STA-SCA bypass, followed by a two-stage endovascular treatment. Another approach is unilateral occlusion of the vertebral artery proximal to the PICA, followed by contralateral vertebral artery occlusion distal to the PICA. The goal in delaying occlusion of the second vertebral artery is to provide the graft with time to mature. Ultimately, one PICA depends on back-flow from the basilar artery, and this demand is thought to help prevent basilar thrombosis, thus maintaining flow from the bypass to the basilar artery and the brainstem-perforating vessels.

CONCLUSION

Recent developments in endovascular techniques now provide additional options for the management of these difficult lesions. Nonetheless, for many lesions, surgical management remains an important and necessary aspect of treatment. An understanding of the unique anatomical considerations and choices regarding surgical access is therefore still paramount.

REFERENCES

1. Anson JA, Lawton MT, Spetzler RF: Characteristics and surgical treatment of dolichoectatic and fusiform aneurysms, *J Neurosurg* 84:185–193, 1996.
2. Higa T, Ujiie H, Kato K, et al: Basilar artery trunk saccular aneurysms: morphological characteristics and management, *Neurosurg Rev* 32:181–191, 2009.
3. Yamaura A, Ise H, Makino H: Treatment of aneurysms arising from the terminal portion of the basilar artery—with special reference to the radiometric study and accessibility of trans-sylvian approach, *Neurol Med Chir (Tokyo)* 22:521–532, 1982.
4. Drake CG, Peerless SJ: Giant fusiform intracranial aneurysms: review of 120 patients treated surgically from 1965 to 1992, *J Neurosurg* 87:141–162, 1997.
5. Peerless SJ, Nemoto S, Drake CG: Acute surgery for ruptured posterior circulation aneurysms, *Adv Tech Stand Neurosurg* 15:115–129, 1987.
6. Sanai N, Tarapore P, Lee AC, et al: The current role of microsurgery for posterior circulation aneurysms: a selective approach in the endovascular era, *Neurosurgery* 62:1236–1249, 2008.
7. Quinones-Hinojosa A, Alam M, Lyon R, et al: Transcranial motor evoked potentials during basilar artery aneurysm surgery: technique application for 30 consecutive patients, *Neurosurgery* 54:916–924, 2004.

8. Cantore G, Santoro A, Guidetti G, et al: Surgical treatment of giant intracranial aneurysms: current viewpoint, *Neurosurgery* 63(Suppl 2): 279–289, 2008.

9. Fiorella D, Kelly ME, Albuquerque FC, et al: Curative reconstruction of a giant midbasilar trunk aneurysm with the pipeline embolization device, *Neurosurgery* 64:212–217, 2009.

10. Hassan T, Ezura M, Takahashi A: Treatment of giant fusiform aneurysms of the basilar trunk with intra-aneurysmal and basilar artery coil embolization, *Surg Neurol* 62:455–462, 2004.

11. Inamasu J, Suga S, Sato S, et al: Long-term outcome of 17 cases of large-giant posterior fossa aneurysm, *Clin Neurol Neurosurg* 102: 65–71, 2000.

12. Kang HS, Oh CW, Han MH, et al: Treatment of a sequential giant fusiform aneurysm of the basilar trunk, *Korean J Radiol* 6:125–129, 2005.

13. Kimura T, Onda K, Arai H: Multiple basilar artery trunk aneurysms associated with fibromuscular dysplasia, *Acta Neurochir (Wien)* 146:79–81, 2004.

14. Lawton MT, Daspit CP, Spetzler RF: Technical aspects and recent trends in the management of large and giant midbasilar artery aneurysms, *Neurosurgery* 41:513–520, 1997.

15. Ponce FA, Albuquerque FC, McDougall CG, et al: Combined endovascular and microsurgical management of giant and complex unruptured aneurysms, *Neurosurg Focus* 17:E11, 2004.

16. Uda K, Murayama Y, Gobin YP, et al: Endovascular treatment of basilar artery trunk aneurysms with Guglielmi detachable coils: clinical experience with 41 aneurysms in 39 patients, *J Neurosurg* 95: 624–632, 2001.

17. Van Rooij WJ, Sluzewski M, Menovsky T, et al: Coiling of saccular basilar trunk aneurysms, *Neuroradiology* 45:19–21, 2003.

18. Greene KA, Marciano FF, Hamilton MG, et al: Cardiopulmonary bypass, hypothermic circulatory arrest and barbiturate cerebral protection for the treatment of giant vertebrobasilar aneurysms in children, *Pediatr Neurosurg* 21:124–133, 1994.

19. Kato Y, Sano H, Zhou J, et al: Deep hypothermia cardiopulmonary bypass and direct surgery of two large aneurysms at the vertebrobasilar junction, *Acta Neurochir (Wien)* 138:1057–1066, 1996.

20. Mack WJ, Ducruet AF, Angevine PD, et al: Deep hypothermic circulatory arrest for complex cerebral aneurysms: lessons learned, *Neurosurgery* 60:815–827, 2007.

21. Spetzler RF, Hadley MN, Rigamonti D, et al: Aneurysms of the basilar artery treated with circulatory arrest, hypothermia, and barbiturate cerebral protection, *J Neurosurg* 68:868–879, 1988.

22. Yu CL, Tan PP, Wu CT, et al: Anesthesia with deep hypothermic circulatory arrest for giant basilar aneurysm surgery, *Acta Anaesthesiol Sin* 38:47–51, 2000.

23. Saito I, Takahashi H, Joshita H, et al: Clipping of vertebro-basilar aneurysms by the transoral transclival approach, *Neurol Med Chir (Tokyo)* 20:753–758, 1980.

24. Bambakidis NC, Kakarla UK, Kim LJ, et al: Evolution of surgical approaches in the treatment of petroclival meningiomas: a retrospective review, *Neurosurgery* 62(Suppl 3):1182–1191, 2008.

25. Hsu FP, Clatterbuck RE, Spetzler RF: Orbitozygomatic approach to basilar apex aneurysms, *Neurosurgery* 56(Suppl):172–177, 2005.

26. Lemole GM Jr, Henn JS, Zabramski JM, et al: Modifications to the orbitozygomatic approach. Technical note, *J Neurosurg* 99:924–930, 2003.

27. Zabramski JM, Kiris T, Sankhla SK, et al: Orbitozygomatic craniotomy. Technical note, *J Neurosurg* 89:336–341, 1998.

28. Inoue Y, Mikami J, Omiya N, et al: Subtemporal transpetrosal approach to ruptured midbasilar trunk aneurysm, *Skull Base Surg* 2:98–102, 1992.

29. Rosenberg SI, Flamm ES, Hoffer ME, et al: The retrolabyrinthine transsigmoid approach to midbasilar artery aneurysms, *Laryngoscope* 102:100–104, 1992.

30. Terasaka S, Itamoto K, Houkin K: Basilar trunk aneurysm surgically treated with anterior petrosectomy and external carotid artery-to-posterior cerebral artery bypass: technical note, *Neurosurgery* 51:1083–1087, 2002.

31. Jafar JJ, Russell SM, Woo HH: Treatment of giant intracranial aneurysms with saphenous vein extracranial-to-intracranial bypass grafting: indications, operative technique, and results in 29 patients, *Neurosurgery* 51:138–144, 2002.

32. Lawton MT, Hamilton MG, Morcos JJ, et al: Revascularization and aneurysm surgery: current techniques, indications, and outcome, *Neurosurgery* 38:83–92, 1996.

33. Nabika S, Oki S, Migita K, et al: Dissecting basilar artery aneurysm growing during long-term follow up—case report, *Neurol Med Chir (Tokyo)* 42:560–564, 2002.

34. Ewald C, Kuhne D, Hassler W: Giant basilar artery aneurysms incorporating the posterior cerebral artery: bypass surgery and coil occlusion—two case reports, *Neurol Med Chir (Tokyo)* 38(Suppl): 83–85, 1998.

35. Wenderoth JD, Khangure MS, Phatouros CC, et al: Basilar trunk occlusion during endovascular treatment of giant and fusiform aneurysms of the basilar artery, *AJNR Am J Neuroradiol* 24:1226–1229, 2003.

36. Ricolfi F, Decq P, Brugieres P, et al: Ruptured fusiform aneurysm of the superior third of the basilar artery associated with the absence of the midbasilar artery. Case report, *J Neurosurg* 85:961–965, 1996.

37. Ali MJ, Bendok BR, Tella MN, et al: Arterial reconstruction by direct surgical clipping of a basilar artery dissecting aneurysm after failed vertebral artery occlusion: technical case report and literature review, *Neurosurgery* 52:1475–1480, 2003.

38. Horie N, Kitagawa N, Morikawa M, et al: Giant thrombosed fusiform aneurysm at the basilar trunk successfully treated with endovascular coil occlusion following bypass surgery: a case report and review of the literature, *Neurol Res* 29:842–846, 2007.

39. Russell SM, Post N, Jafar JJ: Revascularizing the upper basilar circulation with saphenous vein grafts: operative technique and lessons learned, *Surg Neurol* 66:285–297, 2006.

40. Amin-Hanjani S, Ogilvy CS, Buonanno FS, et al: Treatment of dissecting basilar artery aneurysm by flow reversal, *Acta Neurochir (Wien)* 139:44–51, 1997.

SURGICAL REVASCULARIZATION OF THE POSTERIOR CIRCULATION

27

LALIGAM N. SEKHAR; DINESH RAMANATHAN; LOUIS KIM;
DANIAL HALLAM; BASAVARAJ GHODKE

INTRODUCTION

Revascularization of the posterior circulation may be critical in order to prevent a major stroke during the treatment of aneurysms, and certain cases of intractable ischemia and skull base tumors. Aneurysms requiring revascularization generally involve situations not amenable to endovascular surgery such as fusiform or blister aneurysms, origin of vessels from the aneurysm sac, or failure with maximal endovascular interventions. Strokes in the posterior circulation can be devastating, whether they occur due to perforator occlusion, or due to the occlusion of the major arteries. A careful understanding of the anatomy of the patient, the operative approaches, and the techniques of revascularization is needed in order to achieve good outcomes.

SURGICAL ANATOMY AND COLLATERAL CIRCULATION

Most patients have two patent vertebral arteries (VAs), and the left one is usually dominant. In some patients, one of the arteries ends in the PICA, or is occluded by atherosclerotic disease, which makes the inflow situation more tenuous. At the upper end, the posterior communicating arteries connect the ICAs with the PCAs; however, the size of these is variable. When there are two posterior communicating arteries (PCOM) that are 1 mm. or more in size, then the patient may safely tolerate basilar artery (BA)[1] or bilateral VA occlusion, but in patients who have less than optimal collaterals (e.g., only one PCOM of $\geq$1 mm in size), the revascularization must be considered, prior to occlusion. Other variants may include bilateral (or unilateral) fetal PCOMs, fenestrations of the vertebrobasilar junction, persistent trigeminal arteries (with varying degrees of contribution to the upper BA), etc.

In general, younger patients without significant comorbidities such as heart disease, hypertension, or diabetes are able to withstand vascular occlusions better than older patients, who may be smokers and/or have chronic hypertension, diabetes, and hypercholesterolemia. Connective tissue disorders such as Marfan's disease will also need to be taken into account in planning surgery. In patients about to undergo elective surgery, every attempt should be made to modify risk factors. This includes moderate ($<$140 to 160 mm systolic pressure) control of the blood pressure, oral statins to lower cholesterol, and smoking cessation. Patients who may undergo revascularization for ischemia should also be worked up for hypercoagulable disorders.

ENDOVASCULAR ALTERNATIVES

In patients with aneurysms, or ischemic disease, endovascular treatment assisted by endoluminal stents (stent with coiling, or angioplasty followed by a stent) may be an alternative.[2–4] Based on the patient's age and other risk factors, this should be discussed with the patient. Centers where the microsurgical treatment is performed should also have the appropriate endovascular expertise, and collaboration.

ANESTHESIA AND NEURO MONITORING

All patients who undergo general anesthesia for posterior circulation procedures should be managed by a neuroanesthesiologist, with specialized training in bypass procedures. In our center, most such patients are managed under total intravenous anesthesia, to permit the monitoring of somatosensory-evoked potentials (SSEP), and motor-evoked potentials (MEPs). The brainstem-evoked response and some cranial nerve functions (CNs 7, 8, 10, 11, 12) may also be monitored during such procedures.

All patients are maintained on antiplatelet therapy with aspirin 81 mg per oral on the day of surgery, and postoperatively. For all EC-IC bypass grafts, we administer 2000 to

2500 units of heparin intravenously after the clamping of the vessels. During the temporary occlusion of arteries, the patient is placed in burst suppression with propofol. In patients with unruptured aneurysms, ischemia, or basal tumors, blood pressure is raised 20% over the baseline to improve the collateral circulation. If MEP changes during the occlusion, then the BP can be raised further. The BA cannot be clamped longer than 15 minutes without adverse consequences. If prolonged clamping is needed, then the patient should be placed in deep hypothermic circulatory arrest.

SKULL BASE APPROACHES

For operations involving bypass procedures, and for complex posterior circulation aneurysms in general, skull base approaches are essential. The correct approach to use for each case is determined by a careful study of the aneurysm anatomy, along with the landmarks on the skull, and the experience of the surgeon. The most common approaches used are the orbitozygomatic approach, the transpetrosal approach (retrolabyrinthine approach, or partial labyrynthectomy petrous apicectomy approach, and rarely, a total petrosectomy approach), a combined far-lateral retrosigmoid approach, the presigmoid approach (with the division and resuture of the sigmoid sinus in some patients), and the extreme lateral transtubercular approach.[5] Some of the complex approaches take time to develop, and in elective cases, a staged approach is taken, with the approach being performed on one day, and the definitive operation on another day.

BYPASS PROCEDURES

Two types of bypasses are used: in situ bypass procedures and bypass procedures using graft vessels for flow diversion. Bypasses using graft vessels such as the radial artery graft (RAG) and SV graft are generally high flow and can be either EC-IC (connecting extracranial vessel to intracranial vessel) or IC-IC (connecting two intracranial vessels). In general, the type of bypass performed depends upon the need (small vessel replacement needs an in situ or low-flow bypass, whereas large vessel replacement will require a high-flow bypass). The availability of donor and recipient vessels, and graft vessels, is also a factor. A bypass can only replace major vessels, and cannot solve perforator problems. In some patients with unruptured aneurysms, a distal (rather than proximal) occlusion of the aneurysm may be used in order to protect the flow through the perforating vessels. EC-IC bypasses include low-flow bypasses such as the superficial temporal to the superior cerebellar artery, and an occipital (OC) to PICA anastomosis (OC-PICA bypass), and high-flow bypasses that encompass RAGs or SV grafts. The choice between the RAG and the SVG is

based on the size of the available donor vessel (diameter >0.23 cm for the RAG, and 0.3 cm for the SV), the passage of the Allen test for the RAG, and an adequate length available (at least 20 cm) for the SVG. We make this determination on the basis of a preoperative duplex examination. For RAGs, the use of the pressure distension technique has revolutionized the patency rate, by greatly reducing the incidence of postoperative vasospasm (Figure 27–1).[6] High-flow bypasses are generally constructed from the ipsilateral VA, or the ECA, to end in the VA, or the PCA. In one case, the bypass was placed directly into the BA, under deep hypothermic circulatory arrest.

In situ bypasses are technically easier to perform than EC-IC bypasses. In situ bypasses include reimplantation of arteries, short interposition grafts, direct resuture of vessels, and side-to-side anastomosis. Reimplantation of vessels can be done in an end-to-side fashion after the resection of the aneurysm from which the vessel originates. Segmental resection with an interposition graft of similar caliber is performed when an aneurysm involves a segment of a vessel (e.g., fusiform aneurysm). Side-to-side anastomosis in posterior circulation is performed for flow replacement when clipping of aneurysm will result in total occlusion (or critical stenosis) of a small artery. Both the vessels of the anastomosis need to be approximately of the same caliber. Aneurysms involving PICA, AICA, or SCA can be addressed with PICA-PICA to AICA-PICA, or SCA-PICA, anastomosis (Table 27–1).[7,8] Side-to-side anastomosis is a comparatively easier technique to perform for a small-vessel revascularization and generally stays patent (there were no known occlusions in our series) (Figure 27–2).[7]

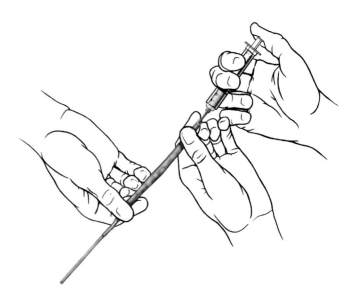

Figure 27–1. Pressure distention technique: distention of the radial artery with saline injection while distally occluding the graft with fingers. *(Courtesy of Laligam Sekhar.)*

Table 27–1. BYPASS PROCEDURES PERFORMED FOR VARIOUS CONDITIONS IN POSTERIOR CIRCULATION.

	Treatment	Total number
Aneurysms		
Basilar tip aneurysms	M2 MCA to P2 PCA with microsurgical clipping (2), ECA to P2 PCA with distal basilar occlusion (1)	3
Midbasilar aneurysms	V3 VA to P2 PCA (SVG or RAG) with distal occlusion of basilar artery	5
Vertebral artery aneurysms	V3 VA to PCA with occlusion of vertebral artery	4
AICA aneurysms	AICA-PICA in situ side-to-side anastomosis	1
PICA aneurysms	OC-PICA anastomosis CCA to PICA RAG with occlusion of PICA (1), PICA to PICA (1)	10
Ischemia		
Vertebral dissections	V3 VA to P2 PCA (SVG or RAG), with occlusion of vertebral artery	3
Tumors		
Chordoma	V3 VA to P3 PCA (SVG or RAG) with gross total resection tumor along with encased portion of vertebral artery	5
Giant cell tumor (foramen magnum)	SVG interposition graft for vertebral artery with gross total resection of tumor	4
Meningioma (foramen magnum)	Vertebral artery resection and anastomosis, and gross total resection of tumor	7

AICA, anterior inferior cerebellar artery; MCA, middle cerebral artery; PCA, posterior cerebral artery; PICA, posterior inferior cerebellar artery; SCA, superior cerebellar artery; VA, vertebral artery.

FOLLOW-UP

After a bypass operation, we perform an indocyanine green (ICG) angiogram to check the patency, and the speed of flow. The patient is monitored with Doppler flow probes in the postoperative period, and a cerebral angiogram is performed on the first postoperative day. In some patients, the postoperative angiogram may be performed the same evening, and may be repeated after 3 to 7 days, to verify aneurysmal thrombosis. Patients are maintained on aspirin 81 mg orally for at least 3 months, and subcutaneous heparin 5000 units twice daily for prophylaxis against deep venous thrombosis for about a week. Further postoperative follow-up examinations can be done by Duplex examinations, and CT angiography. We generally obtain a postoperative angiogram at 12 to 18 months.

CASE EXAMPLES

Patient 1

This 72-year-old woman presented with a subarachnoid hemorrhage (Hunt and Hess 4) secondary to a ruptured basilar tip aneurysm and was initially treated by endovascular coiling. She had various strokes during the hospitalization, and sustained permanent right third nerve palsy, but recovered to be independent for all daily living activities. Follow-up angiograms showed aneurysm recurrence due to coil compaction with the entire aneurysm mass measuring 21 × 19 × 25 mm, causing significant brainstem compression. She had four additional coiling procedures over the previous 5-year follow-up period (see Figures 27–1, 27–2A and 27–2B). Her examination indicated a right third nerve palsy, memory difficulties, and mild gait ataxia, and no other deficits. Her functional status was graded as modified Rankin score (mRS) 2.

During the clipping procedure, with a frontotemporal craniotomy and orbitozygotomy approach because of the coil mass, it was felt that the clip blades might slide onto the right PCA, or both PCAs during the clipping procedure. A RAG bypass surgery was performed from the right middle cerebral artery to the right PCA-P2 segment, under propofol-induced burst suppression, moderate induced hypertension, and mild anticoagulation. Following the bypass, the aneurysm could be clipped, albeit with significant narrowing of the right PCA by the clip due to the "funnel effect" caused by the coils.

The patient suffered a transient neurological decline postoperatively, but recovered significantly with fluid administration. She recuperated in a rehabilitation facility, with recovery to her baseline at about 3 months. An angiogram immediately after the operation showed excellent flow through the bypass into the PCA, and occlusion of the aneurysm (Figure 27–3 and Figures 27–4A and 27–4B). Delayed angiography at 3 months showed sluggish flow through the bypass. Angiography at 18 months postoperatively demonstrated the complete occlusion of the bypass and the aneurysm, but good filling of the right PCA from the BA and through the right PCOM artery (Figures 27–4C and 27–4D). At this time, and at 4 years postoperatively, the patient was independent for activities of daily life. Her gait ataxia was worse than her preoperative baseline, with the patient needing a cane, and not driving. But she was mentally alert with a good memory, and able to go out to restaurants, exercise, and socialize (mRS 2).

Patient 2

A 62-year-old woman presented with progressive deterioration in her daily abilities and difficulty swallowing over a period of 1 year. She had undergone four coiling procedures over a period of 4 years, for an unruptured basilar tip aneurysm

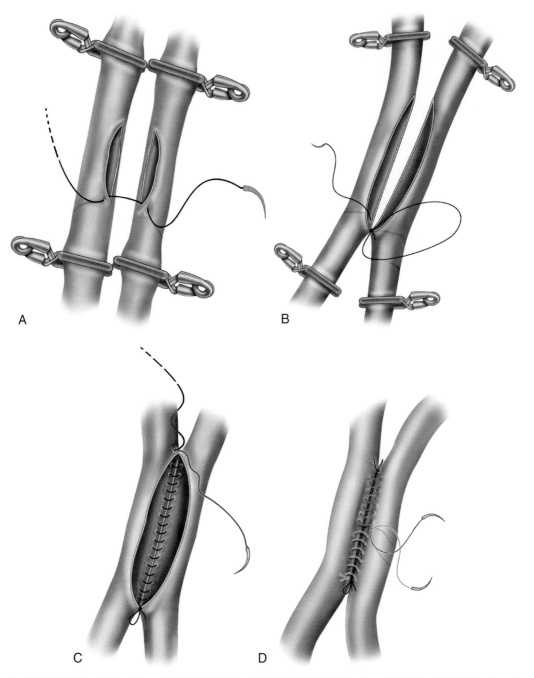

Figure 27–2. A, First suture from outside in to inside out. **B,** After tying the first suture, it is taken to the left wall, and then the suture is run continuously on the posterior wall to reach the other end of the arteriotomy. **C,** A new suture is placed in the upper corner and tied, which is then tied to the end of the first suture. **D,** A suture is started from the inferior corner, and both are tied together. Sutures are then tightened and anastomosis completed, after flushing with heparinized saline.

(Courtesy of Laligam Sekhar.)

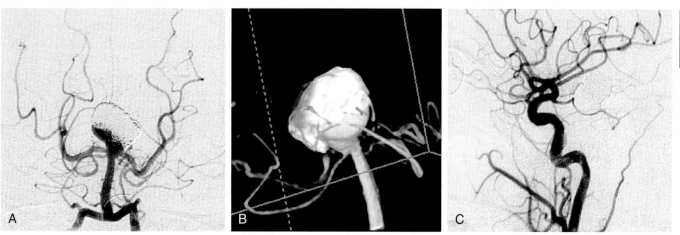

Figure 27–3. A, Preoperative angiogram (AP view) showing the basilar artery with coil compaction and recurrent aneurysm at the tip. **B,** DSA showing the Basilar tip aneurysm preoperatively. **C,** Angiogram right ICA injection lateral view, showing the size of the PCOM preoperatively.

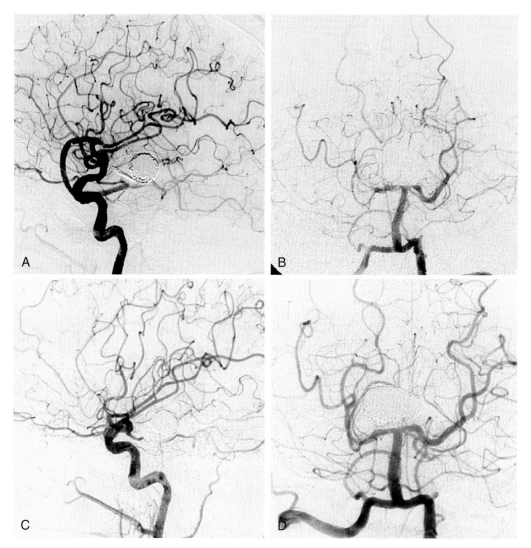

Figure 27–4. A, Immediate postoperative angiogram (right internal carotid angiogram, lateral view) showing the aneurysm completely occluded with the patent bypass and the PCOM. **B,** Immediate postoperative angiogram vertebral injection AP view. Note the filling of the right PCA. **C,** Angiograms 18 months postsurgery (RICA lateral view). Showing the patent PCOM and occluded bypass. **D,** Angiogram 18 months postsurgery (vertebral injection, AP view), showing the aneurysm completely occluded from the circulation. The right PCA is enlarged and filling better compared to immediately after surgery (see Figure 27-2D).

measuring 27 × 22 × 21 mm (Figures 27–5 and 27–6). Her neurological condition had steadily declined. She was unable to swallow liquids, but could swallow solids. On examination, she was awake, was unable to speak, could follow commands intermittently, had right facial paralysis, and had severe right spastic hemiparesis as a result of which she was restricted to a wheelchair. An MRI scan showed a large cyst adjacent to the aneurysm, which was extending into the third and lateral ventricles (see Figure 27–5). The brain cyst had been previously treated using an Ommaya catheter, which had later been fenestrated when clogged. Cerebral angiography demonstrated

continued filling of the aneurysm from the BA (see Figure 27–6A). The patient had a very small PCOM artery (<1 mm) on the left side and a large PCOM artery (≥1 mm) on the right (see Figure 27–6B).

After the endoscopic fenestration of the cyst, the treatment of the aneurysm was done in two stages. The first stage was a transtemporal, transpetrosal approach to the posterior fossa with exposure of V2 and V3 segments of the VA and decompression of sigmoid sinus and facial nerve. This approach was the only one implemented due to the time taken for the procedure (about 6 hours). The second stage of the

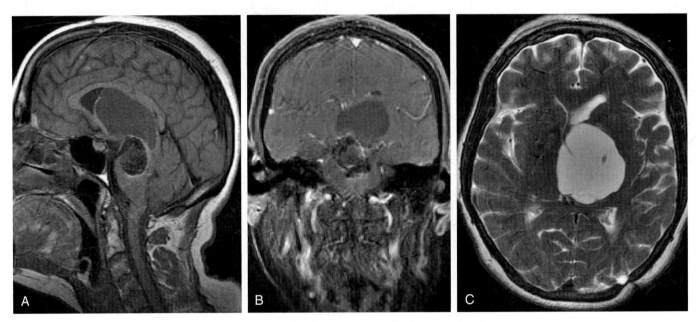

Figure 27–5. MRI scans: sagittal (**A**), coronal (**B**), and axial (**C**) showing the cyst in relation to the giant basilar tip aneurysm.

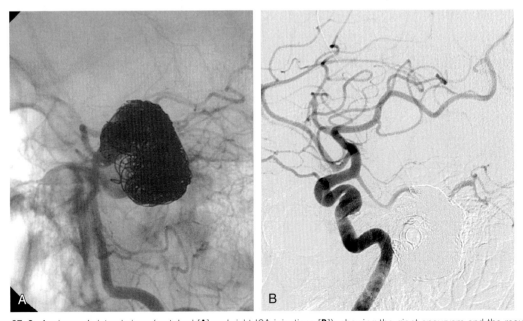

Figure 27–6. Angiogram's lateral views (vertebral [**A**] and right ICA injections [**B**]), showing the giant aneurysm and the recurrence.

operation was performed 3 days afterward and involved the bypass procedure with a SV graft from the VA (V3 segment) to the right PCA (P2 segment), followed by occlusion of the upper BA (Figure 27–7). During this operation, the aneurysm could not be visualized due to the larger coil mass and the brainstem, which was draped around it. The BA was occluded just inferior to the SCA. A saphenous vein was chosen for the graft, since the radial arteries were not available to be used as a bypass conduit.

The patient recovered without any postoperative complications. An immediate postoperative angiogram and an MRI scan showed that the aneurysm remnant filling from the right PCOM artery and through the bypass (Figures 27–8 through 27–10). The graft was widely patent, and the BA terminated at the site of the clip. At 18 months follow-up, the patient had improved marginally from her condition at initial presentation. She was able to converse with a few words, remember and speak with family members, and walk a few steps with assistance with her hemiparesis improved. Angiograms at this time showed a patent graft and partially filling stable aneurysm remnant.

Patient 3

A 17-year-old boy presented with headaches for 3 days, and stabbing eye pain and vomiting for a day. On CT scan, he was found to have a giant aneurysm with hemorrhage measuring 5 × 4.9 × 4.0 (Figure 27–11A-D) centered around the right hippocampus.

The angiogram showed a giant aneurysm arising from the P2 segment of the right PCA also associated with an additional fetal PCOM on the same side (see Figure 27–11A-D). A frontotemporal craniotomy with transsylvian approach was used to dissect the aneurysm, although it was found very difficult to identify proximal and distal vessels. Despite the

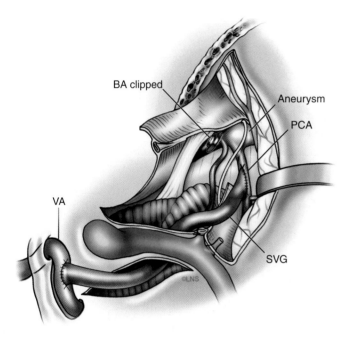

Figure 27–7. Illustration showing the SV graft flowing from the vertebral artery to the P2 segment of the PCA, with the clip on the BA in place.

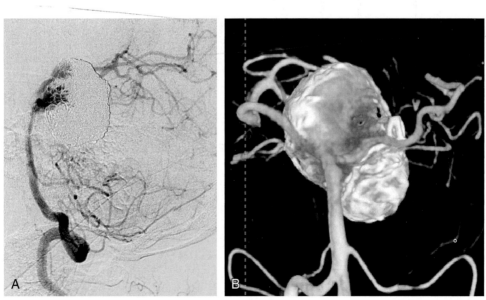

Figure 27–8. A, Angiogram lateral view of the basilar tip aneurysm, showing circulant portion of the previously coiled aneurysm, preoperatively. **B,** 3-D reconstruction angiograms, posterior view of the giant basilar aneurysm.

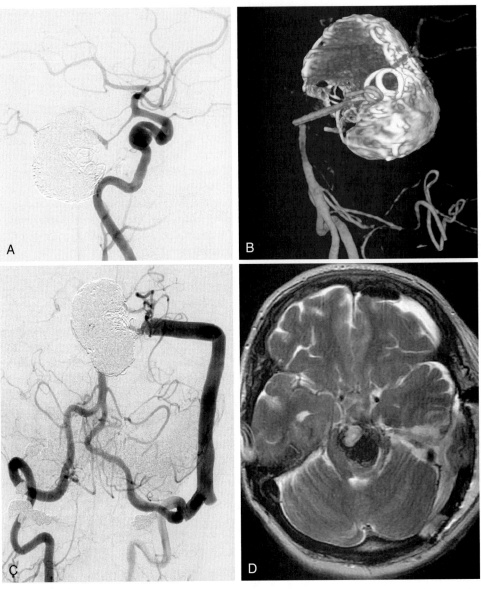

Figure 27–9. **A** to **C,** Day 1 postoperative angiograms and 3-D reconstructions showing the complete exclusion of the aneurysm from the circulation and the vein graft to the PCA from the VA. **D,** MRI axial postoperative showing filling of the aneurysm.

ventriculostomy the brain was found to be rather full and the right temporal gyrus was resected to dissect the aneurysm. Following the puncturing and partial evacuation of blood clots, the aneurysm was clipped and resected completely with a segment of parent vessel (Figure 27–12). Side-to-side anastomosis of the remaining vessel ends was performed, which was later identified as the posterior lateral choroidal branch of the PCA (Figures 27–13 and 27–14).

Postoperatively, the patient recovered steadily with no complications and vision intact. He had headaches due to hydrocephalus, which were treated with lumbar punctures.

Patient 4

A 42-year-old man presented after an automobile accident, after suddenly passing out. The patient had spells of dizziness and problems with memory for 2 years. CTA showed a giant (27 × 13 mm) diffuse fusifom aneurysm of the BA, arising from below the AICA and ending 1 cm inferior to the origin of SUCA (Figure 27–15). Since the anatomy of the aneurysm was not favorable for endovascular coiling (even with stenting), revascularization was planned. Collateral circulation to the BA, distal to the aneurysm was poor. The patient had a

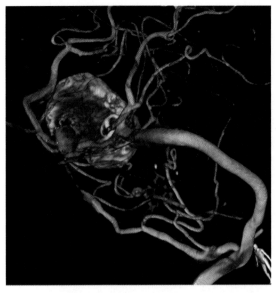

Figure 27–10. 3-D digital subtraction angiograms at 18 months showing the patent vessel graft supplying the PCA and the partially filling aneurysm remnant.

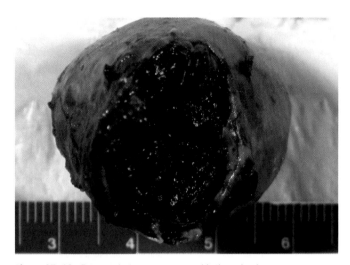

Figure 27–12. Resected giant aneurysm with thrombosis.

Figure 27–11. Preoperative angiograms (lateral [**A**] and AP [**B**]) and vertebral injections (**C** and **D**), showing fusiform aneurysm arising from the P2 segment of the PCA.

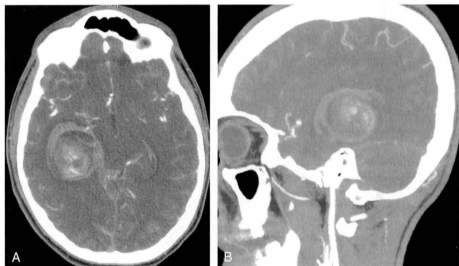

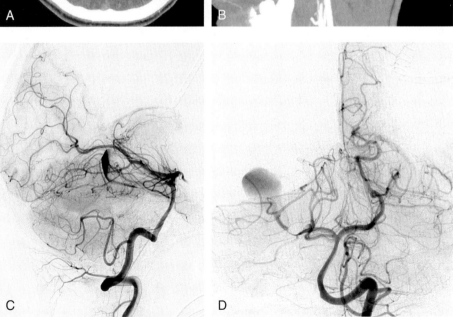

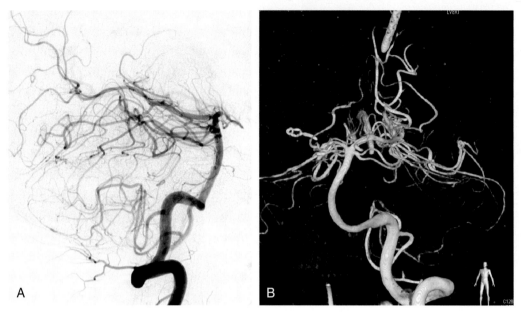

Figure 27–13. A and **B**, Angiograms showing total removal of aneurysm and the clip in place.

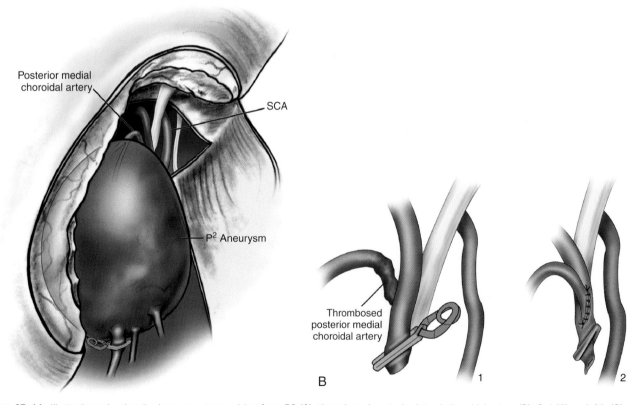

Figure 27–14. Illustrations showing the large aneurysm arising from P2 (**A**), thrombosed posterior lateral choroidal artery (**B**), 3rd (**1**) and 4th (**2**) cranial nerves.
(Courtesy of Laligam Sekhar.)

2 weeks. Follow-up angiograms showed a decrease in graft flow and good flow in the left PCA supplied by an enlarged PCOM.

Patient 5

This 21-year-old man with a known history of collagen vascular disease more prominent on the right side of the body, presented for evaluation of a fusiform aneurysm of the VA (Figures 27–18 and 27–19). Nine years ago, he had a coil embolization of an ICA aneurysm, which resulted in occlusion of the right ICA. The aneurysm measured 1×2.2 cm extending from the V3 region to the origin of the PICA, without involving it. He tolerated the balloon occlusion test well, without symptoms. However, the right PICA was not filling with the left vertebral injections, indicating a need for its revascularization. An OC-PICA anastomosis was performed via a far lateral transtubercular approach with the clip occlusion of the right VA (Figure 27–20). Dissection of the occipital artery as well as performing the approach were tedious because the tissues were not elastic and exuberant. The patient recovered well postoperatively with no neurological deficits (Figures 27–21 through 27–23). He developed a CSF leak from the wound (which was re-explored and resutured) and developed hydrocephalus for which a shunt procedure was performed.

After 40 days, an anterior circulation revascularization was performed with an RAG from the ECA to the M2 segment of the MCA to treat the tenuous nature of blood supply to the right brain, which was dependent on the left ICA (see Figure 27–23). The left VA was chosen, since the right was abnormal, and the right MCA (M2) was found to have a normal caliber and wall thickness during surgery.

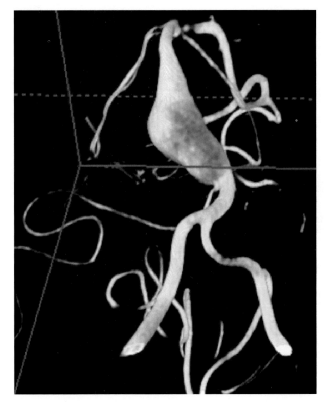

Figure 27–15. Preoperative DSA showing the diffuse fusiform aneurysm.

fetal PCOM on the right side and no PCOM on the left side. Via a transpetrosal approach, a left-sided ECA-PCA bypass was performed with an RAG followed by the distal occlusion of the BA (Figures 27–16 and 27–17). The patient recovered well with no complications and was discharged home in

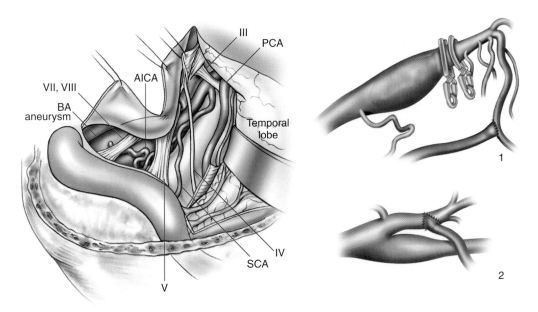

Figure 27–16. Illustration showing the surgical approach with the graft (**1** and **2**) in place.
(Courtesy of Laligam Sekhar.)

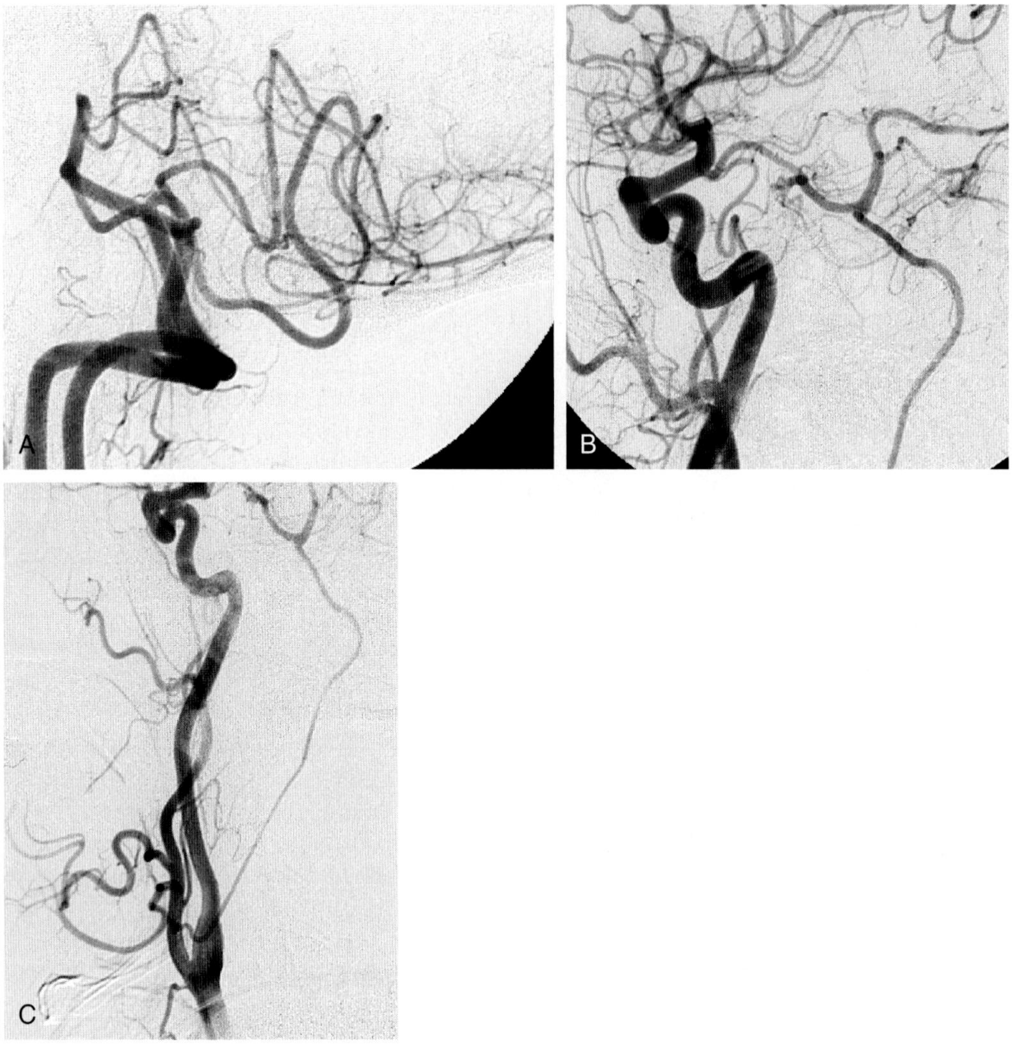

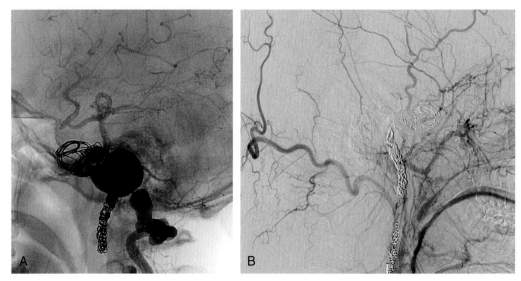

Figure 27–17. A to C, Follow-up angiograms 30 months postsurgery showing enlarged PCOM and patent but narrower graft.

Figure 27–18. A, The aneurysm size and location. **B,** Previously occluded ICA circulation on the right side.

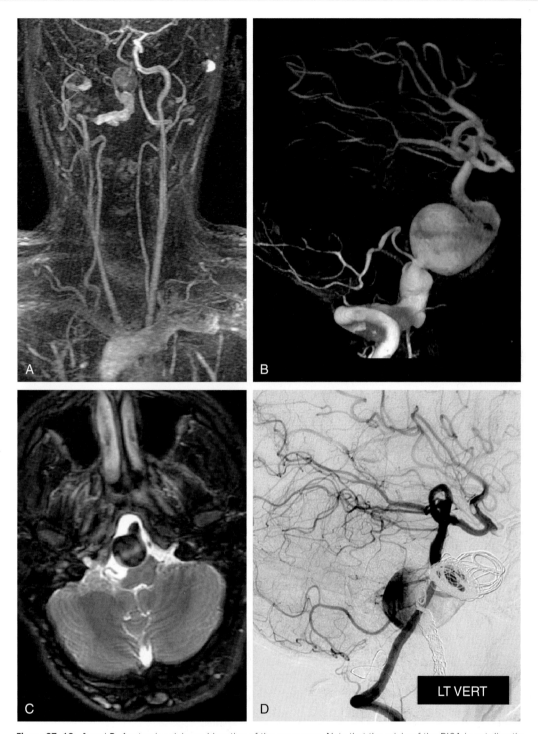

Figure 27–19. **A** and **B,** Anatomic origin and location of the aneurysm. Note that the origin of the PICA is not directly from the aneurysm sac. **C,** MRI showing the filling of the aneurysm. **D,** Angiogram lateral view, vertebral injection showing the aneurysm.

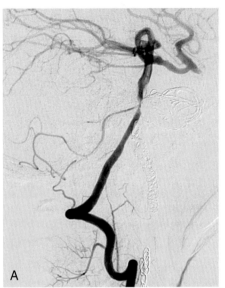

R VA

PICA

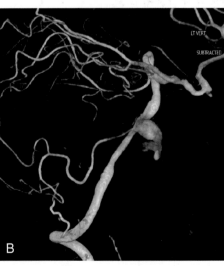

R occipital artery
to PICA bypass

Figure 27–20. Illustration showing the clipping
of vertebral with OC-PICA anastomosis.
(Courtesy of Laligam Sekhar.)

A

B

Figure 27–21. A and **B,** Postoperative angiograms showing complete occlusion of the
aneurysm.

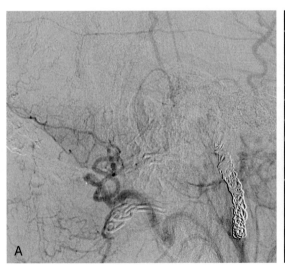

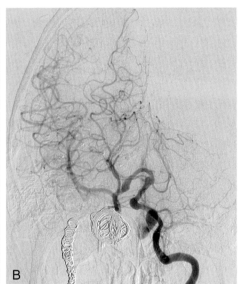

A

B

Figure 27–22. A and **B,** Postoperative angiograms showing complete
occlusion of the aneurysm.

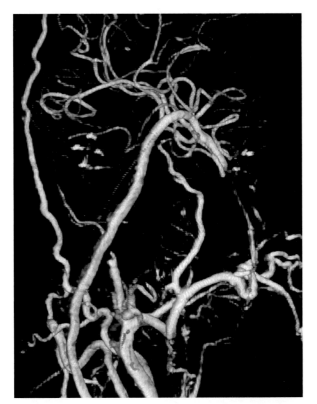

Figure 27–23. Shows RAG graft from the ECA to M2. The OC-PICA anastomosis was occluded after this procedure and the patient was neurologically intact.

Patient 6

A 16-year-old boy had a recurrent giant cell tumor of the lower clivus, C1, occipital condyle, foramen magnum area on the left side, 4 years after initial resection (Figure 27–24). An extreme lateral complete transcondylar approach was performed for a total tumor resection. The tumor was filling the jugular bulb, occluding the sigmoid sinus and encasing the hypoglossal nerve. Gross total resection was pursued meticulously and all extensions of the tumor were removed (Figures 27–24A, 27–25A, and 27-5B). Extracranially, the nondominant left VA was encased by the tumor (Figure 27–26), supplied numerous branches to it, and was damaged during tumor removal. An SV graft was used to replace the affected V3 segment (Figure 27–27). Also, there was an additional area of tumor involvement found at the entrance point of the VA (V3-V4 junction). This segment was resected and the artery primarily resutured (Figure 27–28). He recovered well after surgery and follow-up angiogram confirmed the patency of the VA. Because of the unilateral condylar resection, occiput-C3 fusion was done followed by halo traction. Vocal cord medialization was done later to improve voice quality to compensate for cranial nerve X weakness. The patient remained tumor free 4 years after surgery.

Patient 7

A 10-year-old boy referred for the treatment of a recurrent giant fusiform basilar aneurysm previously coiled two times (Figure 27–29). A right far lateral and transpetrosal approach

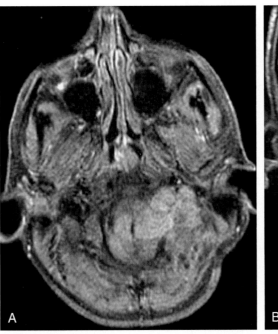
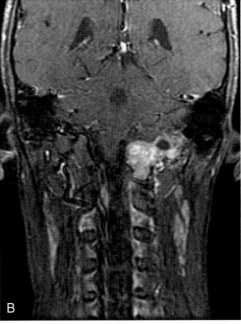

Figure 27–24. MRI (axial [**A**] and coronal [**B**]) showing extensions of the tumor.

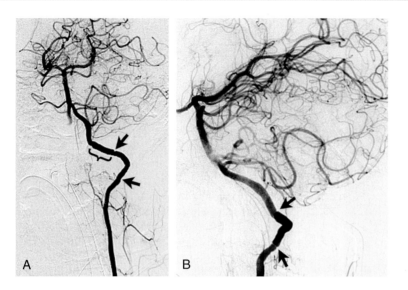

Figure 27–25. A, Postoperative angiogram, AP view, showing SVG (*arrows* pointing to SV graft). **B,** Postoperative angiogram lateral view (*arrow* pointing to SV graft).

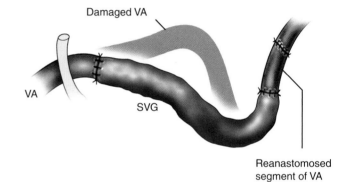

Figure 27–27. SV graft and resection of the stenotic segment and re-anastamosis of V4.
(Courtesy of Laligam Sekhar.)

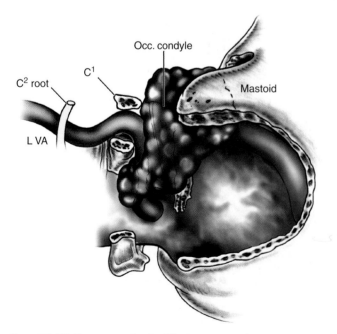

Figure 27–26. Tumor encasing the VA.
(Courtesy of Laligam Sekhar.)

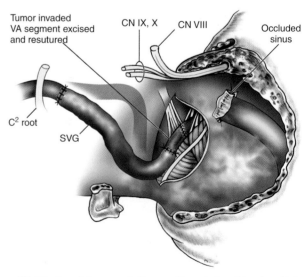

Figure 27–28. Complete removal of tumor with occlusion of the sigmoid sinus.
(Courtesy of Laligam Sekhar.)

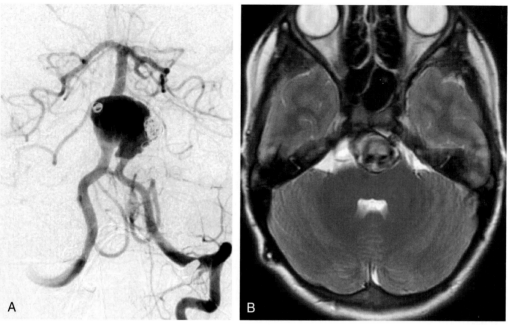

Figure 27–29. A, Fusiform aneurysm with coils inside from previous embolization. **B,** MRI showing the fusiform aneurysm of the BA.

was used to perform SVG bypass from the V3 segment of the VA to the P2 segment of the PCA along with the proximal occlusion of both VAs for complete obliteration of the aneurysm (Figure 27–30). A postoperative MRI and angiograms showed presence of filling from the contralateral VA (see

Figure 27–30). This residual filling was treated with further coil embolizations and the aneurysm was completely obliterated (Figures 27–31 and 27–32). This specific case illustrates the usefulness of endovascular therapy in obliterating minimal remnants, thereby augmenting the success of surgical therapy.

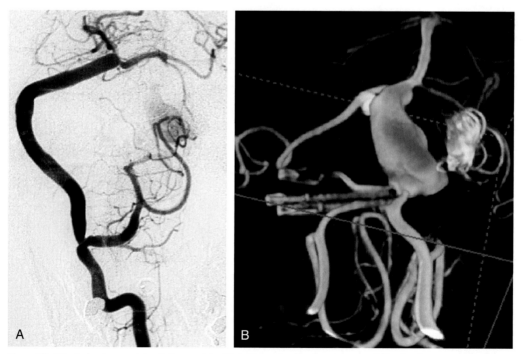

Figure 27–30. A, Angiogram lateral view vertebral injections showing the patent graft flowing from the VA to the P2 PCA. **B,** 3-D reconstruction angiogram showing the proximal clip occlusion and residual filling of the aneurysm from the left VA.

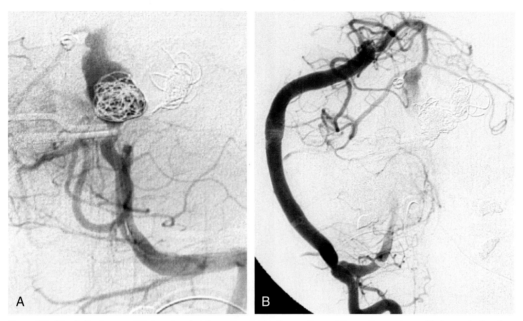

Figure 27–31. A, Angiogram AP view showing the coil embolization performed 3 months postoperatively, occluding flow to the aneurysm. **B,** Angiogram vertebral injection showing the aneurysm completely obliterated by the coiling procedure.

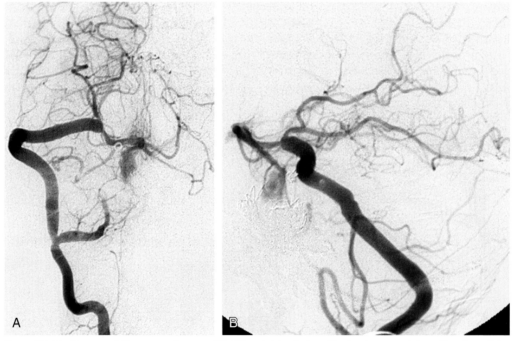

Figure 27–32. One-year follow-up angiograms AP (**A**) and lateral view (**B**) showing complete obliteration of the aneurysm and the patent graft.

RESULTS AND COMPLICATIONS

Tables 27–2 through 27–4 show the results of in situ and EC-IC posterior circulation bypasses in 42 patients (45 bypasses) performed from 1989 to December 2009. All of the bypasses (100%) were patent immediately postsurgery. Two patients had delayed graft occlusion, which was found on angiograms on follow-up visits. One of these patients had an RAG bypass from MCA to P2 PCA bypass for basilar tip aneurysm and the other had an OC-PICA anastomosis with occlusion of the VA (for a giant VA aneurysm dissection).

There were three perioperative deaths and one major stroke (see following for details). The final outcome of the posterior circulation bypass patients was mRS 0-1 in 25 (60%), mRS 2 in nine (21%), mRS 3 in four (10%), mRS 4-5 in one (2%), and mRS 6 in three (7%) of the population (see Table 27–3).

Table 27–2. COMPLICATIONS OF POSTERIOR CIRCULATION BYPASSES FOR ANEURYSMS, TUMORS, AND ISCHEMIA.

Location of Pathology	Bypass	Complications	Management	Outcome (mRS)
Vertebrobasilar aneurysm	VA to PCA (with occlusion of the bilateral vertebral artery)	Aneurysm thrombosis leading to PICA occlusion (brainstem infarction)	None	6
Dissecting PICA aneurysm (PICA 1-PICA 2)	OC-PICA anastomosis, trapping of aneurysm	Intraventricular hemorrhage after shunt placement, patient on anticoagulation for heart valve	None	6
Recurrent osteogenic sarcoma at foramen magnum, contralateral VA occluded, ipsilateral VA tumor encased	SVG interposition graft and PICA-PICA in situ side-to-side anastomosis	Lower cranial nerve palsy, aspiration pneumonia leading to death	None	6
Vertebrobasilar aneurysm	V3 VA to PCA RAG, occlusion of VA, coiling of remaining aneurysm	Small cerebellar peduncle infarction (asymptomatic infarct)	None	1
VA, giant aneurysm, ICA previously occluded for giant aneurysm (Patient 5)	OC-PICA anastomosis with occlusion of the VA, ECA to MCA RAG 2 months later	CSF leak	Reapproximation of sutures	1

Table 27–3. RESULTS OF BYPASS SURGERIES IN POSTERIOR CIRCULATION.

Outcomes (3 to 6 months) of bypasses for mRS of posterior circulation	0, 1	2	3	4, 5	6
Number of patients	25 (60%)	9 (21%)	4 (10%)	1 (2%)	3 (7%)

mRS, Modfied Rankin Score, as evaluated during the postoperative follow-up clinical visits (3- to 6-month period).

Table 27–4. PATENCY RATES OF BYPASSES IN POSTERIOR CIRCULATION.

Time Period Postbypass	Patency of Bypasses	Patency Rate
Immediate postoperative	All patent	100%
Medium- to long-term follow-up (>6 weeks)	Two grafts spontaneously occluded— 1 RAG (one MCA and P2 PCA delayed occlusion), 1 OC-PICA. Both patients asymptomatic with well-developed collateral flow	95%

Among the patients who died, one had a giant vertebrobasilar aneurysm and was treated with an RAG from the VA to P2 PCA and occlusion of both VAs. But the PICA, which was arising from the aneurysm, was not revascularized. He did well initially, but as the aneurysm thrombosed, he developed a PICA thrombosis, leading to infarction and then to respiratory arrest and eventually death. Two of the three patients died due to postoperative ICU complications. (One died due to intraventricular hemorrhage following a shunt procedure 2 days postbypass surgery while on anticoagulation for mechanical heart valves; the other died due to aspiration pneumonia.)

One patient developed a CSF leak (Patient 5), with a good eventual outcome; another patient suffered a perforator-related stroke (cerebellar infarction), which was asymptomatic. Other complications included postoperative subdural hematoma (one patient), which was decompressed, with good clinical outcome.

CONCLUSION

The availability of flow diversion stents (if present studies show them to be safe and effective) will make them the treatment of choice for some complex posterior circulation aneurysms in the future.[2,9] However, various types of bypasses will continue to remain effective options for the treatment of some of these aneurysms. Microsurgeons and endovascular surgeons need to be aware of these options, and work collaboratively in order to achieve the best outcomes for their patients.

REFERENCES

1. Steinberg GK, Drake CG, Peerless SJ: Deliberate basilar or vertebral artery occlusion in the treatment of intracranial aneurysms. Immediate results and long-term outcome in 201 patients, *J Neurosurg* 79:161–173, 1993.
2. Fiorella D, et al: Preliminary experience using the Neuroform stent for the treatment of cerebral aneurysms, *Neurosurgery* 54:6–16, 2004; discussion 16–17.
3. Thorell WE, et al: Y-configured dual intracranial stent-assisted coil embolization for the treatment of wide-necked basilar tip aneurysms, *Neurosurgery* 56:1035–1040, 2005; discussion 1035–40.
4. Wanke I, Gizewski E, Forsting M: Horizontal stent placement plus coiling in a broad-based basilar-tip aneurysm: an alternative to the Y-stent technique, *Neuroradiology* 48:817–820, 2006.
5. Babu RP, Sekhar LN, Wright DC: Extreme lateral transcondylar approach: technical improvements and lessons learned, *J Neurosurg* 81:49–59, 1994.
6. Sekhar LN, et al: Cerebral revascularization using radial artery grafts for the treatment of complex intracranial aneurysms: techniques and outcomes for 17 patients, *Neurosurgery* 49:646–658, 2001; discussion 658–9.
7. Ramanathan D, Hegazy A, Mukherjee S, et al: Intracranial in-situ side-to-side microvascular anastomosis: principles, operative technique and applications, *World Neurosurgery* 2010. In press.
8. Quinones-Hinojosa A, Lawton MT: In situ bypass in the management of complex intracranial aneurysms: technique application in 13 patients, *Neurosurgery* 62(Suppl 3):1442–1449, 2008.
9. Biondi A, et al: Neuroform stent-assisted coil embolization of wide-neck intracranial aneurysms: strategies in stent deployment and midterm follow-up, *Neurosurgery* 61:460–468, 2007; discussion 468–9.

EC-IC AND IC-IC BYPASS FOR GIANT ANEURYSMS USING THE ELANA TECHNIQUE

ALBERT VAN DER ZWAN; TRISTAN P.C. VAN DOORMAAL;
LUCA REGLI; CEES A.F. TULLEKEN

NATURAL HISTORY

Giant intracranial aneurysms, approximately 5% of all intracranial aneurysms, are one of the most challenging lesions in neurosurgery. By definition their fundus size is 2.5 cm or larger, and they are predominantly located in those proximal parts of the vascular tree with high blood flow, such as the internal carotid artery (cavernous and supraclinoid ICA), the proximal middle cerebral artery (MCA), the basilar artery (BA), and vertebral artery (VA). Two-thirds of these aneurysms are located in the anterior circulation and are slightly more common in the female population. Approximately 8% present in the pediatric age, but most commonly they become manifest during the fifth to seventh decades. Most of these aneurysms (20% to 70%) present with rupture and they have the same re-rupture rate as other smaller aneurysms.[1,2] The second most common presentation is the mass effect of the aneurysm causing ocular movement disturbances due to cranial nerve palsies, vision or vision field loss and focal weakness/gait disorders, headaches and seizures. Third, approximately 8% of giant aneurysms present with ischemic syndromes most likely due to embolic phenomena originating from the aneurysm sac to more distally located vascular territories. The natural history of these aneurysms is very poor with high morbidity and mortality rates between 65% to 85% within 2 years after discovery.[1,2]

Therefore, effective treatment of these lesions is lifesaving. However, this asks tremendous and intensive investment in pretreatment diagnostics and considerations regarding the two aims that are the most important in the treatment of giant aneurysms: the permanent exclusion of the aneurysm from the circulation and the relief of mass effect that in some cases also plays a role in symptomatology.

THERAPEUTIC MODALITIES

Many treatment modalities are extensively discussed in literature like Hunterian ligation, endovascular coiling, gluing, stenting, coiling, reconstructive clipping, trapping, and parent vessel replacement bypass surgery, or combinations of these treatment modalities. Reliable comparative analysis of all these treatment modalities, however, is difficult due to small numbers, variable secondary circumstances, and no standardization of results or outcomes.

Endovascular Treatment

As primary clipping can be technically very difficult or impossible, the endovascular approach to these aneurysms has been increasingly popular. Although in smaller aneurysms endovascular treatment has proven to be effective in many cases, the results of endovascular treatment of giant aneurysms are still very disappointing.[3,4] Endovascular Hunterian obstruction in the case of a giant ICA aneurysm of the parent vessel seems to be the most effective and simplest method of treatment. The functionality of the ICA and its intracranial collaterals as the circle of Willis and the leptomeningeals should be thoroughly evaluated before definitive occlusion. Therefore, at our center in patients harboring these aneurysms, first a balloon test occlusion (BTO) of the ICA is performed with venous outflow study to observe if the patient tolerates definitive ICA occlusion. If the patient clinically does not tolerate the occlusion, or if asymmetry in venous outflow is over 1 second, a replacement bypass procedure is planned before definitive ICA occlusion. In more distal giant aneurysms, however, BTO is less reliable due to the complexity of the aneurysm and its afferent arteries. In the explicit review of Parkinson et al., a total of 316 patients with giant aneurysms treated endovascularly using coils, parent vessel occlusion, Onyx®, stenting with or without coil or Onyx® were reviewed. In only 57% of patients was a complete occlusion or cure achieved, with 7.7% mortality and 17.2% major neurological morbidity.[2] In addition, in distally located giant aneurysms the results of endovascular treatment are poor.[4] Endosaccular coiling proves to be an ineffective long-term treatment of these aneurysms due to recanalization and further aneurysm growth. Parent vessel occlusion can be considered, but risks of late ischemia remain relatively large. Selective embolization of these distal giant aneurysms harbors high complication risks (20% mortality). In those cases, especially in more distal giant aneurysms of the MCA, ACA, and PCA where mass effects also play a role in symptomatology, endovascular treatment seems to be less effective.

Parent Vessel Replacement Bypass Surgery

No major reviews on results of flow replacement bypass surgery are available but smaller series are available.[5,6] From these studies the results of parent artery bypass surgery using mostly VSM or radial arterial grafts with consequent trapping or proximal occluding with or without additional endovascular therapy seem to be more promising than the results of endovascular treatment alone.

Before planning bypass surgery it is mandatory to determine the amount of flow to be replaced by the bypass. As most giant aneurysms are located in the more proximal cerebropetal arteries conducting high flows like the ICA, MCA, ACA, BA, and VA, the flow to be replaced by any bypass is most highly dependent on the functional capacity of the Circle of Willis and collaterals as the leptomeningeal vessels, ophthalmic artery, and choroidal plexus. Exact determination of flow needed to replace is therefore hard to make. However, in case of BTO failure in a giant ICA aneurysm, it seems to be safe to choose for a bypass type with potential high flows. In cases of giant MCA, ACA, BA, or VA aneurysms the flows to be replaced in the parent arteries should be determined using single vessel flow MRA flowmetry or multivessel NOVA technique (VasSol®).[7–9] Consequently, partially based on these data a custom made plan for an EC-IC or IC-IC bypass has to be defined to rebuild vascular architecture. The anatomy must be studied in detail to determine which vessels are approachable for bypass grafting. Currently, conventional angiography, and CT perfusion and MRA are used to study this.

Before bypass attachment, intraoperative quantitative flow measurements are performed on different intracerebral arteries using a dedicated flow meter (Transonic®, Ithaca, NY), again to assess the flow, which has to be replaced by the bypass. If we use the superficial temporal artery (STA) as a donor, cut flow is measured before bypass completion to use in the cut flow index.[10]

In aneurysms located more distally, like on the P2 or M3, we measured medium-high flows and replaced the flows using a conventional STA-MCA or STA-PCA bypass based on pre- and intra-operative flow measurements where the aneurysm was trapped. The flows in the bypasses ranged between 30 and 60 cc/min after trapping. In more proximally located aneurysms like the ICA, MCA, BA, and VA, the flows to be replaced can measure up to 180 cc/min. In those cases, a high-flow bypass on the proximal arteries to replace these amounts of flow has to be considered.

It is important here to recall Poiseuille's law, which says that flow varies proportionally to the pressure drop over the bypass, the length of the bypass, and the fourth power of the radius: $Q = \pi\ r4\ P/8\mu L$ (Q = flow rate; r = radius of pipe; P = pressure drop over the pipe; μ = viscosity of fluid; L = length of the pipe). For example, because cortical vessel and the STA have a relatively small diameter, the possible flow through the conventional STA-cortical MCA bypass is limited to 10 to 40 cc/min. Increased flows of 84 to 100 mL/min are possible when the STA is connected to the larger M3.[11] High flows of 130 to 200 cc/min can be achieved when a venous or arterial interponate is used to connect the ECA with the intracranial ICA. So, in cases where higher flows are needed, a more proximal anastomosis should be made. However, anastomosing techniques on more proximally located arteries are technically demanding for surgeons and anesthesiologists. The conventional anastomosing technique with temporal occlusion of the major cerebral arteries theoretically provides an extra risk of ischemia during the classical procedure, and measures to prevent hypothermia and cardiac arrest and pentothal protection are described to minimize this risk. To circumvent this risk, the ELANA technique was developed by our senior author (Tulleken).

THE ELANA TECHNIQUE

The ELANA technique (Figure 28–1) facilitates the construction of an end-to-side anastomosis without temporary occlusion of the recipient artery. It was primarily developed for cerebral augmentative revascularization (1992); however, it turned out that the technique was also quite feasible for creating protective or replacement bypasses.[12–15] A vein (mostly the vena saphena magna, VSM) or artery (radial artery, RA) can be used as the donor vessel. The inner diameter should be minimally 2 mm to enable the laser catheter to pass through the donor vessel. First, depending on the size of the recipient vessel, a platinum ring of 2.6 mm or 2.8 mm is attached to the distal segment of the donor vessel using eight microsutures (see Figures 28–1A through 28–1C). The ring with the attached distal donor segment is subsequently stitched end-to-side to the recipient using again eight microsutures (see Figure 28–1D). This is followed by the passing of the ELANA 2.0® laser suction catheter down the lumen of the open donor vessel. The tip of the catheter is placed against the sidewall of the recipient vessel (see Figure 28–1E and Figure 28–2). After 2 minutes of active suctioning from the dedicated inside portion of the catheter, the laser fibers on the outside of the catheter are activated within 5 seconds. The laser broaches the recipient arterial wall and separates an arteriotomy flap from the recipient (see Figure 28–1F). The suction portion of the catheter maintains contact with the small arteriotomy flap, thus preventing its migration into the lumen of the recipient.

A major advantage of this procedure is the nonocclusive character of the anastomosis, and to our knowledge this is the first nonocclusive anastomosis technique in neurosurgery. Second, for creating this nonocclusive type of anastomosis less intracranial arterial exposure is needed as no temporal clips are used. Third, no measures as hypothermia are needed, as the complete procedure is nonischemic. Fourth, as there is no exposure to the ring and maximally four through-the-vessel-microsutures are

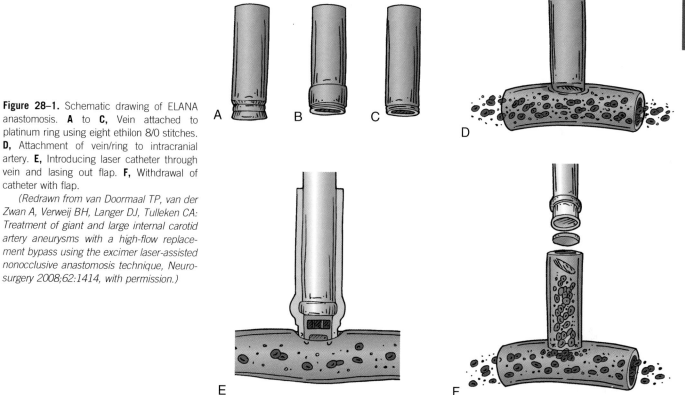

Figure 28–1. Schematic drawing of ELANA anastomosis. **A** to **C,** Vein attached to platinum ring using eight ethilon 8/0 stitches. **D,** Attachment of vein/ring to intracranial artery. **E,** Introducing laser catheter through vein and lasing out flap. **F,** Withdrawal of catheter with flap.

(Redrawn from van Doormaal TP, van der Zwan A, Verweij BH, Langer DJ, Tulleken CA: Treatment of giant and large internal carotid artery aneurysms with a high-flow replacement bypass using the excimer laser-assisted nonocclusive anastomosis technique, Neurosurgery 2008;62:1414, with permission.)

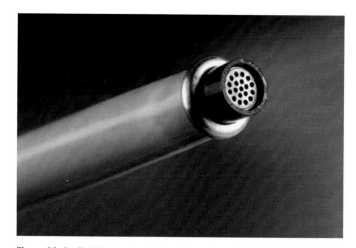

Figure 28–2. ELANA laser catheter tip.

needed, adequate re-endothelialization is achieved.[16] Due to these characteristics safe anastomoses can be made on proximal recipients (ICA, proximal MCA, proximal ACA, P1, and BA) (Figure 28–3A through 28–3E) and various bypass types have been constructed (Figure 28–4). At our institute more than 300 patients and worldwide a large cohort of more than 400 patients were treated using the ELANA technique between 1992 and 2010 with good results and good long-term patency rates (up to 93%). After finalizing the ELANA technique in the form described, we treated 265 patients with large and giant aneurysms since 1999. These aneurysms were located in the cavernous ICA,

supraclinoid ICA, ICA bifurcation, proximal MCA, proximal ACA, BA, and at the VA-BA junction. Although this technique introduces the major advantage of its nonocclusiveness and therefore the absence of intraoperative stress moments of temporal occlusion of major arteries, the technical challenges are mainly formed by the stitching of the donor vessel with the ring on the recipient vessel, most often deep intracranially. Mainly as the result of this part of the procedure, one ELANA anastomosis takes between 90 to 120 minutes, depending on its location and the neurosurgeon's experience.

Therefore, ELANA training sessions organized at our institute are mandatory for future ELANA neurosurgeons. In addition, for every vascular neurosurgeon, regular lab training sessions are obligatory for maintaining and developing adequate microvascular skills using ELANA techniques. Further developments of the ELANA technique will focus on safe, sutureless, and minimally invasive techniques to make this technique easier and consequently shorten the procedure.

PERIOPERATIVE PREPARATION AND MONITORING

Preoperative Flow Measurements

For preoperative planning of surgery, bypass indication, type of bypass and location, and an estimation of the flow to be replaced can be made by using single-vessel flow MRA

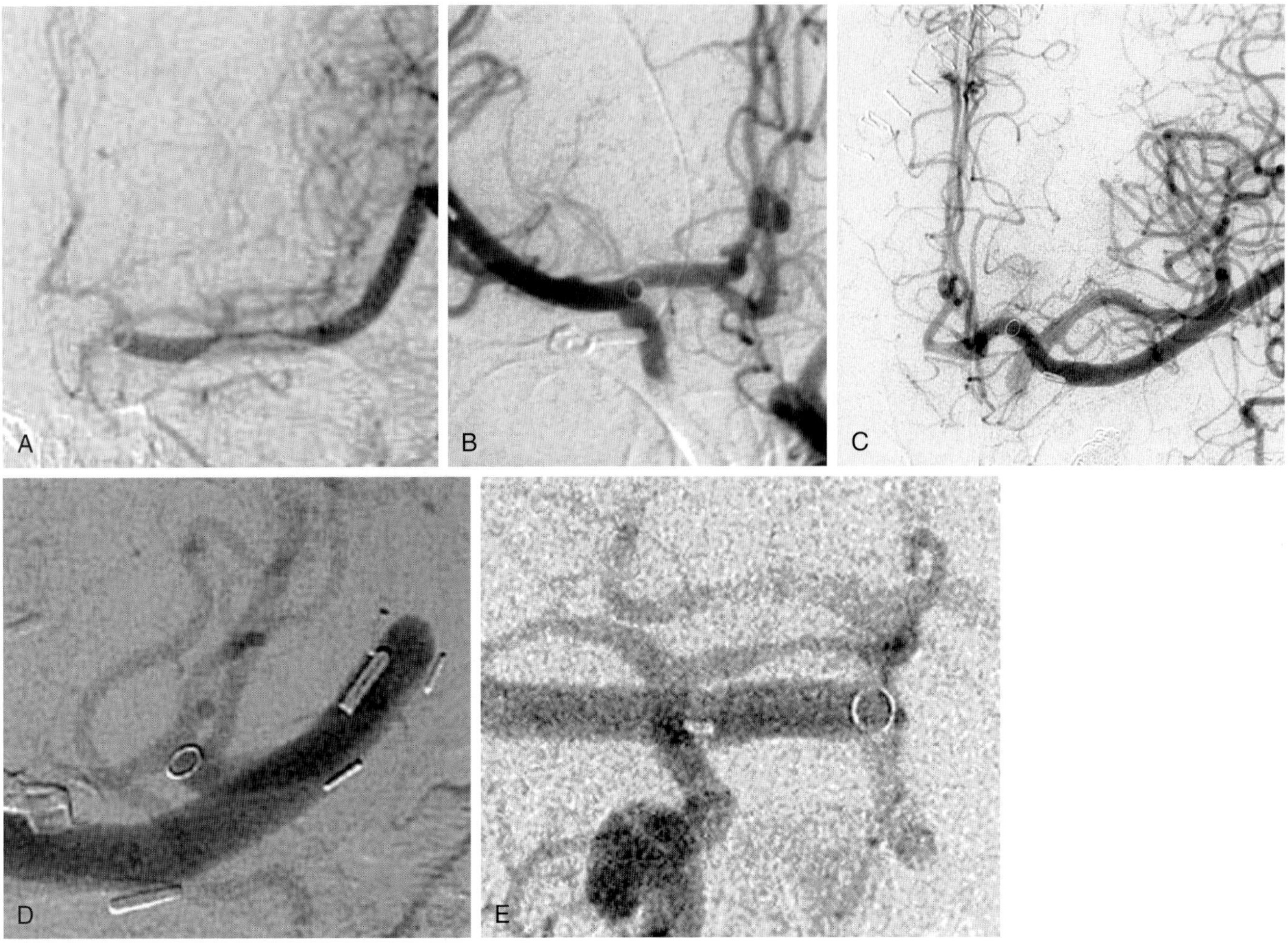

Figure 28–3. Angiography of ELANA anastomoses. **A,** On ICA. **B,** ICA bifurcation. **C,** A1. **D,** MCA bifurcation. **E,** Basilar artery.

flowmetry or multivessel NOVA technique (VasSol®). At our institute, only single-vessel MRA flowmetry is available, and this technique is also used for postoperative evaluation of bypass flow.[9]

Anticoagulation Strategy

Although in the early years of our experience we did not administer anticoagulation medication preoperatively to avoid hemorrhagic complications during surgery, over 4 years ago we began to premedicate patients with acetylsalicylic acid (80 mg/day) 3 days before surgery. Heparin is administered intraoperatively intravenously by bolus injection (1000 IU) at the moment that the bypass is opened. During the rest of the procedure, an extra bolus of 1000 IU heparin is administered approximately every 2 to 3 hours. At the end of the surgery, the median quantity of intraoperatively administered heparin is 2000 IU (range, 1000 to 5000 IU). Postoperatively, all patients receive bypass thrombosis prophylaxis. From 1999 to 2002, this was achieved with 50 g/day dextran 40 (Rheomacrodex; Medisan Pharmaceuticals, Parsippany, NJ) and, from

2002 on, with 15,000 IU/day of heparin. Both of these medications were administered during the 3 days in the intensive care unit. After 3 days, they were stopped, and one daily dose of acetylsalicylic acid (80 mg) was administered. We changed this postoperative protocol over 4 years ago, however, and only acetylsalicylic acid is continued directly after surgery.

Intraoperative Flow Measurements

In all procedures since 1998 we intraoperatively measured flow through parent vessels, distal efferent vessels, and the bypass using a dedicated flow meter (Transonic®, Ithaca, NY).[9] Especially in flow replacement bypass surgery it is important to measure the flow in the artery that is to be replaced. In addition, after bypass completion, it is important to monitor bypass flow during parent vessel occlusion and aneurysm trapment to measure the increase in the flow through the bypass during these maneuvers. Any complication, such as kinking of the bypass, compression of the bypass during closure, or thrombosis of the bypass, can be detected by flow monitoring during the rest of the procedure until the end of closure.

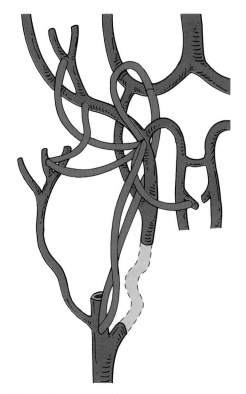

Figure 28–4. Different types of ELANA bypasses.

Intraoperative Near-Infrared Indocyanine Green Video Angiography (ICGA)

Before and after bypass construction as well as during aneurysm trapment or reconstruction, the use of indocyanine green video angiography (ICGA)[17] can be very useful to monitor involvement of perforating arteries. Although this method is not replacing intraoperative DSA, which is not available in

our hospital, it can be very helpful as long as it is taken into account that this method can only be used on those vessels in the field of surgery that are visible, and that deeper vessels are missed.

ELANA EC-IC BYPASS FOR GIANT ANEURYSMS OF THE ICA

Between 1999 and 2009 we operated on 45 patients with giant aneurysms of the cavernous and supraclinoid ICA[18] (Figure 28–5). Mean age was 53 years (standard deviation [SD] 15) and predominantly female (75%). Thirty-two patients (71%) failed occlusion tests, and the remaining patients lacked sufficient collaterals on imaging. Presentation of symptoms included cranial nerve compression signs exclusively in 27 patients (75%) and SAH, with or without cranial nerve compression signs, in 14 patients (31%). In the remaining four patients, no objective symptoms were registered. In all patients the VSM was used for bypass. The vein was cut in half and firstly the ELANA anastomosis was created on the intracranial ICA, ICA bifurcation, or proximal MCA. In a second phase the other half of the vein was used to make a conventional end-to-side anastomosis on the ECA and finally both vein pieces were connected in an end-to-end anastomosis. The mean surgical time for the bypass procedure of all patients was 443 minutes (range, 300 to 750 min). The mean time until catheter vacuum suction—meaning the anastomosis between recipient, platinum ring, and donor vessel was made, but the recipient artery wall was still intact—was 246 minutes (range, 150 to 330 min). During surgery, the recipient artery was never occluded as part of the bypass procedure. With an intact bypass, we proceeded with intraoperative ligation of the ICA

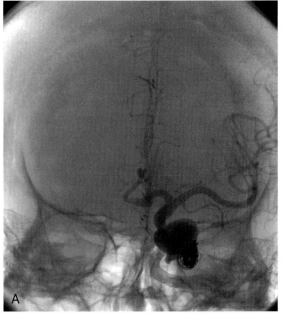
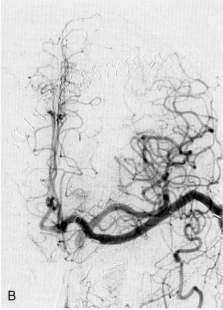

Figure 28–5. Preoperative (**A**) and postoperative (**B**) angiography of a giant aneurysm of the left ICA after unsuccessful previous endovascular treatment. During surgery, an EC-IC bypass from the ECA to the ACA (ELANA) was performed and the ICA proximally occluded.

A

B

if an acute danger of aneurysm bleeding existed or if the compression symptoms increased rapidly before the operation. In the first patients of our series, the ICA was left patent during surgery to prevent ischemic complications. In these patients, we occluded the ICA after surgery with detachable balloons after confirmation that the bypass remained patent for at least 24 hours as demonstrated on contrast imaging. However, at present, we choose for immediate intraoperative occlusion of the ICA, because in the early years five out of 23 patients (22%) had to be re-operated on. In these cases, the bypass occluded within a day due to low bypass flow because the ICA was left open postoperatively, waiting for endovascular occlusion.

A successful patent EC-IC bypass was constructed in 44 out of 45 patients (98%). After ligation of the ICA, a mean intraoperative bypass flow of 102 mL/min (range, 65 to 170 mL/min) was recorded using a flow probe (Transonic®, Ithaca, NY). In 15 patients, magnetic resonance angiography bypass flow measurement was performed after ICA occlusion. A mean flow of 138 ml/min (range, 70 to 180 mL/min) was recorded, demonstrating a powerful replacement EC-IC bypass. Control imaging from all patients in whom we performed intraoperative ICA ligation or postoperative ICA balloon occlusion showed ICA aneurysm thrombosis.

Complications of ELANA Bypass for Giant Aneurysms of the ICA

Two fatal complications (4%) occurred, neither directly related to ELANA application. The first patient died of an air embolism from a central line 1 day postoperatively and the second patient died of an aneurysm rupture 2 days after surgery. Both patients waited for postoperative endovascular final treatment. The last complication again underlines the importance of direct surgical treatment by ligating the ICA after the bypass procedure.

Non-fatal complications, including ischemia due to thrombosis or manipulation of the aneurysm (two patients), aneurysm bleeding before definitive occlusion of the ICA (one patient), ischemia due to thrombosis of the bypass (two patients), occurrence of transient ischemic attacks (TIAs) due to stenosis of the conventional anastomosis in the ECA (one patient), and progressive cranial nerve palsy due to aneurysm thrombosis (two patients) occurred in eight patients (18%).

Bypass Patency of ELANA Bypass for Giant Aneurysms of the ICA

As there is heterogeneity of surgical strategy and indication in the pursuing years, patency data on the whole group are not informative. As in the early years, for safety reasons, we planned to wait with definitive treatment of the aneurysm 1 or more days after bypass surgery. The patency rate in this group was only 71%. The competition between bypass flow

and parent artery flow plays an important role in this. Changing our strategy to immediate (partial) trapping of the parent artery and aneurysm increased patency rates to 93%.

Functional Outcome of ELANA Bypass for Giant Aneurysms of the ICA

Long-term follow-up outcome was defined as favorable if the modified Rankin Scale (mRS) was found to be equal to or higher than the preoperative mRS (mean long-term follow-up: 3.3 years; range, 0.6 to 5.6 years). This was found in 35 patients (78%). Defining patients with a mRS score of 3 (moderate disability, needing help in daily life, but walking without assistance) or worse, 37 patients (82%) of our patient group were independent in the long term. Cranial nerve recovery occurred in 42% of the patients.

Discussion of ELANA Bypass for Giant Aneurysms of the ICA

Comparing these data with the results of currently available endovascular treatment modalities, our results strongly suggest that neurosurgical treatment using ELANA EC-IC bypass neurosurgery is favorable above endovascular treatment. Our changing strategy of directly, intraoperatively ligating the ICA seems to obtain even better results.

ELANA BYPASS FOR GIANT ANEURYSMS OF THE MCA

As MCA giant aneurysms are even more life-threatening lesions prone to rupture compared to giant aneurysms of the ICA, an aggressive therapeutic strategy is even more warranted[1] (Figure 28–6). The preferred treatment is to take the aneurysm completely out of circulation and in some cases even debulking the mass of the aneurysm. The results of filling these MCA aneurysms with coils or glue are mostly disappointing by recanalization, impaction, or sustaining mass effect. Although literature provides many case reports of flow replacement bypasses using the STA as donor end-to-side connected to a small distal MCA branch for reversal of flow in these aneurysms, this technique still demands a temporal MCA occlusion with a theoretical risk of ischemia. In addition there is also a risk of ischemia due to insufficient flow replacement. According to the mathematical model of Hillen et al., there are hemodynamic arguments that, for replacing higher flows in the MCA (up to 120 ml/min), larger diameter bypasses (>2 mm) should be preferred.[19] An intracranial IC-IC bypass should be able to replace the MCA in an orthograde, and therefore, more physiological direction; this approach also minimizes surgical exposure, thus avoiding neck carotid surgery for the donor part of a regular conventional EC-IC bypass.

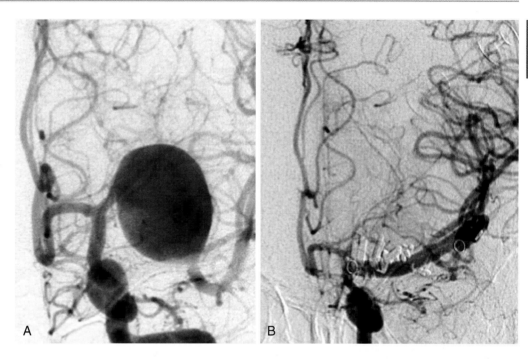

Figure 28–6. Preoperative (**A**) and postoperative (**B**) angiography of patient with a giant aneurysm of the left MCA. ELANA IC-IC bypass (type I) from the ICA to the M1 bifurcation.

Therefore, at our institute, we prefer to treat these aneurysms using IC-IC ELANA replacement bypass followed by trapment of the complete aneurysm after determining the flow to be replaced by combining preoperative (MRI) and intraoperative flowmetry data (Transonic Flow Probe and Flow Meter, Transonic Systems, Ithaca, NY).

Since 1999, we have treated 25 patients with giant aneurysms with a mean diameter of 38 mm (SD, ±12 mm) measured on imaging.[20] The mean age was 45 years (SD ±16 years) and 12 patients were female (48%). All aneurysms were assessed as being not safely clippable or coilable. Preoperative flow measurements were performed as far as possible, as coils previously unsuccessfully delivered into these aneurysms (in six patients, 24%) disturb flow measurements.

In 11 patients (44%), the aneurysm presented with SAH, in three patients (12%) with ischemic stroke, in three patients (12%) with epilepsy, in three patients with TIA (12%), and in four patients with no objective symptoms. Three types of ELANA bypasses were performed in this group of patients, all using the VSM as the bypass graft.

Type I, ICe-ICe: Type I is defined as an IC-IC bypass with proximal and distal anastomoses constructed both using the ELANA technique (ICe-ICe). This type of bypass was performed in 12 patients (36%). The proximal anastomosis was made on the proximal ICA (*n* = 8) or MCA (*n* = 4) depending on reach ability and quality of these proximal arteries. The VSM was cut in half and the anastomosis was constructed on the ICA or MCA. After completion of this anastomosis a temporal clip was placed on the vein. The distal anastomosis was mostly made on the distal MCA (M2, *n* = 10; M3, *n* = 2) using the second half of the VSM, again followed by temporally clipping this vein. The two vein halves were then end-to-end anastomosed and just before finalizing flushed by removing both temporal clips. An example of this type of bypass is shown in Figure 28–6. As no temporal occlusion of any of the vessels is necessary, we prefer to construct this type of bypass.

In three patients the configuration of the aneurysm was very complex with an extra MCA branch originating from the aneurysm. Therefore an extra EC-IC bypass was constructed considering the size of these smaller branches using conventional anastomosing techniques (end-to-side STA-MCA) (Figure 28–7).

Type II, ICe-ICc: Type II is defined as an IC-IC bypass with an ELANA anastomosis on the proximal side and a conventional anastomosis on the distal side, as the distal MCA branch is not always large enough (>2.6 mm) to construct an ELANA anastomosis on (ICe-ICc). This type was constructed in 14 patients (56%). The proximal ELANA anastomosis was made on the ICA (*n* = 10) and on the MCA (*n* = 4). Distal conventional anastomoses were made on the M2 (*n* = 4) and on the M3 (*n* = 10).

Type III, EC-ICe: This type is defined as an EC-IC bypass with an ELANA anastomosis on the distal side (EC-ICe). In two patients (8%) the intracranial ICA or MCA proximal to the aneurysm was not surgically reachable due to aneurysm size. Therefore an EC-IC bypass with a distal ELANA anastomosis on the distal MCA and a proximal anastomosis on the ECA was constructed. This type of flow replacement bypass was described previously in the treatment of internal carotid aneurysms.

Of 59 anastomoses, 40 (68%) were ELANA. In three patients, a second bypass procedure was initiated after the first

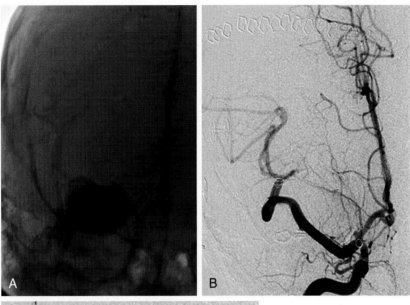

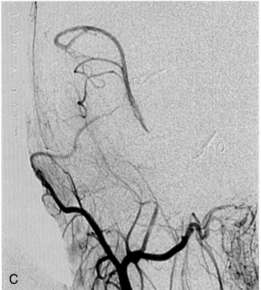

Figure 28–7. Seventeen-year-old boy with giant MCA aneurysm (**A**). An IC-IC ELANA bypass (**B**) and an extra STA-MCA bypass (**C**) were constructed. The MCA aneurysm was completely trapped.

bypass attempt failed. All 40 ELANA attempts resulted in a patent anastomosis with a strong backflow directly after ELANA catheter retraction. In six ELANA anastomoses (15%), the disk of arterial wall, which is normally attached to the tip of the catheter after laser application and catheter retraction (the flap), was not found on the tip. In these patients no adverse events occurred and bypasses were functioning well.

Mean intraoperative flow (±SD) through the 23 IC-IC bypasses before any part of the MCA or aneurysm was occluded was 15 (±10 cc/min). The mean intraoperative flow (±SD) through the IC-IC bypasses after partial or full MCA occlusion, measured at the end of the operation, was 53 (±13 ml/min). The two EC-IC bypasses had a flow before MCA occlusion of 35 (±50 ml/min). These aneurysms were endovascularly treated the next day, and MR flow measurement on the first EC-IC bypass showed that bypass flow had increased from 35 cc/min

(intraoperatively) to 100 cc/min postoperatively and after endovascular occlusion of the parent artery.

In the early phases of our experience, for safety reasons we decided to construct the bypass first and planned the definitive aneurysm endovascular treatment 1 or 2 days postoperatively. However, as we found out, the risks of this strategy are twofold—thrombosis of the bypass and postoperative preendovascular treatment aneurysm bleeding—so our present strategy is total exclusion of the aneurysm from the circulation during the same procedure. This should be performed with clips placed on the MCA proximal of and distal from the aneurysm, thus trapping the aneurysm completely. We succeeded in this in only 11 patients (44%), because in most cases total trapping can be impossible if the complexity of the aneurysm base (e.g., calcification or vessel incorporation) does not allow clip application on the MCA nearby. In that situation, we tried different partial trapping configurations with clips on the proximal and/or distal parts of the MCA, leaving a selection of proximal and/or distal MCA branches patent. We repeatedly measured bypass flow and MCA flow (Transonic flow probe and flow meter; Transonic Systems, Inc., Ithaca, NY) after every temporary and definitive clip placement to monitor sufficient bypass flow. This partial trapping approach was used in 14 patients (56%). In two of these patients, there was still a considerable flow in the aneurysm after distal partial trapping. These remnants, including the parent vessel, were successfully coiled after surgery. However, partial trapping in which the aneurysm itself partially filling also comes with a risk of bleeding of the aneurysm. This occurred in four out of 14 aneurysms (29%) that were partially trapped. In one patient with a large 60-mm MCA fusiform aneurysm where partial trapping was impossible due to calcifications, a balloon occlusion was planned 3 days postoperatively. One day postoperatively, the aneurysm bled and the patient died.

Of special interest were our findings on one patient who was provided with an IC-IC bypass. At that time in the early phase of our experience we decided to plan the definite endovascular treatment 1 day after surgery using detachable balloon as described previously. Surprisingly, the next day, the aneurysm spontaneously thrombosed with the bypass still open. Currently, this is not our strategy, as we consider the risk of thrombosis of the bypass with the parent artery still open too high.

Complications of ELANA Bypass for Giant Aneurysms of the MCA

Hemorrhagic: Besides the fatal aneurismal hemorrhage ($n = 1$, 4%), there were 11 nonfatal complications in nine patients (36%). In three patients, a nonfatal postoperative SAH occurred before endovascular treatment was performed.

Ischemic: Eight ischemic complications occurred in eight patients (32%). Three of these (12%) were due to failure of the distal conventional anastomosis in type II treatment modality. In the first of these three patients, the thrombosis began at the site of the distal conventional anastomosis and the proximal ELANA anastomosis remained patent as was clearly visible on angiography. We decided not to perform a second bypass procedure because of the relatively small neurological deficits (right-hand paresis), which was probably attributable to a large intracerebral and leptomeningeal collateral network also visible on angiography. In the other two patients, an ischemic region was observed at the site of the temporarily occluded recipient distal M2 and M3 branch.

Four patients (16%) experienced minor ischemic symptoms because of the occlusion of small MCA branches leaving the aneurysm as a result of aneurysm thrombosis. However, none of these patients experienced a poor functional outcome (postoperative mRS score higher than preoperative mRS score).

Finally, in one patient (4%) an intraoperative infarct occurred. She was a 22-year-old patient with a left-sided giant MCA aneurysm with only headache symptoms (see Figure 28–6). An IC-IC bypass (type I) was planned and during surgery, when both proximal and distal ELANA anastomoses were constructed and only the final stage of end-to-end anastomosing of the two venous bypass segments was to be finished, a spontaneous hemorrhage of the (until this part) asymptomatic aneurysm occurred at the neck of the aneurysm. The massive bleeding that followed urged us to temporally trap the MCA and the aneurysm to make further finishing of the bypass possible. This turned the procedure from a nonocclusive one into a temporal ischemic procedure and it took us 12 minutes to finish the bypass and remove the temporary clips on the bypass. During this time we checked collateral leptomeningeal capacity by removing the distal clip on the MCA, and there was no backflow indicating that in this patient collateral capacity was minimal. Although the occlusion time was only 12 minutes, which is much shorter than the occlusion time usually necessary for a conventional anastomosis on larger proximal arteries, the patient woke up with right-sided hemiparesis and mild dysphasia. Postoperative CT showed a left-sided putamen infarct, and 2 months were required for full recovery. This incident, together with the three ischemic incidents of the distal conventional anastomoses, clearly shows that conventional anastomosing techniques with temporal occlusion bear significant risk of infarction and that the nonocclusive character of the ELANA anastomosing technique does prevent infarcts in certain patient groups. As there are currently no reliable methods to test leptomeningeal capacity in the treatment of giant MCA aneurysms, we prefer to use the ELANA nonocclusive anastomosing technique in these patients as much as possible.

Bypass Patency of ELANA Bypass for Giant Aneurysms of the MCA

In total, four bypasses occluded because of thrombosis at the distal conventional anastomosis site (16%), and one bypass thrombosed because of a postoperative aneurysm hemorrhage (4%), making short-term bypass patency in 20 (80%) of 25 bypasses. Although long-term follow-up studies are preferred, we could not manage to have a 100% long-term follow-up MRA in all patients. However, of the remaining 22 short-term patent bypasses, two patients after 2 and 3 years show symptomless occlusion of the bypass but with extensive collaterals between the distal MCA branches and the ACA and PCA arterial networks. Long-term patency in this group therefore amounted to 72%.

Functional Outcome of ELANA Bypass for Giant Aneurysms of the MCA

On long-term follow-up (mean, 3.6 years; range, 0.2 to 7.7 years after surgery), 20 patients (80%) had a favorable outcome, meaning that their postoperative mRS score was equal to (10 patients) or higher (10 patients) than their preoperative status. Five patients (20%) had a long-term unfavorable outcome. In four of these patients, the unfavorable outcome was related to surgery (16%). One patient (5%) died 2 months postoperatively of unknown causes. The family refused a postmortem study, but the patency of the bypass of this patient was angiographically confirmed 2 weeks before death.

Defining patients with a mRS score of 3 (moderate disability, needing help in daily life, but walking without assistance) or worse as dependent, long-term independence totaled 16 patients (64%).

Discussion of ELANA Bypass for Giant Aneurysms of the MCA

Comparing the results of these treatments with literature is problematic, as different patient groups and outcome measurements are used. Using GOS scale in our patients we had a good or excellent outcome in 84%. However, this does not take the preoperative status into account. In addition the challenges in the treatment of giant MCA aneurysms are unique and should not be compared with results in the treatment of giant ICA or posterior circulation aneurysms.

It is noteworthy that, in 14 patients in whom the aneurysm was not completely trapped intraoperatively, four aneurysms bled postoperatively (29%). For one patient the bleeding was fatal and in one patient the bypass occluded as the result of this. The outcome of these patients was poor. On the other hand, in 11 patients where complete trapping was possible the minor ischemic complications attributable to trapping or manipulation of the aneurysm did not cause any decrease in long-term functional outcome. The only bypass that on long term occluded after trapping also did not cause any decrease in functional outcome. Retrospectively, this bypass was probably not needed because of the preexisting large collateral flow through intracerebral and leptomeningeal collaterals, as shown on imaging. These differences in the groups with and without direct total trapping suggest that direct total trapping of the aneurysm after bypass construction during the same procedure should be pursued whenever possible. Prevention of hemorrhagic complications probably outweighs the functional decrease caused by ischemic complications.

Although numbers are too small to make reliable comparison possible, it is remarkable that three bypasses occluded because of thrombosis at the site of the conventional anastomoses, and another two patients had an ischemic complication with neurological sequelae owing to temporary occlusion time, which was necessary to construct a peripheral conventional anastomosis. This clearly shows that temporary occlusion of arteries to the brain is accompanied by higher risks.

The phenomenon of the long-term bypass occlusion in two patients with extensive leptomeningeal collaterals with previous successful and patent bypasses reveals that the human cerebral vasculature is dynamic and that it can adapt itself to changing circumstances. After bypass construction, a new equilibrium is slowly established in the MCA flow territory, which varies inter-individually but also intra-individually in time depending on preexisting collaterals and bypass location. The bypass could then function as a slowly fading, nonphysiologic bridge to reach a new physiologic situation with the aid of leptomeningeal and intracerebral collaterals. This hypothesis is supported by earlier reports on leptomeningeal function after MCA occlusion.[21] Although in literature numbers of bypass patencies are often used in the discussions of treatment modalities in giant aneurysms, this finding of long-term occlusion of bypasses without symptomatology, due to extensive collaterals, clearly demonstrates that follow-up in terms of functional outcome as the mRS is much more important.

ELANA BYPASS FOR GIANT ANEURYSMS OF THE ACA

Although we frequently see patients with giant aneurysms of the ACA, it is rarely necessary to use ELANA technique for bypassing these lesions. An example of this is a 61-year-old patient with an SAH and a giant aneurysm of the ACA that was not coilable and because of multicalcifications not easily clippable (Figure 28–8). As there are no possibilities of measuring distal leptomeningeal anastomoses, we decided to perform a IC-IC bypass from the A1 to the proximal A2, and then clipping the aneurysm, including the distal A1 and ACA. Intraoperative flow measurements on the A2 showed a flow of 30 cc/min to be replaced. As the STA in this case was very small we decided to construct an IC-IC bypass and to trap the aneurysm. According to intraoperative flow measurements, initial flow in the bypass with the A1 still open was 15 cc/min but went up to 30 after trapping the aneurysm, including the A1-A2 segment, demonstrating that the bypass functioned as a 100% replacement bypass. The patient recovered very well and is at work (follow-up 40 months), and CTA control after 2 years showed the bypass to be fully patent.

ELANA BYPASS FOR GIANT ANEURYSMS OF THE POSTERIOR CIRCULATION

Giant aneurysms of the posterior circulation are even more challenging than those of the anterior circulation. This is because of the large size of the aneurysm and the little space there is left for the thrombosing and consequently swelling aneurysm. In addition, thrombosing perforators coming out of the aneurysm often cause devastating infarcts in the brainstem with consequent sequelae. Finally, complete trapping is seldom possible, leaving the risk of bleeding of the aneurysm.

We treated 10 patients with a giant aneurysm of the posterior circulation with an ELANA bypass on the BA

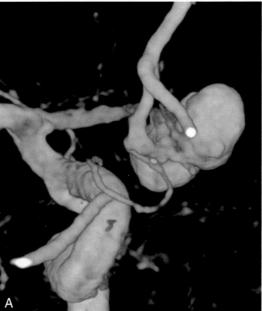

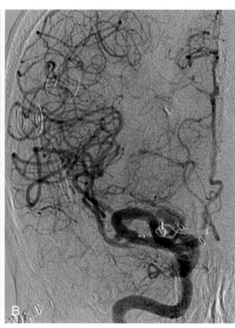

Figure 28–8. Giant aneurysm of the ACA (**A**) and complete trapping of the aneurysm after construction of an ELANA IC-IC bypass from the A1 to the A2 (**B**).

(Figures 28–9A and 28–9B), P1 (Figure 28–9C), P2, or the SCA.[22-24] An example of progressive brainstem ischemia after reversal of flow is the case of a 55-year-old male who suffered a SAH from a giant fusiform BA aneurysm. We constructed an IC-IC bypass from the ICA to the BA, thus creating a large artificial posterior communicating artery (PCom) (Figure 28–9A). Both anastomoses were made using the ELANA technique. The next day both VAs were endovascularly occluded and the flow through the bypass, which first was directed from the P1 to the ICA, now reversed to the posterior circulation supplying the BA vascular territories. The aneurysm slowly thrombosed, but the next day a progressive brainstem ischemia developed with the bypass still patent and the patient died.

A clear example of the risk of aneurysm rupture after reversal of flow treatment and therefore not complete trapping of the aneurysm is a 44-year-old male patient with a giant BA aneurysm and progressive brainstem symptomatology (see Figure 28–9B). He was treated with an EC-IC bypass from the external carotid artery (ECA) to the BA using the ELANA technique for the latter anastomosis. Both VAs were occluded in the same session. Postoperative angiography showed partly thrombosis of the aneurysm due to reversal of flow. The patient was slowly recovering but died after 2 months as the result of a massive SAH from the aneurysm remnant.

Of the group of 10 patients, only two had a good functional outcome (20%). One of these two cases is a 31-year-old female with a history of SAH from a giant basilar aneurysm and unsuccessful coiling of the aneurysm 2 months before. An EC-IC ELANA bypass was constructed from the ECI to the P1 (ELANA anastomosis) (see Figure 28–9C). The intraoperative flow in this bypass was 70 cc/min with the VAs still open, and we planned an endovascular occlusion of the VAs and aneurysm the next day. The aneurysm occluded and the bypass completely took over posterior circulation. MR flowmetry after 2 weeks showed that the flow in the bypass increased to 120 cc/min, and on follow-up (12 years) she had maximum outcome scores and is fully active in daily life.

ELANA PROTECTIVE BYPASS

In patients for whom the possibility of reconstructing the parent artery harboring a large or giant aneurysm is considered a protective bypass, ELANA can be very helpful. After construction of the bypass, the surgeon is able to temporarily occlude the parent artery for a prolonged time for extensive reconstruction of the vascular tree, as the bypass temporarily takes over blood flow. Also, in the case of aneurysm rupture, the neurosurgeon is in complete control; eventually, after several attempts at reconstruction, the decision to permanently trap the aneurysm can easily be made. In this treatment modality, the ELANA anastomosis again has the major advantage of the absence of temporal occlusion of the parent artery and thus the risk of consequent ischemia can be avoided.

At our institute, we have performed 34 protective ELANA bypass procedures since 1994. Of this total, 32 bypasses were patent during further treatment of the aneurysm and 1 was reconstructed in a second procedure. In four patients (12%), the protective bypass turned out to be necessary as a permanent replacement bypass. Outcome parameters of this group of patients are multifactorial determined. Three patients (9%) suffered from a hemorrhagic complication. The intraoperative use of heparin could have played a significant role in this. In two patients (6%), ischemic complications located distally from the aneurysm occurred even without temporal occlusion of the parent artery, suggesting possible embolic sequelae from aneurysm manipulation.

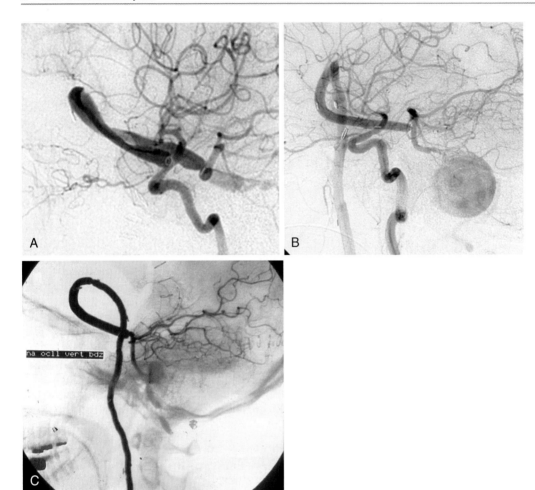

Figure 28–9. A, EC-IC bypass from the ECA (conventional anastomosis) to the BA (ELANA anastomosis). **B,** IC-IC bypass from the ICA (ELANA anastomosis) to the BA (ELANA anastomosis). **C,** EC-IC bypass from the ECA (conventional anastomosis) to the P1 (ELANA anastomosis).

In 29 patients (88%), the functional outcome was favorable (mRs at follow-up < mRs preoperative) at long-term follow-up (mean, 6.0; SD, ≥3.5 years). Complete independence at long-term follow-up was found in 26 patients (79%). These results show that the ELANA technique can be also a valuable tool in difficult-to-clip aneurysms.

CONCLUSION

It is clear that the nonocclusive nature of the ELANA anastomosis technique is a major advantage in flow replacement bypass surgery where large proximal arteries with higher flows need to be replaced or reconstructed, as is mostly the case in giant intracranial aneurysms. In addition, the construction of a deep intracranial anastomosis using the ELANA technique needs less vessel exposure than a conventional technique, as temporal clips that can also disturb the visual field are not needed. This extra advantage facilitates the construction of anastomoses even on P1, P2, SCA, or BA using the transsylvian route only, without major skull base surgery.

Giant and large intracranial aneurysms are a formidable challenge for treatment considering their grim prognosis. To date, endovascular treatment options are still disappointing, and neurosurgical treatment results are by far the most promising. There is no doubt that bypass surgery should be part of the armamentarium of the vascular neurosurgeon who treats these lesions. However, in the treatment of giant aneurysms, conventional bypass techniques are of great value, especially the ELANA bypass technique. Therefore, we recommend that patients with these life-threatening lesions be referred to major highly specialized vascular neurosurgical centers where complete and multidisciplinary treatment options are available.

REFERENCES

1. Barrow DL, Alleyne C: Natural history of giant intracranial aneurysms and indications for intervention, *Clin Neurosurg* 42:214–244, 1995.
2. Drake CG: Giant intracranial aneurysms: experience with surgical treatment in 174 patients, *Clin Neurosurg* 26:12–95, 1979.
3. Parkinson RJ, Eddleman CS, Hunt Batjer H, et al: Giant intracranial aneurysms: endovascular challenges, *Neurosurgery* 59(Suppl 3): S103–S113, 2006.
4. Ross IB, Weil A, Piotin M, et al: Endovascular treatment of distally located giant aneurysms, *Neurosurgery* 47:1147–1153, 2000.

5. Jafar JJ, Russel SM, Woo HH: Treatment of giant intracranial aneurysms with saphenous vein extracranial-to-intracranial bypass grafting: indications, operative technique, and results in 29 patients, *Neurosurgery* 51:138–144, 2002; discussion 144–146.

6. Sekhar LN, Kalavakonda C: Cerebral revascularization for aneurysms and tumors, *Neurosurgery* 50:321–331, 2002.

7. Bakker CJ, Kouwenhoven M, Hartkamp CJ: Accuracy and precision of the time-averaged flow as measured by non-triggered 2D phase-contrast angiography, *Magn Reson Imaging* 13:959–965, 1995.

8. Charbel FT, Hoffman WE, Misra M, et al: Ultrasonic perivascular flow probe: technique and application in neurosurgery, *Neurol Res* 20:439–442, 1998.

9. van der Zwan A, Tulleken CA, Hillen B: Flow quantification of the non-occlusive excimer laser-assisted EC-IC bypass, *Acta Neurochir (Wien)* 143:647–654, 2001.

10. Amin-Hanjani S, Du X, Mlinarevich N, et al: The cut flow index: an intraoperative predictor of the success of extracranial-intracranial bypass for occlusive cerebrovascular disease, *Neurosurgery* 56(Suppl 1):75–85, 2005.

11. Alaraj A, Ashley WW Jr, Charbel FT, et al: The superficial temporal artery trunk as a donor vessel in cerebral revascularization: benefits and pitfalls, *Neurosurg Focus* 24:E7, 2008.

12. Tulleken CA, Hoogland P, Slooff J: A new technique for end-to-side anastomosis between small arteries, *Acta Neurochir Suppl (Wien)* 28:236–240, 1979.

13. Tulleken CA, Verdaasdonk RM, Berendsen W, et al: Use of the excimer laser in high-flow bypass surgery of the brain, *J Neurosurg* 78:477–480, 1993.

14. Tulleken CA, Verdaasdonk RM: First clinical experience with Excimer assisted high flow bypass surgery of the brain, *Acta Neurochir (Wien)* 134:66–70, 1995.

15. Tulleken CA, Verdaasdonk RM, Beck RJ, et al: The modified excimer laser-assisted high-flow bypass operation, *Surg Neurol* 46:424–429, 1996.

16. Streefkerk HJ, Kleinveld S, Koedam EL, et al: Long-term reendothelialization of ecximer laser-assisted nonocclusive anastomoses compared with conventionally sutured anastomoses in pigs, *J Neurosurg* 103:328–336, 2005.

17. Raabe A, Beck J, Gerlach R, et al: Near-infrared indocyanine green video angiography: a new method for intraoperative assessment of vascular flow, *Neurosurgery* 52:132–139, 2003; discussion 139.

18. van Doormaal TP, van der Zwan A, Verweij BH, et al: Treatment of giant and large internal carotid artery aneurysms with a high-flow replacement bypass using the excimer laser-assisted nonocclusive anastomosis technique, *Neurosurgery* 62:1411–1418, 2008.

19. Hillen B, Hoogstraten HW, Post L: A mathematical model of the flow in the circle of Willis, *J Biomech* 19:187–194, 1986.

20. van Doormaal TP, van der Zwan A, Verweij BH, et al: Treatment of giant middle cerebral artery aneurysms with a flow replacement bypass using the excimer laser-assisted nonocclusive anastomosis technique, *Neurosurgery* 63:12–20, 2008.

21. Harvey J, Rasmussen T: Occlusion of the middle cerebral artery: an experimental study, *AMA Arch Neurol Psychiatry* 66:20–29, 1951.

22. Tulleken CAF, Streefkerk HJN, van der Zwan A: Construction of a new posterior communicating artery in a patient with poor posterior fossa circulation: technical case report, *Neurosurgery* 50:415–419, 2002.

23. Tulleken CA, van der Zwan A, van Rooij WJ, et al: High-flow bypass using nonocclusive excimer laser-assisted end-to-side anastomosis of the external carotid artery to the P1 segment of the posterior cerebral artery via the sylvian route. Technical note, *J Neurosurg* 88:925–927, 1998.

24. Streefkerk HJ, Wolfs JF, Sorteberg W, et al: The ELANA technique: constructing a high flow bypass using a non-occlusive anastomosis on the ICA and a conventional anastomosis on the SCA in the treatment of a fusiform giant basilar trunk aneurysm, *Acta Neurochir (Wien)* 146:1009–1019, 2004.

ENDOVASCULAR TECHNIQUES FOR GIANT INTRACRANIAL ANEURYSMS

SABAREESH K. NATARAJAN; ALEXANDER A. KHALESSI;
SHADY JAHSHAN; ADNAN H. SIDDIQUI; L. NELSON HOPKINS;
ELAD I. LEVY

INTRODUCTION

Giant aneurysms (fundus diameter ≥25 mm) comprise approximately 5% of the intracranial aneurysms in most published series.[1-5] These lesions are slightly more common in women. Approximately two thirds are in the anterior circulation and one-third in the posterior circulation.[1] The proportion of patients who present with rupture varies between 20% and 70%, with rebleeding rates similar to those seen for smaller aneurysms in patients presenting with subarachnoid hemorrhage (SAH).[3,5,6] Other presenting signs and symptoms are related to mass effect and ischemic syndromes. Ischemic syndromes are seen in fewer than 10% of giant aneurysms.[3,4]

Giant aneurysms include saccular-shaped aneurysms with a demonstrable neck and fusiform-shaped aneurysms, which are fusiform dilatations of the entire vessel wall with a segmental defect in the parent artery.[4] Saccular aneurysms are thought to develop from smaller saccular aneurysms at points of maximal hemodynamic stress, such as flow vector points or intracranial bifurcations. Fusiform aneurysms are thought to arise from atherosclerotic degeneration of the vessel wall that leads to aneurysmal defects in the parent vessel. They often involve entire segments of a first- or second-order intracranial vessel and incorporate branches and perforators.

NATURAL HISTORY

The natural history of a giant intracranial aneurysm, once diagnosed, is poor. Drake[6] observed a group of 31 patients with untreatable intracranial aneurysms and found a mortality rate of 66% at 2 years and >80% at 5 years. In the first International Study of Unruptured Intracranial Aneurysms (ISUIA), the relative risk of rupture of an unruptured giant aneurysm when compared to an unruptured aneurysm <10 mm in size was 59.0 ($p <$ 0.001).[7] In the second ISUIA, 55 giant aneurysms were observed without treatment and the 5-year cumulative rupture risk by

location was 6.4% in the cavernous carotid artery, 40% in other segments of the internal carotid artery (ICA), anterior cerebral artery, anterior communicating artery (AComA), and middle cerebral artery (MCA), and 50% in the posterior communicating artery (PComA) and posterior circulation.[8] In the same study, giant aneurysms were treated with open surgery in 80 patients and endovascular methods in 55 patients. In the surgical group, the chances of poor outcomes (defined as a modified Rankin Scale [mRS] score of 3-5, or an impaired cognitive outcome) were 25% to 35% in the anterior circulation and 45% in the posterior circulation. In the endovascular group, the chances of poor outcomes were 12% to 15% in the anterior circulation and 40% in the posterior circulation. In giant aneurysms, a high-risk natural history is associated with a higher treatment risk. Accordingly, a decision to treat or not may in part be based on the decisions of patients and their physicians about whether risk is preferable immediately or over time; decisions might also be strongly influenced by the patient's age and presence of medical comorbidities and aneurysmal mass effect.

SURGICAL MANAGEMENT

The two goals of surgical treatment of giant aneurysms are permanent exclusion of the aneurysm from the circulation with possible preservation of distal blood flow and release of mass effect. Reconstructive or deconstructive microsurgical techniques are used. Reconstructive techniques include direct clipping of the aneurysm neck and aneurysmorrhaphy (reconstruction of the vessel using redundant aneurysm sac or graft material). Deconstructive techniques include proximal (Hunterian) ligation and trapping of the aneurysmal segment with or without bypass.

Clipping of the aneurysm neck is generally seen as the best treatment strategy if it is feasible. The results of giant aneurysm surgery have been augmented by (1) use of operative instrumentation and technology, including microscopes, endoscopes, and intraoperative indocyanine green angiography; (2) cerebral protection strategies, such as improvements in anesthetic and intensive care management, cranial base approaches, intraoperative monitoring, hypothermia, adenosine-induced circulatory arrest, and cardiac bypass procedure; (3) preoperative imaging, including 3-D CT or MRA to assess aneurysm geometry, intraluminal thrombus, branches, and perforating vessels, and relationship to the skull base; 6-vessel 3-D angiography to assess the vascular anatomy and availability of donor superficial temporal artery vessels; and balloon occlusion testing with adjunctive measures to assess collaterals for use of temporary occlusion or deconstructive techniques; and (4) intraoperative techniques, such as the use of tandem clips to reinforce the wide aneurysm neck and clip reconstruction of the vessel branch points incorporated in the aneurysm fundus or neck, decompression of the aneurysm by needle puncture, or opening the dome of the aneurysm after flow arrest, performing advanced EC-IC bypass procedure (including ELANA or IC-IC bypass techniques) to preserve distal blood flow.

A meta-analysis by Raaymakers et al.[3] that examined the outcome of surgical treatment for unruptured aneurysms in studies from 1970 to 1996 showed posterior circulation aneurysms to have a 9.6% mortality and 37.9% morbidity and anterior circulation aneurysms to have a 7.4% mortality and 26.9% morbidity. The early reports of Drake[6] and the more modern surgical series of Lawton et al.,[9,10] Samson et al.,[11] Surdell et al.,[12] Piepgras et al.,[13] Hanel et al.,[14] and Sekhar et al.[15–17] have shown improvement in the morbidity and mortality associated with surgically treating these lesions. Most surgical series report an operative mortality of at least 6% and a major morbidity of at least 20%. The results of endovascular therapies should always be compared to these surgical series.

ENDOVASCULAR THERAPY

Although the advances made in microsurgical management have reached a plateau in recent years, the endovascular management of giant intracranial aneurysms and all intracranial aneurysms in general is still evolving. The relative importance of surgery and endovascular strategies and their relative merits in terms of safety, effectiveness, ease of use, and durability are being studied. These techniques can be combined in certain situations to augment the advantages and nullify the disadvantages of either modality. Training of aneurysm specialists in both endovascular and microsurgical techniques would stimulate strategies involving both these modalities in a complementary fashion with an aim to decrease overall morbidity and mortality.

Endovascular Techniques

Endovascular techniques can be generally divided into reconstructive and deconstructive techniques. Reconstructive techniques preserve flow through the parent vessel while excluding the aneurysm from pulsatile blood flow and include the following: (1) primary coiling with or without balloon remodeling; (2) stenting with or without coiling; (3) polymer embolization with or without stenting; and, (4) more recently, parent vessel reconstruction and flow diversion. Deconstructive techniques exclude the aneurysm and the parent vessel from the circulation and include the following: (1) coil occlusion of the parent vessel and (2) detachable balloon trapping and N-butyl cyanoacrylate (nBCA) (glue) embolization after an EC-IC bypass of the vessel to be sacrificed or, rarely, after a negative balloon occlusion test in a patient whose medical condition is too fragile for any other therapy.

Currently, the most common factor for choosing endovascular therapy is anticipated surgical morbidity. A staged approach may be performed in patients with high-grade SAH, occluding the site of the hemorrhage and then planning definitive treatment once the patient has recovered. However, this is not a strategy that is universally accepted. Decision making should be done after careful discussions at an experienced center with a multidisciplinary team including microvascular surgeons, endovascular surgeons, anesthetists, and critical care specialists who specialize in treating intracranial aneurysms. Combination surgical and endovascular procedures planned on a collaborative basis have also been reported on an individual basis.

PREOPERATIVE IMAGING

Catheter-based angiography, 3-D CT imaging, and MR angiography are helpful in confirming the diagnosis and/or consideration of an endovascular, surgical, or combination therapy approach. The performance of a six-vessel 3-D diagnostic cerebral angiogram is crucial before final decisions about treatment options are made. Catheter-based angiography provides critical information regarding not only the anatomic and morphologic features of the lesion but also the potential for collateral circulation should vessel occlusion be entertained as a treatment option. Cross-compression views can aid in determining the patency of PComAs and AComAs, as appropriate. In addition, potential donor arteries for surgical bypass can be assessed. Multiple angiographic projections or 3-D angiography can be extremely useful at delineating the relevant pathological anatomy. Balloon test occlusion is performed concurrently if permanent vessel occlusion (endovascular or surgical) is considered as a treatment option or as a bailout maneuver. Currently, microsurgical and endovascular deconstructive strategies without a bypass are used only for bailout when other treatment options are not available; this is because all the tests for collateral supply after temporary occlusion have false-negative results and a 16% to 20% chance of an ischemic event exists after carotid sacrifice, even if balloon occlusion tests were negative.[18,19] If surgical bypass is planned, endovascular sacrifice should be performed promptly after the surgical procedure to minimize the risk of graft thrombosis owing to low flow.

3-D CT angiography provides valuable information regarding the relative composition of the aneurysm (thrombus or calcifications) and provides delineation of some anatomic aspects of the aneurysm and any additional aneurysms. The technique is quick, noninvasive, and can aid in decision making (surgical versus endovascular versus combination therapy) in acute emergencies, such as when dealing with a concomitant hemorrhage that is producing significant mass effect. However, this technique is dependent on the quality of 3-D image reconstruction; and suboptimal imaging quality can lead to misinterpretation, especially when the aneurysm is intimately associated with bony structures or multiple surgical clips or coils. MR angiography is useful for screening but typically not for treatment decision making. MR imaging can be quite useful to evaluate for intra-aneurysmal thrombus, mass effect, edema, and any potentially associated ischemic lesions.

ANESTHESIA

At our center, we prefer to perform endovascular procedures under conscious sedation so that we can conduct neurologic examinations intermittently. Avoidance of general anesthesia also reduces the cardiovascular risk of the overall procedure. However, if a complication does occur, the potential exists for further harm until the patient's airway can be secured and additional maneuvers (e.g., ventriculostomy, further embolization) can be performed. One must be prepared to intubate at a moment's notice. Not all patients are candidates for conscious sedation because of poor neurologic status, young age, excessive anxiety, or inability to lie still. General anesthesia offers the advantages of control of the airway as well as reduction or elimination of patient movement during the procedure. General anesthesia is routinely used at most centers.

ANTIPLATELET THERAPY

Patients scheduled to undergo elective stent or flow-diversion device placement receive aspirin (325 mg by mouth daily) and clopidogrel (75 mg by mouth daily) for a minimum of 4 days before the procedure. Those undergoing stenting on a more urgent basis receive aspirin (650 mg by mouth) and clopidogrel (600 mg by mouth) 4 hours before the procedure. If stenting is performed as an emergency bailout maneuver, we administer an intravenous bolus dose of glycoprotein IIb-IIIa inhibitor (180 mg/kg eptifibatide at our institution) and then clopidogrel (600 mg by mouth) and aspirin (650 mg by mouth) immediately after the procedure. Eptifibatide (2 mg/kg/min) is continued as an intravenous drip for 4 hours after the procedure to allow the clopidogrel to reach therapeutic levels of platelet inhibition. In the rare case of a patient with an acutely ruptured aneurysm undergoing stent placement, the glycoprotein IIb-IIIa inhibitor can be given after the stent

is in place and the first or second coil is in proper position. All patients with a stent or flow-diversion device are placed on clopidogrel (75 mg daily) for 3 months and aspirin (325 mg daily) for life. Patients who do not have stent placement are kept on aspirin for life.

ANTICOAGULATION THERAPY

Proper decision making regarding periprocedural systemic anticoagulation is essential when using complex endovascular techniques for aneurysm treatment. We routinely administer heparin (an intravenous bolus of 50 to 70 units/kg) to obtain an activated coagulation time of 250 to 300 seconds before catheterization of intracranial vessels for elective and emergent patients, except those with SAH. Anticoagulation therapy is used more judiciously in patients with SAH. In these patients, we typically administer a 25- to 35-unit/kg bolus of heparin after the first coil is placed successfully, followed by a similar bolus after intra-aneurysmal flow is reduced. The effect of the heparin is allowed to wear off after the procedure, unless there is evidence of intraprocedural wire perforation or contrast extravasation, in which case the heparin is reversed during or after the procedure with protamine sulfate.

For patients with SAH, CT examination is performed immediately before treatment to assess for latent intracerebral hemorrhage (whether caused by aneurysm rebleeding or ventriculostomy placement), because such hemorrhage will prevent our use of stents or glycoprotein IIb-IIIa antagonists. Because of the degree of systemic anticoagulation, the arterial access site is typically secured by use of a closure device at the conclusion of the procedure.

Before the procedure, preferably the previous day, the patient should be assessed and all the available imaging studies reviewed in preparation for the case. Decisions about overall strategy should be made ahead of time to permit accurate device selection and smooth and efficient performance during the case. Considerations should include choice of access vessel, endovascular technique (i.e., primary coiling versus stent-assisted or balloon-assisted coiling), and device types and sizes.

ENDOVASCULAR ACCESS

The route for endovascular access, including the iliofemoral artery anatomy, arch anatomy, and supra-aortic vessel, needs to be assessed to decide on the access site and the devices that would facilitate safe access and provide a stable platform for intracranial therapies. Brachial or radial artery access may be considered if there is a disease in the iliofemoral arterial segments or descending aorta. Patients with giant aneurysms have a greater likelihood of having an atherosclerotic arch or tortuous and elongated supra-aortic vessel, especially in cases with associated collagenopathies. In such cases, special devices to access difficult arch anatomy, a carotid cutdown in the neck, or a cutdown of the extracranial vertebral artery (VA) as it traverses over the posterior arch of C1 could be used to access the intracranial vasculature.

GUIDE CATHETER SELECTION

A stable guide catheter platform is critical for endovascular treatment of giant aneurysms. We are increasingly using the Neuron™ Intracranial Access System (Penumbra, Alameda, CA) as the guide catheter. This device is more stable the farther distally it is placed. The two guide catheters previously used most often were the Envoy® (Codman and Shurtleff, Inc., Raynham, MA) and the Guider Softip™ XF guide catheter (Boston Scientific, Natick, MA). A 6-French (F) 90-cm Cook Shuttle® (Cook, Bloomington, IN) also provides a large, stable platform for intervention. The guide catheter can be placed directly or by use of an exchange method in patients with tortuous anatomy, atherosclerosis, or fibromuscular dysplasia. We often use a "tower of power" where the Neuron is placed through a large guide catheter for added stability and distal access.

PARENT VESSEL SACRIFICE

The key step in the sacrifice of a large vessel, such as the ICA or the VA, is the temporary arrest of proximal flow to prevent inadvertent embolization into the cerebral vasculature during the procedure. In general, the vessel should be occluded either at or immediately proximal to the lesion. Vessel occlusion can be accomplished with detachable coils or detachable balloons. Although detachable balloons are not commercially available in the United States at the present time, they are available in Europe and Japan.

Coil Occlusion of the Parent Vessel

For vessel occlusion with coils, guide catheter access to the parent vessel is established. A single 6-F, 90-cm sheath has an inner diameter large enough to accommodate two microcatheters. Under roadmap guidance, the microcatheter to be used for coil deployment is positioned in the vessel where occlusion is planned. A nondetachable balloon is positioned in the proximal segment of the vessel.

The balloon is inflated, and temporary flow arrest is confirmed with gentle injection of contrast material through the guide catheter under fluoroscopy. The first coil is deployed. The 0.018-inch system 3-D coils with a diameter approximately twice that of the vessel are usually effective. Prior to detachment, the balloon is briefly deflated to confirm that the first coil is stable. If there is no movement of the first coil with restoration of flow, the balloon is re-inflated and the first

coil is detached. Additional coils are deployed as necessary to achieve tight packing of several centimeters of the vessel. The balloon is then deflated, and final angiographic images are obtained. Liquid embolic agents, especially nBCA, can be used as an adjunct to coil occlusion.

Detachable Balloon Embolization

The Goldvalve™ detachable balloon (Acta Vascular/Nfocus Neuromedical, Santa Clara, CA) is available in most of the world outside of the United States, and the vendor is working on obtaining approval for the North American market. Complete stasis of flow can be achieved more quickly with balloons than with coils, but the balloons require a little more preparation. Occlusion of an artery with detachable balloons should always be undertaken with two balloons, placed end to end, with the proximal balloon functioning as a "safety" balloon to minimize the chance of distal migration of the balloons.

A large guide catheter is required, often 7- or 8-F (or a 6- or 7-F, 90-cm sheath). A balloon size is chosen that is slightly larger than the diameter of the vessel to be occluded. The balloons are attached to their recommended delivery catheters. If the guide catheter is large enough, it is preferable to advance the two balloons simultaneously through the guide catheter and into the vessel in order to limit the risk of premature detachment. Ideally, the balloons should be positioned in a relatively straight segment of the vessel. When in proper position, the balloons are inflated with contrast material. If they are properly sized, they will flatten out and elongate as they are inflated. When the balloon position and stability appear to be satisfactory, the distal balloon is detached by slowly, gently pulling back on the balloon catheter.

PARENT VESSEL PRESERVATION

Coil Embolization

Some giant aneurysms may have a configuration amenable to pure endovascular coiling alone. The best angiographic projection of the aneurysm neck and parent vessel, or vessels, should be obtained. Placement of the microcatheter in a deep position and use of a larger microcatheter that will reduce catheter back-out may be helpful to improve the degree of coil packing. Ideally, 0.018-inch system coils should be used initially to provide the most stable framework from which to coil the bulk of the aneurysm. We prefer to continue to deposit sequentially smaller 3-D coils as feasible to increase the chances of good coverage of the aneurysm neck. Several series of results after simple coiling of giant aneurysms have been reported. Overall, the rate of complete occlusion is approximately 40%, and the rate of near-complete occlusion is approximately 66.7%.[20-23] An extremely high recanalization rate of 40% to 60% that required retreatment was noted even in patients in whom complete occlusion was achieved during the primary procedure. With time, most aneurysms reopen by coil compaction, coil migration into intraluminal thrombus, or dissolution of intraluminal thrombus resulting in luminal enlargement.[20–23] Clearly, according to these results, coil embolization alone typically is well tolerated clinically, but it is not sufficient to provide a complete and durable long-term result in most patients.

Balloon-Assisted Coil Embolization

The use of balloons to occlude the aneurysm neck during coiling of wide-necked aneurysms was first described in 1994 by Moret et al.[24] A 6-F or larger guide catheter is required to accommodate both a balloon catheter and a microcatheter. A microcatheter is placed into the aneurysm fundus, and a balloon catheter is centered over the aneurysm neck. The balloon is subsequently inflated during placement of a coil and then deflated intermittently in between coils to allow antegrade flow. Sequential inflations and deflations are performed as additional coils are placed, until the aneurysm is completely coiled, at which point the balloon is removed. The concept is that the balloon prevents distal embolization and conforms the coil mass to the shape of the balloon and that the coil mass shape becomes stable, thereby protecting the parent artery as the individual coils interlock. Care must be taken during the initial insertion of a coil to form a loop directing the distal end of the coil away from the aneurysm fundus to limit the risk of aneurysm perforation during balloon inflation (Figures 29–1 through 29–3).

Forty to 50 coils can be required to fill a giant aneurysm, leading to 40 to 50 cycles of balloon inflations, for which the risk may be prohibitive. In addition, the ability to protect the parent artery lumen by means of balloon occlusion during the coiling procedure, especially when there is extensive fusiform dilation, is minimal. Temporary balloon occlusion exposes the patient to an increased risk of cerebral ischemia resulting from thromboembolic complication and vessel rupture. The increase in thromboembolic complications occurs because of stasis of blood or temporary occlusion of local perforating end arteries covered by the balloon. The risk of vessel rupture stems from the compliant design of most balloons used for these purposes and is associated with dramatic changes in volume and pressure in the balloon with minimal inflation volume changes. Soeda et al.[25] reported that the occurrence of diffusion-weighted imaging (DWI) lesions was significantly associated with the use of balloon remodeling. In that series, DWI was positive in 73% of all patients receiving a remodeling procedure, as compared to 49% in the control group. Other authors demonstrated lower rates of DWI lesions in 20% of patients treated with remodeling but did not provide a control group.[26] Overall procedural balloon-assisted coiling morbidity and mortality range from 0% to 20.4% in all aneurysms. No results for specific series of balloon-assisted coiling for giant aneurysms have been reported.[27]

At our center, balloon assistance is used for cases of ruptured wide-necked giant aneurysms in which the use of antiplatelet agents is contraindicated and for those patients in whom the deployment of a stent is not feasible. The number of patients in the second category is decreasing as more deliverable self-expanding intracranial microstents (SEIM) become available. We currently use the HyperGlide and HyperForm balloons (Covidien Vascular Therapies, Mansfield, MA) for these patients having limited options.

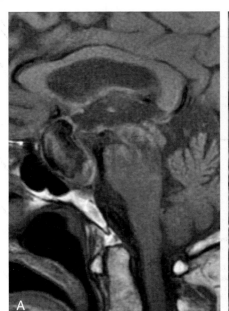
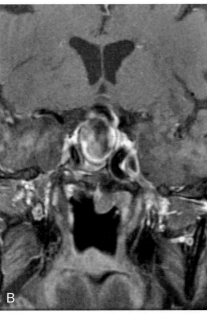
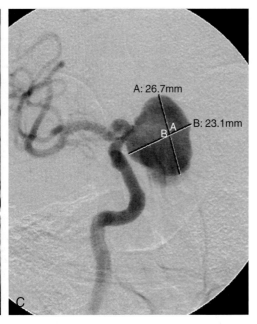

Figure 29–1. This 69-year-old woman presented with a giant aneurysm masquerading as a pituitary adenoma. Sagittal (**A**) and coronal (**B**) MR images showing a mass lesion near the pituitary region. **C,** Right ICA injection showing a giant ICA aneurysm. She underwent near-complete coiling with the balloon-assisted technique.

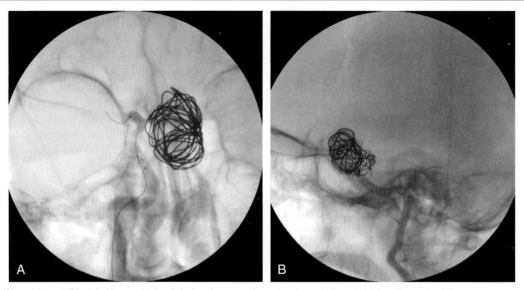

Figure 29–2. AP (**A**) and lateral (**B**) plain X-rays obtained during the procedure showing a balloon bridging the neck of the aneurysm.

Balloon-Assisted Liquid Agent Embolization

Onyx HD-500 (ev3) embolization for the treatment of intracranial aneurysms is still investigational. Onyx is comprised of ethylene vinyl alcohol (EVOH) copolymer dissolved in dimethyl sulfoxide (DMSO) and suspended in micronized tantalum powder (to provide contrast for visualization under fluoroscopy). The EVOH copolymer is infused through a microcatheter into an aqueous environment; the DMSO diffuses outward into the surrounding tissue, allowing the material to precipitate into a spongy, space-occupying cast. Onyx embolization of aneurysms requires a balloon-assisted technique to permit infusion of the material into the aneurysm without embolization into the distal circulation. All devices must be compatible with DMSO.

The patients receive a loading dose of aspirin and clopidogrel before the procedure (as described for stent-assisted coiling). A deflated, compliant DMSO-compatible balloon (HyperGlide) is placed in the parent vessel adjacent to the aneurysm. A DMSO-compatible microcatheter (Rebar, ev3) is navigated into the aneurysm. The balloon is inflated, and contrast material is gently injected through the microcatheter to confirm that the balloon has made an adequate seal over

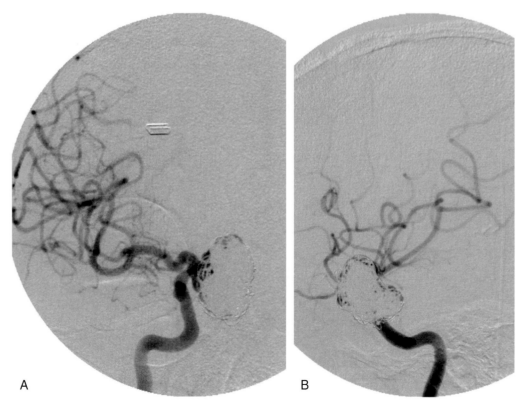

Figure 29–3. Follow-up angiogram obtained 3 years later shows no recurrence of the aneurysm. AP (**A**) and lateral (**B**) projections of right ICA injection.

the aneurysm neck. After the microcatheter is primed with DMSO, a Cadence Precision Injector syringe (ev3) is filled with Onyx and attached to the hub of the microcatheter. Onyx is injected under fluoroscopic observation at a rate of approximately 0.1 ml per minute or slower. The injection is continued and paused after each incremental volume of approximately 0.2 to 0.3 ml has been administered to allow the material to polymerize and to allow temporary balloon deflation. Several sequential re-inflations and injections may be necessary.

At the completion of the embolization, with the balloon deflated, the microcatheter syringe is decompressed by aspiration of 0.2 ml of Onyx left in the catheter; this prevents dribbling of Onyx material during the removal of the microcatheter. Prior to removal of the microcatheter, 10 minutes are allowed to elapse to permit the Onyx material to set within the aneurysm. For microcatheter removal, the balloon should be inflated a final time to stabilize the Onyx mass as the microcatheter is withdrawn. The patient should be kept on a dual antiplatelet regimen with aspirin and clopidogrel for 1 month after the procedure.

In a multicenter study conducted by Molyneux et al.,[28] permanent neurologic morbidity was 8.3% (eight of 97 patients), with two procedural deaths. In large and giant aneurysms, procedural time was long (up to 6 hours). Delayed occlusion of the carotid artery occurred in nine of 100 (9%) patients. At 12 months' follow-up of 53 patients, 38 (72%) large and giant aneurysms were completely angiographically occluded. Retreatment was performed in nine instances. Although some single-center studies show slightly better results,[29] in our opinion, the relatively high complication rate and high rate of delayed carotid artery occlusion do not justify this treatment in patients with unruptured aneurysms who cannot tolerate carotid artery occlusion. At present, the short-term results of Onyx occlusion for large and giant aneurysms are not better than those for selective coil occlusion, and the immediate and delayed complication rate is probably higher.

STENT-ASSISTED COILING

Intracranial stenting for aneurysm therapy has undergone a remarkable evolution over the past decade. The devices themselves, as well as the manner in which they are applied, have changed dramatically. Initially utilized exclusively as adjunctive devices to simplify (or, in some cases, to allow) the treatment of wide-necked aneurysms, stents have become increasingly used to achieve flow redirection and vascular remodeling in an attempt to augment the durability of endovascular treatments. The newest generations of intracranial microstents have surpassed their predecessors, evolving into stand-alone devices designed to cure aneurysms without other embolic materials.

In the early 1990s, we described the application of stents to treat experimental aneurysms.[30] The basic principles of stent-supported therapy delineated by early experiments are (1) parent vessel protection by preventing coil prolapse[30] and (2) parent vessel remodeling providing a scaffold for neointimal growth and producing flow-diversion that may facilitate and maintain

aneurysm thrombosis.[31,32] Balloon-expanding coronary stents were used initially to support coiling of wide-necked intracranial aneurysms.[33–40] These stents were of limited benefit due to their rigid nature and the challenges involved in their delivery and deployment within the tortuous cerebrovasculature. The newer generation of balloon-mounted stents designed specifically for intracranial use (Pharos, Micrus Endovascular, Sunnyvale, CA) are more stable than the predicate devices designed for coronary applications and have indications for the treatment of both cerebral aneurysms and intracranial atherosclerosis.[41–44]

SELF-EXPANDING INTRACRANIAL MICROSTENTS (SEIMS)

Presently, there are two SEIMs designed specifically for stent-assisted coiling of wide-necked intracranial aneurysms available in the United States: the Neuroform3™ stent (Boston Scientific) and the Enterprise™ Vascular Reconstruction Device (Codman and Shurtleff, Inc., Raynham, MA). Each device consists of a self-expanding nitinol stent that is deployed in the parent vessel adjacent to the aneurysm neck; the stent then acts as a scaffold to hold coils in place inside the aneurysm. Both devices are extremely navigable (compared to delivery of balloon-mounted coronary stents [BMC]); and the Enterprise presents several benefits over the Neuroform including reconstrainability, a lower profile delivery system, and a technically less-complicated deployment mechanism. If sized appropriately, SEIMs automatically expand to appose the walls of the parent artery, even within very tortuous vascular segments. In addition, these devices have the ability to differentially expand to accommodate adjacent vascular segments that vary significantly in diameter. The anatomic distortion of the vessel that is created by the insertion of these devices is minimized by their flexibility and conformability. The superelastic properties of the SEIM result in the device exerting a small chronic outward radial force against the vessel wall, which stabilizes the device in vivo.

The introduction of these devices led to a marked increase in the number of stent-assisted aneurysm treatments performed and greatly broadened the scope of lesions that were amenable to endovascular therapy. As practitioners gained experience with SEIMs, novel approaches to more complex lesions were innovated and the sophistication of endovascular reconstruction increased.[45–52] Over the past decade, stenting has become a standard adjunctive technique used to facilitate the treatment of giant and complex aneurysms.

Recently, SEIM have begun to be viewed not only as adjunctive devices to support coiling but also as tools that could potentially support the long-term durability of coil embolization—particularly for difficult cases in which the aneurysm is prone to recurrence. This is because stents have several possible effects on the physiology and biology of the aneurysm–parent vessel complex. These effects include the following: (1) alteration of the parent vessel configuration, thus possibly a change in the intra-aneurysmal flow dynamics;

(2) disruption of the inflow jets; (3) reduction in the vorticity and wall shear stress on the aneurysm wall and reduction of the water-hammer effect of the pulsatile blood flow that causes coil compaction by the tines of the stents; and (4) providing a scaffolding and stimulus for the overgrowth of endothelial and neointimal tissue across the neck of the aneurysm, creating a matrix for "biological remodeling" across the aneurysm neck.

NEUROFORM STENT

The Neuroform stent comes from the manufacturer preloaded in a 3-F microdelivery catheter. A "stabilizer" catheter, which is also preloaded in the microdelivery catheter, is then used to stabilize and deploy the stent as the microdelivery catheter is withdrawn. The stent consists of a fine wire mesh that cannot be seen during standard fluoroscopic imaging; however,

each end of the stent is equipped with four radiopaque platinum marker bands. This device comes in sizes ranging between 2.5 and 4.5 mm in diameter and 10 and 30 mm in length. The diameter recommended by the manufacturer for placement is 0.5 mm greater than the largest diameter of the parent artery to be stented. The length is chosen such that the stent extends for at least 5 mm proximal and distal to the aneurysm neck. The struts composing the stent measure approximately 60 microns in thickness. The interstices of the fully expanded stent are large enough to accommodate a microcatheter tip that is 2.5 F or smaller (realistically, <2.0 F) for coiling. When the stent is placed in curved anatomy (in experimental models), the stent cells are prone to opening, producing gaps in stent coverage along the outer curvature of the vessel.[53,54] These gaps could conceivably lead to incomplete coverage of the aneurysm neck and coil prolapse from the aneurysm into the parent artery during embolization (Figures 29–4 through 29–8).

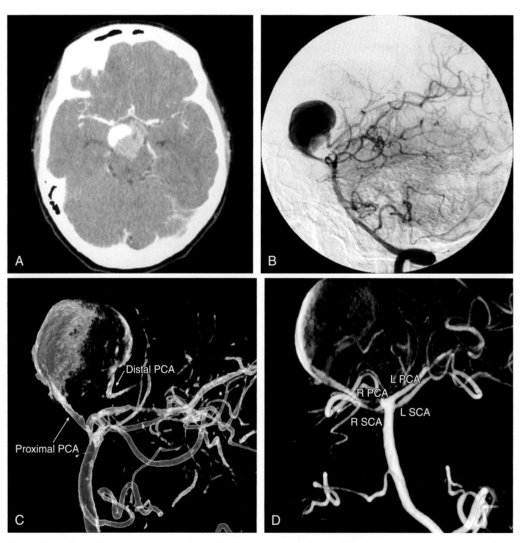

Figure 29–4. This 43-year-old woman presented with severe headaches and a giant partially thrombosed fusiform aneurysm of the right posterior cerebral artery (PCA). Axial contrast CT image (**A**) and right VA injection angiographic image (**B**) showing the aneurysm. **C** and **D,** Three-dimensional reconstructions of the angiogram showing the detailed anatomy.

29

Figure 29–5. A 4- × 30-mm Neuroform3 stent was inserted from the top of the basilar artery (BA) into the right PCA, across the neck of the aneurysm (**A**). The aneurysm was coiled through the stent tines (**B**). The patient was sent home on aspirin and clopidogrel.

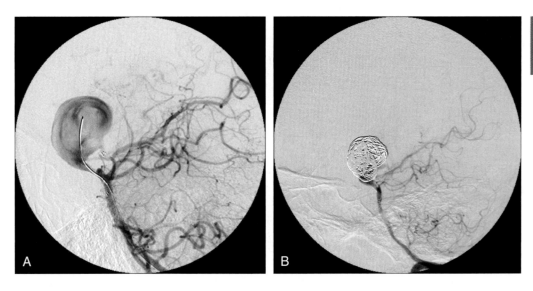

Figure 29–6. The patient presented 10 days later with dysarthria and expressive aphasia. **A,** Non-contrast CT scan. CT perfusion imaging showed increased mean transit time (**D**) and decreased cerebral blood flow (**C**) without a cerebral blood volume lesion (**B**), which was suggestive of a large region of the left MCA territory ischemia, without a completed infarct.

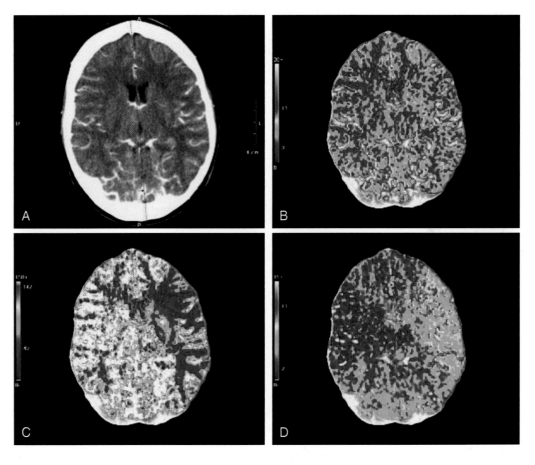

The microcatheter and microwire (0.010-inch or 0.014-inch) are navigated, using a roadmap, past the aneurysm. The microwire is removed and replaced with an exchange-length 0.014-inch microwire with a soft, J-shaped distal curve. The microdelivery catheter containing the Neuroform stent is threaded onto the exchange-length wire and advanced across the neck of the aneurysm. The stabilizer catheter is then held firmly in place as the microdelivery catheter is pulled back over the stabilizer and microwire, so that the stent is unsheathed. As the stent expands, the marker bands can be

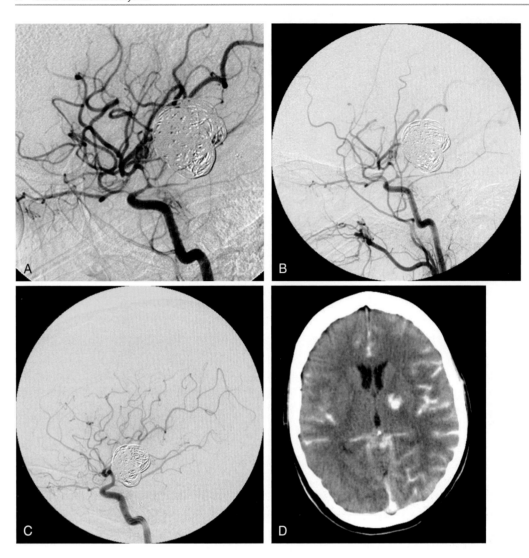

Figure 29–7. Angiography showed spasm of the left ICA and PComA (**A** and **B**) that resolved completely after balloon angioplasty and verapamil injection (**C**). Post-therapy, the patient had a dense right hemiplegia and global aphasia, and the CT scan showed a left basal ganglia intracranial hemorrhage and an SAH (**D**). She had a prolonged hospital course and was sent for inpatient rehabilitation therapy with a right hemiparesis (grade 3/5), and improving expressive aphasia, and she was following commands.

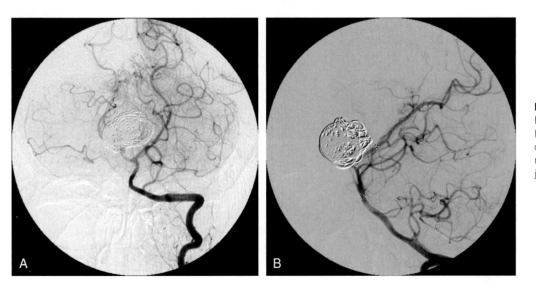

Figure 29–8. At 6 months, she had recovered completely, and her follow-up angiogram showed complete occlusion of the aneurysm. AP (**A**) and lateral (**B**) projections of left VA injection.

seen to spread. The microdelivery catheter and stabilizer are then removed over the exchange-length wire. A standard-length microcatheter is then advanced over the microwire until it is past the stent. The exchange-length microwire is then removed and replaced with a standard-length microwire. The microwire and microcatheter are then guided through the stent and into the aneurysm for coiling.

ENTERPRISE STENT

The Enterprise stent comes preloaded with a delivery wire, and both the stent and wire are enclosed within a plastic sheath (the "dispenser loop"). The delivery wire has three radiopaque zones: the proximal wire, the "stent-positioning marker" (which indicates where the undeployed stent is loaded and runs the length of the stent), and the distal tip. The Enterprise measures 4.5 mm in diameter when unconstrained, and as

such, is only indicated for use in vessels measuring between 2.5 and 4 mm in diameter. The device comes in 14-, 22-, 28-, and 37-mm lengths. The struts of the Enterprise, like those of the Neuroform, are approximately 60 microns thick. The stent struts cannot be seen on standard fluoroscopy; each end of the four platinum marker bands can be seen, but these are considerably more difficult to see compared with the markers on the Neuroform stent. The interstices of the fully expanded Enterprise stent are large enough to accommodate a microcatheter tip with an outer diameter size of ≤2.3 F for coiling (Figures 29–9 and 29–10).

The closed-cell design of the Enterprise stent makes it reconstrainable. This design also prevents the stent from splaying open along the outer curvature of vascular bends and results in the incorporation of each cell into the entire device structure, making the individual cells more durable and less likely to become damaged during attempted traversal of the device with a microcatheter. At the same time, the loss of segmental flexibility created by the continuous closed-cell structure may result in

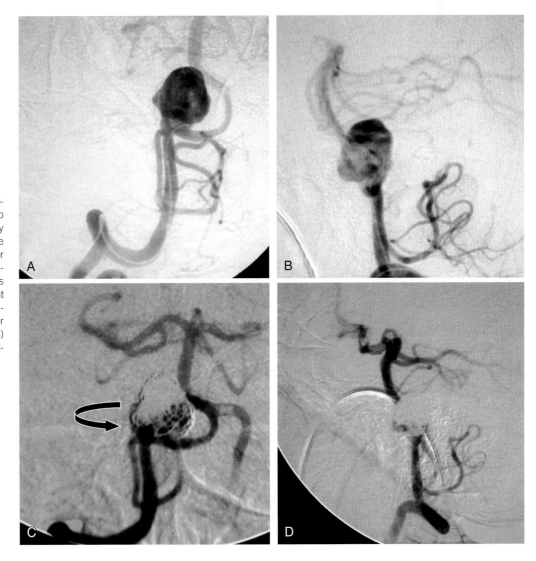

Figure 29–9. This 67-year-old woman presented with a thunderclap headache and SAH. Angiography revealed a giant aneurysm in the right VA that involved the posterior inferior cerebellar artery (PICA) origin. AP (**A**) and lateral (**B**) projections of right VA injection. She underwent partial coiling to protect the aneurysm and returned 1 month later for a follow-up angiogram. AP view (**C**) and lateral view (**D**) showed a residual neck (*arrow* in C).

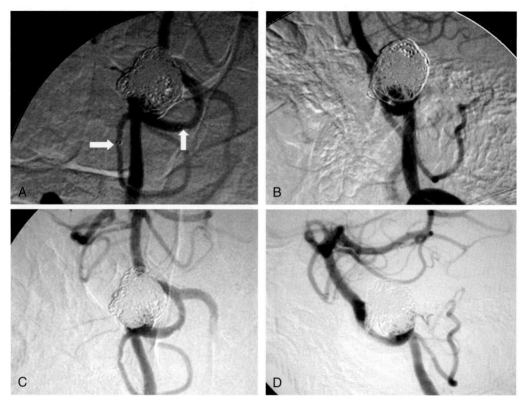

Figure 29–10. Owing to the sharp turn in the right VA (*arrows*) and the direct angle from the portion of the right VA distal to the aneurysm into the right PICA, retrograde catheterization of the right VA was done from the left VA; and an Enterprise stent (*arrows* showing stent tines) was inserted from the right VA into the right PICA to bridge the neck of the aneurysm: AP view (**A**) and lateral view (**B**). Coiling of the remnant was done through the stent tines to achieve complete occlusion of the aneurysm: AP view (**C**) and lateral view (**D**).

the device "kinking" or forming a "cobra-head" configuration around tight vascular curves, potentially resulting in poor vessel wall apposition and suboptimal parent vessel protection.[45,53] The interstices between the stent struts are also smaller and less deformable in some anatomic configurations, making microcatheter traversal more difficult in some situations. Finally, although the closed-cell structure provides higher radial resistive force (i.e., resistance to outward compression once deployed), it also exerts less chronic outward force (i.e., outward pressure upon the vessel wall), potentially making it more prone to migration during attempted catheterization of the aneurysm or, in some anatomic configurations, spontaneously.[55]

A Prowler Select Plus microcatheter (2.9 F or 2.3 F proximal or distal outer diameter; 0.021-inch inner diameter; Codman Neurovascular) and microwire (0.010-inch or 0.014-inch; Codman Neurovascular) are navigated past the aneurysm using a roadmap. The tip is positioned at least 12 mm distal to the aneurysm neck. The microwire is removed, and the Enterprise stent is inserted into the Prowler Select Plus microcatheter by placing the tip of the dispenser loop in the rotating hemostatic valve and advancing the delivery wire. The delivery wire can be advanced without fluoroscopy, until the marker on the wire is at the rotating hemostatic valve. The marker on the delivery wire is 150 cm from the distal tip. The delivery wire and stent are then navigated into

position across the aneurysm neck. The stent is deployed by holding the delivery wire firmly in place while carefully retracting the microcatheter. If the stent position is not satisfactory, advancing the microcatheter may recapture the stent. Stent recapture (i.e., pulling the stent back into the microcatheter) may be done provided that <80% of the stent has been deployed. If the proximal end of the stent-positioning marker is still within the microcatheter, it is possible to recapture the stent. The stent should be recaptured only once. If further repositioning is needed, the stent is removed and a new one used. The microwire and microcatheter are then guided through the stent and into the aneurysm for coiling. The ability to recapture the stent, as well as enhanced navigability, are distinct advantages with the Enterprise.

INDICATIONS FOR SEIMS

The current indications for SEIMs for the treatment of aneurysms include stent-assisted coil embolization, rescue during coil embolization, and balloon-assisted coiling followed by stenting.

Stent-assisted coil embolization. The most common technique is trans-stent coiling in which an SEIM is placed across the aneurysm neck, and coil embolization is performed after microcatheter manipulation. Trans-stent coiling may be performed at the time of the initial procedure or during a second procedure ("staged technique"), typically 4 to 8 weeks after stenting. Some operators prefer the staged technique to allow endothelialization of the stent prior to attempted coiling. The advantages are that the stent is more stable after endothelialization, and the clopidogrel therapy is most often discontinued before coiling. Another technique used is a jailing technique in which a microcatheter is placed inside the aneurysm before stent deployment.[56] This technique is less favored, because there is a chance of displacement of the microcatheter during stent placement and even a higher chance of coil stretching or breakage because the coil can get caught between the stent and the vessel wall.

Rescue during coil embolization. If detached coils or the entire mass of coils prolapse into the parent vessel during the procedure, the stent is placed in the vessel either to re-position the coils back in the aneurysm lumen or tack up the coils against the vessel wall and thus prevent further migration and distal emboli.[57,58]

Balloon-assisted coiling followed by stenting. Some operators prefer balloon-assisted coiling followed by SEIM deployment because (1) the aneurysm neck-parent vessel interface is best seen during balloon-assisted coiling, (2) this approach allows adjustment of the coil mass to configure the coils to the neck of the aneurysm and thus allows denser packing, (3) the balloon pins the microcatheter and allows easier recatheterization if the microcatheter is displaced, and (4) if intraprocedural perforation of the aneurysm occurs, the balloon can be inflated to cause temporary flow arrest and allow time for reversal of heparin and/or further coiling to secure the bleeding.

ADVANCED SEIM TECHNIQUES USED IN GIANT ANEURYSMS

Advanced techniques of SEIM stenting include the balloon anchor, Y-stent, waffle-cone, trans–Circle of Willis, and balloon in-stent. These are unique approaches to complex lesions.

Balloon anchor technique. This technique is useful for the treatment of wide-necked aneurysms having a dominant flow jet that constantly directs any device used for distal vessel access into the aneurysm (Figures 29–11 and 29–12). This, coupled with the inability to achieve stable distal purchase of the access after it is obtained, often leads to abortion of the procedure. In a case treated with this technique at our center, distal parent vessel access was obtained by allowing the microwire to follow the local hemodynamics into a giant ICA aneurysm and around its dome into the distal vessel. An over-the-wire balloon inflated in the distal vessel followed by gentle retraction of the balloon catheter and microwire allowed only a wire bridge across the aneurysm neck, thereby allowing the stent catheter to be brought up in a standard fashion.

Y-stent. This technique is most commonly used for bifurcation aneurysms arising from the basilar tip or carotid terminus (carotid T). Two stents are placed, with the first extending out one limb of the bifurcation and the second introduced through the interstices of the first stent and extending into the other limb of the bifurcation. This configuration forms a "Y"-shaped construct at the bifurcation and provides very robust support for the coil embolization of terminal aneurysms.[46,51,52] This Y-stent technique has also been applied to treat MCA aneurysms[51] and AComA aneurysms.

Waffle-cone. In cases in which the application of the Y-stent technique is not feasible, a stent may be deployed from the parent artery directly into the aneurysm (i.e., "intra-extra-aneurysmal stent placement") to achieve parent artery protection[59] (Figure 29–13). Using this technique (called the waffle-cone technique because of the appearance of the stent-coil combination after treatment), a single stent can be used to stabilize an intra-aneurysmal coil mass.[59] However, the final construct redirects flow into the terminal aneurysm sac and actually disrupts flow into the bifurcation branches. One might expect that such a construct could lead to high rates of recanalization. In addition, if this technique fails or leads to recanalization, other available means of treatment (surgical clipping, endovascular therapy with balloon remodeling, or Y-stent reconstruction) (see Figures 29–13C and 29–13D) are made considerably more difficult, if not impossible.

Trans–Circle of Willis stenting. In some cases where Y-stenting is not feasible for terminal aneurysms, a stent can be placed across the circle of Willis from P1 to P1 via the PComA, from A1 to M1 via the AComA, or from the ipsilateral A1 to contralateral A1 via the AComA.[49] This technique provides a means by which to achieve protection of both limbs of the bifurcation with a single SEIM.

Balloon in-stent technique. In a circumferential fusiform aneurysm with a large parent artery defect, a BMC to bridge the proximal and distal vessels and a microcatheter placed outside the stent before balloon inflation can be used for coiling of the aneurysm around the BMC. The main disadvantages are the difficulty in tracking the BMCs through the intracranial vasculature and the possibility of prolapse of the coil mass into the lumen of the stent. SEIMs cannot be used for this purpose as they tend to overexpand into the saccular component of the aneurysm, making it a challenge for the operator to ascertain whether the embolization coils are being placed within the parent artery or within the saccular component of the aneurysm. In addition, the SEIMs are easily damaged and displaced; such migration can result in displacement of one end of the stent into the saccular component of the aneurysm. The recent development of flow-diverting devices has essentially obviated the need to perform this technique.

FLOW-DIVERTING DEVICES

The concept of parent vessel reconstruction is quickly advancing with the very recent development of dedicated flow-diverting endovascular constructs designed for intracranial

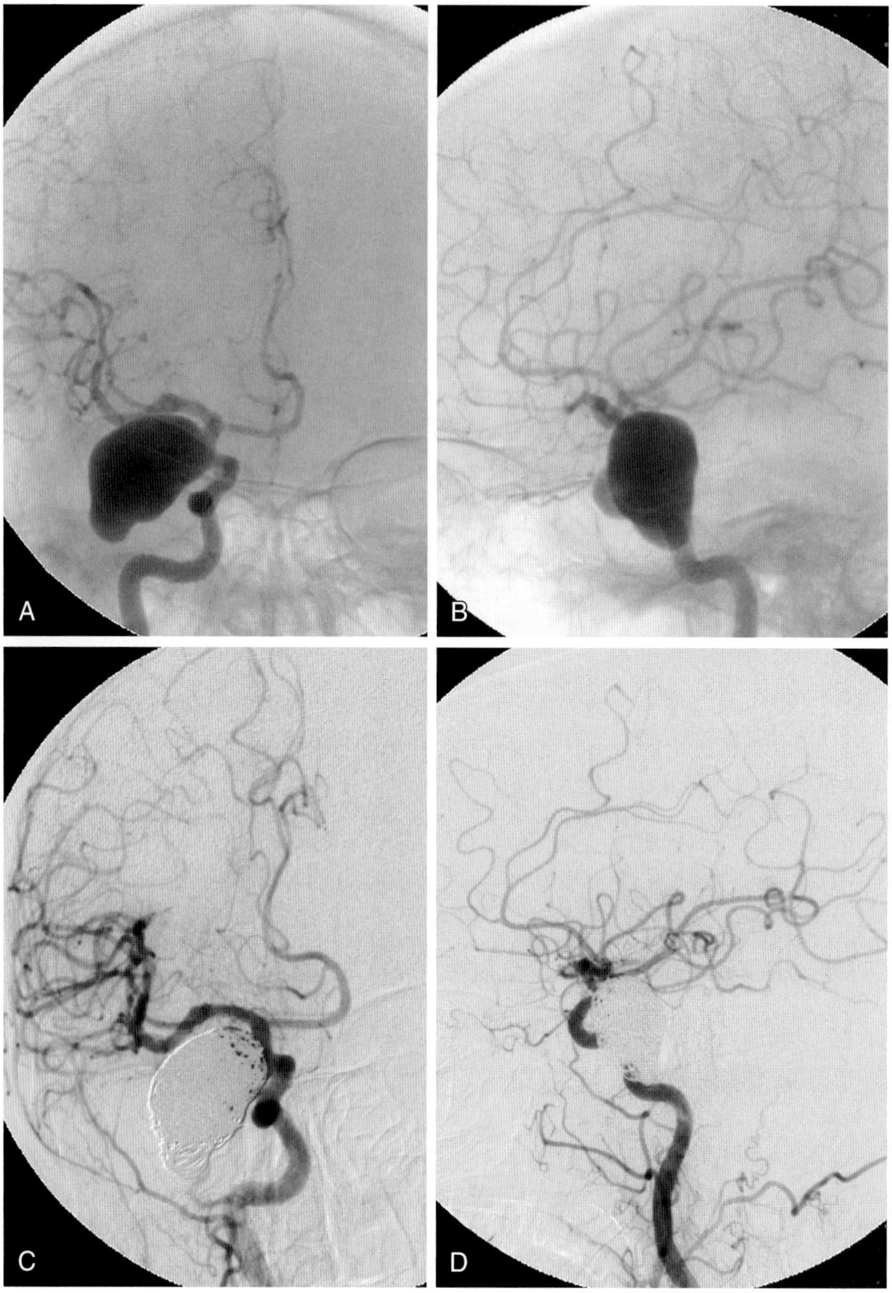

Figure 29–11. Right ICA angiograms showing giant ICA aneurysm before (**A,** AP view; **B,** lateral view) and after (**C,** AP; **D,** lateral) coiling.

use. These devices primarily target parent vessel reconstruction, rather than endosaccular occlusion, as the means by which to achieve definitive aneurysm treatment. Thus, these devices can be used also in aneurysms with a fusiform component and a segmental aneurysmal defect in the parent vessel. Currently, these flow-diverting devices are high metal surface area coverage, stent-like constructs that are designed to provide enough flow redirection and endovascular remodeling to induce aneurysm thrombosis without the use of additional endosaccular occlusive devices (i.e., coils). At the same time, the pore size of the constructs is large enough to allow for

the continued perfusion of branch vessels and perforators arising from the reconstructed segment of the parent vessel.[60] Large or giant size or the presence of intra-aneurysmal thrombus, both of which are factors typically associated with coil compaction and aneurysm recurrence, are not an issue with the flow-diverting devices, because no endosaccular coils are placed. In fact, once the diseased segment is reconstructed and the construct fully endothelialized, the aneurysm and the diseased vascular segment could be considered "definitively" treated with the typical mechanisms of aneurysm recurrence or regrowth being essentially eliminated. In addition, as a

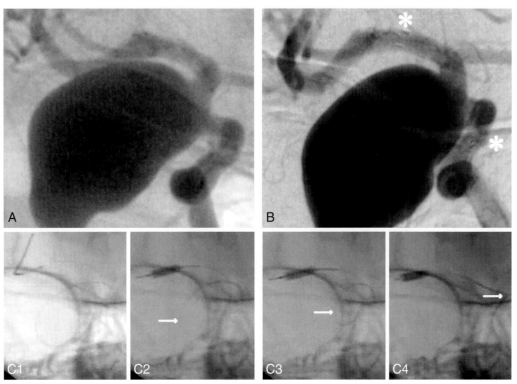

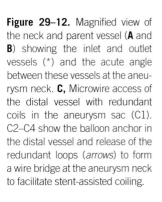

Figure 29–12. Magnified view of the neck and parent vessel (**A** and **B**) showing the inlet and outlet vessels (*) and the acute angle between these vessels at the aneurysm neck. **C,** Microwire access of the distal vessel with redundant coils in the aneurysm sac (C1). C2–C4 show the balloon anchor in the distal vessel and release of the redundant loops (*arrows*) to form a wire bridge at the aneurysm neck to facilitate stent-assisted coiling.

purely "extrasaccular" treatment strategy, no direct catheterization or manipulation of the aneurysm sac is required, possibly reducing the likelihood of procedural rupture and potentially improving the safety of endovascular aneurysm treatment. The Pipeline Embolization device (PED; ev3) represents the first flow-diversion device used in humans. We have recently used the SILK flow-diverting device (BALT Extrusion, Montmorency, France). Multiple other flow-diverting devices are currently under development and in testing.

PIPELINE EMBOLIZATION DEVICE

The pipeline embolization device (PED) is a cylindrical, stent-like construct composed of 48 braided strands of cobalt chromium and platinum. The device is packaged within an introducer sheath collapsed upon a delivery wire. The device is loaded into and delivered via the hub of a 0.027-inch internal diameter microcatheter that has been positioned across the neck of the aneurysm. Initially collapsed within the delivery sheath or microcatheter, the device is elongated approximately 2.5 times its deployed length when expanded to nominal diameter. As it is deployed, the device foreshortens toward its nominal length (which it achieves only if allowed to expand fully to its nominal diameter). Currently, the available devices range from 2.5 to 5 mm in diameter (in 0.25-mm increments) and 10 to 20 mm in length (in 2-mm increments). The deployed device is very flexible and conforms to the normal

parent anatomy, even in very tortuous vascular anatomy (Figures 29–14 through 29–19).

When fully expanded, the PED provides approximately 30% metal surface area coverage. When deployed in a parent artery smaller than the nominal diameter of the device, the PED cannot fully expand, and as such, it deploys longer than its nominal length and yields a lesser metal surface area coverage. To augment surface area coverage, several devices can be overlapped, or an individual device can be deployed with forward pressure on the microcatheter. To achieve coverage of vessel defects measuring more than 20 mm in length, multiple devices can be telescoped to reconstruct longer segments of the cerebrovascular anatomy. The tremendous versatility of the device essentially allows the operator to achieve reconstructions of most any segment of the cerebrovascular anatomy and allows some control of the metal surface coverage of different regions of the conglomerate construct. This control over the length, shape, and porosity of the final reconstructed vessel allows the operator to build a "customized" implant for each patient treated.

Accurate control and one-to-one responsiveness of the microcatheter and delivery system are critical for accurate device deployment; for this reason, stable guiding catheter access is essential. After the guiding catheter platform is in place, a 0.027-inch internal microcatheter is manipulated across the lesion under fluoroscopic roadmap control. Once in position, the first PED is introduced into the hub of the microcatheter using the provided loading sheath. The device is advanced through the microcatheter, until it is visualized

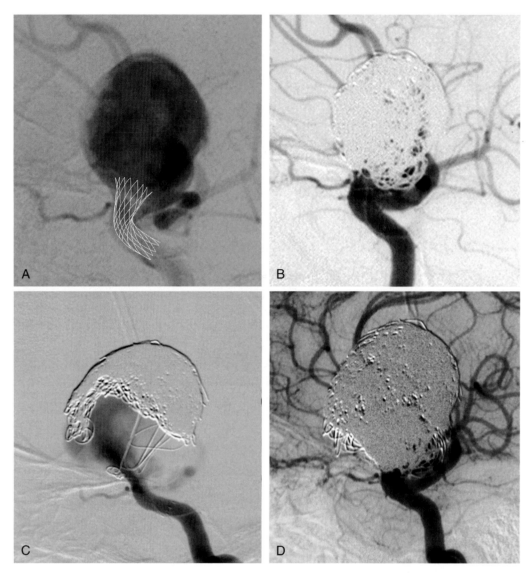

Figure 29–13. Lateral digital subtraction angiogram (left ICA injections) depicting a giant, left ophthalmic artery aneurysm in a 75-year-old woman (at the time of initial presentation) at various stages over the 4-year treatment course. **A,** Initial treatment in which a Neuroform stent (Boston Scientific) was directly deployed into the aneurysm neck (the waffle-cone technique is demonstrated with the superimposed cartoon). **B,** Subsequent coiling. **C,** Recent treatment (4 years later). Note the jet of flow into the aneurysm. The coil mass is compacted and rides up at the dome of the aneurysm, with some coil strands attached to the distal stent tines of the waffle-cone stent. **D,** The final result is acceptable as palliation. Careful follow-up is warranted.

fluoroscopically across the aneurysm neck. The delivery wire is then stabilized as the microcatheter is gently retracted. After the distal aspect of the device is exposed, the PED will begin to expand and ultimately come free of the "capture coil" mechanism, which secures the PED to the delivery wire. When the distal aspect of the PED comes off of the delivery wire, the application of gentle pressure to the delivery wire, which gradually "backs out" the microcatheter, typically results in deployment of the remainder of the device. The distal aspect of the PED is then freed from the capture coil, and the delivery wire becomes steerable and can be selectively navigated into a preselected large branch vessel during the final stages of deployment. Once fully deployed, the microcatheter is navigated over the delivery wire to recapture the wire and re-establish

microcatheter position through the lumen of the deployed construct and within the normal segment of the parent artery distal to the aneurysm neck defect. At this point, control angiography can be performed and additional devices placed as needed.

To date, the PED has been implanted in more than 80 patients for the treatment of intracranial aneurysms— 39 have been in the context of clinical studies, the Pipeline Embolization Device in the Intracranial Treatment of Aneurysms (PITA) trial or the single-center "Budapest post-PITA study." The remainder have been performed under provisions for compassionate use for aneurysms that were otherwise untreatable or had failed numerous other conventional treatments.[61]

The PITA trial, a single-arm 31-patient clinical safety study, included wide-necked saccular aneurysms and aneurysms that had failed prior endovascular coiling (Nelson PK: Stent for Treatment of Intracranial Aneurysms. Presentation, AANS/CNS Cerebrovascular Section Meeting, International Stroke Conference, New Orleans, LA, February 20–22, 2008). The majority of aneurysms in the study were large and wide-necked, with an average aneurysm sac diameter of 11.5 mm and an average neck width of 5.8 mm. The device was delivered successfully in 100% of the cases with a 6% rate of periprocedural complications (two strokes, no deaths). At the 6-month follow-up evaluation, 93% (28 of 30) of the lesions demonstrated complete angiographic occlusion. This unprecedented rate of complete angiographic occlusion at follow-up surpasses any of the reported occlusion rates for aneurysms after endovascular therapy and far exceeds those reported for large or wide-necked lesions.

The PED has also been used to successfully treat nonsaccular (fusiform or circumferential) aneurysms. Three such cases have been performed by Fiorella et al.[62] in North America under a Food and Drug Administration compassionate-use exemption. All three lesions, which were judged to be untreatable with existing endovascular or open surgical technologies, were angiographically cured with PED, without technical or neurologic complications. In two cases, eloquent perforators or side-branch vessels were covered by the PED construct; and in both cases, these remained patent at angiographic follow-up. Two of these patients now have more than 1 year of

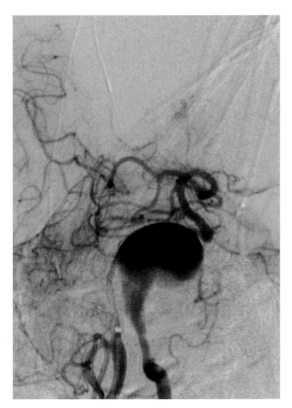

Figure 29–14. This 66-year-old man presented with symptoms suggestive of brainstem compression from this giant fusiform BA trunk aneurysm extending into the intracranial right VA. He failed balloon occlusion testing.

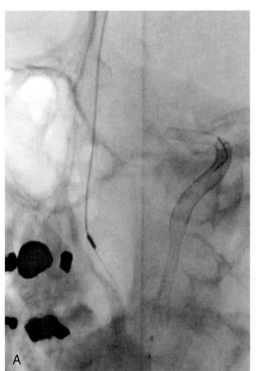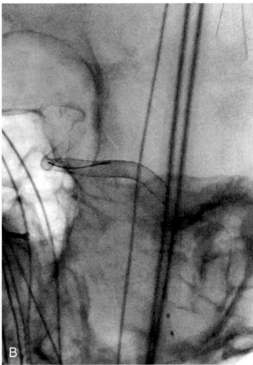

Figure 29–15. After the induction of general anesthesia, 9 Pipeline (Covidien Vascular Therapies, Mansfield, MA) devices advanced through the right VA (access through the right groin) were used to reconstruct the BA from the right VA: AP view (**A**) and lateral view (**B**). The left VA was accessed through the left groin.

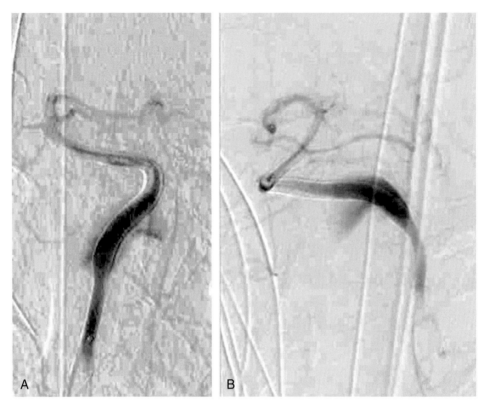

Figure 29–16. Microinjection after deploying the construct showed minimal contrast flow into the aneurysm: AP view (**A**) and lateral view (**B**).

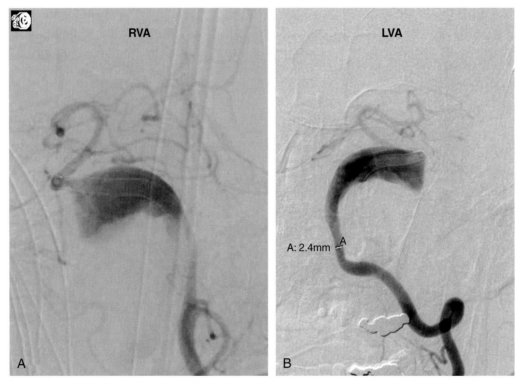

Figure 29–17. Bilateral VA injections showed competing flow around the Pipeline construct. **A,** RVA, right vertebral artery. **B,** LVA, left vertebral artery.

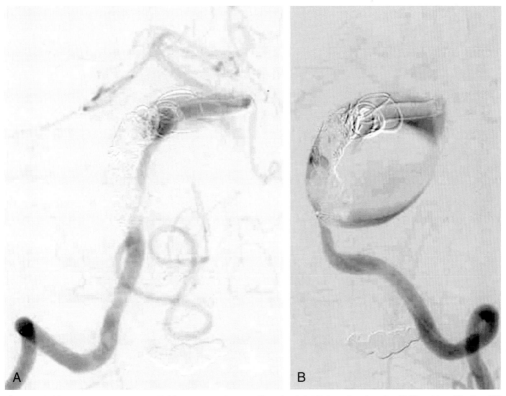

Figure 29–18. Complex coils and nBCA were used to sacrifice the left VA just distal to the PICA origin: AP view (**A**) and lateral view (**B**). This caused contrast stasis around the Pipeline construct.

clinical and angiographic follow-up and remain angiographically cured of their lesions and are without neurological symptoms.[62]

SILK FLOW-DIVERTING DEVICE

The SILK device is similar to the PED and has 48 braided wires (44 nitinol and four platinum). It is available in diameters of 2.0 to 5.5 mm (in 0.5-mm increments) and lengths of 15 to 40 mm (also in 5-mm increments). The SILK device shortens by at least 50% when deployed. It comes prepackaged with a delivery system comprised of a delivery wire and an introducer and a reinforced microcatheter for placement (Vasco+21 2.4 F for devices 2 to 4.5 mm in diameter and 3 F for devices 5 to 5.5 mm in diameter, preshaped with a multipurpose distal curve). The SILK device is preloaded on the delivery wire inside the introducer. After microcatheter access to the aneurysm has been obtained, working projections and vessel measurements are taken for device sizing. The SILK device is transferred from the introducer into the hub of the microcatheter using a Y connector and by gently advancing the delivery wire. The SILK device is positioned past the aneurysm neck at least 1.5 times the diameter of the parent vessel. A gentle push is given on the delivery wire until the distal

radiopaque end is out of the distal marker on the microcatheter. Withdrawing the microcatheter to deploy the SILK device to approximately 1 cm creates a distal anchor of the SILK device on the vessel wall. This manipulation ensures that the SILK device does not move distally, because the wire struts of the SILK may cause damage to the vessel wall. After the SILK is deployed to approximately 1 cm, the distal tip is positioned by simultaneously pulling on the catheter and on the delivery wire. It is possible to move the SILK device by pulling the delivery wire, as long as the distal ring of the catheter does not superimpose the radiopaque marker on the delivery wire. If SILK repositioning is required, the catheter is gently advanced over the deployed SILK, the system is repositioned, and the device is re-deployed in the new location. The SILK is fully deployed when the marker of the delivery wire lines up with the distal ring of the catheter. It is then impossible to resheath the SILK. The delivery wire is pushed until its marker overpasses the catheter's marker by a minimum of 2 mm, when it completely detaches. Once detached, the SILK proximal tip might be not fully deployed (particularly in a curve). The most effective technique is to push the proximal end with the microcatheter and make the device open. The microcatheter is positioned distal to the stent to maintain access through the stent before removal of the delivery wire. The main advantages of the SILK device over the PED is better translatability of the one-to-one movement of the microcatheter and

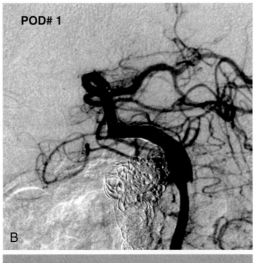

POD# 1

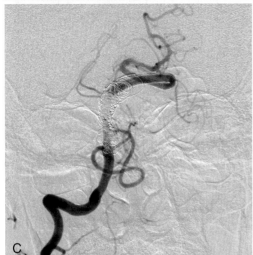

A

POD# 1

B

C

D

Figure 29–19. Angiogram performed the next day (POD# 1) showing complete occlusion of the aneurysm and reconstruction of the right VA and BA with the Pipeline construct: AP view (**A**) and lateral view (**B**). Angiogram at 3 months: AP view (**C**) and lateral view (**D**).

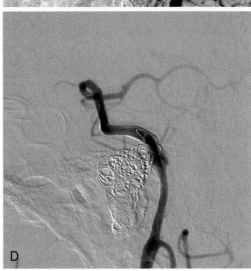

the delivery system and the ability to recapture and reposition the system even up to 90% deployment. The ability to recapture a flow-diverting device in our experience is very important. These devices require frequent repositioning as they foreshorten during deployment, and we very often get to know what the final position of the stent would be only after partial deployment (Figures 29–20 through 29–22).

The international SILK registry (Personal communication, BALT Extrusion, September 2009) includes a total of 68 patients with 69 aneurysms (12 giant aneurysms), of which 46 are saccular and 23 are fusiform, and does not include the two patients treated in the United States. Stent deployment was considered suboptimal in 14 of 71 stents deployed (19.7%), of which four had parent artery occlusion during the procedure (three parent artery occlusions were permanent and resulted in neurological deficit in one of the patients). At the 3-month follow-up evaluation, three more patients had parent artery occlusion and all three had permanent deficits. Only 38 (55%) aneurysms were followed up; and of these, only 19 (50%) were completely occluded at delayed (1 year) follow-up. The overall morbidity and mortality was 10%.

There are key technical issues associated with flow-diverting devices. The working views should allow the unambiguous and continuous visualization of a suitable distal branch vessel into which to navigate the tip of the delivery wire during device delivery, as well as the targeted distal and proximal landing zones for the device deployment; thus, continuous visualization of the parent artery–aneurysm neck interface is less important. Visualization of the aneurysm dome is irrelevant, as endosaccular reconstruction is not attempted. Accurate measurement of the parent artery landing zones both distal and proximal to the targeted aneurysm is absolutely essential for optimized device sizing and adjusting metal surface coverage of the device. Complete aneurysm occlusion is not achieved at the completion of the procedure. The procedure is stopped when there is stasis of contrast material persisting into late phases of angiography that can sometimes be visualized as an "eclipse sign." If the aneurysm is large and circumferential, the device construct, if visualized in a "down-the-barrel" projection, may create a negative defect within the pool of static contrast filling the aneurysm. In cases in which the neck of the aneurysm is wide and there is an inflow

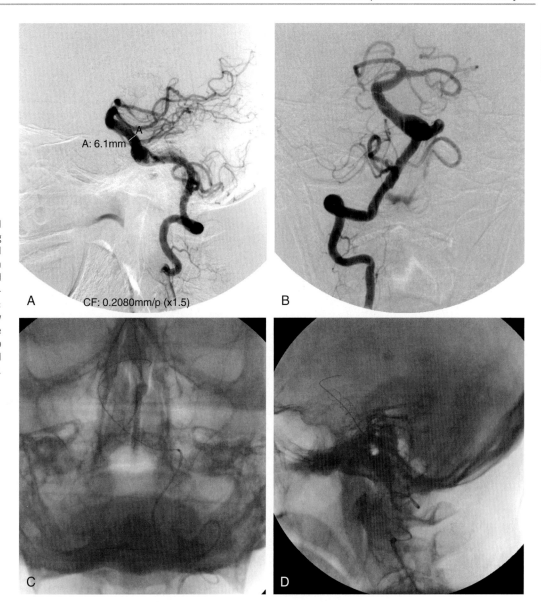

Figure 29–20. This 75-year-old man presented with increasing instability, gait disturbance, and imbalance requiring ambulation with a walker. Imaging revealed a fusiform aneurysm of the vertebrobasilar junction and BA: AP view (**A**) and lateral view (**B**), angiographic projections. He underwent stenting with a Leo stent scaffold: AP view (**C**) and lateral view (**D**), lateral plain films.

jet into the aneurysm, the proximal end of the device has a potential to prolapse into the aneurysm. In such cases, it is very important to maintain distal microwire access to deploy a second device and reconstruct the neck. In certain cases, SEIMs, such as the Enterprise or the Leo (BALT Extrusion), can be used as a scaffold inside which the flow-diverting device is constructed.

The main limitations of the flow-diverting devices, when compared with the SEIMs, include the efficacy and safety of their use in bifurcation aneurysms—as there is a potential for jailing of one limb of the bifurcation—and a lack of data regarding the safety of these devices in vessels rich with eloquent perforators. The available data in experimental animal models and in humans, especially with the PED, suggest that coverage with a single device is safe.

COVERED STENTS

A family of balloon-mounted stents covered with nonporous membranes (typically, polytetrafluoroethylene [PTFE]), developed for the treatment of coronary artery rupture (JoStent coronary stent graft, JoMed International, Helsingborg, Sweden; Symbiot, Boston Scientific), has been used in a very limited capacity as flow-diversion devices to treat intracranial aneurysms. However, these devices are extremely rigid and very difficult (often impossible) to deliver through the tortuous cerebrovascular anatomy and are not indicated for intracranial use. Unlike the SEIMs and the aforementioned flow-diverting devices, covered stents are completely nonporous and cause immediate and complete occlusion of perforator or branch

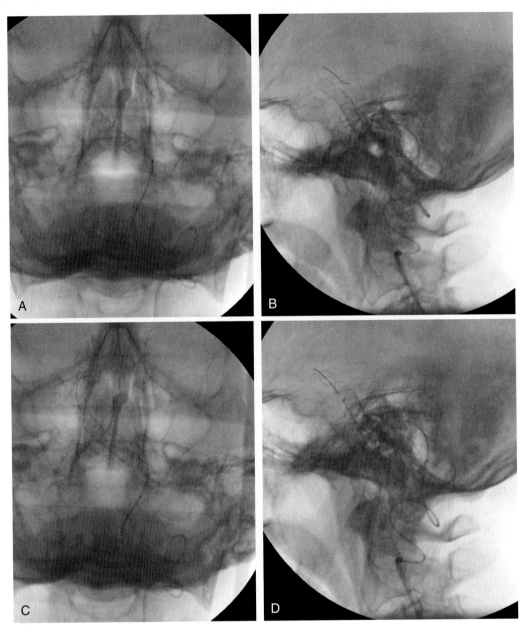

Figure 29–21. Plain films showing two SILK devices: AP view (**A**) and lateral view (**B**), after first SILK device; AP view (**C**) and lateral view (**D**) after second SILK device.

vessels that they cover. This design feature limits the application of these devices to segments of the cerebrovascular anatomy that do not contain important branch vessels—typically, the petrous and cavernous segments of the ICA. Another limitation is the potential for leakage of blood around the outside of the stent and into the aneurysm. However, should an endoleak occur, an angioplasty can often be performed to achieve better stent apposition and complete exclusion of the aneurysm from the circulation.

Newer generations of balloon-expandable covered, partially covered, and semiporous covered stents are currently under development, with modifications designed to overcome the aforementioned limitations of the predicate devices.

The Willis covered stent (Micro-port, Shanghai, China) is built upon a cobalt chromium platform that incorporates a very thin layer of PTFE into its structure, designed to maximize its flexibility and deliverability. The limited clinical data available for the use of this stent in humans has been encouraging.[63–65] The endovascular clip system (eCLIPs, Evasc Medical Systems, Vancouver, BC, Canada) is a partially covered, balloon-expandable stent that is designed such that the covered portion can be oriented to selectively cover an aneurysm neck,[66] while leaving the remainder of the endoluminal surface of the parent artery uncovered, thus potentially allowing continued perfusion of regional perforators while occluding the aneurysm.

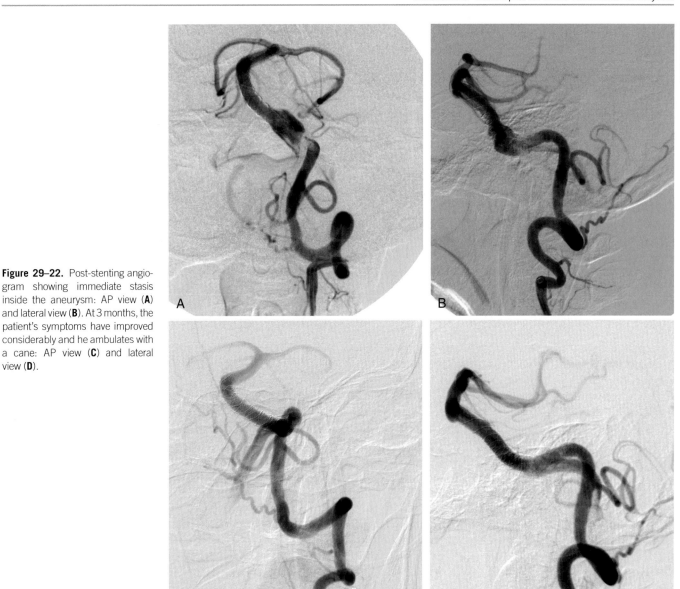

Figure 29–22. Post-stenting angiogram showing immediate stasis inside the aneurysm: AP view (**A**) and lateral view (**B**). At 3 months, the patient's symptoms have improved considerably and he ambulates with a cane: AP view (**C**) and lateral view (**D**).

COMPLICATION AVOIDANCE AND MANAGEMENT

Reduction of endovascular complications in the treatment of giant aneurysms lies primarily in prevention, because many complications are not readily treatable. Proper patient selection, assessing the most reasonable approach to each particular aneurysm, and careful attention to detail are keys to avoiding complications. At institutions in which these complex lesions are treated, an honest assessment must be made in terms of the locally available treatment techniques and their relative risks at that institution (whether they are surgical, endovascular, or combination approaches).

Vessel or Aneurysm Perforation

Extrusion of the microwire, microcatheter, or a coil is the most common mechanism of vessel or aneurysm perforation. Ruptured aneurysms have a higher chance of perforations than unruptured aneurysms. An abrupt rise in blood pressure or intracranial pressure or a sudden slowing of the heart rate should prompt the immediate performance of a guide catheter angiogram to confirm whether a perforation has occurred. The extruding device may occlude or partially occlude the perforation and, hence, should not be pulled back immediately. The heparin is immediately reversed with 1 mg/100 units of protamine. If the microcatheter has perforated the aneurysm wall, a coil can be partially deployed into the subarachnoid space;

the microcatheter can be pulled back slightly until the microcatheter tip is inside the aneurysm again; and then the remaining portion of the coil can be deployed within the aneurysm. Alternatively, a second microcatheter can be navigated into the aneurysm to continue coiling the aneurysm. After the aneurysm is secured, a ventriculostomy may be necessary, particularly if the patient remains hypertensive. Once the perforation is controlled, an immediate cranial CT scan is warranted.

Thromboembolism

Procedure-related thromboembolic complications occur in 2.5% to 11% of intracranial aneurysms treated by coil embolization, with permanent deficits in 2.5% to 5.5% of patients. The main mechanisms are platelet-rich thrombus formation on devices, thrombus formation at the anode during electrolytic coil detachment, and slowing of flow in the parent vessel due to vasospasm or occlusion of the guide catheter. Guide catheter angiograms should be done frequently to monitor for evidence of thrombosis, such as a filling-defect within the parent vessel adjacent to the aneurysm neck or vessel dropout. Most thrombotic material that appears during coiling is likely to be platelet-rich; therefore, the infusion of a glycoprotein IIb-IIIa inhibitor is the first approach. Thrombolysis or snare-assisted clot retrieval can be used if necessary.

Difficult Stent System Delivery

A stable and distal guiding catheter position within the cervical artery leading to the target lesion is important. It is advantageous to use a triaxial system consisting of a 6-F long sheath and a standard inner 6-F guiding catheter (e.g., Envoy or a 6-F Neuron guiding catheter) for delivery of the stent. Often, the 6-F Neuron guiding catheter can be manipulated into the cavernous segment of the ICA.

Having microwire access well distal to the targeted delivery zone facilitates the delivery. The largest branch vessel is first catheterized with a standard small, 1.7-F (outer diameter) microcatheter (e.g., SL-10, Boston Scientific) over a standard 0.014-inch microwire. Following catheterization and a microcatheter run to exclude the possibility of a distal wire perforation, the microcatheter can be exchanged over a 0.014-inch exchange length, 300-cm microwire for the stent delivery system.

A significant "step-off" between the 0.014-inch guidewire and the 0.027-inch lumen of the delivery catheter, especially with the Neuroform stent, allows the catheter to catch on any changes in the vessel contour, particularly if positioned along the outer curvature of the artery (e.g., branch vessel orifices like the ophthalmic artery and in situ stent struts). A useful technique in this situation is the "balloon-bounce" maneuver in which a hypercompliant balloon (HyperGlide, ev3) is placed side by side with the stent delivery system.

Gentle inflation of the balloon deflects the stent delivery system away from the "step-off," allowing navigation of the delivery system more distally.

In wide-necked aneurysms, the stent system may prolapse into the aneurysm or drive the exchange wire into the aneurysm fundus. Stable distal microwire access and use of balloon-assisted coiling followed by stenting may help to avoid these difficulties. Depending on the anatomy, retrograde delivery of the stent device through the Circle of Willis can also be attempted.

In aneurysms arising from dolichoectatic vertebrobasilar vessels where the parent arteries measure >5 mm in diameter, no SEIMs are large enough to accommodate the parent artery. Larger coronary or biliary stenting systems may be useful in these situations. However, the delivery of these stents often requires direct surgical access of the extracranial VA.

Difficult Stent Deployment

The SEIMs can be difficult to deploy, especially the Neuroform due to its coaxial over-the-wire delivery system. The delivery system should be delivered beyond the targeted lesion and withdrawn back to remove redundancy from the system. Active flushing of heparinized saline through the rotating hemostatic valve minimizes friction within the system. The stent deployment is started in a distal nontortuous segment and pulled back to the tortuous target site to complete the deployment. A 0.017-inch coil pusher could be used to deliver the device if over-the wire delivery is difficult. In general, the delivery and deployment mechanism of the Enterprise overcomes many of the issues presented by the Neuroform.

Stent Misplacement

The delivery system can shift during deployment, either because of an unstable delivery catheter position within tortuous anatomy or during a difficult deployment due to "binding" within the system, resulting in stent misplacement. When the stent is malpositioned, if the stent does not provide sufficient coverage of the aneurysm neck, a second device can be deployed to bridge the neck. If there is partial coverage of the neck, coiling without prolapse of the coil mass may be possible as the dimension of the neck may have been reduced by the misplaced stent. A second device may be used if necessary. If the stent is misplaced in a hazardous position, retrieval using commercially available foreign-body retrieval devices may be attempted.

Spontaneous delayed stent migration after proper placement has been observed only with the Enterprise.[55] The closed-cell structure of the device results in its ability to migrate when placed into vessels of discrepant caliber. The force of the stent in the smaller vessel is transmitted to the part of the stent in the larger vessel, and the device can "watermelon seed" into the larger artery.

Coil Stretching through the Stent

During trans-stent coil embolization, the microcatheter may become "kicked out" of the aneurysm, leaving the embolization coil exposed and directly in contact with the stent. During attempts to re-catheterize the aneurysm or manipulate the coil, the coil can lose its integrity and begin stretching. If manipulation of the coil continues after stretching, the coil can actually break off within the microcatheter. The stretched, broken coil can become an embolic risk, within the parent artery and possibly embolize downstream into the cerebrovasculature. When a coil becomes unraveled to the point that it can no longer be advanced or withdrawn, the unraveled, elongated coil can extend for a long distance (≥ 1 to 2 m). Three recommended salvage maneuvers are (1) a microsnare is used to grasp and withdraw the stretched coil (the "monorail snare technique"), (2) the elongated portion of coil can be withdrawn from the parent vessel and secured in an extracranial vessel, and (3) the elongated portion of coil can be withdrawn all the way to the femoral artery and secured there. An SEIM can be deployed to "pin" the proximal aspect of the damaged, aberrant coil against the parent artery, thus preventing distal migration and reducing the exposed surface area available for thromboembolus formation.

In-stent Stenosis

Delayed in-stent stenosis following implantation of a Neuroform stent represents a relatively uncommon ($\sim 5\%$) event.[67] Neuroform-induced in-stent stenosis is usually asymptomatic; and, in more than half of the cases reported, spontaneously regressed at angiographic follow-up.[67] Only in rare cases does this stenosis progress to the point where it can actually produce significant luminal compromise, perfusion failure, and clinical symptoms that may lead to ischemic stroke.

Hemorrhage

Most hemorrhagic complications at the groin puncture site occur at the femoral access site during the immediate postprocedural period. A meticulous technique should be applied to gain access with a micropuncture system, and the puncture site should be amenable to the use of closure devices because the patient will be receiving antiplatelet agents. Extracerebral bleeding complications (e.g., gastrointestinal bleeding) are also a potential issue but are minimized to some extent by the limited duration of the required dual antiplatelet therapy.

Imaging Follow Up

Given the high recurrence and retreatment rates associated with simple coiling in giant aneurysms, regular follow-up imaging is essential to monitor exclusion of the aneurysm from the circulation. Conventional angiography represents the only technique that provides a reliable assessment of the stented parent artery. As in-stent stenosis usually develops within 6 months, a 6-month conventional angiography is performed for assessment of the stented parent artery. Short echo time (TE) MR angiography sequences have been designed specifically to assess aneurysms after endovascular therapy.[68] This sequence is designed to minimize susceptibility artifacts related to the coil mass and stents. Although very effective for imaging of the coil mass and assessing residual aneurysm, MR is limited to some extent for evaluation of the parent artery after stenting. CT angiography is of use in those cases treated with stenting alone, as the stents themselves produce much less artifact than the embolization coils.

At 6 months after stent-supported coiling, we perform a follow-up conventional angiogram and specialized short TE MR angiography sequences. Provided that the examinations correlate, this MR angiogram functions as a baseline for subsequent comparison at 12 to 15 months and at 3 and 5 years. Should the coil mass appear stable, it is possible that all of these follow-up evaluations can be performed with MR angiography alone, with any evidence of increasing flow or contrast enhancement within the coil mass prompting conventional angiography.

Results of Endovascular Therapy

Most of the reported results of the endovascular management of giant aneurysms pertain to treatment via either parent vessel occlusion or simple coiling. We reported a series of 38 patients with 39 giant aneurysms treated between December 2001 and July 2007 in which stent-assisted coiling was used in 25 patients at some point during at least one treatment session.[69] At the last angiographic follow-up examination (mean, 21.5 months; standard deviation [SD], ± 22.9 months), 95% or higher and 100% occlusion rates were documented in 64% and 36% of aneurysms, respectively, with parent vessel preservation maintained in 74%. Twenty percent of treatment sessions resulted in permanent morbidity; death within 30 days occurred after 8% of treatment sessions. An average of 1.9 sessions (SD, ± 1.1) were required to treat each aneurysm, with a resulting cumulative per-patient mortality of 16% and morbidity of 32%. At the last known clinical follow-up examination (mean, 24.8 months; SD, ± 24.8 months), 24 (63%) patients had Glasgow Outcome Scale scores of 4 or 5 (good or excellent), 10 patients had worsened neurological function from baseline (26% morbidity), and 11 had died (29% mortality). Although the results in this series are comparable to microsurgical series, the endovascular technology used in this series has been outdated with the introduction of the Enterprise stent and dedicated flow-diversion devices.

THE FUTURE

Advances in endovascular techniques and understanding of the physiology of aneurysm growth and the biology of parent vessel reconstruction with stents has made endovascular treatment of giant aneurysms one of the mainstream options for giant aneurysms in locations with prohibitively high risks of rupture and considered high risk for microsurgical treatment. Careful evaluation of the recently developed devices and techniques should be performed prospectively in multicenter studies involving experienced centers. Dual training in endovascular and microsurgical techniques at specialized aneurysm centers is essential in developing the skills of decision making and managing these complex patients with acceptable morbidity and mortality.

The current market is proliferating with numerous flow-diverting devices that are being designed and tested by multiple endovascular device manufacturers. The preliminary experience with the PED shows promise, although long-term results and the ability of these devices to preserve perforators and branch vessels need to be studied in detail. Asymmetric covered stents that can be positioned in such a way that they occlude only the circumference of the parent vessel involved by the aneurysm neck are being developed.[70,71] In the future, stents with custom-made covers based on the morphology of the aneurysm neck-parent vessel interface may be available. Advances in endovascular device technology and imaging may allow the design of newer stents with increasing trackability and easy deployment in the tortuous cerebrovasculature. Stents specifically designed for terminal bifurcation aneurysms are being developed that will allow aneurysm occlusion with preservation of flow in both branches. Stents and systemic drugs that accelerate stent and orifice endothelialization need to be developed to reduce the duration of antiplatelet therapy, increase aneurysm occlusion rates, and allow more widespread use of these stents for ruptured aneurysms.

CONCLUSION

Recent advances in endovascular parent vessel reconstruction and flow diversion have allowed treatment of giant aneurysms previously considered untreatable by endovascular techniques with acceptable morbidity and mortality. Although the durability of these treatment modalities needs to be studied, we anticipate that advancements in endovascular techniques and technology will soon allow durable occlusion of an increasing number of these aneurysms with morbidity and mortality that is comparable to or lower than the rates associated with microsurgical techniques.

REFERENCES

1. Locksley HB: Natural history of subarachnoid hemorrhage, intracranial aneurysms and arteriovenous malformations. Based on 6368 cases in the cooperative study, J Neurosurg 25:219–239, 1966.
2. Morley TP, Barr HW: Giant intracranial aneurysms: diagnosis, course, and management, Clin Neurosurg 16:73–94, 1969.
3. Raaymakers TW, Rinkel GJ, Limburg M, et al: Mortality and morbidity of surgery for unruptured intracranial aneurysms: a meta-analysis, Stroke 29:1531–1538, 1998.
4. Choi IS, David C: Giant intracranial aneurysms: development, clinical presentation and treatment, Eur J Radiol 46:178–194, 2003.
5. Khanna RK, Malik GM, Qureshi N: Predicting outcome following surgical treatment of unruptured intracranial aneurysms: a proposed grading system, J Neurosurg 84:49–54, 1996.
6. Drake CG: Giant intracranial aneurysms: experience with surgical treatment in 174 patients, Clin Neurosurg 26:12–95, 1979.
7. International Study of Unruptured Intracranial Aneurysms Investigators: Unruptured intracranial aneurysms—risk of rupture and risks of surgical intervention. International Study of Unruptured Intracranial Aneurysms Investigators, N Engl J Med 339:1725–1733, 1998.
8. Wiebers DO, Whisnant JP, Huston J 3rd, et al: Unruptured intracranial aneurysms: natural history, clinical outcome, and risks of surgical and endovascular treatment, Lancet 362(9378):103–110, 2003.
9. Lawton MT, Quinones-Hinojosa A, Sanai N, et al: Combined microsurgical and endovascular management of complex intracranial aneurysms, Neurosurgery 62(Suppl 3):1503–1515, 2008.
10. Lawton MT, Spetzler RF: Surgical strategies for giant intracranial aneurysms, Acta Neurochir Suppl 72:141–156, 1999.
11. Samson D, Batjer HH, Kopitnik TA Jr: Current results of the surgical management of aneurysms of the basilar apex, Neurosurgery 44:697–704, 1999.
12. Surdell DL, Hage ZA, Eddleman CS, et al: Revascularization for complex intracranial aneurysms, Neurosurg Focus 24:E21, 2008.
13. Piepgras DG, Khurana VG, Whisnant JP: Ruptured giant intracranial aneurysms. Part II. A retrospective analysis of timing and outcome of surgical treatment, J Neurosurg 88:430–435, 1998.
14. Hanel RA, Spetzler RF: Surgical treatment of complex intracranial aneurysms, Neurosurgery 62(Suppl 3):1289–1297, 2008.
15. Mohit AA, Sekhar LN, Natarajan SK, et al: High-flow bypass grafts in the management of complex intracranial aneurysms, Neurosurgery 60(Suppl 1):ONS105–ONS123, 2007.
16. Sekhar LN, Stimac D, Bakir A, et al: Reconstruction options for complex middle cerebral artery aneurysms, Neurosurgery 56(Suppl 1):66–74, 2005.
17. Evans JJ, Sekhar LN, Rak R, et al: Bypass grafting and revascularization in the management of posterior circulation aneurysms, Neurosurgery 55:1036–1049, 2004.
18. Larson JJ, Tew JM Jr, Tomsick TA, et al: Treatment of aneurysms of the internal carotid artery by intravascular balloon occlusion: long-term follow-up of 58 patients, Neurosurgery 36:26–30, 1995.
19. Origitano TC, al-Mefty O, Leonetti JP, et al: Vascular considerations and complications in cranial base surgery, Neurosurgery 35:351–363, 1994.
20. Sluzewski M, Menovsky T, van Rooij WJ, et al: Coiling of very large or giant cerebral aneurysms: long-term clinical and serial angiographic results, AJNR Am J Neuroradiol 24:257–262, 2003.
21. Gruber A, Killer M, Bavinzski G, et al: Clinical and angiographic results of endosaccular coiling treatment of giant and very large intracranial aneurysms: a 7-year, single-center experience, Neurosurgery 45:793–804, 1999.
22. van Rooij WJ, Sluzewski M: Coiling of very large and giant basilar tip aneurysms: midterm clinical and angiographic results, AJNR Am J Neuroradiol 28:1405–1408, 2007.
23. Murayama Y, Nien YL, Duckwiler G, et al: Guglielmi detachable coil embolization of cerebral aneurysms: 11 years' experience, J Neurosurg 98:959–966, 2003.
24. Moret J, Pierot L, Boulin A, et al: "Remodeling" of the arterial wall of the parent vessel in the endovascular treatment of intracranial aneurysms (abstr S83). Proceedings of the 20th Congress of the European Society of Neuroradiology, Neuroradiology 36(Suppl 1):S83, 1994.
25. Soeda A, Sakai N, Sakai H, et al: Thromboembolic events associated with Guglielmi detachable coil embolization of asymptomatic cerebral aneurysms: evaluation of 66 consecutive cases with use of diffusion-weighted MR imaging, AJNR Am J Neuroradiol 24:127–132, 2003.
26. Albayram S, Selcuk H, Kara B, et al: Thromboembolic events associated with balloon-assisted coil embolization: evaluation with

diffusion-weighted MR imaging, *AJNR Am J Neuroradiol* 25:1768–1777, 2004.

27. Kurre W, Berkefeld J: Materials and techniques for coiling of cerebral aneurysms: how much scientific evidence do we have? *Neuroradiology* 50:909–927, 2008.

28. Molyneux AJ, Cekirge S, Saatci I, et al: Cerebral Aneurysm Multicenter European Onyx (CAMEO) trial: results of a prospective observational study in 20 European centers, *AJNR Am J Neuroradiol* 25:39–51, 2004.

29. Weber W, Siekmann R, Kis B, et al: Treatment and follow-up of 22 unruptured wide-necked intracranial aneurysms of the internal carotid artery with Onyx HD 500, *AJNR Am J Neuroradiol* 26:1909–1915, 2005.

30. Szikora I, Guterman LR, Wells KM, et al: Combined use of stents and coils to treat experimental wide-necked carotid aneurysms: preliminary results, *AJNR Am J Neuroradiol* 15:1091–1102, 1994.

31. Wakhloo AK, Schellhammer F, de Vries J, et al: Self-expanding and balloon-expandable stents in the treatment of carotid aneurysms: an experimental study in a canine model, *AJNR Am J Neuroradiol* 15:493–502, 1994.

32. Wakhloo AK, Tio FO, Lieber BB, et al: Self-expanding nitinol stents in canine vertebral arteries: hemodynamics and tissue response, *AJNR Am J Neuroradiol* 16:1043–1051, 1995.

33. Han PP, Albuquerque FC, Ponce FA, et al: Percutaneous intracranial stent placement for aneurysms, *J Neurosurg* 99:23–30, 2003.

34. Lanzino G, Wakhloo AK, Fessler RD, et al: Efficacy and current limitations of intravascular stents for intracranial internal carotid, vertebral, and basilar artery aneurysms, *J Neurosurg* 91:538–546, 1999.

35. Lylyk P, Ceratto R, Hurvitz D, et al: Treatment of a vertebral dissecting aneurysm with stents and coils: technical case report, *Neurosurgery* 43:385–388, 1998.

36. Malek AM, Halbach VV, Phatouros CC, et al: Balloon-assist technique for endovascular coil embolization of geometrically difficult intracranial aneurysms, *Neurosurgery* 46:1397–1407, 2000.

37. Mericle RA, Lanzino G, Wakhloo AK, et al: Stenting and secondary coiling of intracranial internal carotid artery aneurysm: technical case report, *Neurosurgery* 43:1229–1234, 1998.

38. Sekhon LH, Morgan MK, Sorby W, et al: Combined endovascular stent implantation and endosaccular coil placement for the treatment of a wide-necked vertebral artery aneurysm: technical case report, *Neurosurgery* 43:380–384, 1998.

39. Wilms G, van Calenbergh F, Stockx L, et al: Endovascular treatment of a ruptured paraclinoid aneurysm of the carotid siphon achieved using endovascular stent and endosaccular coil placement, *AJNR Am J Neuroradiol* 21:753–756, 2000.

40. Higashida RT, Smith W, Gress D, et al: Intravascular stent and endovascular coil placement for a ruptured fusiform aneurysm of the basilar artery. Case report and review of the literature, *J Neurosurg* 87: 944–949, 1997.

41. Freitas JM, Zenteno M, Aburto-Murrieta Y, et al: Intracranial arterial stenting for symptomatic stenoses: a Latin American experience, *Surg Neurol* 68:378–386, 2007.

42. Kurre W, Berkefeld J, Sitzer M, et al: Treatment of symptomatic high-grade intracranial stenoses with the balloon-expandable Pharos stent: initial experience, *Neuroradiology* 50:701–708, 2008.

43. Mocco J, Darkhabani Z, Levy EI: Pharos neurovascular intracranial stent: elective use for a symptomatic stenosis refractory to medical therapy, *Catheter Cardiovasc Interv* 74:642–646, 2009.

44. Zenteno MA, Santos-Franco JA, Freitas-Modenesi JM, et al: Use of the sole stenting technique for the management of aneurysms in the posterior circulation in a prospective series of 20 patients, *J Neurosurg* 108:1104–1118, 2008.

45. Benndorf G, Klucznik RP, Meyer D, et al: "Cross-over" technique for horizontal stenting of an internal carotid bifurcation aneurysm using a new self-expandable stent: technical case report, *Neurosurgery* 58 (Suppl 1):ONS–E172, 2006.

46. Chow MM, Woo HH, Masaryk TJ, et al: A novel endovascular treatment of a wide-necked basilar apex aneurysm by using a Y-configuration, double-stent technique, *AJNR Am J Neuroradiol* 25:509–512, 2004.

47. Cross DT 3rd, Moran CJ, Derdeyn CP, et al: Neuroform stent deployment for treatment of a basilar tip aneurysm via a posterior communicating artery route, *AJNR Am J Neuroradiol* 26:2578–2581, 2005.

48. Fiorella D, Albuquerque FC, Masaryk TJ, et al: Balloon in-stent technique for the constructive endovascular treatment of "ultra-wide necked" circumferential aneurysms, *Neurosurgery* 57:1218–1227, 2005.

49. Kelly ME, Turner R, Gonugunta V, et al: Stent reconstruction of wide-necked aneurysms across the circle of Willis, *Neurosurgery* 61(Suppl 2):249–255, 2007.

50. Moret J, Ross IB, Weill A, et al: The retrograde approach: a consideration for the endovascular treatment of aneurysms, *AJNR Am J Neuroradiol* 21:262–268, 2000.

51. Sani S, Lopes DK: Treatment of a middle cerebral artery bifurcation aneurysm using a double Neuroform stent "Y" configuration and coil embolization: technical case report, *Neurosurgery* 57(Suppl 1):E209, 2005.

52. Thorell WE, Chow MM, Woo HH, et al: Y-configured dual intracranial stent-assisted coil embolization for the treatment of wide-necked basilar tip aneurysms, *Neurosurgery* 56:1035–1040, 2005.

53. Ebrahimi N, Claus B, Lee CY, et al: Stent conformity in curved vascular models with simulated aneurysm necks using flat-panel CT: an in vitro study, *AJNR Am J Neuroradiol* 28:823–829, 2007.

54. Hsu SW, Chaloupka JC, Feekes JA, et al: In vitro studies of the Neuroform microstent using transparent human intracranial arteries, *AJNR Am J Neuroradiol* 27:1135–1139, 2006.

55. Kelly ME, Turner RD 4th, Moskowitz SI, et al: Delayed migration of a self-expanding intracranial microstent, *AJNR Am J Neuroradiol* 29:1959–1960, 2008.

56. Hanel RA, Boulos AS, Sauvageau EG, et al: Stent placement for the treatment of nonsaccular aneurysms of the vertebrobasilar system, *Neurosurg Focus* 18:E8, 2005.

57. Fiorella D, Albuquerque FC, Han P, et al: Preliminary experience using the Neuroform stent for the treatment of cerebral aneurysms, *Neurosurgery* 54:6–17, 2004.

58. Lavine SD, Larsen DW, Giannotta SL, et al: Parent vessel Guglielmi detachable coil herniation during wide-necked aneurysm embolization: treatment with intracranial stent placement: two technical case reports, *Neurosurgery* 46:1013–1017, 2000.

59. Horowitz M, Levy E, Sauvageau E, et al: Intra/extra-aneurysmal stent placement for management of complex and wide-necked-bifurcation aneurysms: eight cases using the waffle cone technique, *Neurosurgery* 58(Suppl 2):ONS–258–ONS-262, 2006.

60. Kallmes DF, Ding YH, Dai D, et al: A new endoluminal, flow-disrupting device for treatment of saccular aneurysms, *Stroke* 38:2346–2352, 2007.

61. Fiorella D, Kelly ME, Turner RDI, et al: Endovascular treatment of cerebral aneurysms, *Endovascular Today* (June):53–64, 2008. Available at www.evtoday.com/PDFarticles/0608/EVT0608_06.php Accessed January 5, 2009.

62. Fiorella D, Woo HH, Albuquerque FC, et al: Definitive reconstruction of circumferential, fusiform intracranial aneurysms with the pipeline embolization device, *Neurosurgery* 62:1115–1121, 2008.

63. Li MH, Li YD, Gao BL, et al: A new covered stent designed for intracranial vasculature: application in the management of pseudoaneurysms of the cranial internal carotid artery, *AJNR Am J Neuroradiol* 28: 1579–1585, 2007.

64. Li MH, Zhu YQ, Fang C, et al: The feasibility and efficacy of treatment with a Willis covered stent in recurrent intracranial aneurysms after coiling, *AJNR Am J Neuroradiol* 29:1395–1400, 2008.

65. Wang JB, Li MH, Fang C, et al: Endovascular treatment of giant intracranial aneurysms with Willis covered stents: technical case report, *Neurosurgery* 62:E1176–1177, 2008.

66. Marotta TR, Gunnarsson T, Penn I, et al: A novel endovascular clip system for the treatment of intracranial aneurysms: technology, concept, and initial experimental results. Laboratory investigation, *J Neurosurg* 108:1230–1240, 2008.

67. Fiorella D, Albuquerque FC, Woo H, et al: Neuroform in-stent stenosis: incidence, natural history, and treatment strategies, *Neurosurgery* 59:34–42, 2006.

68. Wallace RC, Karis JP, Partovi S, et al: Noninvasive imaging of treated cerebral aneurysms, part I: MR angiographic follow-up of coiled aneurysms, *AJNR Am J Neuroradiol* 28:1001–1008, 2007.

69. Jahromi BS, Mocco J, Bang JA, et al: Clinical and angiographic outcome after endovascular management of giant intracranial aneurysms, *Neurosurgery* 63:662–675, 2008.

70. Ionita CN, Paciorek AM, Dohatcu A, et al: The asymmetric vascular stent: efficacy in a rabbit aneurysm model, *Stroke* 40:959–965, 2009.

71. Ionita CN, Paciorek AM, Hoffmann KR, et al: Asymmetric vascular stent: feasibility study of a new low-porosity patch-containing stent, *Stroke* 39:2105–2113, 2008.

FUSIFORM INTRACRANIAL ANEURYSMS: MANAGEMENT STRATEGIES

30

DUKE SAMSON; BABU G. WELCH

INTRODUCTION

Even in the 21st century, fusiform or nonsaccular aneurysms of the intracranial circulation remain a challenge to neurosurgical therapies. This is due, in part, to the fact that these lesions commonly involve more than 180 degrees of the parent artery circumference, do not arise from arterial bifurcations, and frequently incorporate the origins of multiple distal vessels. It is intuitive to think of these lesions in the category of giant aneurysms but important to realize that the "small" fusiform aneurysm can be similarly daunting to the most accomplished cerebrovascular neurosurgeon.

In reviewing treatises of the past decade[1,2] on this topic, it is clear that neuroimaging represents major progress in the understanding of these lesions. The contributions of rotational digital subtraction angiography (R-DSA), computed tomographic angiography (CT-A), and MRI have refined the preoperative understanding of this vascular lesion and further clarified the interaction with the surrounding parenchyma. While diagnostic radiology provides an improved ability to formulate a surgical plan, the rapid evolution of endovascular techniques has changed the role of the cerebrovascular surgeon in the management of fusiform intracranial aneurysms. Endovascular vessel reconstruction and flow diversion techniques have, in many cases, provided a viable alternative in the management of fusiform aneurysms.[3–6] Despite these improvements, many such lesions are "beyond the reach" of endovascular devices and encourage cooperation between surgical and endovascular specialists to execute the best possible management of this complex disease.[7–11] To be part of this multidisciplinary team, the modern cerebrovascular surgeon must be able to demonstrate proficiency in the use of intracranial bypass techniques.

As this text focuses on the use of cerebral revascularization techniques, this chapter will utilize case material to discuss the strategies employed in the management of complex fusiform aneurysms that were not amenable to primary reconstruction. A stepwise approach of radiographic characterization, surgical planning, and intraoperative evaluation will be employed in devising a strategy to address these complex lesions using EC-IC and IC-IC bypass techniques with or without endovascular adjuncts.

THE THOUGHT PROCESS

In developing a management strategy for any aneurysm of the intracranial circulation, the ultimate goals of aneurysm exclusion and maintenance of parent vessel flow remain the same. Thorough preoperative evaluation, adequate surgical exposure, meticulous intraoperative inspection, and control of the proximal and distal vasculature are key steps in attaining theses goals. All surgical strategies should include a postoperative evaluation of aneurysm occlusion and distal blood flow. The fusiform aneurysm increases the complexity of surgical repair by circumferential involvement of the parent vessel and involvement of the origins of distal vessels. In larger lesions, mass effect, partial thrombosis, and poor wall malleability frequently preclude direct vessel reconstruction and encourage the use of cerebral bypass techniques.

The best question for the surgeon to ask is not "What can I do?" but "What should I do . . . with what I have?" It is important to understand not only one's limitations but also the ability of the operative team to adapt intraoperatively. Additional questions including "Is complete surgical exclusion of the aneurysm possible/necessary with an acceptable morbidity?" or "Can combination with endovascular adjuncts serve to reduce the potential morbidity of the surgery?" should also be asked in the formulation of a management strategy. A thorough evaluation of potential causes of the aneurysm can assist in responding to these questions.

PREOPERATIVE UNDERSTANDING

Potential Causes

Although many factors may contribute to their development, fusiform aneurysms are generally suspicious for a dissecting etiology that may or may not have an atherosclerotic component.[12-14] The presence of intramural hemorrhage has been observed in both acute and chronic lesions.[14] The contribution of infection, heritable arteriopathy, neoplasia, radiation, or previous cerebrovascular surgery should be considered when formulating a treatment strategy.[1,12,15-18] The location of the aneurysm may also suggest the etiology of the aneurysm and modify the management strategy. For example, fusiform aneurysms of the distal anterior circulation aneurysms are more likely to be related to trauma or infection, while a fusiform aneurysm of the vertebrobasilar junction frequently has an atherosclerotic component.

Radiological Evaluation

Historically, the preoperative understanding of fusiform aneurysm anatomy has been limited to the images provided by subtraction angiography. Despite the existence of noninvasive technologies, the visualization of blood flow during semiocclusive testing (Alcock's maneuver, cross-compression) and provocative testing (trial balloon occlusion) that are possible during angiography make this an indispensible tool in the evaluation of the fusiform aneurysms. This is especially important where bypass may be employed. Digital subtraction angiography with three-dimensional (3-D) reconstruction provides a circumferential view of the lesion in question. Newer CT-A reconstruction techniques are the method of choice for understanding aneurysm relationships with the skull base. It is important not to underestimate aneurysm wall calcifications that are also best visualized using this modality. Magnetic resonance imaging is most useful in detailing the aneurysms interaction with the brain parenchyma. By demonstrating associated edema, displacement of brain structures by the larger aneurysms, and demonstration of partial thrombosis within the aneurysm, MRI observations can drastically change the approach to the aneurysm. This knowledge allows a better prediction of operative risk and can suggest difficulty with postoperative recovery. An appreciation of the strengths and weaknesses of these radiographic modalities allows the modern cerebrovascular surgeon to better anticipate surgical difficulty and plan accordingly.

Trial Balloon Occlusion (TBO)

The use of trial balloon occlusion (TBO) should be a routine consideration in the management of all fusiform aneurysms. The substantial pathology of the arterial wall increases the possibility of permanent wall injury and need for parent vessel occlusion as a salvage during the procedure. In many institutions, the necessity and type of bypass (high-, mid-, low-flow) are determined by information obtained from the results of a protocol including this technique.[19] Although 80% of patients may tolerate ICA or nondominant vertebral artery occlusion,[20-23] a 20% chance of morbidity is unacceptable. Our

technique of utilizing clinical examination and single photon emission computed tomography (SPECT) has been previously published.[24] Since the introduction of the balloon occlusion technique by Matas,[25] significant changes in endovascular technology have allowed safer and more precise placement of a compliant balloon in an area that more closely mimics clip placement. This precise placement has produced more reliable results. Anecdotal experiences of balloon occlusion of the inflow to fusiform aneurysms have been discussed (personal communication) but not reported. The use of provocative measures such as EEG and hypotension in an attempt to further improve predictive values has been reported with up to a 95% correlation with successful vessel sacrifice.[19,26-28]

SURGICAL CONSIDERATIONS BY LOCATION

Middle Cerebral Artery

Fusiform aneurysms in the MCA have an uncertain natural history. In addition to being a common location for rupture, a concurrent risk for ischemia and symptoms attributed to mass effect also exists. Although data from the International Study of Unruptured Intracranial Aneurysms (ISUIA) noted a 5-year cumulative risk of 40% in giant lesions of the anterior circulation,[29] as an isolated group, the relative risk of rupture for the middle cerebral artery appears to be inversely proportional to growth. In a retrospective meta-analysis of spontaneous fusiform aneurysms of the middle cerebral artery, Day et al. emphasized that the risk of ischemia and mass effect was higher in the larger lesions than the risk of rupture.[15] As a group these lesions are exposed more superficially, are less likely to be endovascular candidates, and are frequently treated by primary reconstruction.[30] When bypass options are entertained, the strategy should minimize the number of vascular territories at risk even if a staged procedure is necessary. Reliance on collateral circulation in this location is a gamble for the patient.

Case 1: Calcified lesion of proximal M2

A 55-year-old male presented with a 3-month history of progressive left hand numbness. MRI and MRA suggested an 18 × 14 × 11 mm fusiform, right middle cerebral artery aneurysm that involved the origin of the insular M2 branch as well as subsequent exiting M3 branches. These findings were confirmed by CTA, which further clarified significant mural calcifications (Figure 30–1). Both CTA and R-DSA (Figure 30–2) made it clear that the multiple M3 vessels originating from the dome of the aneurysm would require the use of at least two bypass conduits to maintain the patency of these vessels if the aneurysm was to be obliterated.

Preoperatively, a plan was made for the use of the ipsilateral superficial temporal artery (STA) and lesser saphenous vein as possible bypass conduits. The use of both STA branches was

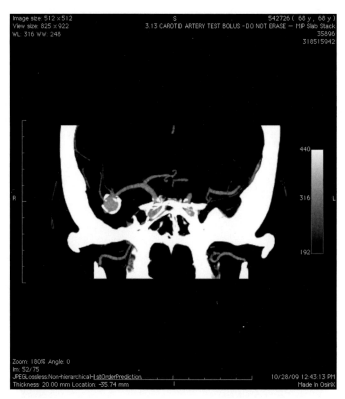

Image size: 512 × 512
View size: 825 × 922
WL: 316 WW: 248

S
3.13 CAROTID ARTERY TEST BOLUS - DO NOT ERASE — MIP Slab Stack

542726 (68 y , 68 y)
35896
318515942

440

316

192

R

L

Zoom: 180% Angle: 0
Im: 52/75
JPEGLossless.Non-hierarchical.1stOrderPrediction
Thickness: 20.00 mm Location: -35.74 mm

10/28/09 12:43:13 PM
Made In OsiriX

Figure 30–1. Sagittaly reformatted CTA demonstrates the significant mural calcifications.

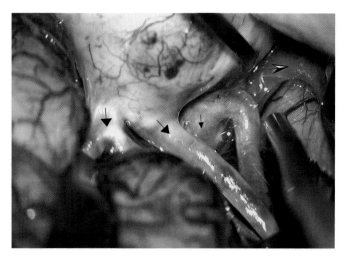

Figure 30–3. Intraoperative image of the aneurysm originating from the insular M2 branch (*small black arrow*) with M3 branches leaving the aneurysm dome (*large black arrows*). The fortuitous positioning of the late anterior temporal branch (*black/white arrow*) made it available for a side-to-side anastomosis.

After establishing patency of the bypassed segments, primary clipping of the aneurysm was prevented by the mural calcifications. The aneurysm was opened and tandem clips were placed for complete occlusion that was confirmed by postoperative angiography (Figure 30–5).

Case 2: Metastatic cardiac myxoma of the M1 bifurcation

A 34-year-old, right-handed woman presented with episodic left hemisphere transient ischemic attacks (TIAs). A previous "stroke" at age 4 was followed by an operation on her heart for treatment of atrial myxoma. Evidence of previous ischemia and calcifications were visualized in the left sylvian fissure (Figure 30–6). Coronal CT reconstructions revealed the partially calcified wall of the lesion (Figure 30–7A). Angiography demonstrated a large, left-sided fusiform aneurysm involving a distal M1 segment and all exiting M2 segments. The proximal

also a consideration. Intraoperative evaluation of the aneurysm confirmed the radiographic anatomy (Figure 30–3). The close proximity of a large anterior temporal artery made it possible to include an in situ, side-to-side anastomosis to an M3 vessel with the treatment options. A cut-flow of 20 cc/min was measured in the frontal branch of the STA. This was thought to be more than adequate to supplement ultrasonic flow measurements of 13 cc/min (Charbel microflow probe, Transonic Systems) noted at the medial M3 trunk. The side-to-side anastomosis was chosen for the lateral M3 branch (Figure 30–4) due to the inadequate length of the parietal STA branch.

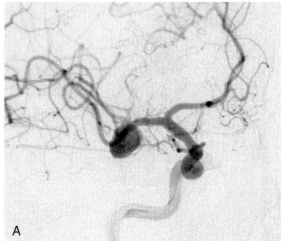

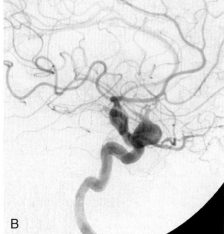

A

B

Figure 30–2. A and **B**, Oblique images of the right internal carotid artery clarify the origination of the M3 vessels from the aneurysm dome.

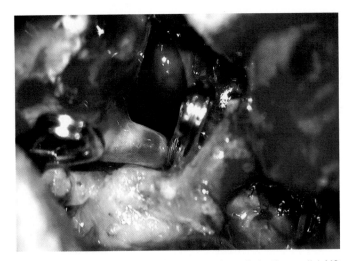

Figure 30–4. Superficial temporal artery anastomosis to the medial M3 trunk in the foreground (covered with cotton). Both aneurysm clips serve to occlude the aneurysm outflow. Sutures in the background mark the side-to-side anastomosis.

M1 segment containing the origins of the lateral lenticulostriate vessels was unaffected (Figure 30–7B).

With the likelihood of metastatic cardiac myxoma, a complete excision of the distal middle cerebral artery and proximal M2 vessels was planned via a left frontotemporal craniotomy. A right radial artery was harvested to serve as the conduit for the EC-IC bypass from the external carotid artery. After complete exposure of the left MCA from the origin of lateral lenticulostriate vessels to distal normal M2 branches (Figure 30–8 and Figure 30–9A), one M2 was amputated from the aneurysm and sutured, end to side, to the radial artery graft 2 cm from its distal tip (Figure 30–9B, 1). A temporary clip was placed on the radial graft distal to this anastomosis and the second M2 insular branch was amputated and sutured to the distal tip of the radial artery graft (Figure 30–9B, 2). Then temporary clips were placed on the M1 segment distal to the origin of the lenticulostriate vessels and a second clip on the third M2, just distal to its origin. The aneurysm was

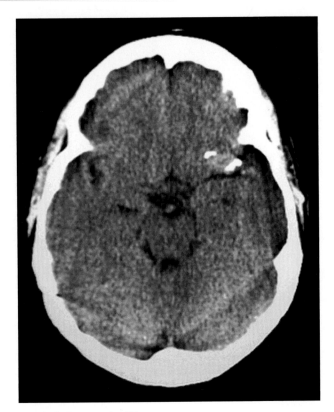

Figure 30–6. Preoperative CT scan.

then excised and removed from the field. A short radial artery interposition graft was placed (end to end) between the M1 and remaining M2 (Figure 30–9B, 3).

Immediate postoperative angiography demonstrated opacification of the two insular M2 segments via the EC-IC bypass (Figure 30–10). Significant spasm of the radial graft was clear. The more proximal M2 segment filled in continuity with the native M1. Clinically, the patient had a brief exacerbation of her mild expressive aphasia, but had returned to her preoperative level of functioning with 3 days. No clinical changes were noted at a 5-year follow-up examination.

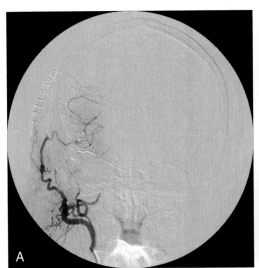
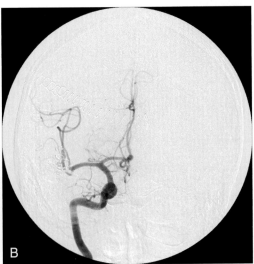

Figure 30–5. Postoperative angiography demonstrating patency of the EC-IC (**A**) and IC-IC (**B**) anastomoses.

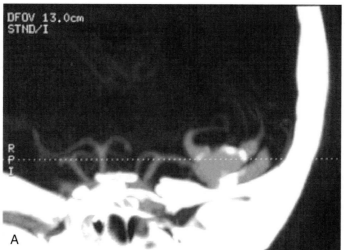
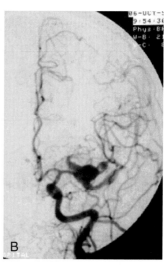

Figure 30–7. Coronal CT reconstructions (**A**) demonstrate mural calcifications, while angiography clarifies the fusiform involvement of all M2 branches (**B**).

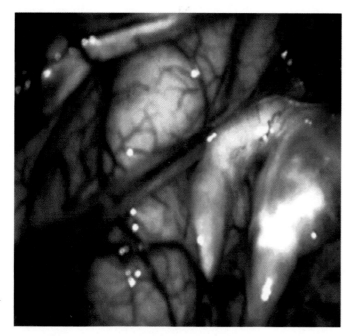

Figure 30–8. Intraoperative visualization of a myxomatous lesion of the middle cerebral artery. Note the characteristically thickened and iridescent walls.

Learning points

The MCA lesions presented here represent cases where disease pathology required complete trapping and exclusion of a necessary arterial segment. Thorough preoperative evaluation of the imaging allowed for multiple reconstructive options to be available in surgery. In Case 1, the intraoperative evaluation and blood-flow measurements (Transonic Systems) suggested robust collateral flow during proximal occlusion of the aneurysm. The ability to use a single STA to supply two exiting branches was also suggested by these flow measurements.

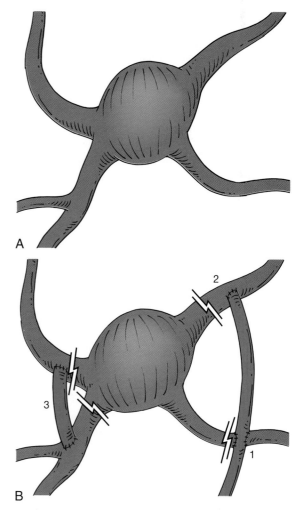

Figure 30–9. A, Schematic representations of the clip strategy. **B,** The order of anastomosis creation is delineated by 1, 2, 3. Breakpoints indicate clip placement.

(Courtesy of Sule K. Welch.)

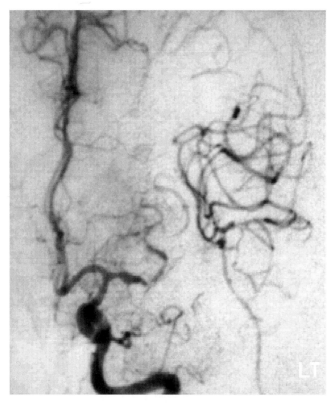

Figure 30–10. Intraoperative angiography of completed bypass with exclusion of the fusiform aneurysm.

Although the "double-barrel bypass"[30] would have, similar to Case 2, put less vascular territory at risk, the orientation of the vessels exiting the calcified aneurysm would not allow for a tension-free anastomosis of the second STA. Although an in situ anastomosis was performed, preparation of the radial artery for interposition grafting might have minimized vascular risk and provided a conduit with a better size match than the saphenous vein that was available.

In Case 2, it is important to emphasize the utility of addressing vascular beds individually. The use of the cervical radial artery bypass allowed for "tying in" each bed serially such that no more than 20 minutes of occlusion was permitted per arterial territory. Previous studies have confirmed a significant increase in operative morbidity when temporary occlusion persists for longer than 19 minutes.[31] The postoperative spasm of the radial artery, noted in Case 2, is a reported liability of the radial artery bypass. This occurred despite use of the pressure distension technique that has been described by Sekhar, et al.[32] Endovascular angioplasty should be considered should medical blood pressure manipulation not succeed in improving the clinical exam.

Anterior Cerebral Artery

Aneurysms of the anterior cerebral arteries have unique characteristics when discussed in the context of fusiform lesions. A distinction between proximal and distal groups is useful for the purposes of surgical approach and the variance in surgical options. The more common proximal, or anterior communicating (AComm), aneurysms frequently arise on the side of the dominant A1 vessel and incorporate the exiting, ipsilateral A2 vessel. As they are uniquely situated, the effects of changes in flow between the hemispheres, the growth of these aneurysms may involve distal circulations bilaterally. Complex anatomical relationships with hypothalamic perforators, accessory supply to the pericallosal region ("third A2"), and the recurrent artery of Huebner necessitate a detailed preoperative understanding of radiologic anatomy prior to surgical treatment. Despite the inherently fusiform characteristics of the more proximal lesions, primary clip reconstruction is commonly possible via pterional or subfrontal approach without removal of the orbital rim.

Similar to their proximal counterparts, distal aneurysms of the anterior circulation commonly involve the origins of the exiting vessels. Detailed analysis by Lehecka et al.[33] revealed a broad base, wider than the parent artery, in 68% of patients, and 94% of patients had a branch origin at the base. The same group revealed that 52% of these lesions were associated with another aneurysm.[34] More distally located lesions commonly supply well-collateralized vascular beds. TBO testing, in an elective situation, may reveal that vessel sacrifice is the less morbid therapy for the more distal anterior circulation aneurysm. When this is not feasible, the anatomic arrangement of the distal anterior cerebral vascular is favorable for side-to-side, in situ reconstruction.

Case 3: Fusiform aneurysm of a singular anterior cerebral artery

A 15-year-old female was found to harbor a 3.7-cm fusiform aneurysm in the parasellar region following MRI work-up of precocious puberty and right hemianopsia (Figure 30–11).

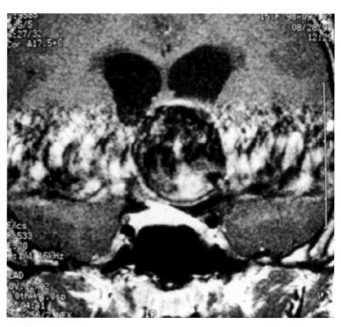

Figure 30–11. Coronal image of a large pulsatile lesion above the left cavernous internal carotid artery.

CT imaging suggested no mural calcifications. Initial angiography suggested a giant left ICA bifurcation aneurysm with bilateral anterior cerebral arteries filling only from a left carotid injection (Figure 30–12). Based on these findings, direct clipping of this lesion was planned via a left frontotemporal craniotomy. No bypass was planned.

Upon exposure, a fusiform aneurysm of the entire left A1 segment was identified (Figure 30–13). The ICA bifurcation and left A1-A2 junction were nonpathologic. Preparations were made to harvest a portion of lesser saphenous vein. The aneurysm was excised and a short saphenous vein graft was used as an interposition graft (Figure 30–14). Postoperative angiography demonstrated a widely patent graft with good filling of both A2 segments (Figure 30–15). There was no neurological deficit postoperatively.

Learning points

In-depth, preoperative evaluation of the patient's unique anatomical situation using the diagnostic techniques outlined previously will minimize, but not eliminate, intraoperative surprises of the type encountered in this patient. When extensive operative exposure reveals unexpected morphology, the cerebrovascular team must be capable of responding with treatment options that are optimal for the pathology that is encountered. In this situation, a definitive reconstruction procedure was not reasonable, and the diseased A1 segment represented the patient's sole angiographically visible supply of both distal anterior cerebral territories, making A1 sacrifice alone untenable.

The major branches of the anterior cerebral system are infrequent sites of fusiform aneurysms, but, despite their depth, represent excellent candidates for the use of bypass techniques when this pathological process is encountered. The normal vessels are generally of relatively uniform caliber, have few branch points and a minimum of interval small branches, and are

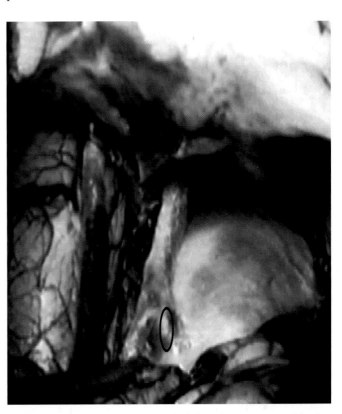

Figure 30–13. Intraoperative image depicting the aneurysm originating from just distal to the A1 origin. The ellipse is where the A1 enters the aneurysm.

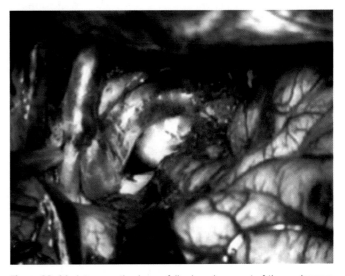

Figure 30–14. Intraoperative image following placement of the saphenous vein interposition graft.

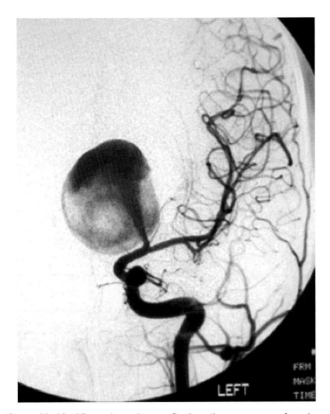

Figure 30–12. AP angiography confirming the presence of a large aneurysm at the bifurcation of the distal internal carotid artery. No A1 segment is visualized.

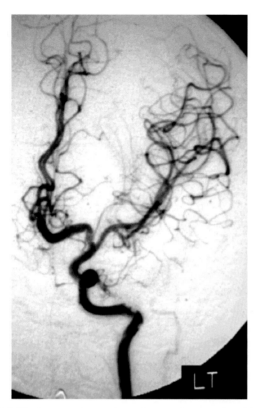

Figure 30–15. Postoperative angiography revealing a patent A1 without aneurismal involvement.

located in a single anatomical plane. An appropriately sized segment of STA or lesser saphenous vein will provide ample length to serve as an interposition graft, and the anastomotic technique (almost always end to end) requires between four and six 10-0 nylon sutures.

Proximal Internal Carotid Artery

Involvement of the proximal ICA is common in discussions of the subgroup of fusiform aneurysms.[1,2,7,11,16] Because of the relationship to the anterior clinoid process, close association with the optic apparatus, and common mural calcifications, fusiform ophthalmic aneurysms represent a unique challenge to the basic concepts of proximal control, adequate visualization, and clip application. For these reasons, carotid occlusion following TBO evaluation should remain a part of the treatment plan despite the best of intentions. Patient age, visual complaints, and marginal TBO results are relevant in the decision to selectively include bypass in the surgical treatment of fusiform aneurysms of this region.

Case 4: Enlarging ophthalmic aneurysm

A 57-year-old female presented with progressive visual loss in her right eye and enlargement of a known right ophthalmic aneurysm over the preceding year. A large left ophthalmic aneurysm had been treated by carotid sacrifice 5 years earlier.

Angiographic evaluation revealed a 2-cm multilobulated, partially thrombosed, fusiform aneurysm of the proximal ICA (Figure 30–16). Prompt clinical failure of a TBO confirmed the need for creation of a high-flow bypass. In an attempt to minimize the carotid occlusion time, the Excimer Laser Assisted Non-Occlusive Anastomosis (ELANA) technique[35,36] was used to perform a saphenous vein bypass graft from the proximal external carotid to the ipsilateral M2 artery (Figure 30–17 and Figure 30–18). No carotid occlusion was necessary to create the intracranial anastomosis. The ICA was sacrificed, intraoperatively, proximal to the posterior communicating artery (distal) and at the cervical ICA (proximal). Intraoperative angiography confirmed the absence of aneurysm opacification (Figure 30–19). The patient noted improved right eye vision and is functioning at her preoperative baseline at 1.5 years follow-up.

Learning points

In the case of a growing fusiform aneurysm of the proximal ICA, a component of progressive visual loss strongly suggests that surgical decompression be part of the treatment strategy. Despite the existence of some literature and clinical experience suggesting equivalence between surgical and endovascular therapies in similar circumstances,[11,37,38] the size of the lesion and presence of a pre-existing visual field deficit minimize our enthusiasm for endovascular approaches to this problem. The previous contralateral ICA sacrifice and the significant clinical changes during TBO eliminated the option of Hunterian ligation from the treatment strategy. The presence of STA

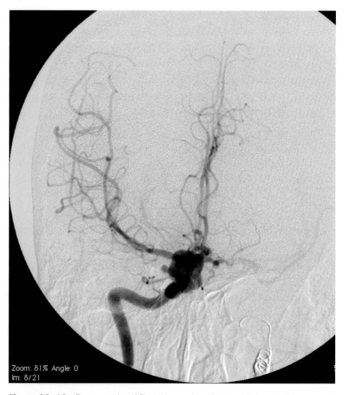

Figure 30–16. Preoperative AP angiography of a multilobulated aneurysm of the proximal right ICA. Note the endovascular sacrifice of the contralateral ICA.

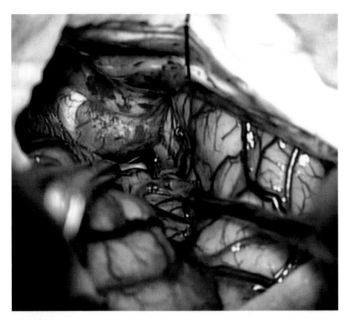

Figure 30–17. Intraoperative image along the right sylvian fissure depicting a large aneurysm producing significant distortion of the right optic nerve. The suction device is pointing at the temporal M2 branch that was used for the saphenous vein anastomosis.

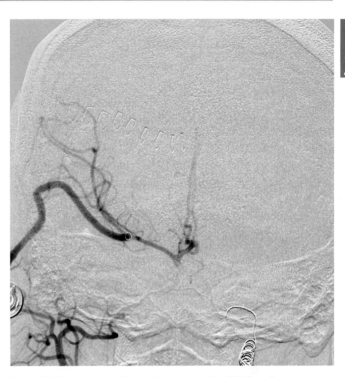

Figure 30–19. Intraoperative angiography verifies EC-IC graft patency and without filling of the ophthalmic aneurysm.

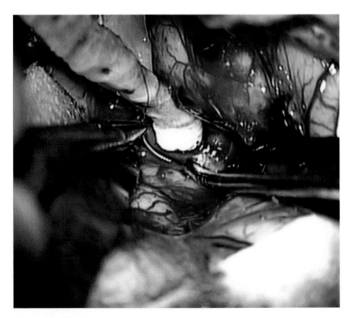

Figure 30–18. Anastomosis of the saphenous vein is being performed. A platinum ring has been placed within the everted vein cuff.

collaterals to the ophthalmic artery suggested that carotid sacrifice that involved this vessel would not further endanger the patient's vision. Although clip reconstruction should be the treatment of choice, the significant vessel wall involvement clarified by R-DSA and optic nerve displacement (see Figure 30–17) support a deconstructive option with bypass.

The ELANA technique has been well described in the literature[35,36,39,40] and is slowly becoming available to more

cerebrovascular surgeons. The adequate caliber of the M2 vessel (~2.3 mm) and the demonstrated need for carotid replacement increase the likelihood of success with the procedure. The use of a nonocclusive technique was ideal based on this patient's blood flow needs.

Posterior Circulation

When discussing fusiform aneurysms of the posterior circulation, the giant and highly morbid transitional[41] or dolichoectatic lesions involving the vertebral and basilar arteries are a common focus. Treatment of these lesions is often deconstructive and no consensus exists in the cerebrovascular community regarding an appropriate treatment strategy with or without the addition of bypass. Aneurysms of the proximal vertebral artery are more commonly managed by bypass techniques and will be the focus of discussion for this section.

There is little disagreement that the proximal intracranial vertebral artery (VA) is prone to traumatic dissection and frequently affected by atherosclerotic changes. The classification of nonatherosclerotic and fusiform aneurysms by Mizutani and colleagues heavily concentrated on the vertebrobasilar region and provides a good clinicopathological discussion on these lesions.[42] Heightened awareness of acute stroke attributed to pathology in this region has increased the number of these lesions that present for neurosurgical consultation.

In the current era, many of the posterior circulation lesions that present for surgical discussion are "out of reach" of endovascular technology. Limitations include the common size discrepancies between the vertebral and branching vessels that constrain manipulations of endovascular equipment (i.e., catheters within stents) as well as the presence of important perforating vessels (i.e., anterior spinal artery). The proximal VA is unique in a discussion on bypass due to both the vessel sizes and the smaller working corridor provided. The average VA is approximately 3 mm in diameter, the posterior inferior cerebellar artery measures between 1.2 and 1.7 mm. An added complexity in this region is the close relationship between the lower cranial nerves that are frequently distorted by a growing aneurysm. Surgical strategies here generally include the use of a midline or far lateral suboccipital approach. Resection of the occipital condyle is tailored to the extent of anterior or medial access that is desired. Close attention should be given to initial patient positioning and maximal bony exposure.

Case 5: Aneurysm of the proximal PICA

A 46-year-old male presented with an MRI showing symptomatic infarct of the right cerebellum (Figure 30–20). Subsequent angiographic workup revealed a fusiform aneurysm of the right posterior inferior cerebellar (PICA) artery that demonstrated enlargement following a 6-week period of convalescence on antiplatelet therapy (Figure 30–21). Although conservative medical management was discussed, surgical repair of the vessel was recommended and accepted as the next course of therapy.

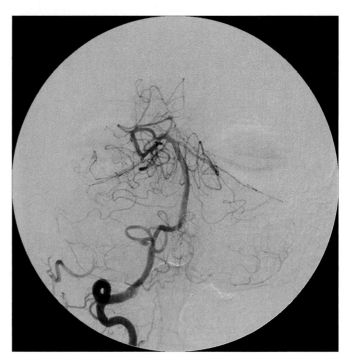

Figure 30–21. AP injection of the right vertebral artery revealed PICA aneurysm distal to the origin from the vertebral artery.

Based on the angiographic anatomy, surgical options included direct clip reconstruction, aneurysm excision with primary anastomosis, OA-PICA bypass, or PICA-PICA bypass. The OA was harvested before a far lateral suboccipital craniectomy was performed. Intraoperative evaluation revealed redundancy of the PICA distal to the fusiform aneurysm that was located on the first PICA segment proximal to lateral medullary perforators (Figure 30–22). This redundancy allowed for the reimplantation of the PICA at a more proximal location on the ipsilateral VA. A previously unseen perforator just distal to the aneurysm made the primary anastomosis a difficult

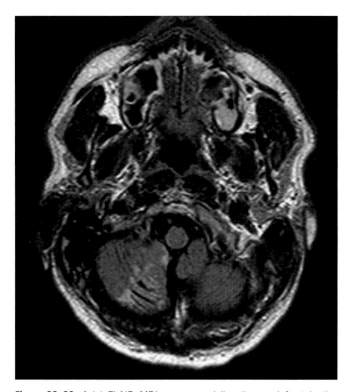

Figure 30–20. Axial FLAIR MRI sequence delineating an infarct in the distribution of the PICA.

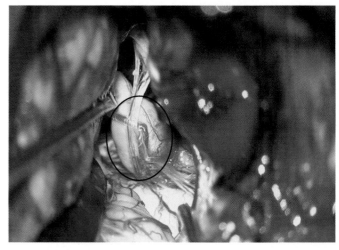

Figure 30–22. Intraoperative image of the proximal PICA aneurysm (*ellipse*) as exposed via a right suboccipital, far lateral craniectomy. The VA is seen to the right of the aneurysm.

exercise. Doppler flow and indocyanine green angiography (ICG-A) findings of graft patency were confirmed by subsequent angiography (Figure 30–23).

Learning points

The preceding case demonstrates a viable option for the management of a proximal PICA lesion that was of dissecting etiology. Intraoperative visualization clearly revealed arterial dissection, as the etiology for both lesions involved the PICA proximal to the telovelotonsillar, or fourth segment. As established literature exists concerning the stroke risk involved when PICA is occluded proximal to this segment,[30,43,44] the need for bypass techniques should be expected when addressing aneurysms at this level. In Case 5, the redundancy of the PICA distal to the aneurysm allowed for reimplantation of the PICA on the proximal VA and placed only the ipsilateral PICA territory at ischemic risk. It was fortunate that the involved perforators had a length to allow for mobilizing the PICA vessel proximally. Similar ischemic risks would have resulted from the use of OA-PICA anastomosis but the concern for a tension-free repair limited this as an option.

Unpublished experience from this institution includes radiographic documentation of continued dissection and aneurysm formation beyond a "repaired" segment. This argues the case for complete exclusion of injured vascular tissue where possible as well as close postoperative, and delayed, imaging follow-up of arterial dissections. IC-IC bypass techniques with the use of radial artery grafting can facilitate reaching this goal.[45] Although the use of a PICA-PICA bypass[30,46,47] would be appropriate in this case, the potential exposure of

two vascular territories to ischemic risk generally places this as a third bypass option for pathologies of the VA that involve the PICA.

Combined Microvascular and Endovascular Approaches

In developing a management strategy for the fusiform aneurysm, treatment options should include the discussion of both endovascular and microsurgical techniques. In their discussion of combined operative and endovascular approaches from 1998, Hacein-Bey and colleagues appropriately emphasize the conviction that a "prospective evaluation" of lesion complexities and appreciation of the complementary nature of surgical and endovascular techniques offers the best chance for reducing treatment morbidity and improving long-term outcomes.[7] While both of these techniques provide reconstructive and deconstructive options, current endovascular technology is more limited by vessel size, while surgical techniques are limited by vessel location. As the notion of becoming a complete cerebrovascular surgeon increasingly involves endovascular training, it is likely that combined approaches to complex aneurysms will only increase in frequency.

Case 6: Traumatic aneurysm of the middle cerebral artery

A 26-year-old male with a history of multiple concussive injuries related to football was found to harbor a fusiform aneurysm of the left MCA at an outside institution. "Clip reconstruction was not possible" at the time of the surgery, and wrapping and acrylic application was performed. The patient developed a seizure disorder and recovered from a right hemiparesis following this surgery. He presented to our institution, 2 years later, with refractory seizures, an intermittent aphasia, and growth of the known aneurysm (Figure 30–24).

The patient's medical history strongly suggested the possibility of traumatic aneurysm of the left MCA that involved, on separate aneurysm lobes, the origins of the M2 trunks. The lobulated angiographic appearance was associated with a pattern of contrast stasis suggestive of a pseudoaneurysmal component that, along with previous surgical exposure, increased the difficulty of gaining proximal control and diminished the possibility of primary clip reconstruction via a pterional approach. Based on these observations, a strategy of temporal M2 bypass and proximal endovascular reconstruction of the insular M2 branch was devised to allow for aneurysm embolization.

A complex surgical approach was further complicated by the failure of the initial left STA-M2 bypass. This required a return to the operating room for harvest of the occipital artery that was tunneled subcutaneously in a second attempt at bypass of the temporal M2. Angiographic confirmation of OA-M2 bypass patency allowed for initial embolization of the distal aneurysm (Figure 30–25) that was followed 6 weeks later by the stent-assisted endovascular reconstruction of the

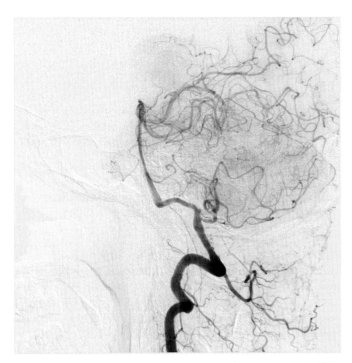

Figure 30–23. Postoperative angiography confirming patency of the PICA vessel that is located just proximal to a stump of the original PICA.

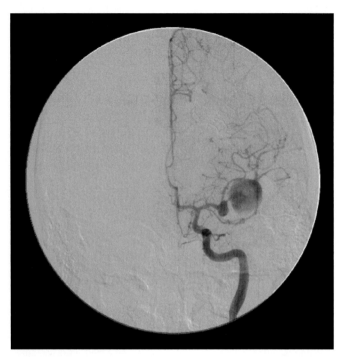

Figure 30–24. AP injection of the left ICA demonstrating a multilobulated aneurysm of the distal MCA. The smaller lobe involves the origin of the insular M2 branch, while the larger lobe distorts the proximal trunk of the temporal M2 branch prior to an M3 bifurcation.

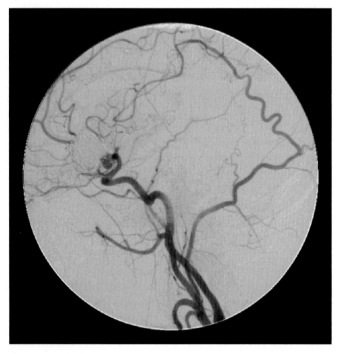

Figure 30–25. Lateral common carotid injection confirms the OA-M3 bypass filling the circulation distal to the coil mass that was the larger lobe of the aneurysm.

insular M2 artery and complete embolization of the aneurysm (Figure 30–26). A transient postoperative hemiparesis resolved and the patient returned to his preoperative baseline at 3 months of follow-up.

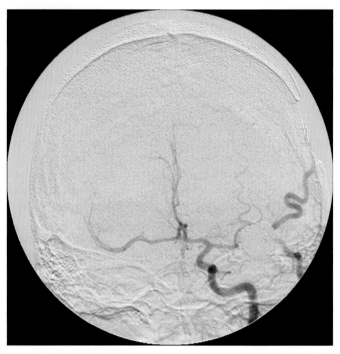

Figure 30–26. Complete occlusion of the aneurysm was possible once an endovascular reconstruction device was placed to maintain the patency of the insular M2 branch.

Learning points

Although similar to Cases 1 and 2 in therapeutic strategy, this case was further complicated by the poor access to the proximal aspect of the aneurysm. When proximal control is limited by previous surgery, excessive mural calcifications or aneurysm thrombosis, the advantages of endovascular technology should be appreciated. In the case of failure of the initial graft, it is important to understand the alternative options that existed. In this case, these included a radial artery direct bypass from the external carotid artery as demonstrated in Case 2 versus an interposition graft from the STA trunk using this same conduit. The decision to use the OA was based on observations of the angiographic anatomy and the presence of a sizeable donor vessel. It is highly likely distal occlusion of the aneurysm facilitated the long-term coil obliteration that was observed in such a large lesion.

CONCLUSION

In his 1944 publication, *Intracranial Arterial Aneurysms*, Walter Dandy proclaimed that "intracranial aneurysms…are now added to the lengthening line of lesions that are curable by surgery."[48] Since that time, the methods by which the cerebrovascular surgeon excludes an aneurysm from the circulation while maintaining parent vessel flow have been refined by evolutions in microvascular technique, radiological imaging, and a better comprehension of cerebral hemodynamics. The relatively infrequent occurrence of fusiform aneurysms in the aneurysm population accounts for less standardized management of these lesions. This does not change the need for adherence to established principles of surgical exposure, microvascular technique, and maintenance of proximal and distal control. The fusiform aneurysm increases the importance of preoperative evaluation and thorough intraoperative inspection while increasing the probability that bypass will contribute to a favorable surgical outcome.

When a bypass becomes part of the treatment strategy of fusiform aneurysms, it is helpful to understand the benefits and disadvantages of the EC-IC, IC-IC, interposition, and reimplantation alternatives that define "the bypass" and are described in this text. The ability to intraoperatively evaluate and quantitate blood flow as a final determinant of bypass conduit should not be underestimated in its significance.[49] It is essential for the modern cerebrovascular surgeon to realize that bypass alternatives are not exclusionary of one another in the management of fusiform aneurysms. These options should be creatively considered, along with endovascular techniques, to provide an elegant solution to the problem of the fusiform aneurysm.

REFERENCES

1. Drake CG, Peerless SJ: Giant fusiform intracranial aneurysms: review of 120 patients treated surgically from 1965 to 1992, *J Neurosurg* 87:141–162, 1997.
2. Sundt TM, et al: Giant intracranial aneurysms, *Clin Neurosurg* 37:116–154, 1991.
3. Fiorella D, et al: Curative reconstruction of a giant midbasilar trunk aneurysm with the pipeline embolization device, *Neurosurgery* 64:212–217, 2009; discussion 217.
4. Hauck EF, et al: Stent/coil treatment of very large and giant unruptured ophthalmic and cavernous aneurysms, *Surg Neurol* 71:19–24, 2009; discussion 24.
5. Van Rooij WJ, Sluzewski M: Endovascular treatment of large and giant aneurysms, *Am J Neuroradiol* 30:12–18, 2008.
6. Lylyk P, et al: Curative endovascular reconstruction of cerebral aneurysms with the pipeline embolization device: the Buenos Aires experience, *Neurosurgery* 64:632–642, 2009; discussion 642–643; quiz N6.
7. Hacein-Bey L, et al: Complex intracranial aneurysms: combined operative and endovascular approaches, *Neurosurgery* 43:1304–1312, 1998; discussion 1312–1313.
8. Lawton MT, et al: Combined microsurgical and endovascular management of complex intracranial aneurysms, *Neurosurgery* 52:263–274, 2003; discussion 274–275.
9. Lawton MT, et al: Combined microsurgical and endovascular management of complex intracranial aneurysms, *Neurosurgery* 62(Suppl 3):1503–1515, 2008.
10. Hoh BL, et al: Combined surgical and endovascular techniques of flow alteration to treat fusiform and complex wide-necked intracranial aneurysms that are unsuitable for clipping or coil embolization, *J Neurosurg* 95:24–35, 2001.
11. Hoh BL, et al: Results after surgical and endovascular treatment of paraclinoid aneurysms by a combined neurovascular team, *Neurosurgery* 48:78–89, 2001; discussion 89–90.
12. Anson JA, Lawton MT, Spetzler RF: Characteristics and surgical treatment of dolichoectatic and fusiform aneurysms, *J Neurosurg* 84:185–193, 1996.
13. Moffie D: Fusiform aneurysm of intracranial arteries, *Psychiatr Neurol Neurochir* 71:85–91, 1968.
14. Nakatomi H, et al: Clinicopathological study of intracranial fusiform and dolichoectatic aneurysms: insight on the mechanism of growth, *Stroke* 31:896–900, 2000.
15. Day AL, et al: Spontaneous fusiform middle cerebral artery aneurysms: characteristics and a proposed mechanism of formation, *J Neurosurg* 99:228–240, 2003.
16. Park S, et al: Intracranial fusiform aneurysms: its pathogenesis, clinical characteristics and management, *J Kor Neurosurg Soc* 44:116, 2008.
17. Morris B, et al: Cerebrovascular disease in childhood cancer survivors: a children's oncology group report, *Neurology* 73:1906–1913, 2009.
18. Horowitz MB, et al: Multidisciplinary approach to traumatic intracranial aneurysms secondary to shotgun and handgun wounds, *Surg Neurol* 51:31–41, 1999; discussion 41–42.
19. Surdell DL, et al: Revascularization for complex intracranial aneurysms, *Neurosurg Focus* 24:E21, 2008.
20. Abud DG, et al: Venous phase timing during balloon test occlusion as a criterion for permanent internal carotid artery sacrifice, *AJNR Am J Neuroradiol* 26:2602–2609, 2005.
21. Dare AO, et al: Failure of the hypotensive provocative test during temporary balloon test occlusion of the internal carotid artery to predict delayed hemodynamic ischemia after therapeutic carotid occlusion, *Surg Neurol* 50:147–155, 1998; discussion 155–156.
22. Vazquez Anon V, et al: Balloon occlusion of the internal carotid artery in 40 cases of giant intracavernous aneurysm: technical aspects, cerebral monitoring, and results, *Neuroradiology* 34:245–251, 1992.
23. Miller JD, Jawad K, Jennet B: Safety of carotid ligation and its role in the management of intracranial aneurysms, *J Neurol Neurosurg Psychiatry* 40:64–72, 1977.
24. Eckard DA, Purdy PD, Bonte FJ: Temporary balloon occlusion of the carotid artery combined with brain blood flow imaging as a test to predict tolerance prior to permanent carotid sacrifice, *AJNR Am J Neuroradiol* 13:1565–1569, 1992.
25. Matas RI: Testing the Efficiency of the Collateral Circulation as a Preliminary to the Occlusion of the Great Surgical Arteries, *Ann Surg* 53:1–43, 1911.
26. Graves VB, et al: Endovascular occlusion of the carotid or vertebral artery with temporary proximal flow arrest and microcoils: clinical results, *AJNR Am J Neuroradiol* 18:1201–1206, 1997.
27. Mathis JM, et al: Temporary balloon test occlusion of the internal carotid artery: experience in 500 cases, *AJNR Am J Neuroradiol* 16:749–754, 1995.
28. Standard SC, et al: Balloon test occlusion of the internal carotid artery with hypotensive challenge, *AJNR Am J Neuroradiol* 16:1453–1458, 1995.
29. The International Study of Unruptured Intracranial Aneurysms Investigators: Unruptured intracranial aneurysms: natural history, clinical outcome, and risk of surgical and endovascular treatment, *Lancet* 362:103–110, 2003.
30. Lawton MT, et al: Revascularization and aneurysm surgery: current techniques, indications, and outcome, *Neurosurgery* 38:83–92, 1996; discussion 92–94.
31. Samson D, et al: A clinical study of the parameters and effects of temporary arterial occlusion in the management of intracranial aneurysms, *Neurosurgery* 34:22–28, 1994; discussion 28–9.
32. Sekhar LN, et al: Cerebral revascularization using radial artery grafts for the treatment of complex intracranial aneurysms: techniques and outcomes for 17 patients, *Neurosurgery* 49:646–658, 2001; discussion 658–659.
33. Lehecka M, et al: Anatomic features of distal anterior cerebral artery aneurysms: a detailed angiographic analysis of 101 patients, *Neurosurgery* 63:219–228, 2008; discussion 228–229.
34. Lehecka M, et al: Distal anterior cerebral artery aneurysms: treatment and outcome analysis of 501 patients, *Neurosurgery* 62:590–601, 2008; discussion 590–601.
35. Langer DJ, et al: Excimer laser-assisted nonocclusive anastomosis. An emerging technology for use in the creation of intracranial-intracranial and extracranial-intracranial cerebral bypass, *Neurosurg Focus* 24:E6, 2008.

36. Streefkerk HJ, et al: The excimer laser-assisted nonocclusive anasto-mosis practice model: development and application of a tool for practicing microvascular anastomosis techniques, *Neurosurgery* 58 (Suppl 1):ONS148–ONS156, 2006; discussion ONS148–ONS156.

37. Day AL: Aneurysms of the ophthalmic segment. A clinical and anato-mical analysis, *J Neurosurg* 72:677–691, 1990.

38. Ferguson GG, Drake CG: Carotid-ophthalmic aneurysms: visual abnormalities in 32 patients and the results of treatment, *Surg Neurol* 16:1–8, 1981.

39. Streefkerk HJ, Bremmer JP, Tulleken CA: The ELANA technique: high flow revascularization of the brain, *Acta Neurochir Suppl* 94:143–148, 2005.

40. Streefkerk HJ, et al: The ELANA technique: constructing a high flow bypass using a non-occlusive anastomosis on the ICA and a conven-tional anastomosis on the SCA in the treatment of a fusiform giant bas-ilar trunk aneurysm, *Acta Neurochir (Wien)* 146:1009–1019, 2004; discussion 1019.

41. Flemming K, et al: History of radiographically defined vertebrobasilar nonsaccular intracranial aneurysms, *Cerebrovasc Dis* 20:270–279, 2005.

42. Mizutani T, et al: Proposed classification of nonatherosclerotic cerebral fusiform and dissecting aneurysms, *Neurosurgery* 45:253–259, 1999; discussion 259–260.

43. Ali MJ, et al: Trapping and revascularization for a dissecting aneurysm of the proximal posteroinferior cerebellar artery: technical case report and review of the literature, *Neurosurgery* 51:258–262, 2002; discus-sion 262–263.

44. Hudgins RJ, et al: Aneurysms of the posterior inferior cerebellar artery. A clinical and anatomical analysis, *J Neurosurg* 58:381–387, 1983.

45. Sanai N, Zador Z, Lawton MT: Bypass surgery for complex brain aneur-ysms: an assessment of intracranial-intracranial bypass, *Neurosurgery* 65:670–683, 2009; discussion 683.

46. Ausman JI, et al: Posterior inferior to posterior inferior cerebellar artery anastomosis combined with trapping for vertebral artery aneurysm. Case report, *J Neurosurg* 73:462–465, 1990.

47. Lemole GM, et al: Cerebral revascularization performed using posterior inferior cerebellar artery–posterior inferior cerebellar artery bypass. Report of four cases and literature review, *J Neurosurg* 97:219–223, 2002.

48. Dandy WE: *Intracranial Arterial Aneurysms*, Ithaca, NY, 1944, Comstock.

49. Amin-Hanjani S, et al: The utility of intraoperative blood flow measure-ment during aneurysm surgery using an ultrasonic perivascular flow probe, *Neurosurgery* 62(Suppl 3):1346–1353, 2008.

V

SKULL BASE TUMORS

DECISION-MAKING STRATEGIES FOR EC-IC BYPASS IN THE TREATMENT OF SKULL BASE TUMORS

31

PHILIPP TAUSSKY; WILLIAM COULDWELL

INTRODUCTION

Since the first EC-IC bypass operation by Donaghy and Yasargil, both the technique and indications have evolved.[1] Initially, an EC-IC bypass procedure was used to augment blood flow in the context of a high-grade stenosis or atherosclerotic occlusion of the carotid artery or a proximal segment of the middle cerebral artery.[2–4] The indications for an EC-IC bypass have evolved, however, to include its use in the context of acute flow replacement. Replacement may be indicated in the treatment of complex aneurysms not amenable to clipping where parent artery ligation is needed or as part of a radical skull base tumor resection with resection of the carotid artery.[5–8] Skull base surgery techniques have evolved over the last two decades, and their applications have offered radical tumor resection. In cases of tumors involving the anterior skull base, a radical surgical resection will often include resection of the carotid artery encased or infiltrated by the tumor. Often surgical decision making will need to address the option of preserving the carotid artery at the cost of a subtotal tumor resection versus resection of the carotid artery to achieve a radical tumor removal.[9,10] Furthermore, in cases of radical tumor resection and sacrifice of the carotid artery, there is controversy relating to the option of revascularization by means of an EC-IC bypass. In this chapter, we address the surgical decision making for EC-IC bypass in the treatment of skull base tumors.

INDICATIONS FOR CAROTID ARTERY SACRIFICE

Benign Tumors

Many anterior and middle fossa skull base tumors, including meningiomas, pituitary adenomas, nerve sheath tumors, and juvenile angiofibromas, are of a benign nature.[11,12] Even these benign tumors may encase the internal carotid artery (ICA), however, and carotid sacrifice may become a consideration in surgical resection. Hirsch and colleagues[13] developed a grading system to describe the involvement of the C4 segment of the ICA in meningiomas of the cavernous sinus. The grading system defines three grades: (1) tumor partially encases the ICA, (2) tumor completely encases the ICA without narrowing it, and (3) tumor completely encases and narrows the ICA.

Several authors have demonstrated safe removal of meningiomas encasing the ICA. In a recent series, Abdel-Aziz and colleagues[14] achieved a total resection in 22 of 24 patients whose tumors were scored as Hirsch grade 1. In 14 patients with tumors graded Hirsch grade 2 or 3, an incomplete resection was achieved with 0% mortality. DeMonte and colleagues[15] achieved a total resection in 31 of 41 patients with skull base meningiomas, preserving the ICA in all patients.

Tumor dissection off the ICA can be achieved in cases in which an arachnoid membrane separates the tumor and the vessel. This appears to be true in many cases, even those involving tumors of Hirsch grade 3.[9,16] In those cases where the carotid artery cannot be dissected free completely, the residual tumor may be thinned out using microsurgical technique.[17] The residual tumor can then be treated with stereotactic radiotherapy techniques with excellent local control.[18,19]

Before the widespread use of radiosurgery for residual tumor, attempts at radical tumor resection with sacrifice of the ICA and revascularization provided modest benefit in terms of recurrence rate. Sen and Sekhar[20] reported their experience with 17 patients with skull base meningiomas in whom the ICA was resected and a bypass was performed. A gross total resection was achieved in 13 patients, and recurrence rates were 8% after total removal and 25% after subtotal resection. Compared with current series in which the carotid artery was preserved and radiosurgery was used as an adjuvant, these results appear to offer no substantial benefit in terms of tumor recurrence.[14–16,21]

Since carotid resection and bypass reconstruction involve an additional complication risk of 7% to 10%, carotid artery sacrifice and revascularization seem to offer little additional benefit in the treatment of benign skull base tumors at the time of the initial resection.[9,17,20,22] Although gross total resection is the goal of surgery, results do not indicate worse outcome in patients with residual tumor treated by radiosurgery and closely followed clinically and radiologically.[18,19,21,23]

As a result, cerebral revascularization is currently not indicated for most benign skull base tumors. We note two possible exceptions to this rule. One is for patients with complete carotid occlusion due to tumor encasement and with neurologic symptoms or progressive tumor growth. Moreover, in patients with tumor encasement of the carotid in whom no local tumor control can be achieved despite surgical and radiotherapeutic measures, we recommend salvage surgery with carotid artery sacrifice and revascularization.[3,9,24]

Malignant Skull Base Tumors

Malignant skull base tumors are a pathologically diverse group of neoplasms. The most frequent malignant skull base tumors are summarized in Table 31-1.[25] The treatment of malignant skull base tumors involves a different surgical approach than is used for benign tumors. Malignant tumors tend to invade adjacent anatomical structures, and they may metastasize to remote organs and thus cause death. Because of their ability to directly invade vessel walls, they may cause rupture of the carotid artery due to tumor invasion.[26,27]

The primary goal of surgical treatment in these malignancies is complete removal with tumor-free margins to control local disease.[10,28,29] Radical surgical resection, including carotid artery sacrifice, is considered the only treatment option offering cure or long-term survival for these patients.[30,31] Other nonsurgical treatment options, especially radiotherapy and chemotherapy, offer only palliative treatment, with almost no long-term survivors.[30–33]

Malignant skull base tumors tend to not only encase but actively infiltrate and invade the walls of the carotid artery.[10,28] This is in marked contrast to benign tumors, which encase the carotid artery but often leave an arachnoid plane between tumor and artery.[16] Therefore, gross total resection of malignant skull base tumors involving the carotid artery can only be achieved in most cases by carotid artery resection and carotid sacrifice.[9,10,17,28] Other options, such as peeling the tumor off the carotid adventitial wall, often leave the wall weakened and thus increase the potential risk of rupture while failing to achieve a gross total resection.[28,34]

Carotid artery involvement can be determined preoperatively by MRI with a sensitivity of close to 100%.[35,36]

Although the specificity for the evaluation of carotid infiltration by the tumor is only 85% for MRI, and computed tomography (CT) scanning is associated with a false-positive rate of 94%,[35] in most cases, the decision to sacrifice the carotid artery with tumor resection can be made preoperatively.

The risk of radical surgical resection, including carotid artery sacrifice, must be viewed in the context of the dismal prognosis of patients suffering from malignant skull base tumors.[10] Although the morbidity and mortality of carotid artery resection remains significant,[10,29,37,38] these risks must be carefully weighed against the significant morbidity and mortality of carotid artery involvement in this patient population. Most contemporary studies report a mortality rate of about 7% and a neurologic morbidity rate of up to 17% with carotid artery resection,[29,37,38] but the risk of carotid artery rupture is reported at around 18% and tends to happen within 6 months of carotid invasion.[34,39,40] Reports mention mortality rates at 40% and morbidity at 60% in instances of carotid rupture.[41,42] For this reason, most surgeons believe carotid artery resection followed by revascularization is a safer option than carotid preservation.[9,10,28]

Carotid artery resection not only lowers the possible complication rate from vessel invasion by tumor, it also offers the only option of an oncologic resection and the only chance for survival.[28] This is of particular significance in malignant tumors involving the cavernous sinus, where carotid artery sacrifice allows en bloc resection with disease-free margins.[43,44]

While overall prognosis remains grim in patients suffering from malignant skull base tumors, an international collaborative study group showed radical resection with negative margins to be highly predictive of overall survival. Residual tumor is also highly associated with tumor recurrence.[45–47]

EVALUATION AND INDICATION OF CAROTID REVASCULARIZATION AFTER CAROTID RESECTION

After the decision has been made to resect the carotid artery, the option of an EC-IC bypass needs to be addressed. The indication for cerebral revascularization remains controversial, and decision making involves two different positions. The universal approach favors revascularization for all patients who have undergone carotid sacrifice, whereas the selective approach strives to evaluate those patients in need of flow replacement.

Carotid resection without revascularization involves a significant risk of ischemic complications, with mortality ranging from 0% to 31% and a neurologic morbidity of 0% to 45%.[10,28,48,49] Various diagnostic measures have been developed to select those patients in whom a bypass is necessary to guarantee adequate perfusion after carotid sacrifice.[3,50–52]

Normal cerebral blood flow is maintained at approximately 54 ml/100 g/min,[53] over a wide range of blood pressure values.

Table 31-1. MOST COMMON MALIGNANT TUMORS OF THE ANTERIOR SKULL BASE.
Adenoid cystic carcinoma
Adenocarcinoma
Sarcoma
Squamous cell carcinoma
Esthesioneuroblastoma
Chondrosarcoma
Malignant meningioma

To cause neuronal dysfunction, cerebral blood flow must drop below 20 ml/100 g/min. Permanent cell damage is expected if values drop below 15 ml/100 g/min.[53] Physiological responses to decreased cerebral blood flow include autoregulatory vasodilation and an increase in the oxygen extraction fraction.[54,55] Autoregulatory vasodilation reflects cerebrovascular reserve, which is a significant indicator of ischemic events.[56] An increase in oxygen extraction fraction by hypoperfused neurons is also termed "misery perfusion," and is of special importance in patients with chronic hypoperfusion such as those with atherosclerotic stenosis or occlusion of the carotid artery.[57] Evaluation of these compensatory mechanisms is of importance in identifying patients in whom carotid artery sacrifice would result in critical hypoperfusion and ischemic neurologic events.[4]

Balloon test occlusion (BTO) of the ICA is considered to be the gold standard to assess collateral circulation before occlusion of the carotid artery.[3,58,59] This usually includes a 20- to 30-minute period of carotid balloon occlusion and a clinical neurologic examination. Those patients whose neurologic status changes during balloon occlusion are considered to have poor autoregulatory reserve and would not tolerate carotid sacrifice without neurologic deficits. The predictive value of BTO, however, is not without limitations. Approximately 10% of patients passing the BTO have decreased hemispheric blood flow as measured by stable xenon CT.[60] About 5% of patients passing the BTO will develop neurologic deficits in the early postoperative period.[61,62]

This has led investigators to modify the BTO to include functional studies, including perfusion imaging, pharmacological-induced hypotension with electroencephalographic monitoring, and stump pressure measurements.[55,63] Most commonly, a BTO is paired with an acetazolamide challenge to assess cerebrovascular reserve.[59,64,65] Acetazolamide is a carbonic anhydrase inhibitor that crosses the blood-brain barrier (BBB) slowly and acts as a cerebral vasodilator. Peak cerebral blood flow augmentation occurs after 10 to 15 minutes, and a 30% to 60% increase is considered to indicate a physiological change.[66] A pathologic cerebrovascular reserve has been defined as a <10% increase in absolute cerebral blood flow as well as a change of <10 ml/100 g/min.[66,67]

Jain and colleagues[68] have suggested that patients who demonstrate good cerebrovascular reserve during BTO and acetazolamide testing using CT perfusion imaging would tolerate carotid sacrifice without neurologic deficits. Patients with asymmetric cerebral blood flow and pathologic response to acetazolamide would need a revascularization procedure after carotid resection. Because the study included only eight patients, however, it may not be valid to extrapolate the results.

Studies involving perfusion MRI in the context of BTO may not adequately predict patients with pathologic cerebrovascular reserve and those who will develop neurologic deficits later.[69] Overall, historic stroke risks ranging from 1.4% to 1.9% annually have been reported in patients after carotid sacrifice.[70,71] Moreover, altered flow dynamics through the Circle of Willis after carotid sacrifice may be contributing to de novo aneurysm formation.[17]

Failure to adequately predict patients who will develop delayed neurologic complications after carotid sacrifice and risk of de novo aneurysm formation have led many surgeons to be generous with the indications for bypass surgery after carotid sacrifice. The risk of carotid sacrifice without revascularization, specifically the reported mortality rate of about 7% and neurologic morbidity rate of up to 17%, should be weighed against the complication rate of bypass surgery, for which a morbidity rate of 3% to 7% and no mortality have been reported.[4,9] The senior author has adopted this latter approach. This is especially true in younger patients, where many authors espouse a universal approach for all patients undergoing a bypass procedure after carotid sacrifice.[3,10,17]

The decision about the nature of bypass to be performed (high flow or low flow, such as superficial artery to middle cerebral artery) is also controversial.[7] There are few prospective studies on which to base a decision. It is the senior author's preference to perform a high- or moderate-flow interpositional (saphenous vein or radial artery) bypass when a carotid artery is to be sacrificed acutely with the resection of a skull base tumor. More recently, we have preferred an M2 or M3 recipient anastomosis site as an alternative to a proximal internal distal recipient carotid anastomosis site to specifically avoid lenticulostriate artery ischemia with cross-clamping of the proximal carotid during the distal anastomosis.[72]

ILLUSTRATIVE CASE

The patient is a 51-year-old woman with a history of multiple surgeries for recurrent atypical skull base meningioma of the right sphenoid wing and anterior clinoid process with invasion of the right cavernous sinus. Adjuvant therapies, including radiosurgery and chemotherapy, failed to provide local control (Figure 31-1). The pathologic analysis indicated an atypical meningioma progression. The patient showed progressive tumor on sequential follow-up and worsening of her cavernous sinus deficit. As a result, a decision was made to undertake a radical en-bloc resection of the cavernous sinus. Preoperative evaluation including BTO showed patent cross-flow through the anterior communicating artery. Because of the patient's young age, however, we decided to perform cerebral revascularization by means of a high-flow submandibular external carotid artery to middle cerebral artery bypass using a saphenous vein graft. The technical aspects of this high-flow bypass have been published previously.[72,73]

Intraoperative bypass patency was assessed by indocyanine green videoangiography. Postoperative CTA, showed patent bypass (Figure 31-2). Postoperatively, the tumor bed was radiated stereotactically, and there has been local tumor control in the 1-year follow-up period.

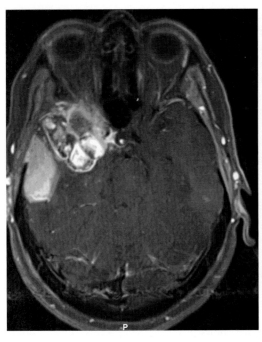
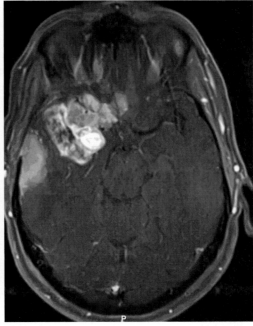

Figure 31-1. Axial MR images demonstrating recurrent tumor of the anterior clinoid with invasion of the right cavernous sinus.

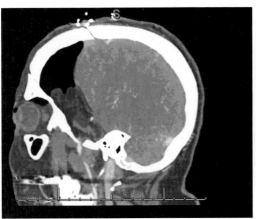
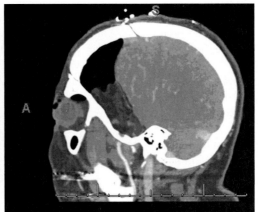

Figure 31-2. Postoperative CT angiography demonstrating good flow through the saphenous vein bypass graft in the submandibular region entering the skull base.

CONCLUSION

Anterior skull base tumors frequently encase or infiltrate the ICA. In cases in which tumors cannot be safely resected off the carotid artery, a surgical decision needs to be made whether a tumor should be resected subtotally or whether the carotid artery should be sacrificed and resected to achieve a gross total resection. The first factor that must be weighed in this decision is the histopathologic character of the involved tumor. Some benign tumors can often be completely resected while preserving the carotid artery. Malignant skull base tumors, however, often invade the carotid artery adventitial wall, and in these cases tumors can only be radically resected by sacrificing the carotid artery. Revascularization after carotid artery resection, however, is controversial. Some authors

therefore advocate a universal approach, in which all patients undergo EC-IC bypass after carotid sacrifice. Others have tried to identify patients with pathologic cerebrovascular reserve after carotid resection by combining a BTO with functional imaging and acetazolamide testing.

REFERENCES

1. Donaghy RM: The history of microsurgery in neurosurgery, *Clin Neurosurg* 26:619–625, 1979.
2. Hayden MG, Lee M, Guzman R, et al: The evolution of cerebral revascularization surgery, *Neurosurg Focus* 26(5):E17, 2009.
3. Vajkoczy P: Revival of extra-intracranial bypass surgery, *Curr Opin Neurol* 22:90–95, 2009.
4. Mendelowitsch A, Taussky P, Rem JA, et al: Clinical outcome of standard extracranial-intracranial bypass surgery in patients with symptomatic atherosclerotic occlusion of the internal carotid artery, *Acta Neurochir (Wien)* 146:95–101, 2004.

5. Evans JJ, Sekhar LN, Rak R, et al: Bypass grafting and revascularization in the management of posterior circulation aneurysms, *Neurosurgery* 55:1036–1049, 2004.

6. Amin-Hanjani S, Chen PR, Chang SW, et al: Long-term follow-up of giant serpentine MCA aneurysm treated with EC-IC bypass and proximal occlusion, *Acta Neurochir (Wien)* 148:227–228, 2006.

7. Liu JK, Couldwell WT: Interpositional carotid artery bypass strategies in the surgical management of aneurysms and tumors of the skull base, *Neurosurg Focus* 14(3):e2, 2003.

8. Fitzpatrick BC, Spetzler RF, Ballard JL, et al: Cervical-to-petrous internal carotid artery bypass procedure. Technical note, *J Neurosurg* 79:138–141, 1993.

9. Lawton MT, Spetzler RF: Internal carotid artery sacrifice for radical resection of skull base tumors, *Skull Base Surg* 6:119–123, 1996.

10. Feiz-Erfan I, Han PP, Spetzler RF, et al: Salvage of advanced squamous cell carcinomas of the head and neck: internal carotid artery sacrifice and extracranial-intracranial revascularization, *Neurosurg Focus* 14(3):e6, 2003.

11. Borges A: Skull base tumours Part II. Central skull base tumours and intrinsic tumours of the bony skull base, *Eur J Radiol* 66:348–362, 2008.

12. Borges A: Skull base tumours part I: imaging technique, anatomy and anterior skull base tumours, *Eur J Radiol* 66:338–347, 2008.

13. Hirsch WL, Sekhar LN, Lanzino G, et al: Meningiomas involving the cavernous sinus: value of imaging for predicting surgical complications, *AJR Am J Roentgenol* 160:1083–1088, 1993.

14. Abdel-Aziz KM, Froelich SC, Dagnew E, et al: Large sphenoid wing meningiomas involving the cavernous sinus: conservative surgical strategies for better functional outcomes, *Neurosurgery* 54:1375–1383, 2004; discussion 1383–4.

15. DeMonte F, Smith HK, al-Mefty O: Outcome of aggressive removal of cavernous sinus meningiomas, *J Neurosurg* 81:245–251, 1994.

16. Al-Mefty O: Clinoidal meningiomas, *J Neurosurg* 73:840–849, 1990.

17. Wolfe SQ, Tummala RP, Morcos JJ: Cerebral revascularization in skull base tumors, *Skull Base* 15:71–82, 2005.

18. Iwai Y, Yamanaka K, Ikeda H: Gamma Knife radiosurgery for skull base meningioma: long-term results of low-dose treatment, *J Neurosurg* 109:804–810, 2008.

19. Igaki H, Maruyama K, Koga T, et al: Stereotactic radiosurgery for skull base meningioma, *Neurol Med Chir (Tokyo)* 49:456–461, 2009.

20. Sen C, Sekhar LN: Direct vein graft reconstruction of the cavernous, petrous, and upper cervical internal carotid artery: lessons learned from 30 cases, *Neurosurgery* 30:732–742, 1992; discussion 742–3.

21. Couldwell WT, Kan P, Liu JK, et al: Decompression of cavernous sinus meningioma for preservation and improvement of cranial nerve function. Technical note, *J Neurosurg* 105:148–152, 2006.

22. Bulsara KR, Patel T, Fukushima T: Cerebral bypass surgery for skull base lesions: technical notes incorporating lessons learned over two decades, *Neurosurg Focus* 24(2):E11, 2008.

23. Walsh MT, Couldwell WT: Management options for cavernous sinus meningiomas, *J Neurooncol* 92:307–316, 2009.

24. Eliason JL, Netterville JL, Guzman RJ, et al: Skull base resection with cervical-to-petrous carotid artery bypass to facilitate repair of distal internal carotid artery lesions, *Cardiovasc Surg* 10:31–37, 2002.

25. Hentschel SJ, Vora Y, Suki D, et al: Malignant tumors of the anterolateral skull base, *Neurosurgery* 66:102–112, 2010; discussion 112.

26. Witz M, Korzets Z, Shnaker A, et al: Delayed carotid artery rupture in advanced cervical cancer—a dilemma in emergency management, *Eur Arch Otorhinolaryngol* 259:37–39, 2002.

27. Kane KK: Carotid artery rupture in advanced head and neck cancer patients, *Oncol Nurs Forum* 10:14–18, 1983.

28. Aslan I, Hafiz G, Baserer N, et al: Management of carotid artery invasion in advanced malignancies of head and neck comparison of techniques, *Ann Otol Rhinol Laryngol* 111:772–777, 2002.

29. Katsuno S, Ishiyama T, Sakaguchi M, et al: Carotid resection and reconstruction for advanced cervical cancer, *Laryngoscope* 107:661–664, 1997.

30. Bourhis J, Fortin A, Dupuis O, et al: Very accelerated radiation therapy: preliminary results in locally unresectable head and neck carcinomas, *Int J Radiat Oncol Biol Phys* 32:747–752, 1995.

31. De Crevoisier R, Bourhis J, Domenge C, et al: Full-dose reirradiation for unresectable head and neck carcinoma: experience at the Gustave-Roussy Institute in a series of 169 patients, *J Clin Oncol* 16:3556–3562, 1998.

32. Taussky D, Dulguerov P, Allal AS: Salvage surgery after radical accelerated radiotherapy with concomitant boost technique for head and neck carcinomas, *Head Neck* 27:182–186, 2005.

33. Huguenin P, Glanzmann C, Taussky D, et al: Hyperfractionated radiotherapy and simultaneous cisplatin for stage-III and -IV carcinomas of the head and neck: long-term results including functional outcome, *Strahlenther Onkol* 174:397–402, 1998.

34. Kennedy JT, Krause CJ, Loevy S: The importance of tumor attachment to the carotid artery, *Arch Otolaryngol* 103:70–73, 1977.

35. Langman AW, Kaplan MJ, Dillon WP, et al: Radiologic assessment of tumor and the carotid artery: correlation of magnetic resonance imaging, ultrasound, and computed tomography with surgical findings, *Head Neck* 11:443–449, 1989.

36. Rothstein SG, Persky MS, Horii S: Evaluation of malignant invasion of the carotid artery by CT scan and ultrasound, *Laryngoscope* 98:321–324, 1988.

37. Snyderman CH, D'Amico F: Outcome of carotid artery resection for neoplastic disease: a meta-analysis, *Am J Otolaryngol* 13:373–380, 1992.

38. Katsuno S, Takemae T, Ishiyama T, et al: Is carotid reconstruction for advanced cancer in the neck a safe procedure? *Otolaryngol Head Neck Surg* 124:222–224, 2001.

39. Hiranandani LH: The management of cervical metastasis in head and neck cancers, *J Laryngol Otol* 85:1097–1126, 1971.

40. Huvos AG, Leaming RH, Moore OS: Clinicopathologic study of the resected carotid artery. Analysis of sixty-four cases, *Am J Surg* 126:570–574, 1973.

41. Razack MS, Sako K: Carotid artery hemorrhage and ligation in head and neck cancer, *J Surg Oncol* 19:189–192, 1982.

42. Porto DP, Adams GL, Foster C: Emergency management of carotid artery rupture, *Am J Otolaryngol* 7:213–217, 1986.

43. Saito K, Fukuta K, Takahashi M, et al: Management of the cavernous sinus in en bloc resections of malignant skull base tumors, *Head Neck* 21:734–742, 1999.

44. al-Mefty O: Management of the cavernous sinus and carotid siphon, *Otolaryngol Clin North Am* 24:1523–1533, 1991.

45. Gil Z, Patel SG, Cantu G, et al: Outcome of craniofacial surgery in children and adolescents with malignant tumors involving the skull base: an international collaborative study, *Head Neck* 31:308–317, 2009.

46. Gil Z, Patel SG, Singh B, et al: Analysis of prognostic factors in 146 patients with anterior skull base sarcoma: an international collaborative study, *Cancer* 110:1033–1041, 2007.

47. Gil Z, Abergel A, Leider-Trejo L, et al: A comprehensive algorithm for anterior skull base reconstruction after oncological resections, *Skull Base* 17:25–37, 2007.

48. Rao G, Suki D, Chakrabarti I, et al: Surgical management of primary and metastatic sarcoma of the mobile spine, *J Neurosurg Spine* 9:120–128, 2008.

49. Konno A, Togawa K, Iizuka K: Analysis of factors affecting complications of carotid ligation, *Ann Otol Rhinol Laryngol* 90(3 Pt 1): 222–226, 1981.

50. Kato K, Tomura N, Takahashi S, et al: Balloon occlusion test of the internal carotid artery: correlation with stump pressure and 99mTc-HMPAO SPECT, *Acta Radiol* 47:1073–1078, 2006.

51. Tomura N, Omachi K, Takahashi S, et al: Comparison of technetium Tc 99m hexamethylpropyleneamine oxime single-photon emission tomograph with stump pressure during the balloon occlusion test of the internal carotid artery, *AJNR Am J Neuroradiol* 26:1937–1942, 2005.

52. Gupta DK, Young WL, Hashimoto T, et al: Characterization of the cerebral blood flow response to balloon deflation after temporary internal carotid artery test occlusion, *J Neurosurg Anesthesiol* 14:123–129, 2002.

53. Masamoto K, Tanishita K: Oxygen transport in brain tissue, *J Biomech Eng* 131:074002, 2009.

54. Derdeyn CP, Videen TO, Yundt KD, et al: Variability of cerebral blood volume and oxygen extraction: stages of cerebral haemodynamic impairment revisited, *Brain* 125(Part 3):595–607, 2002.

55. Vagal AS, Leach JL, Fernandez-Ulloa M, et al: The acetazolamide challenge: techniques and applications in the evaluation of chronic cerebral ischemia, *AJNR Am J Neuroradiol* 30:876–884, 2009.

56. Kleiser B, Widder B, Hackspacher J, et al: Comparison of Doppler CO2 test, patterns of infarction in CCT, and clinical symptoms in carotid artery occlusions, *Neurosurg Rev* 14:267–269, 1991.

57. Baron JC, Bousser MG, Rey A, et al: Reversal of focal "misery-perfusion syndrome" by extra-intracranial arterial bypass in hemodynamic cerebral ischemia. A case study with 15O positron emission tomography, *Stroke* 12:454–459, 1981.

58. Okamoto Y, Inugami A, Matsuzaki Z, et al: Carotid artery resection for head and neck cancer, *Surgery* 120:54–59, 1996.

59. Lorberboym M, Pandit N, Machac J, et al: Brain perfusion imaging during preoperative temporary balloon occlusion of the internal carotid artery, *J Nucl Med* 37:415–419, 1996.

60. Linskey ME, Jungreis CA, Yonas H, et al: Stroke risk after abrupt internal carotid artery sacrifice: accuracy of preoperative assessment with balloon test occlusion and stable xenon-enhanced CT, *AJNR Am J Neuroradiol* 15:829–843, 1994.

61. Higashida RT, Halbach VV, Dowd C, et al: Endovascular detachable balloon embolization therapy of cavernous carotid artery aneurysms: results in 87 cases, *J Neurosurg* 72:857–863, 1990.

62. Vazquez Anon V, Aymard A, Gobin YP, et al: Balloon occlusion of the internal carotid artery in 40 cases of giant intracavernous aneurysm: technical aspects, cerebral monitoring, and results, *Neuroradiology* 34:245–251, 1992.

63. Morioka T, Matsushima T, Fujii K, et al: Balloon test occlusion of the internal carotid artery with monitoring of compressed spectral arrays (CSAs) of electroencephalogram, *Acta Neurochir (Wien)* 101(1–2):29–34, 1989.

64. Segal DH, Sen C, Bederson JB, et al: Predictive value of balloon test occlusion of the internal carotid artery, *Skull Base Surg* 5:97–107, 1995.

65. Adams GL, Madison M, Remley K, et al: Preoperative permanent balloon occlusion of internal carotid artery in patients with advanced head and neck squamous cell carcinoma, *Laryngoscope* 109:460–466, 1999.

66. Yonas H, Darby JM, Marks EC, et al: CBF measured by Xe-CT: approach to analysis and normal values, *J Cereb Blood Flow Metab* 11:716–725, 1991.

67. Piepgras A, Schmiedek P, Leinsinger G, et al: A simple test to assess cerebrovascular reserve capacity using transcranial Doppler sonography and acetazolamide, *Stroke* 21:1306–1311, 1990.

68. Jain R, Hoeffner EG, Deveikis JP, et al: Carotid perfusion CT with balloon occlusion and acetazolamide challenge test: feasibility, *Radiology* 231:906–913, 2004.

69. Michel E, Liu H, Remley KB, et al: Perfusion MR neuroimaging in patients undergoing balloon test occlusion of the internal carotid artery, *AJNR Am J Neuroradiol* 22:1590–1596, 2001.

70. Roski RA, Spetzler RF, Nulsen FE: Late complications of carotid ligation in the treatment of intracranial aneurysms, *J Neurosurg* 54:583–587, 1981.

71. Voris HC: Complications of ligation of the internal carotid artery, *J Neurosurg* 8:119–131, 1951.

72. Couldwell WT, Liu JK, Amini A, et al: Submandibular-infratemporal interpositional carotid artery bypass for cranial base tumors and giant aneurysms, *Neurosurgery* 59(4 Suppl 2):ONS353–ONS359, 2006; discussion ONS359–ONS360.

73. Couldwell WT, Zuback J, Onios E, et al: Giant petrous carotid aneurysm treated by submandibular carotid-saphenous vein bypass. Case report, *J Neurosurg* 94:806–810, 2001.

INTRACRANIAL VENOUS REVASCULARIZATION

32

MARC SINDOU; JORGE ALVERNIA

INTRODUCTION

Ignoring the cerebral venous system (CVS) during surgery would entail disastrous consequences; therefore, thorough knowledge of venous anatomy and physiology is of prime importance in intracranial neurosurgery.[1–8]

There is no doubt that many harmful events after intracranial surgery are related to iatrogenic venous damages. They manifest as locally developed edema, regional or diffuse brain swelling—some being fatal because of uncontrollable intracranial hypertension—or devastating hemorrhagic infarcts that are erroneously attributed to so-called defaults in hemostasis.

Tumors—especially meningiomas—that invade major dural sinuses (superior sagittal sinus, torcular, transverse sinus) confront the surgeon with a dilemma: leave the fragment invading the sinus and experience a relatively high risk of recurrence, or attempt total removal with or without venous reconstruction and expose the patient to a potentially greater operative danger. Radical removal implies preservation or repair of the venous circulation.

Given that 20% of the patients presenting with intracranial hypertension due to venous thrombosis develop threatening manifestations, restoration of the venous flow may contribute to the cure of these diseases.

Before surgery a detailed preoperative study, including venous angio-MR, and, if necessary, DSA with late venous phases, helps to determine optimal surgical strategy. A sustained effort to respect the venous system, especially the so-called "dangerous veins," is an obligation for the surgeon. Reconstruction or restoration of the venous circulation, especially the major dural sinuses, may be of importance in particular situations.

THE "DANGEROUS" VENOUS STRUCTURES

The Dural Venous Sinuses

The superior sagittal sinus (SSS), a major dural sinus, has three parts. The anterior third receives the prefrontal afferent veins (Figure 32–1). It is generally admitted that its sacrifice is well tolerated. Actually, severe mental disorders, personality changes, or loss of recent memory with a general slowing of thought processes and activity, or even akinetic mutism, may occur if sacrificed. The mid-third receives the voluminous cortical veins of the central group. Interruption of this portion entails high risks of (bilateral) hemiplegia and akinesia. The posterior third, as well as the torcular Herophili, which receives the straight sinus, drains a considerable amount of blood. Interruption would inevitably provoke potentially fatal intracranial hypertension.

The lateral sinuses (LS) ensure symmetric drainage in only 20% of the cases. In extreme cases, one LS (most often the right one) may drain the SSS in totality and the other the straight sinus.

The transverse sinus (TS) may be atretic on one side, the remaining sigmoid sinus (SS) draining the inferior cerebral veins (i.e., the Labbé system). The SS drains the posterior fossa; it receives the superior and the inferior petrosal sinuses. When the sigmoid segment of the LS is atretic, the TS with its affluents drains toward the opposite side.

All of these anatomical configurations have surgical implications and must be taken into account before considering interrupting sinuses.[9–11]

The Deep Veins of the Brain

The deep veins of the brain drain toward the venous confluent of Galen (Figure 32–2). The term *venous confluent* is appropriate since, in addition to the two internal cerebral veins, the Galenic system receives the two basilar veins of Rosenthal, and also veins from the corpus callosum, the cerebellum (mainly the vermian precentral vein), and the occipital cortex.

A good knowledge of deep veins is important for surgery in the lateral ventricles, third ventricle, and pineal region. There is general agreement that the sacrifice of the vein of Galen or of one of its main tributaries should be considered high risk, although animal experiments and a few reported clinical observations have shown otherwise.

Regarding the precentral vermian vein, it is generally accepted, and we agree, that its sacrifice to approach the pineal region is without danger.[1–3]

355

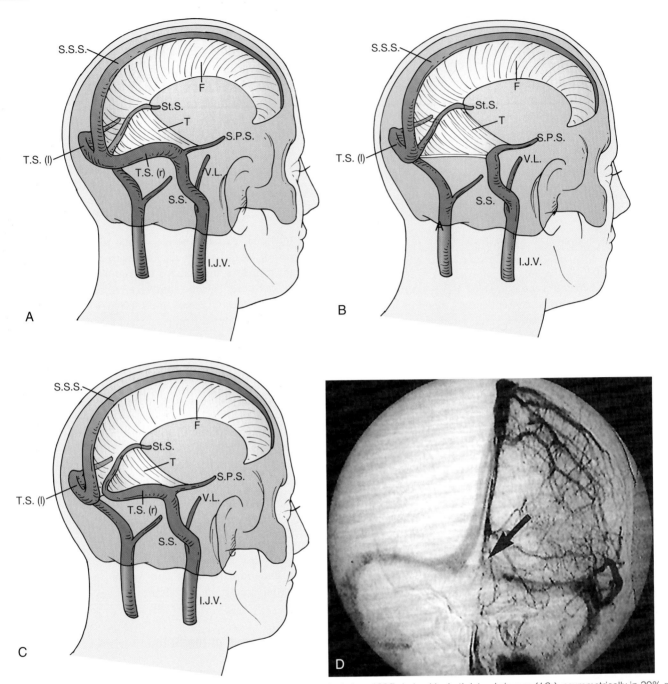

Figure 32–1. Anatomical variations of major venous sinuses. **A,** Superior sagittal sinus (*SSS*) drained by both lateral sinuses (*LS*s), asymmetrically in 20% of cases or asymmetrically in 55%. When asymmetrical ("unbalanced system"), the predominant LS draining is usually the right one. **B,** SSS and straight sinus (*StS*) draining through one LS, here the left because the right transverse sinus (*TS*) is absent. Ligation or injury of the left LS would entail the risk of interrupting SSS drainage of the right sigmoid sinus (*SS*), the risk of interrupting drainage of the superior petrosal sinus (*SPS*) and the vein of Labbé (*VL*). **C,** In 25% of cases, one TS entirely drains the SSS, and the other entirely drains the StS. In cases of "split system," sacrifice of either LS would be extremely dangerous. **D,** Angiogram (*DSA*), AP view, showing a split system, with SSS draining to the right LS, and StS to the left (*arrow*); this configuration is the most common. F, falx; IJV, internal jugular vein; T, tentorium.

The Superficial Veins

Any of the superficial veins of a certain caliber presumably have a functional role. The superficial veins belong to three "systems": the midline afferents to the SSS, the inferior cerebral afferents to the TS, and the superficial sylvian afferents to the cavernous sinus (Figure 32–3). These three systems are strongly interconnected, but there is considerable variability among patients. The main anastomotic veins are Trolard to the SSS, Labbé to the TS, and great superficial sylvian, all of them bearing important surgical implications.

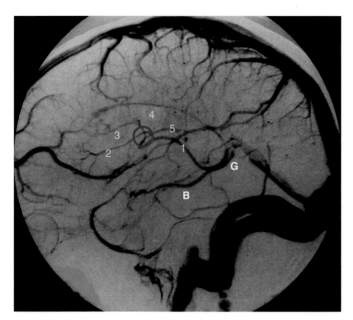

Figure 32–2. Deep cerebral veins and landmarks of the interventricular venous confluent (IVC). DSA by carotid injection, venous phase, lateral view. The interventricular venous confluent (circle) is formed by confluence of the septal vein (2), caudate vein (3, 4), and thalamo-striate vein (5). Confluence gives rise to the internal cerebral vein (1). On the lateral view, the confluent has an almost constant situation and corresponds to the interventricular foramen of Monro. This point may contribute a useful anatomical imaging reference. Confluence of internal cerebral veins and basilar veins (B) gives the Galen vein (G).

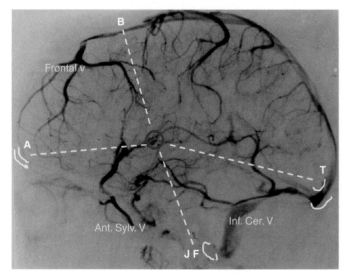

Figure 32–3. Superficial veins involved in (supratentorial) skull base approaches. Three groups of veins can be distinguished—middle afferent frontal, inferior cerebral (i.e., the Labbé system), and anterior sylvian (ASV). These three groups can be delimited by three "triangles": the triangle that corresponds to the frontal veins is delineated by the three following landmarks—interventricular venous confluent (IVC), bregma (B), and anterior limit of anterior cranial fossa (A); the triangle corresponding to the inferior group is delineated by the IVC, torcular (T), and jugular foramen (JF); and the triangle corresponding to the anterior sylvian group is delineated by IVC and A and JF landmarks. Skull base approaches must be designed so that prominent venous drainage(s) is respected.

- Midline afferent veins are met during interhemispheric approaches. Sacrifice of the midline central group is risky.[1,2,12]
- Inferior cerebral veins that channel into the basal sinuses are met in the skull base approaches. Necessary respect of the Labbé vein, especially in the dominant hemisphere, is mandatory to avoid posterior hemispheric infarction.[1,2,4]
- The superficial sylvian vein is formed by anastomosis of the temporosylvian veins. This sylvian system is connected with the midline veins upward, and the juxtabasal temporal veins downward. It enters predominantly the cavernous sinus, either directly or through the sphenoparietal sinus. Sacrificing the superficial sylvian vein is risky when it is of large caliber and poorly anastomosed.[1,2,4]

Intracranial approaches, especially skull base ones, must be prepared taking into account the organization of the superficial venous system (see Figure 32–3).[7,13,14]

Veins of the Posterior Fossa

Sacrifice would expose the cerebellum to swelling or infarction. The conventional statement that the superior petrosal vein, especially when voluminous, can be interrupted without danger needs to be reconsidered. Our experience is that this venous complex should be respected.[1]

AVOIDANCE OF VENOUS OCCLUSIONS DURING SURGERY

The role played by venous occlusions during surgery in the occurrence of postoperative hemorrhagic infarcts is undeniable.[1-3,7] Retraction of the brain provokes local congestion by compressing the cortical venous network, reduction in venous flow by stretching the bridging veins, and thrombosis of veins if compression of the retractor is prolonged.[15] Excessive brain retraction can be avoided by specially designed approaches and limited opening of the dura, obeying two principles, including the minimally invasive opening and bone removal associated with craniotomy at the base of the skull. Keyhole approaches or limited opening of the dura prevent excessive retraction and consequently avulsing veins.

A bridge vein acting as a limitation may occur. To be preserved, the vein has to be dissected free from the arachnoid and cortex at a length of 10 to 20 mm.[16] When an important vein ruptures, its reconstruction may be considered either by resuturing or by using the silicone tubing technique.[17]

Wounds made in a vein wall are common. Rather than coagulating the vein, hemostasis can be attempted by simply wrapping the wall with a small piece of Surgicel (Johnson and Johnson Medical, Viroflay, France). If this is insufficient, a very localized microcoagulation with a sharp bipolar forceps or by placing a single suture with a 10-0 nylon thread is recommended. In cases with a large defect, a patching repair can be performed.[18,19] In all cases, whatever the technique used, hemostasis quality has to be checked by jugular compression at the neck.

TUMORS INVADING THE MAJOR DURAL SINUSES

The study of long-term results in our series of 100 consecutive patients affected by meningiomas involving a major dural sinus, and in whom we *attempted radical removal and venous repair*,[20] led us to the following conclusions. The low recurrence rate of 4% in our series, followed over a 3- to 23-year period (mean

8 years), supports resecting not only the tumor portion outside the sinus, but also the fragment invading the sinus. When radical removal is attempted, we consider venous reconstruction mandatory when the sinus is incompletely occluded, and potentially useful even in cases with complete occlusion. The goal is to restore the flow that might be compromised by impairment of the compensatory collateral channels (Figure 32–4). The traditional belief that radical removal of meningiomas with a totally occluded sinus is not dangerous must be reconsidered.[21-24] In our series, the three patients who died (all three from brain swelling) had a meningioma that totally occluded the sinus and was wholly removed without any restoration of the sinus circulation.[20]

This is not surprising, as surgical access basically involves the destruction of some to all of the collateral pathways that naturally developed to compensate the sinus occlusion.

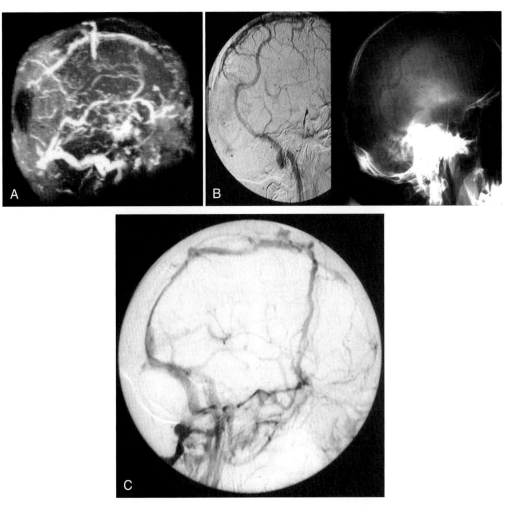

Figure 32–4. Collateral circulation in superior sagittal sinus (SSS) occlusion. **A,** Parasagittal meningioma totally occluding posterior third of SSS (Type VI; venous MR, lateral view). There is a complete stop at posterior third of the SSS. Drainage of SSS is mainly extracranial through transosseous emissary channels. If compromised by surgical approach, such collaterals could lead to acute brain swelling. **B,** Parasagittal meningioma totally occluding posterior third of SSS (Type VI). There is a major intraosseous (i.e., diploic) channel from SSS to sigmoid sinus. DSA angiography, venous phase, lateral view, showing SSS occlusion and venous channel (*left*). Plain X-ray prior to surgery may help to identify bony channel so that bone flap can be designed respecting main collateral pathway(s) (*right*). **C,** Parasagittal meningioma totally occluding mid-third of SSS (Type VI).

Therefore, restoring the venous circulation at end of surgery may reduce brain swelling. Furthermore, patching or bypassing did not increase the morbidity rate in our series.[20]

To guide in surgical decision making, we introduced a *meningioma classification* comprised of six types according to degree of sinus invasion[1,22] (Figure 32–5). This simplified classification was developed after the ones introduced by Merrem,[25] Krause,[26] and Bonnal and Brotchi.[27]

Our classification follows: Type 1, meningioma is simply attached to the outer surface of the sinus wall; Type II, lateral recess is invaded; Type III, ipsilateral wall is invaded; Type IV, both ipsilateral wall and roof are invaded; Type V, sinus is totally occluded, but contralateral wall is free of invasion; and Type VI, sinus is totally invaded with no walls free of invasion.

Based on this classification, surgery should be attempted in the following ways:

Type I: Excision of the outer layer, leaving a clean inner layer.

Type II: Removal of the intraluminal fragment through the recess, and then repair of the defect by resuturing the recess edges or by closing it with a (narrow) patch.

Type III: Resection of the invaded wall and repair with patch (preferably fascia temporalis).

Type IV: Resection of the invaded wall and roof, and reconstruction with patch.

Type V: This type can be formally differentiated from Type VI only by direct surgical exploration of the sinus lumen. Because the opposite wall to the tumor side is free of tumor, it is possible to reconstruct the resected invaded walls with patch.

Type VI: Removal of the entire involved portion of the sinus and restoration of the venous flow with a venous bypass. The site of bypass is on the SSS for meningiomas involving the SSS, between the SSS and the (external) jugular vein for meningiomas totally occluding the posterior third and/or the torcular, and between the TS and the external jugular vein for meningiomas involving the TS.

Surgery on the intracranial venous system is greatly facilitated by obeying the following technical aspects. The semi-sitting (lounging) position allows a good venous return, with a low risk of air embolism (1% in our series). Skin flap and craniotomy should extend across the midline to permit visualization of both sides of the sinus, and some 3 cm outside the margins of the occluded sinus. Approach should consider cutaneous, pericranial, and/or diploic, as well as dural venous pathways, which might be compromised during the approach. These collateral pathways can be identified on preoperative imaging (venous angio-MR and DSA with venous phases) (see Figure 32–4). Then the dura is incised in a circumferential manner around the margin of the tumor, followed by an incision along the border of the corresponding portion of the sinus. Under the microscope, attachment of the meningioma to the wall of the sinus and to the neighboring falx is deinserted by using the bipolar coagulation forceps. Then, after dural devascularization, an "intracapsular" debulking is carried out so that the meningioma can be dissected under the microscope from the underlying cortex.

Because of frequent discrepancies between images and anatomical lesions, the sinus should be explored through a short incision to disclose any intrasinusal fragment. Control of the venous bleeding from the lumen of the sinus, can be easily obtained by plugging/packing small pledgets of Surgicel (Figure 32–6). Balloons or shunts with inflatable balloons should not be used because they do not pass easily through the sinus septa and may disrupt the sinus endothelium. Vascular clamps or aneurysm clips should be avoided because they may injure the sinus walls and afferent veins.

For *patching*, locally harvested dura mater or fascia temporalis (better than pericranium) is rigid enough to enable blood to flow inside and to use as patches. Technical steps are described in Figures 32–7 and 32–8. Also, in appropriate selective cases plasty can be performed by reflexing flap from falx.[1,28]

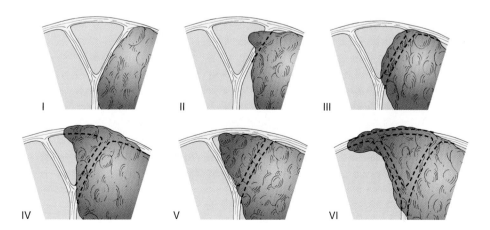

Figure 32–5. Classification of meningiomas involving the major dural sinuses. This personal classification was conceived in six types, according to degree of sinus invasion, for parasagittal meningiomas. It may also be applied to meningiomas involving the torcular and the lateral sinuses.

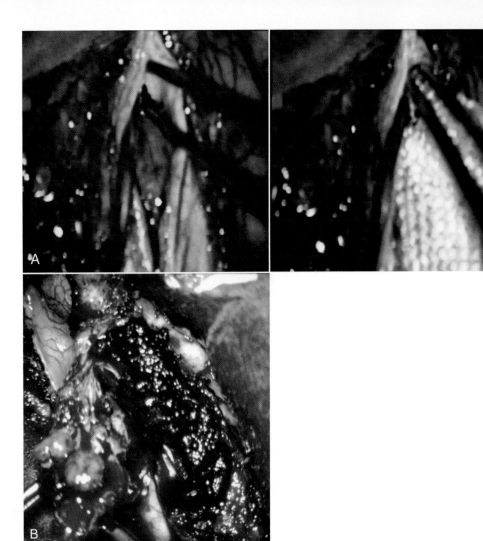

Figure 32–6. Blood control of sinus. **A,** Midline meningioma totally occluding the sinus (Type VI). After opening the roof of the sinus, the anterior margin of the intrasinusal fragment is seen (*left*). To achieve blood control proximally to the tumor, a piece of Surgicel is plugged into the sinus lumen (*right*). **B,** Left meningioma invading the ipsilateral wall of the sinus and partially occluding its lumen (Type III). For achieving resection of the invaded wall (visible on the image), the lumen is packed with Surgicel to ensure blood control. Then the defect will be repaired by patching with a piece of fascia temporalis (not shown).

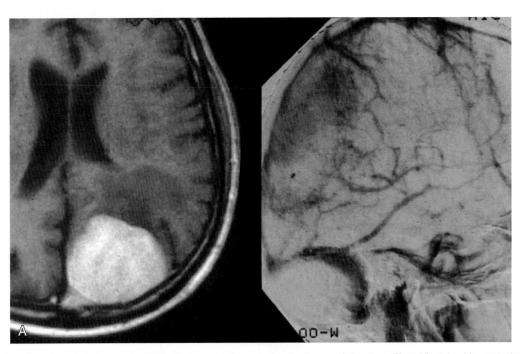

Figure 32–7. Patching technique in SSS parasagittal meningioma totally occluding the lumen of the sinus (Type V), right side, posterior third. **A,** MRI-T1 sequence with gadolinium (*left*) and preoperative angiogram (DSA), venous phase, lateral view (*right*), showing total interruption of circulation in posterior third.

(*Continued*)

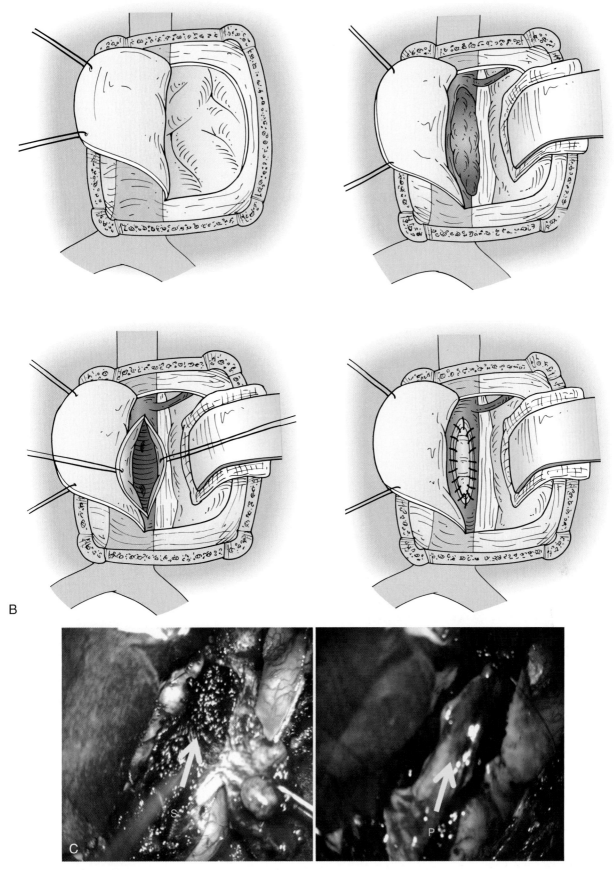

Figure 32–7.—cont'd B, Surgical steps (schematic drawings). *Upper left*: meningioma exposed. *Upper right*: tumor outside of sinus removed, ipsilateral wall invaded. *Lower left*: intraluminal fragment removed; inner aspect of the contralateral wall of the sinus visible, wall intact, ostia of two afferent veins entering the sinus also visible. Control of blood will be achieved by packing of Surgicel (not shown). *Lower right*: reconstruction of resected (right) wall by means of patch made of fascia temporalis sutured with two hemirunning sutures. **C,** Operative views showing resection of invaded wall, blood control being achieved with packed Surgicel (*left*), and patching with fascia temporalis (*right*).

(*Continued*)

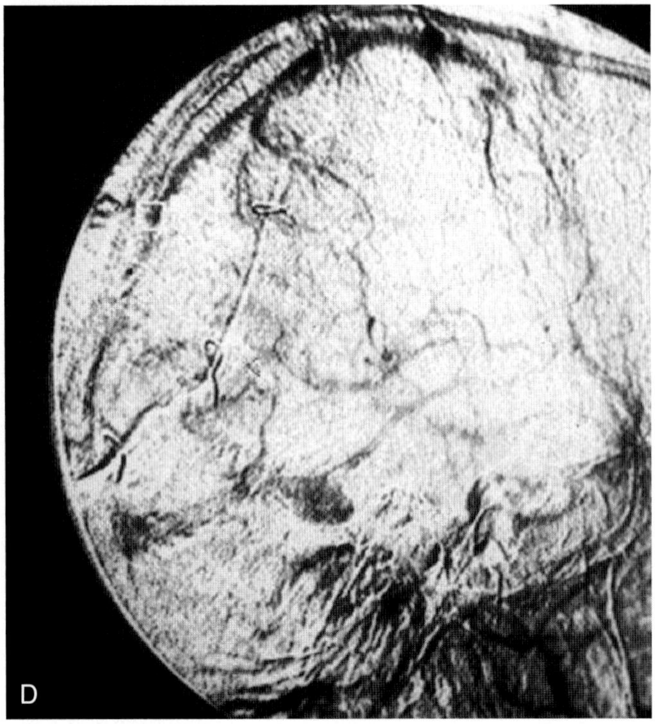

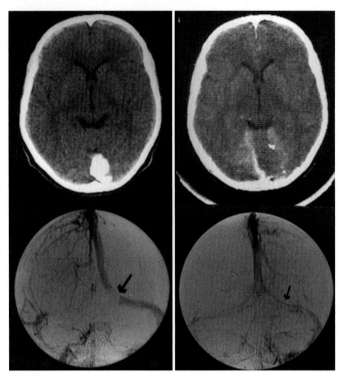

Figure 32–7.—cont'd D, Control angiogram (DSA) at 3 weeks after surgery, which demonstrates patency of posterior third.

Figure 32–8. Torcular meningioma (Type IV); resection and patching. *Left:* Preoperative axial CT-scan and AP view of venous phase of DSA show the meningioma occluding, totally the right transverse sinus and subtotally the left one. Surgery (not shown) was performed in sitting position, and the tumor outside the venous confluence was removed; the invaded (inferior and left lateral) walls of the venous confluence were resected. Venous control was achieved by packing Surgicel into the lumens. Tumor fragments inside the sinus were extracted. The resected wall defect was reconstructed with a patch harvested from healthy neighboring dura. *Right:* Postoperative axial CT-scan and AP view of venous phase of DSA 2 weeks after surgery, demonstrate tumor removal and patency of both the right and the left (*arrow*) transverse sinuses.

In cases with totally invaded sinus, *bypassing* procedures can be indicated to restore venous flow. Bypasses may be performed either immediately after removal of the occluded portion, using end-to-end anastomoses (Figure 32–9), or prior to its removal with end-to-side anastomoses (Figure 32–10). The graft should be an autologous vein: when a long graft (>10 cm) is required, the median saphenous (see Figure 32–10), or the external jugular vein when only a short graft is necessary (see Figure 32–9). GORE-TEX prosthesis should be avoided; in our six cases in whom it was used, the bypass thrombosed within the first week. Five of the thromboses were asymptomatic, but one was accompanied with an acute, but fortunately reversible, comatose state. Technical details for bypassing are provided in Figures 32–9 and 32–11. Suturing on the sinus is performed using two hemirunning sutures, with Prolene 8-0 thread (Laboratoire Ethnor, Neuilly-sur-Seine, France).

Reconstruction or reimplantation of veins may be attempted, if veins are important, such as the Labbé veins (Figure 32–12)[29] or the afferent veins of the central group of the SSS (Figure 32–13).[30–32]

To avoid clotting, we consider *postoperative anticoagulation mandatory* for at least 3 months, until re-endothelization occurs. This strategy did not increase hemorrhagic complications in our series.[20] Heparinotherapy is administered as soon as the morning after surgery and for the following 3 weeks, at dosages to double the coagulation time. Coumadin is then administered over the next 2 or 3 months until the (hypothetical) end of sinus, patch, graft, or endothelization.

Long-term patency of venous repair remains an unsolved problem (Table 32–1). The fact that all of the patients who had a graft that thrombosed (with the exception of one with a GORE-TEX tube) remained asymptomatic does not mean that venous reconstruction was useless. One can postulate that venous repair provides time for compensatory venous pathways to develop. Importantly, the three patients who died of brain swelling all had meningiomas with Type VI sinus invasion that had been totally resected without venous flow restoration.

In brief, achieving radical removal requires temporarily interrupting the sinus circulation; this process can be easily performed with pledgets of Surgicel. Resected walls should be repaired with patching; a graft harvest from adjacent dura, fascia-lata, or preferably fascia temporalis, appears adequate. For performing bypasses, only autologous grafts should be utilized: the external jugular vein for short grafts and the median saphenous vein for longer ones. According to our study patching

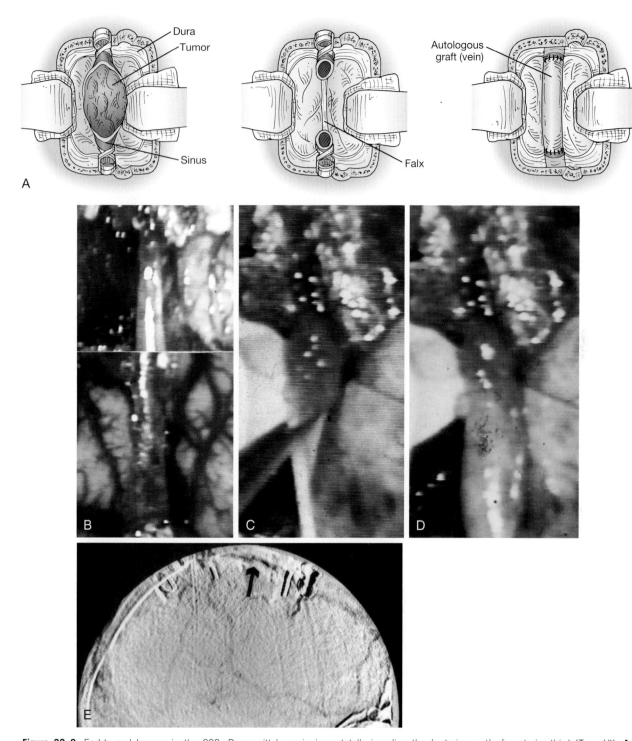

Figure 32–9. End-to-end bypass in the SSS. Parasagittal meningioma totally invading the (anterior part) of posterior third (Type VI). **A,** Schematic drawings of surgical steps. At left, tumor is exposed. At center, meningioma together with the invaded portion of the sinus is removed. At right, circulation is restored with a venous autologous graft from external jugular vein, sutured using end-to-end anastomoses. **B,** Operative views (taken from videotape) after completion of the bypass. **C** and **D,** Positive patency test (using forceps). **E,** Postoperative angiogram (DSA) at 2 weeks postop; venous phase, lateral view, showing patent bypass (*arrow*).

or bypassing to restore venous flow does not increase morbidity rate. Postoperative anticoagulation early and for at least 3 months is to us mandatory, until re-endothelization occurs.

In conclusion, we do not pretend that all tumors invading the major dural sinuses must be radically resected and the sinus systematically repaired. The literature discusses numerous cons[33–35] and pros.[36–43] Ultimately, the decision must be made after weighing benefits and risks. Before deciding to perform a radical removal with restoration of venous circulation, especially for those located in the mid-third portion of the sinus, alternatives

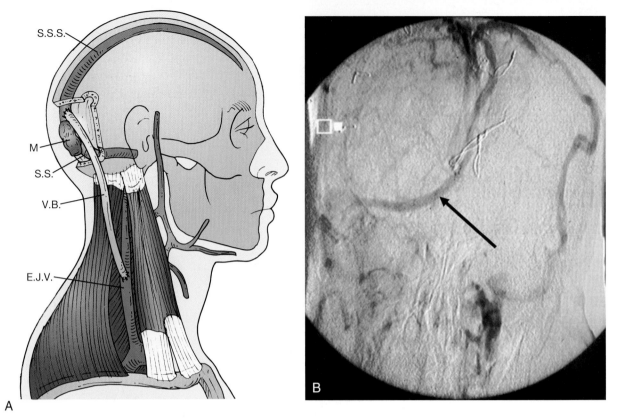

Figure 32–10. Torcular meningioma totally occluding the venous confluence (Type VI); long sino-jugular bypass. Clinical presentation was severe intracranial hypertension syndrome with headaches, papilledema, and dementia. **A,** The venous hypertension was treated by performing an autologous bypass from the posterior third of SSS to the external jugular vein, using as an autologous graft the median saphenous vein (20-cm length). **B,** Bypass was patent as shown on DSA angiography at 2-week follow-up (*arrow*). Patient experienced recovery.

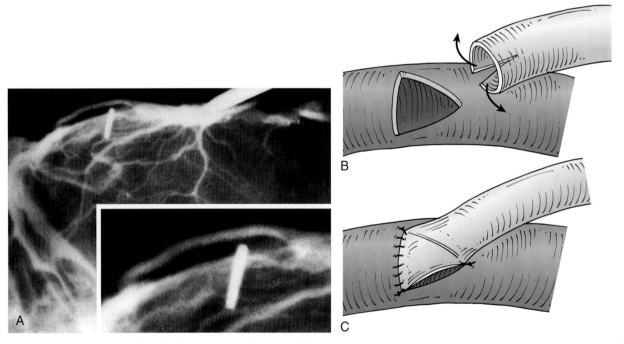

Figure 32–11. Bypass on the SSS sinus (with end-to-side anastomoses); operative technique. **A,** The procedure was introduced in humans in 1980,[44] after experimental work in dogs in 1976.[46] **B,** After exposure of the superficial wall (roof) of the sinus at the portion to be grafted, a sinusotomy is performed by removing an equilateral triangle of wall. Sinus hemostasis is achieved by plugging a small pledget of Surgicel into its lumen. The extremity of the graft is enlarged by a longitudinal cut. **C,** End-to-side anastomosis is performed as follows: triangulation with three stitches, and then running suture or interrupted stitches with an 8-0 thread on each of the three sides of the sinusotomy. Removal of the pledget of Surgicel before completing the last suture(s) must not be forgotten.

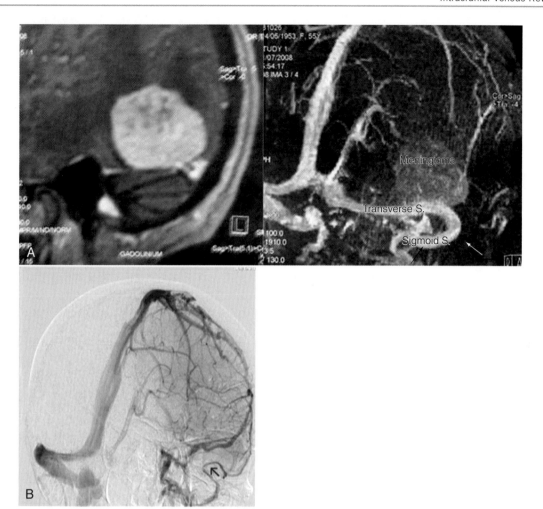

Figure 32–12. Reconstruction of vein of Labbé in temporo-occipital meningioma invading transverse sinus. **A,** Preoperative MRI (*left*) and MR venography (*right*) show tumor invasion of the left TS, and total occlusion of the vein of Labbé (VL) (*arrow*). *Technique and postoperative course (not shown):* After removal of the tumor, except the piece attached to TS and VL, the lumens of both the TS and the VL were explored. The tumor tissue inside was removed along with the invaded venous walls, that is, the superior wall of TS and lateral wall of VL. Control of venous bleeding was achieved by plugging small pledgets of Surgicel inside the lumens. Then venous reconstruction of both TS and VL was performed using one piece of patient's own healthy dura, with two hemirunning sutures (Prolene 8-0). Postoperative course was uneventful. Postoperatively 15,000 units/24 h continuous IV heparin was administered for 4 days; then 2 × 7500 UI/3 ml low-molecular-weight heparin was given subcutaneously for 8 days. Then oral antivitamin K agent was prescribed for use at home for 3 months. Control MRI at 3 months after discharge demonstrated total removal without any remnant. **B,** Venous phase of postoperative DSA shows blood flow in the reconstructed vein of Labbé draining into the distal portion of the left transverse and the sigmoid sinuses (*arrow*).

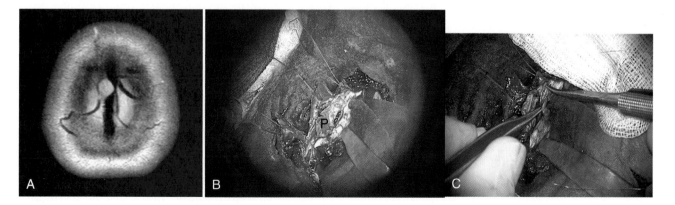

Figure 32–13. Reimplantation of afferent central veins to the superior sagittal sinus. **A,** Right-sided, mid-third, parasagittal meningioma (Type III) on MRI. **B,** After removal of the meningioma, resection of the invaded wall and extraction of the intrasinusal fragment. The dural defect is repaired using a patch harvested from fascia temporalis (P). Note hemostasis of the sinus with Surgicel packing. **C,** Suture of the patch using two hemirunning sutures.

(Continued)

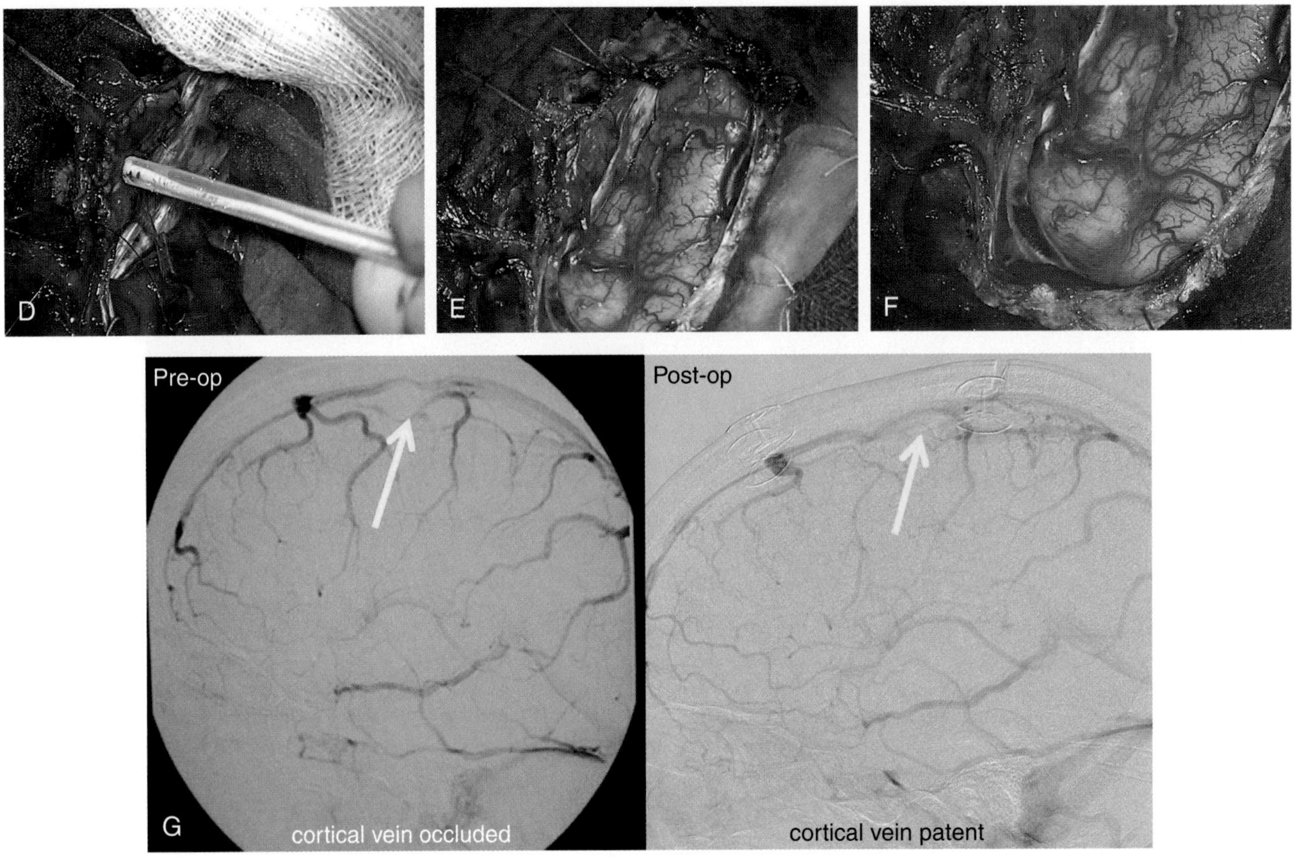

Figure 32–13.—cont'd D, Control of patency of the patched sinus with Doppler probe. Note the two reimplanted afferent central veins clamped. **E,** General view of the sinus repaired with reimplantation of the afferent veins, after declamping the veins. **F,** Patent aspect of the two reimplanted afferent veins at higher magnification. **G,** Pre- (*left*) and postoperative (*right*) DSA showing afferent veins patent.

Table 32–1. PATENCY OF VENOUS RECONSTRUCTIONS IN OUR SERIES.

Angiographic Control Surgical Modality	Total	Angiography	Patent Yes	No
Resection of intraluminal fragment within lateral recess plus resuture	8	8	8	0
Resection of invaded wall plus patch (fascia)	19	15	13	2
Resection of invaded portion plus bypass with saphenous vein	11	10	7	3
Resection of invaded portion plus bypass with external jugular vein	1	1	1	0
Resection of invaded portion plus bypass with GORE-TEX®	6	6	0	6
Total	46	40	29	11

should be discussed. For large tumors, the alternative is primary surgery to shave the tumor from the sinus and, if the tumor grows, adjuvant radiosurgery or radiotherapy. For very small meningiomas, radiosurgery can be the first option, with secondary surgery if tumor growth is not controlled.

SURGICAL RESTORATION OF VENOUS FLOW FOR INTRACRANIAL HYPERTENSION FROM VENOUS OCCLUSION

Chronic intracranial hypertension can be due to venous occlusion of the posterior third of the SSS, torcular, predominant LS, or internal jugular vein. The most frequent causes of "chronic" occlusion of dural sinuses follow: (1) fibrosis after infectious thrombophlebitis and/or cruoric thromboses[44] (Figure 32–14); (2) damage or ligation after trauma or surgery; (3) tumor totally occluding the posterior third of the SSS[1,20] (see Figure 32–10); and (4) dural arteriovenous fistulas accompanying (lateral) sinus thrombosis (Figure 32–15).[1,45]

Intracranial hypertension cannot always be controlled efficiently with antiedema therapy. Lumboperitoneal CSF shunting, which appears to be a simpler technique, is not without pitfalls and complications. In the order of 20% of cases, progressive severe loss of vision and/or encephalopathy develops. Therefore, venous revascularization by sino-jugular bypass—implanted proximally to the occlusion and directed to the jugular venous system (external or internal jugular vein)—can be the solution.[44] The good long-term clinical

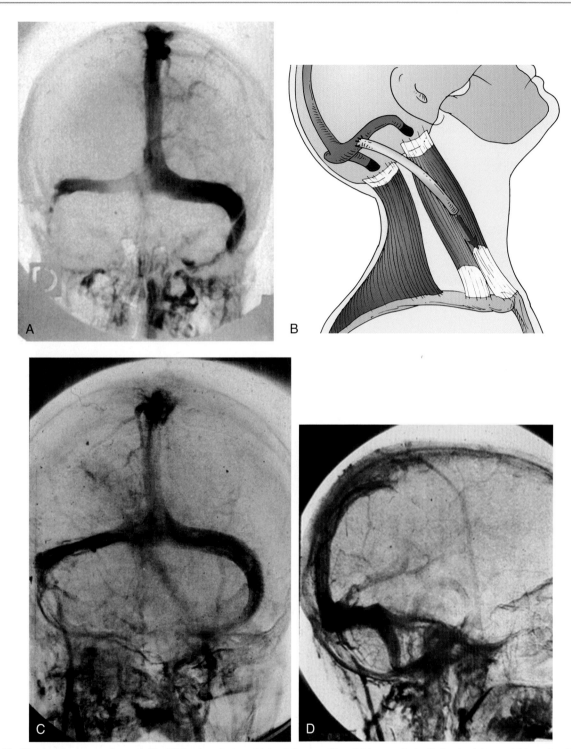

Figure 32–14. Sino-jugular bypass for postotitic bilateral occlusion of lateral sinuses. The child presented with benign intracranial hypertension syndrome characterized by severe evolving loss of vision due to papilledema. **A,** Preoperative angiography, venous phase, AP view, showing bilateral sigmoid sinus thrombosis. **B,** Schematic drawing of the transverse-jugular bypass between right transverse sinus (end-to-side anastomosis) and right external jugular vein (end-to-end anastomosis). **C** and **D,** Postoperative angiography, venous phase, AP view and lateral view, showing patency of bypass with median saphenous graft from transverse sinus to external jugular vein, right side.

results observed in our series of five cases of sino-jugular bypasses argue in favor of this procedure as a logical treatment in these circumstances.

The original surgical technique was described in detail in 1980[44] and briefly more recently in 2000.[1] This graft, which must generally be a long one, has to be harvested from the median saphenous vein.

In a study of 11 patients (five cases from our institution and six from the literature), the patency rate was 82%; there was no mortality or morbidity. The receiver vein was the

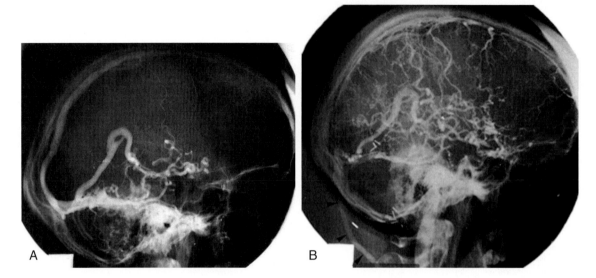

Figure 32–15. Sino-jugular bypass for intracranial hypertension due to bilateral thrombosis of transverse sinuses, with right dural arteriovenous fistula (AVF). **A,** Preoperative angiogram (lateral view) showing occlusion of the right transverse sinus. The dural AVF is clearly visible with retrograde filling of the sagittal and straight sinuses. **B,** Postoperative angiogram (lateral view) showing complete surgical removal of AVF and patent sino-jugular bypass (*arrowhead*).

internal jugular vein in five cases (four patent), and the external jugular vein or a branch in six cases (five patent). These overall results demonstrate the technical feasibility of restoring venous outflow with sino-jugular bypasses achieved with autologous venous grafts. Early and prolonged postoperative anticoagulant therapy is an important adjunct for patency. Absence of neurological complications may be explained by the fact that the bypass is entirely extradural.

CONCLUSION

During surgery dangerous intracranial veins and sinuses have to be scrupulously respected, or reconstructed if necessary, especially in tumor surgery. This is one of the most important things that we have learned from our everyday experience during the past 30 years of performing surgeries. As a matter of fact, prognosis of intracranial operations lies in the preservation of not only the arterial supply, but also the venous drainages. This implies that neurosurgeons must have a strong knowledge of anatomy and physiology of the venous circulation. It also suggests that the surgeon must enter the operating room with all useful information on the intracranial venous system of each individual patient; these data should be available on the imaging screen. Consequently, our neuroradiology colleagues should be full partners in the everyday work of neurosurgeons.

Acknowledgment

We are grateful to Mrs. Sabrina Derkaoui for her secretarial assistance.

REFERENCES

1. Sindou M, Auque J: The intracranial venous system as a neurosurgeon's perspective. Review, *Adv Tech Stand Neurosurg* 26:131–216, 2000.
2. Auque J, editor: Venous sacrifice in neurosurgery: risk, assessment and management, *Neurochirurgie* 42(Suppl 1): 1–136, 1996.
3. Sindou M, Auque J, Jouanneau E: Neurosurgery and the intracranial venous system, *Acta Neurochir (Wien)* 94(Suppl):1686–1692, 2005.
4. Al-Mefty O, Krist AF: The dangerous veins. In Hakuba A, editor: *Surgery of the Intracranial Venous System. Proceedings of First International Workshop on Surgery of the Intracranial Venous System, September 1994*, Tokyo, 1996, Springer-Verlag, pp 36–42.
5. Schmidek HH, Auer LM, Kapp JP: The cerebral venous system. Review, *Neurosurgery* 17:663–678, 1985.
6. Hakuba A, editor: *Surgery of the Intracranial Venous System. Proceedings of the First International Workshop on Surgery of the Intracranial Venous System, Osaka, September 1994*, Tokyo, 1996, Springer-Verlag.
7. Malis LI: Venous involvement in tumor resection. In Hakuba A, editor: *Surgery of the Intracranial Venous System. Proceedings of the First International Workshop on Surgery of the Intracranial Venous System, Osaka, September 1994*, Tokyo, 1996, Springer-Verlag, pp 281–288.
8. Yasargil MG: *Microneurosurgery, vol 1. Microsurgical Anatomy of the Basal Cisterns and Vessels of the Brain, Diagnostic and Studies*, Stuttgart, New York, 1984, Thieme.
9. Alaywan M, Sindou M: Surgical anatomy of the lateral sinus approaches in the sigmoid region. In Hakuba A, editor: *Surgery of the Intracranial Venous System. Proceedings of the First International Workshop on Surgery of the Intracranial Venous System, Osaka, September 1994*, Tokyo, 1996, Springer-Verlag, pp 63–72.
10. Sindou M, Alaywan F, Hallacq P: Main dural sinuses surgery, *Neurochirurgie Suppl* 1:45–87, 1996.
11. Sindou M, Hallacq P: Venous reconstruction in surgery of meningiomas invading the sagittal and transverse sinuses, *Skull Base Surg* 8:57–64, 1998.
12. Kanno T, Kasama A, Shoda M, et al: pitfall in the interhemispheric translamina terminalis approach for the removal of a craniopharyngioma. Significance of preserving draining veins. Part I. Clinical study, *Surg Neurol* 32:111–115, 1989.

13. Samii M: *Skull Base Surgery. Anatomy, Diagnosis and Treatment. Proceedings of the First International Skull Base Congress, Hannover, 1992*, Basel, 1994, Karger.

14. Sindou M, Emery E, Acevedo G, et al: Respective indications for orbital rim, zygomatic arch and orbito-zygomatic osteotomies in the surgical approach to central skull base lesions. Critical, retrospective, review in 146 cases, *Acta Neurochir* 143:967–975, 2001.

15. Kasama A, Kanno TA: pitfall in the interhemispheric translamina terminalis approach for the removal of a craniopharyngioma. Significance of preserving draining veins. Part II. Experimental study, *Surg Neurol* 32:116–120, 1989.

16. Sugita K, Kobayashi S, Yokoo A: Preservation of large bridgings veins during brain retraction. Technical note, *J Neurosurg* 57:856–858, 1982.

17. Sakaki T, Morimoto T, Takemura K, et al: Reconstruction of cerebral cortical veins using silicone tubing. Technical note, *J Neurosurg* 66:471–473, 1987.

18. Donaghy RM, Wallman LJ, Flanagan MJ, et al: Sagittal sinus repair. Technical note, *J Neurosurg* 38:244–248, 1973.

19. Kapp JP, Gielchinsky I, Deardourff SL: Operative techniques for management of lesions involving the dural venous sinuses, *Surg Neurol* 7:339–342, 1977.

20. Sindou M, Alvernia J: Results of attempted radical tumor removal and venous repair in 100 consecutive meningiomas involving the major dural sinuses, *J Neurosurg* 105:514–525, 2006.

21. Oka K, Go Y, Kimura H, et al: Obstruction of the superior sagittal sinus caused by parasagittal meningiomas: the role of collateral venous pathways, *J Neurosurg* 81:520–524, 1994.

22. Sindou M: Meningiomas invading the sagittal or transverse sinuses, resection with venous reconstruction, *J Clin Neurosci* (Suppl):8–11, 2001.

23. Waga S, Handa H: Scalp veins as collateral pathways with parasagittal meningiomas occluding the superior sagittal sinus, *Neuroradiology* 11:199–204, 1976.

24. Sindou M, Hallacq P: Microsurgery of the venous system in meningiomas invading the major dural sinuses. In Hakuba A, editor: *Surgery of the Intracranial Venous System. Proceedings of the First International Workshop on Surgery of the Intracranial Venous System, Osaka, September 1994*, Tokyo, 1996, Springer-Verlag, pp 226–236.

25. Merrem G: Die parasagittalen Meningeome. Quoted in Fedor Krause memorial lecture, *Acta Neurochir* 23:203–216, 1970.

26. Krause F: Operative Frilegung der Vierhügel, nebst Beobachtungen über Hirndruck und Dekompression, *Zentralbl Neurochir* 53: 2812–2819, 1926.

27. Bonnal J, Brotchi J: Surgery of the superior sagittal sinus in parasagittal meningiomas, *J Neurosurg* 48:935–945, 1978.

28. Masuzawa H: Superior sagittal sinus plasty using falx flap in parasagittal meningioma, *Noshinkei Geka* 5:707–713, 1977.

29. Guclu B, Sindou M: Reconstruction of vein of Labbé in temporo-occipital meningioma invading transverse sinus: technical report, *Acta Neurochir* 152:941–945, 2010.

30. Menovsky T, De Vries J: Cortical vein end-to-end anastomosis after removal of a parasagittal meningioma, *Microsurgery* 22:27–29, 2002.

31. Murata J, Sawamura Y, Saito H, et al: Resection of a recurrent parasagittal meningioma with cortical vein anastomosis: technical note, *Surg Neurol* 48:592–597, 1997.

32. Steiger HJ, Reulen HJ, Huber P, et al: Radical resection of superior sagittal sinus meningioma with venous interpostion graft and reimplantation of the rolandic veins. Case report, *Acta Neurochir (Wien)* 100:108–111, 1989.

33. Di Meco F, Li KW, Casali C, et al: Meningiomas invading the superior sagittal sinus: surgical experience in 108 cases, *Neurosurgery* 55:1263–1274, 2004.

34. Logue V: Parasagittal meningiomas, *Adv Tech Stand Neurosurg* 2:171–198, 1975.

35. Brotchi J, Patay Z, Baleriaux D: Surgery of the superior sagittal sinus and neighbouring veins. In Hakuba A, editor: *Surgery of the Intracranial Venous System. Proceedings of the First International Workshop on Surgery of the Intracranial Venous System, Osaka, September 1994*, Tokyo, 1996, Springer-Verlag, pp 207–219.

36. Bederson JB, Eisenberg MB: Resection and replacement of the superior sagittal sinus for treatment of a parasagittal meningioma: technical case report, *Neurosurgery* 37:1015–1019, 1995.

37. Bonnal J: Conservative and reconstructive surgery of the superior longitudinal sinus, *Neurochirurgie* 52:147–172, 1982.

38. Bonnal J, Brotchi J, Stevenaert A, et al: Excision of the intrasinusal portion of rolandic parasagittal meningiomas, followed by plastic surgery of the superior longitudinal sinus, *Neurochirurgie* 17:341–354, 1971.

39. Bonnal J, Buduba C: Surgery of the central third of the superior sagittal sinus. Experimental study, *Acta Neurochir* 30:207–215, 1974.

40. Hakuba A: Reconstruction of dural sinus involved in meningiomas. In Al-Mefty O, editor: *Meningiomas*, New York, 1991, Raven Press, pp 371–382.

41. Hakuba A, Huh CW, Tsujikawa S, et al: Total removal of a parasagittal meningioma of the posterior third of the sagittal sinus and its repair by autogenous vein graft. Case report, *J Neurosurg* 51:379–382, 1979.

42. Nagashima H, Kobayashi S, Takemae T, et al: Total resection of torcular herophili hemangiopericytoma with radial artery graft case report, *Neurosurgery* 36:1024–1027, 1995.

43. Sekhar LN, Tzortzidis FN, Bejjani GK, et al: Saphenous vein graft bypass of the sigmoid sinus and jugular bulb during the removal of glomus jugular tumors. Report of two cases, *J Neurosurg* 86:1036–1041, 1997.

44. Sindou M, Mercier P, Bokor J, et al: Bilateral thrombosis of the transverse sinuses: microsurgical revascularization with venous bypass, *Surg Neurol* 13:215–220, 1980.

45. Schmid-Elsaesser R, Steiger HJ, Yousry T, et al: Radical resection of meningiomas and arteriousvenous fistulas involving critical dural sinus segments: Experience with intraoperative sinus pressure monitoring and elective sinus reconstruction in 10 patients, *Neurosurgery* 41:1005–1018, 1997.

46. Sindou M, Mazoyer JF, Fischer G, et al: Experimental bypass for sagittal sinus repair. Preliminary report, *J Neurosurg* 44:325–330, 1976.

Note: Page numbers followed by *f* indicate figures and followed by *t* indicate tables.